the parent's guide to
play

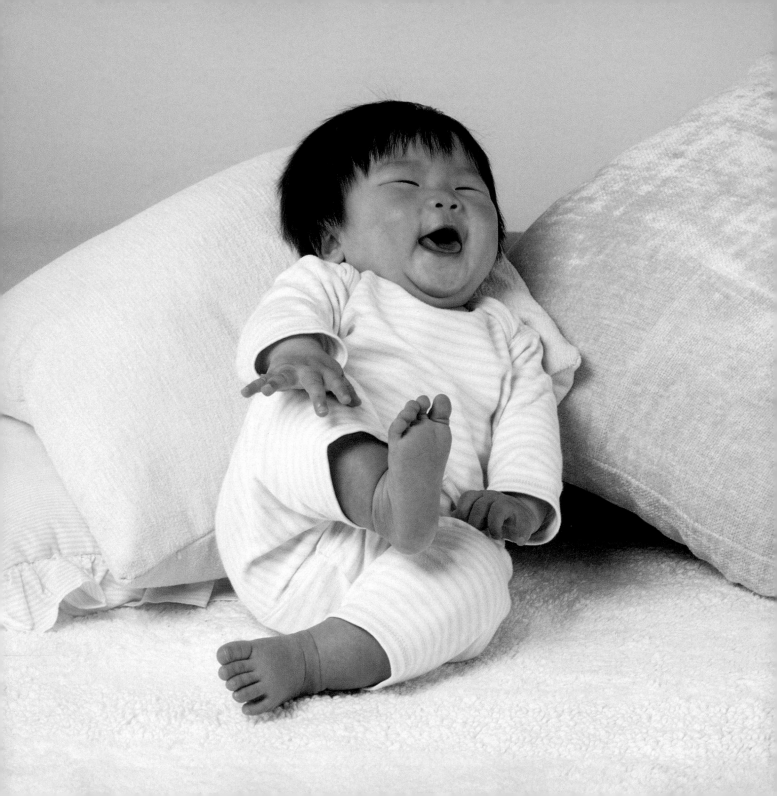

GYMBOREE PLAY & MUSIC

the parent's guide to

play

Consulting Editors

Dr. Wendy S. Masi
Dr. Roni Cohen Leiderman

FIREFLY BOOKS

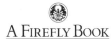

GYMBOREE. PLAY&MUSIC

Produced by Weldon Owen Inc.,
814 Montgomery Street, San Francisco, California 94133,
in collaboration with the Gymboree Corporation, Inc.,
500 Howard Street, San Francisco, California 94105

A FIREFLY BOOK

Published by Firefly Books Ltd. 2006

First printing

Publisher Cataloging-in-Publication Data (U.S.)

   The parent's guide to play / consulting editors, Wendy S.
Masi and Roni Cohen Leiderman.
[304] p. : photos. ;   cm.
Includes index.
ISBN-13: 978-1-55407-205-7 (pbk.)
ISBN-10: 1-55407-205-0 (pbk.)
1. Play - Miscellanea. 2. Creative activities and seat work.
I. Masi, Wendy S. II. Leiderman, Roni Cohen. III. Title.
649.5 dc22   HQ782.M367 2006

Published in the United States by
Firefly Books (U.S.) Inc.
P.O. Box 1338, Ellicott Station
Buffalo, New York 14205

CONSULTING EDITORS
Dr. Wendy S. Masi
Dr. Roni Cohen Leiderman

EDITORIAL ADVISER
Dr. Marilyn Segal

GYMBOREE PLAY & MUSIC PROGRAMS
Chief Executive Officer: **Lisa Harper**
Product Manager: **Lisa Biasotti**
Play & Music Sr. Program Developer: **Helene Silver Freda**

WELDON OWEN INC.
Chief Executive Officer: **John Owen**
Chief Operating Officer & President: **Terry Newell**
Chief Financial Officer: **Christine E. Munson**
Vice President & Publisher: **Roger Shaw**
Vice President, International Sales: **Stuart Laurence**

Cover Photograph: Chris Shorten
Cover Design: Colin Wheatland

Printed in Singapore

SPECIAL NOTE ON SAFETY PRECAUTIONS

At Gymboree, we encourage parents to become active play partners with their children. As you enjoy these enriching activities with your child, please make safety your priority. While the risk of injury during any of these activities is low, take every precaution to ensure your child is as safe as possible.

   To reduce the risk of injury, please follow these guidelines: Do not leave your child unattended, even for a brief moment, during any of the activities in this book; be particularly cautious when participating in the activities involving water because of the risk of drowning; ensure that your child does not place in his or her mouth any small objects (even those depicted in the photos) as some may pose a choking hazard and could be fatal if ingested; make sure crayons, markers, and other writing and crafts materials are nontoxic and have been approved for use by children under three years of age.

   Throughout this book, we have suggested guidelines to the age-appropriateness of each activity; however, it is up to you to assess your own child's suitability for a particular activity before attempting it. Ability, balance, and dexterity vary considerably from child to child, even for children of the same age.

   While we have made every effort to ensure that the information is accurate and reliable, and that the activities are safe and workable when an adult is properly supervising, we disclaim all liability for any unintended, unforeseen, or improper application of the recommendations and suggestions featured.

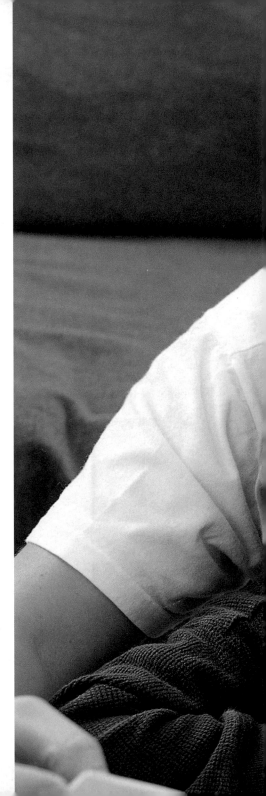

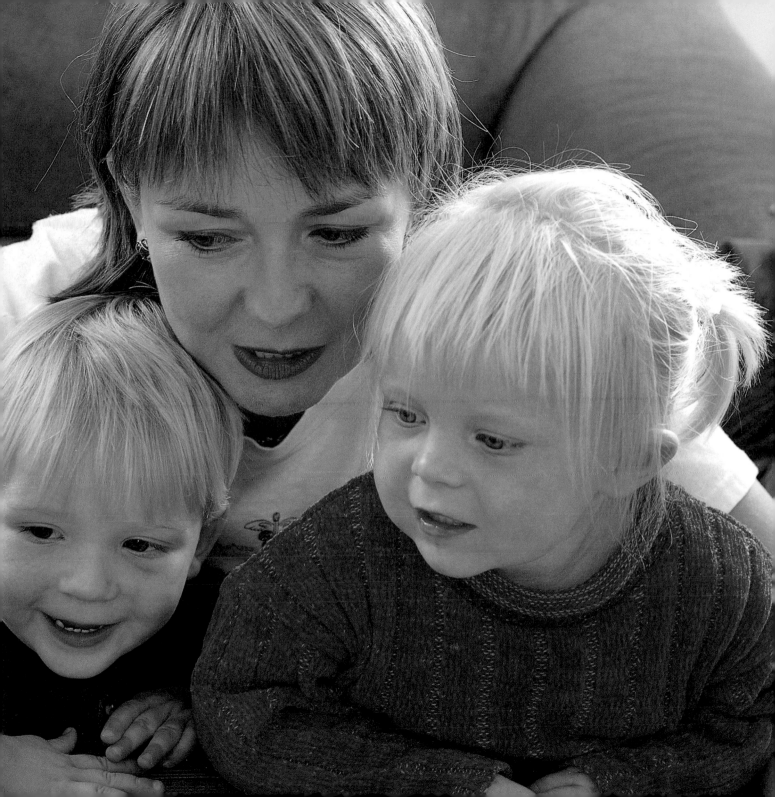

CONTENTS

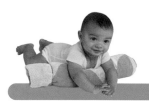

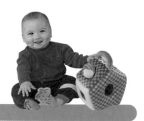

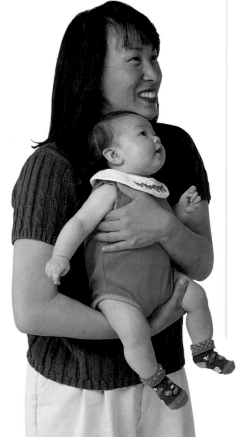

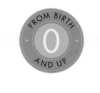

continued on next page ➤

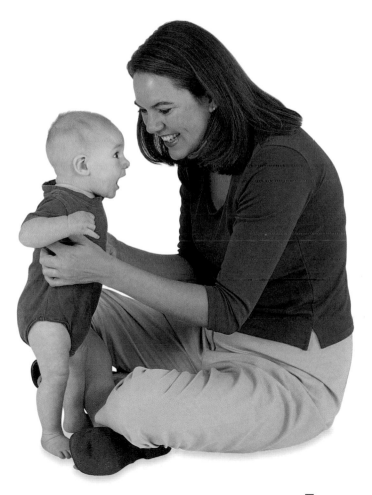

CONTENTS

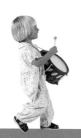
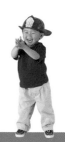

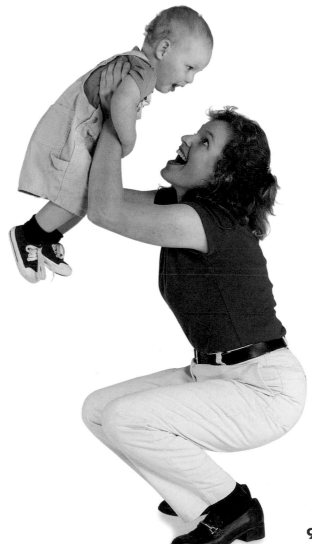

TYPES OF ACTIVITIES

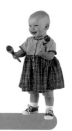

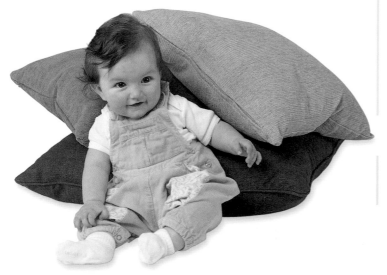

continued on next page ➤

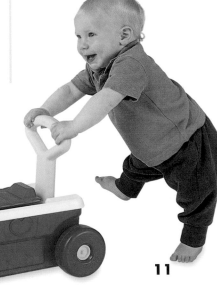

11

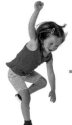
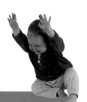

TYPES OF ACTIVITIES

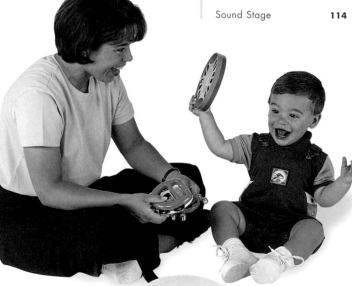

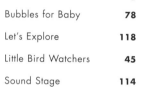

13

FOREWORD

DR. WENDY S. MASI AND DR. RONI COHEN LEIDERMAN

WE HAVE SPENT more than thirty years researching infancy and child development, playing with babies and toddlers, and talking with their parents—and we have loved every minute of it. Between us we have raised six children, making us keenly aware of the challenges and the incredible joy and pride of parenthood. We have learned that most parents want the same thing for their children: a happy and fulfilling life. And we have learned there are many paths leading to that goal.

We firmly believe in the power of nurturing and a positive, playful approach to parenting. This belief is reconfirmed daily by newly released scientific research demonstrating that brain development is strongly influenced by the kinds of early experiences our children receive. A newborn's brain is only 25 percent developed, but by the time your child is three, more than 90 percent of her brain development will be complete.

To achieve his or her greatest potential, your child needs you to provide a variety of interesting learning experiences. Gymboree, America's foremost provider of parent-and-child play programs, developed its "play with a purpose" philosophy to teach parents that the most important way for young children to learn is through play. Through active, hands-on play, your child will learn language, develop problem-solving skills, and master social relationships. Of course, parents benefit from play, too. What can compare to the elation you experience when your baby mimics you and claps for the first time, or your toddler sings and dances to songs?

This book, created by the Gymboree Play and Music experts, is a wonderful resource for parents, a compilation of activities and songs to inspire you to interact with your child on a whole new level. The interchanges you share will support your child's physical, emotional, and cognitive development, and will help establish a loving, joyful connection. You are your child's first and most important teacher, treasured companion, and playmate. Rejoice in her every discovery and celebrate each remarkable achievement.

Have fun with your child and enjoy these incredible years. You know you are getting your child off to a great start.

Dr. Wendy S. Masi   Dr. Roni Cohen Leiderman

PLAYING WITH YOUR BABY

WHEN YOU FIRST bring a new baby home, your thoughts are usually full of the practical matters: how to keep your baby clean, warm, and well-fed; where to store the tiny diapers and clothes; how the car seat and stroller actually work; and getting some sleep.

Once the necessities are taken care of, there's something further that even the littlest baby needs in order to thrive: warm, playful interactions with the caretakers around him. Dozens of studies in recent years have shown that a child's sense of self-

esteem and his ability to form close emotional ties with others greatly depends upon the quality of his bond with his parents. This bond can be enhanced by close, loving play. Indeed, for babies who cannot yet go to school or read a book, play is the primary way they learn.

THE INCREDIBLE FIRST YEAR

During the first 12 months, babies undergo a profound mental, physical, and social awakening. They learn to recognize their families, the cabinet with the crackers, and the playground with the big slide. They learn to support their heads, use their hands, roll over, sit, crawl, stand, and—in some cases—walk. And long before they are ready to speak, they understand a range of human communication, from body language (the quick head shake that discourages further food throwing) to some of the words you say. At the same time, they learn how to communicate their needs and feelings through their very own baby language.

The greatest task in the first year is the development of a baby's trust. Your baby needs to know

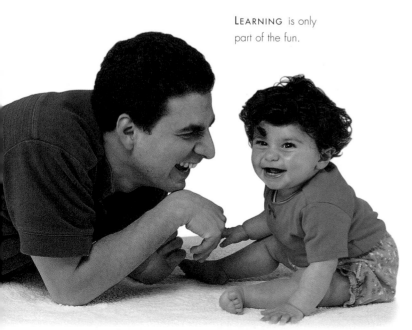

LEARNING is only part of the fun.

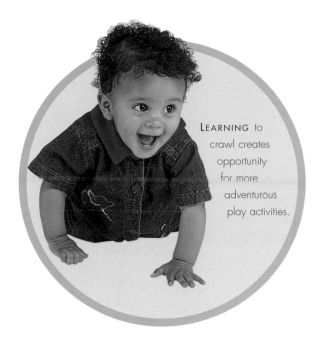

LEARNING to crawl creates opportunity for more adventurous play activities.

later intellectual, emotional, and physical life depends upon the kinds and amount of stimulation she receives in her earliest years.

Such talk of stimulation and mental development has a tendency to sound awfully dry. Play, however, comes naturally to most babies—and to most parents. Inspire yourself by remembering babies aren't born knowing how much fun the world can be, and you get to show them.

ALL KINDS OF PLAY

Babies don't know right away that stuffed animals are for hugging or that peekaboo games provide riotous good fun, or that pinwheels sparkle as they spin. Bringing games and toys to your baby, along

that his physical needs for food and warmth will be fulfilled, that his environment is safe, and, most important, that his caretakers will cherish him and nourish his own budding feelings of love. Hugging, kissing, rocking, and smiling are ways of cultivating this trust. So is introducing your baby to the simple joys of all different kinds of play.

Interacting with your child is vitally important throughout his life, of course. But in the first year play can be especially important and rewarding. Researchers estimate that 50 percent of a human's brain development occurs in the first six months of life; 70 percent is complete by the end of the first year. While much of this development has to do with genetic heritage, a good portion of a child's

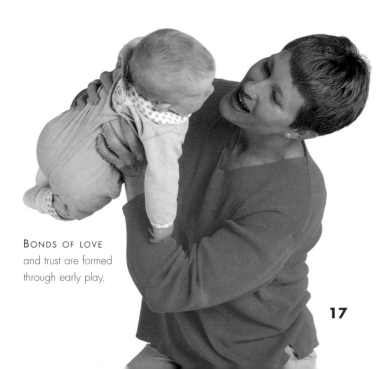

BONDS OF LOVE and trust are formed through early play.

with your attention, laughter, and encouragement, lets both of you share in the explorations.

Another task for parents during this first year is to tune in to their babies as individuals. Play, even "stimulating" play, isn't really about force-feeding experiences, but is rather about understanding your baby's temperament: her likes and dislikes and her tolerance for and ability to adapt to stimulation. Some babies love to be rocked back and forth, while others strongly object. Some like to be chased; others are uncomfortable with such rowdiness. Respond to your baby's cues and follow her lead.

Babies have distinct cycles of rest and activity, attention and inattention. The best time for active play—swatting at toys, rolling balls, or knocking over blocks—is when your baby is receptive and

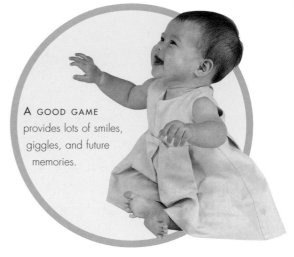

A GOOD GAME provides lots of smiles, giggles, and future memories.

alert. Opt for more passive play—listening to songs or snuggling up with a book—when he is subdued. Both types are important. It's the timing that counts.

Spontaneity can make play even more fun and rewarding, and you'll find opportunities at every turn. Add peekaboo games to diaper changes to minimize squirming. Play "I'm gonna get you" as you're leaving the house together and you'll get out the door quicker—and in probably better humor. Burst into song in the car and your baby's fussing may turn into giggles.

Viewed this way, play becomes less about achieving accomplishments and more about creating relationships. When you play with your baby, you're engaging in intimate activities that help him master certain skills while also creating a loving and joyful bond.

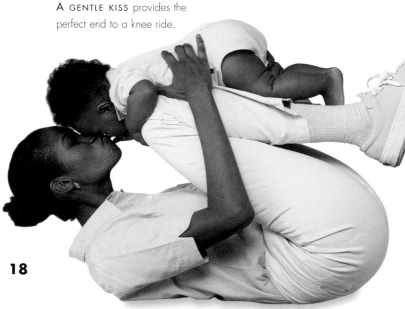

A GENTLE KISS provides the perfect end to a knee ride.

The following activities are grouped chronologically in three-month age ranges that match key stages in a baby's development. These are general guidelines only, as there is a wide range of developmental differences among children.

FROM BIRTH AND UP

At first glance, your newborn may seem unable to do much. But he is actually taking in volumes of information about his world through all his senses. In these early months he will make steady gains in his ability to control his muscles. Sometime in his second month his tightly closed fists may begin to open. Then he'll swipe at objects. Play isn't so much about lively activity as it is about sensory exploration—giving him objects to watch, listen to, and touch.

3 MONTHS AND UP

The second three months of your baby's life introduce the dawn of her sense of control over her world, however elementary. No longer a passive newborn, your baby is stronger and more active. She can now use her hands to reach out and pull objects into her world and then drop them, or put them in her mouth as a means of exploration. These activities are learning experiences through which she develops all kinds of skills along with her sense of self.

6 MONTHS AND UP

By now, your baby is a charmingly social creature, one who laughs and calls out to garner attention or provoke a response. He's also a mobile baby, one who can roll over, creep, crawl, or pull himself up to get what he wants. He will test his emerging fine motor skills by carefully bringing his thumb and forefinger together, fiddling with labels or crumbs. He's starting to understand that an object exists even when it isn't visible. Such conceptual developments make peekaboo and other hiding games possible.

9 MONTHS AND UP

At this age, even those babies who aren't yet walking are beginning to look and act like toddlers. Games that allow your baby to practice gross motor skills—crawling, pulling himself up to stand, toddling across the floor, or climbing—are particularly appealing to him now, because mobility is his main objective. Fine motor skills are equally important to him. He may insist on turning the pages of a book or stacking up a pile of his own. This is the beginning of the "do it myself" stage.

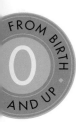

SWAYING, SWAYING

LAPS AND LULLABIES

SKILLSPOTLIGHT

The sensory stimulation *provided by this activity—the sound of your voice, the feel of your hands, and the sight of your face—can reassure and soothe your baby. This activity may even put her to sleep. And as she approaches three months, your smiles and words may inspire her to coo and grin socially in return.*

Body Awareness	✔
Listening	✔
Visual Development	✔

SHE LOVES TO HEAR your voice, she loves to feel your touch, and she loves to be rocked rhythmically from side to side. You can combine all three of these soothing elements by using your lap as a cradle and your voice as a lullaby. Sit in a chair with your baby lying on your thighs, her feet pointing toward your stomach. Cradle her head with your hands and gently sway your body from side to side as you talk or sing to her.

GAZING INTO HER EYES as you sway from side to side—that's what builds the deepest ties.

20

POM-POM PLAY

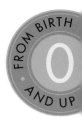

FROM BIRTH
0
AND UP

A TOUCH AND SIGHT GAME

BABIES AREN'T BORN knowing how to visually track an object or how objects move through space. Such developments take time. This gentle game will engage his attention, stimulate his senses, and eventually make him smile.

• Gather together some large brightly colored pom-poms or small plush toys. Get the baby's attention by holding the toy twelve to fifteen inches above his face. Slowly move the toy from side to side, keeping pace with his ability to track the object with his eyes.

• Try slowly lifting the object up and down so he can watch it moving from near to far. Touch the toy to his torso, or use it to stroke his face and arms. Of course, you shouldn't leave the baby unattended with small objects.

SKILL SPOTLIGHT

Watching a brightly colored *object move from side to side and up and down helps strengthen your baby's eye muscles so that he can track objects and focus at different distances, a skill that requires "visual convergence," or having the two eyes working to-gether. Feeling the pom-poms gently touch his torso, face, and limbs lets him explore textures.*

✔ **Tactile Stimulation**

✔ **Visual Development**

✔ **Visual Tracking**

A TINY YELLOW POM-POM is intriguing to a baby, especially when it brushes his skin.

21

INFANT MASSAGE

TOUCHING TO RELAX

SKILL SPOTLIGHT

Touch is deeply reassuring *for infants, especially if it's done calmly and gently. A mild massage stimulates your baby's circulation, sense of touch, and awareness of her body. Looking at and talking to your baby helps to strengthen your all-important emotional bond.*

Body Awareness	✔
Emotional Development	✔
Social Development	✔
Tactile Stimulation	✔

CULTURES AROUND THE WORLD have practiced various forms of infant massage for thousands of years. Classes and books are available on this topic, but you can do very simple forms of massage at home with your baby, too. Find a warm room or a sunny spot on the bed or carpet, and a time when you're relaxed and your baby is receptive. Take off all her clothes and rub oil between your hands to prevent friction and make the massage pleasing. Use a vegetable-based oil, such as grapeseed or safflower oil; avoid baby oil and other petroleum-based products.

• Using a milking motion, gently squeeze down each arm and leg. Then move your hands from the center of her torso out to the sides. Or softly brush your fingertips over her skin. Speak or sing to her at the same time.

• Place your fingers on her temples and make very small, gentle circles. Then place your fingertips in the middle of her forehead and draw them slowly along her eyebrows. Try gently moving your thumbs along the bridge of her nose, down around her nostrils, and to the corners of her mouth.

SHE LOVES TO FEEL YOUR TOUCH, see your eyes, and hear your voice.

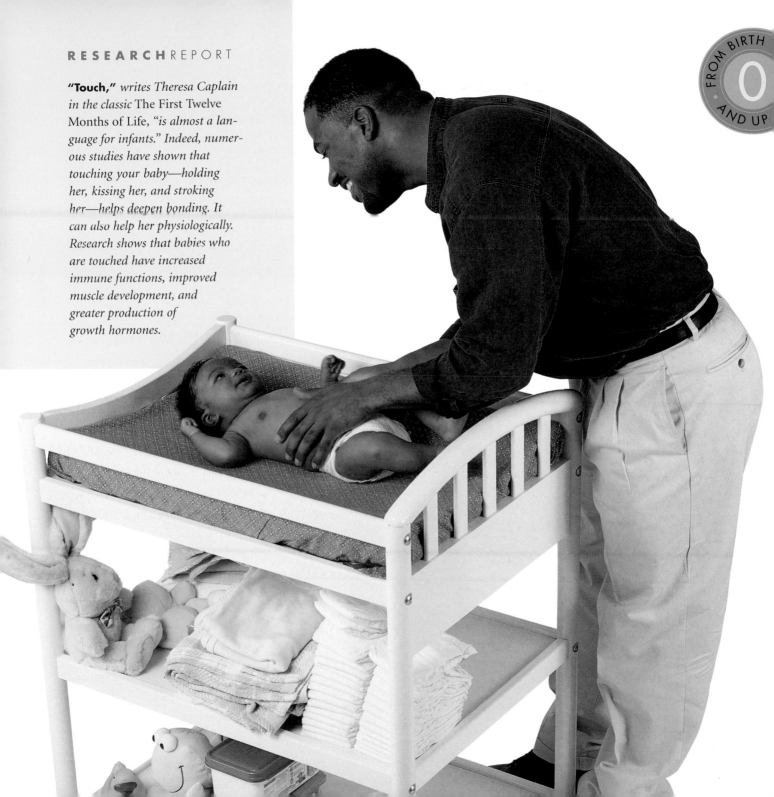

RESEARCH REPORT

"Touch," *writes Theresa Caplain in the classic* The First Twelve Months of Life, *"is almost a language for infants." Indeed, numerous studies have shown that touching your baby—holding her, kissing her, and stroking her—helps deepen bonding. It can also help her physiologically. Research shows that babies who are touched have increased immune functions, improved muscle development, and greater production of growth hormones.*

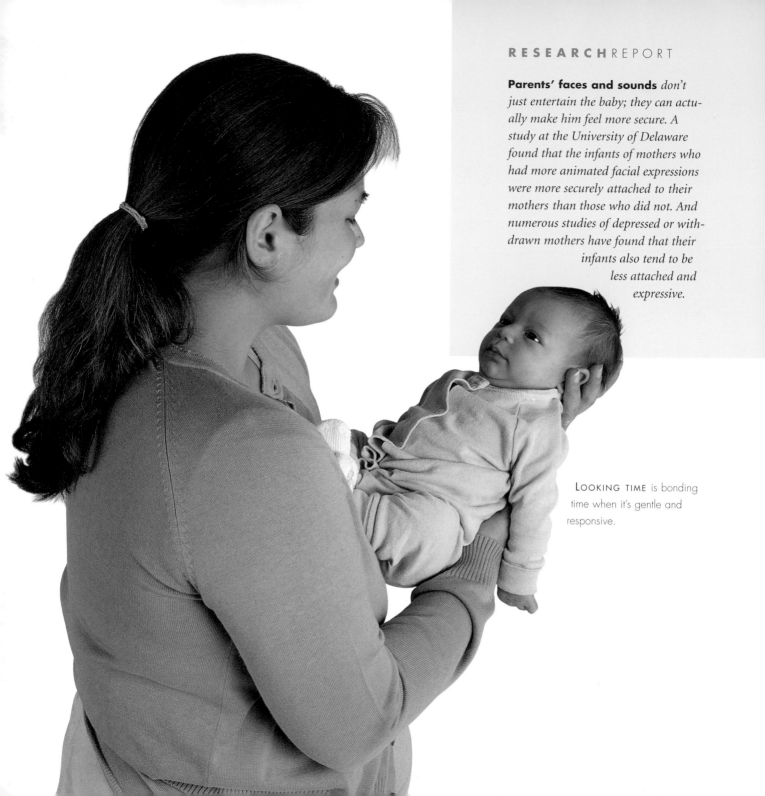

RESEARCHREPORT

Parents' faces and sounds *don't just entertain the baby; they can actually make him feel more secure. A study at the University of Delaware found that the infants of mothers who had more animated facial expressions were more securely attached to their mothers than those who did not. And numerous studies of depressed or withdrawn mothers have found that their infants also tend to be less attached and expressive.*

LOOKING TIME is bonding time when it's gentle and responsive.

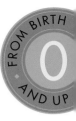

FACIAL EXPRESSIONS

LOOKING, LEARNING, LOVING

NOT ALL THE ACTIVITIES you do with your baby have to be vigorous—or even active. Quiet time is equally important. Babies, especially newborns, are easily overstimulated. And intimacy between parent and child depends as much on touch and eye contact as it does on giggles, tickles, and toys. In other words, time spent simply gazing into your baby's eyes is time well spent, as it allows the two of you a chance to relax and bond.

• Choose a time when your infant is alert and receptive. Cradle him in your arms, prop him up on your knees, or lay him down on the changing table or a soft blanket on the floor.

• When he's looking at you, gaze into his eyes. Speak or sing his name softly. Introduce him to some facial expressions: a smile, an opened mouth, raised eyebrows, a stuck-out tongue. Then go back to simply looking at him and saying his name softly.

• Your baby may surprise you by imitating your expressions; even the littlest babies will sometimes mirror the face of a caregiver. But if he grows restless or turns away repeatedly, stop the activity. Babies need to withdraw from intense interactions to process all they've experienced.

IF YOUR BABY ENJOYS THIS ACTIVITY, also try Who Is That?, page 30.

SKILLSPOTLIGHT

You may have noticed *that your baby began scanning your face—or moving his eyes from your hairline to your chin— almost as soon as he was born. That's evidence that faces are very, very important to young babies. Having time in which he can simply look at your face and its expressions lets him begin to make important attachments and learn social cues for affection.*

✔	**Emotional Development**
✔	**Listening**
✔	**Social Development**
✔	**Visual Development**

25

LULLABIES

IT'S HARD TO SAY why simple melodies soothe infants, but generation upon generation of parents have sung songs to their little ones, and generation upon generation of little ones have thus been lulled. Lots of lullabies just seem to beg babies to fall asleep, but any quiet song, sung lovingly, can induce sleep, or at least settle an overstimulated baby.

CRADLE SONG

 Brahms' Lullaby

Lullaby, and good night—
go to sleep little baby.
Close your eyes now
sweetly rest.
May your slumbers be blessed.
Close your eyes now
sweetly rest.
May your slumbers be blessed.

WHETHER IT COMES from an older sibling or a parent, a tender song is a time-honored way of calming infants.

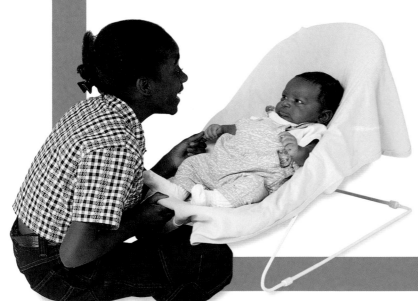

HUSH, LITTLE BABY

Hush, little baby, don't say a word,
Papa's gonna buy you a mockingbird.

And if that mockingbird won't sing,
Papa's gonna buy you a diamond ring.

If that diamond ring turns brass,
Papa's gonna buy you a looking glass.

If that looking glass gets broke,
Papa's gonna buy you a billy goat.

If that billy goat don't pull,
Papa's gonna buy you a cart and bull.

If that cart and bull turn over,
Papa's gonna buy you a dog named
Rover.

If that dog named Rover don't bark,
Papa's gonna buy you a horse and cart.

If that horse and cart fall down,
you'll still be the sweetest little
baby in town.

ALL THE PRETTY HORSES

Hush a bye, don't you cry,
go to sleep little baby.

When you wake, you shall have
all the pretty little horses.

Blacks and bays, dapples and grays,
all the pretty little horses.

Hush a bye, don't you cry,
go to sleep little baby.

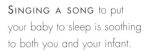

SINGING A SONG to put
your baby to sleep is soothing
to both you and your infant.

27

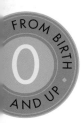

FROM BIRTH
AND UP

HANKIE WAVE

A TRACKING GAME

SKILL SPOTLIGHT

Watching the cloth wave *back and forth at this age will boost your baby's ability to visually track and focus on objects. But by three months, she won't be able to resist reaching out and trying to grab the cloth. And by six months, she'll be gumming the cloth as soon as she gets it into her tiny grasp.*

Listening	✔
Visual Stimulation	✔

ONE OF THE BEST-KEPT SECRETS about playing with young babies is that you don't always need fancy toys with electronic bells and whistles. In fact, sometimes just a cloth, handkerchief, or colorful scarf will do. Place your baby on her back on the floor or changing table. Hold a scarf, handkerchief, or lightweight cloth about twelve inches over her head. Bring it close to her, then lift it farther away, and bring it down again. Sing to her or call her name as you wave the cloth.

A SCARF OR CLOTH creates a tickling breeze and an intriguing visual object for your little one to follow.

28

CRYING AND COLIC

YOUR BABY'S CRY will become as familiar to you as the shapes of his toes. That won't make dealing with it any easier. Some days you'll feel nothing but sympathy; other days your patience will be pushed to its limits.

Babies cry in response to unpleasant experiences, including hunger, loneliness, fatigue, pain, or being chilled or overheated. Some researchers also believe that at three to six weeks, some babies start crying in the early evening simply to let off steam after a long day.

A "colicky" baby cries more persistently and more often than others. Researchers don't know the cause of colic. Colicky babies may have immature digestive systems, or they may just have a harder time dealing with the world's stimuli. Whatever the cause, even the most loving parents can feel inadequate, anxious, or even angry when faced with the nonstop, shrill cries of a colicky baby.

Some people may tell you to let your baby "cry it out." Most pediatricians these days would disagree.

Comforting your baby—or at least trying to comfort him—shows him that he can count on you to respond and that distress eventually ends.

What you can do for your baby: If burping, changing, or feeding your baby doesn't help, try motion (such as walking with the baby in a stroller or front pack, or rocking, dancing, or swinging). Fresh air can quiet a crying baby. And young babies often appreciate being swaddled.

What you can do for yourself: Try to catch up on missed sleep. Fatigue makes parents more vulnerable to depression and short tempers, which can make it hard to respond wholeheartedly to your baby's cries. Ask someone else to watch the baby while you take a shower or go out for a walk. Don't feel you're abandoning your baby. Think of it as replenishing your diminished resources. ■

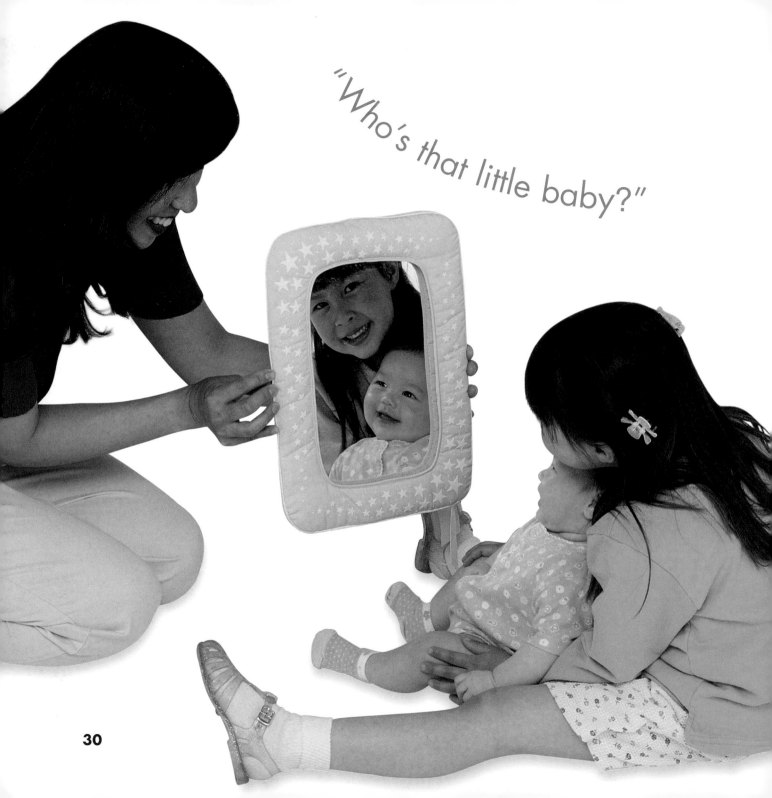

"Who's that little baby?"

WHO IS THAT?

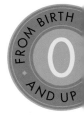

FROM BIRTH
0
AND UP

SELF-REFLECTIONS

NEWBORNS ARE MORE ATTUNED to real human faces than to any other visual object, including rattles, geometric shapes, or even drawings of human faces. In her earliest weeks, a baby stares at faces even though she doesn't know that they, like her, are human. That means she'll be fascinated by her own tiny reflection in a handheld mirror—even though she'll have no idea who it is. Hold a mirror up so your baby can see her reflection. Point at the baby in the mirror, and say her name. As she grows older her reflection will prompt that first sign of sociability—the infant's impish grin.

A MIRROR PROVIDES a fun-filled play experience for the whole family.

SKILLSPOTLIGHT

A baby won't recognize herself in the mirror until she's around fifteen months old. But even in her earliest months, gazing at herself in the mirror helps her learn to visually focus and track as well as to explore the social nature of faces. Eventually, it will help her identify herself as both a baby and a unique being.

✔	**Emotional Development**
✔	**Social Development**
✔	**Visual Development**

IF YOUR BABY ENJOYS THIS ACTIVITY, also try Facial Expressions, page 24.

31

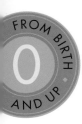

AIRPLANE BABY

SOARING TO NEW HEIGHTS

SKILLSPOTLIGHT

Parents around the world *have spent many long hours comforting colicky babies by swinging them gently back and forth in an "air-plane" hold. The steady pressure along the baby's tummy provides soothing warmth and tactile input. And with every passing week she'll practice lifting her head, neck, and shoulders so that she can look around and widen her baby's-eye view.*

Tactile Stimulation	✔
Trust	✔
Upper-Body Strength	✔

YOU MAY ALREADY have discovered that a classic "airplane" or "football" hold calms your baby when she's gassy, overwhelmed, or just tired. Combining a swinging or swaying motion and a rhythmic song with that firm hold around her belly can be even more calming. Just support your baby, tummy down, by holding her under her chest and belly with one or both of your arms. (But always be sure to support a newborn's head.) Then swing her gently to and fro while singing a song.

WITH A LITTLE BIT OF WIND in her little bit of hair and with Mommy's arm supporting her, she's soaring like a glider.

TICKLE-ME TEXTURES

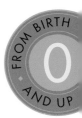

FROM BIRTH
0
AND UP

TELLING TACTILE TALES

NEWBORNS DON'T ALWAYS LIKE to be undressed because the air feels cold on their skin. Older babies often fuss during diaper changes because they don't want to be restrained. You can turn changing time into play and learning time by providing your baby with interesting tactile experiences.

• Gather several objects with different textures. Try swatches of velvet and corduroy, feathers, or a clean sponge dampened with warm water.

• Gently rub an object across your baby's skin and watch for her response. Try a different object. Look for clues that indicate her preferences.

• This is an activity that can entertain your baby for many months. Sometime after her ninth month, she may find the texture toys and hold them out for you to tickle her with!

SKILLSPOTLIGHT

Your baby's skin *is about as alive to touch now as it ever will be because touch is one of the baby's primary ways of exploring the world. This activity introduces her to a wide range of the world's textures. It also gives you a chance to practice recognizing and responding to her body language. Such attuned responses help build her sense of security as she witnesses her needs being taken care of.*

✔	**Body Awareness**
✔	**Social Development**
✔	**Tactile Stimulation**

THE FEATHERY TEXTURE makes her squirm with pleasure.

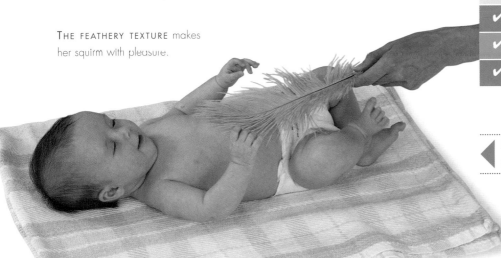

IF YOUR BABY ENJOYS THIS ACTIVITY, also try Infant Massage, page 22.

CRADLE SONGS

YOUR BABY won't actually giggle at a tickle until he's about three months old. Tactile games will intrigue him, however, and will boost his budding awareness of his own body. And incorporating silly songs or chants will appeal to his innate fascination with the human voice.

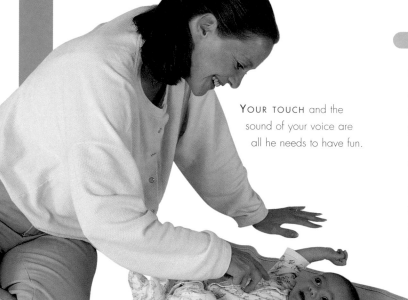

YOUR TOUCH and the sound of your voice are all he needs to have fun.

DID YOU EVER SEE A LASSIE

Did you ever see a lassie,
a lassie, a lassie,
did you ever see a lassie
go this way and that?
walk your fingers slowly back and forth
across baby's body

Go this way and that way,
go this way and that way,
did you ever see a lassie
go this way and that?
walk your fingers slowly back and forth
across baby's body

YANKEE DOODLE

Yankee Doodle went to town
a-riding on a pony;
stuck a feather in his cap
and called it macaroni.

Yankee Doodle keep it up,
Yankee Doodle dandy;
mind the music and the step
and with the girls be handy.

TWINKLE, TWINKLE LITTLE STAR

Twinkle, twinkle little star,
hold hands up, opening and closing fists
how I wonder what you are!

Up above the world so high,
point upward
like a diamond in the sky.
*create a diamond with thumbs
and forefingers*

Twinkle, twinkle little star,
open and close fists
how I wonder what you are!

LITTLE PETER RABBIT

 to the *tune* of "John Brown's Body"

Little Peter Rabbit had a fly
upon his nose.
touch baby's nose

Little Peter Rabbit had a fly
upon his nose.
touch baby's nose

Little Peter Rabbit had a fly
upon his nose.
touch baby's nose

And he flipped it,
and he flopped it
*"shoo" fly near
baby's face*

till it flew away.
make flying motion

HEARING A SIMPLE SONG when in Daddy's arms is always a delight.

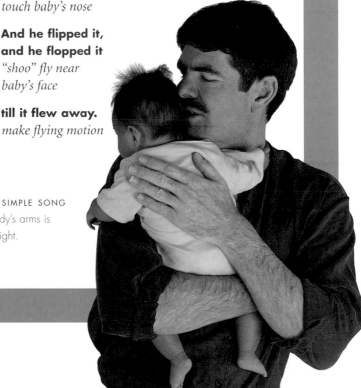

GETTING ORGANIZED

WHEN YOUR BABY is born, your home is filled with the presence of a precious new being. It also gets filled with a whole lot of baby "stuff." It's not just the crib, stroller, and changing table you bought before the baby's due date. Before you know it, your home will also be bursting with everything from tiny clothes and diapers to bottles and toys.

Having a perfectly tidy house isn't the top priority of most new parents. But adapting your expectations and household organizing systems should be. Remember that you can't get as much done as you did in pre-baby days. Be flexible. Make lists, but don't berate yourself for not completing every task.

At your fingertips: Diapers, diaper wipes, rash ointment, and clothing should be kept within arm's reach of the changing table so you don't leave the baby unattended. And baby washcloths, soaps, and towels should be close by at bath time.

Put like with like: You can use baskets or plastic boxes to keep toys sorted. Keeping clothes organized by size and season—all of the things that fit now in the top drawer, and all of the things that are too big but might fit by summer in another—also helps. Having a system makes it easier for you—and any other caretakers—to find the right clothes quickly.

For a rainy, or later, day: You don't have to put out every toy, book, and article of clothing you receive. Toys meant for an eighteen-month-old can be stored; you'll be glad to have some fresh toys when the time comes. Older-baby clothing can be sorted and tucked away in a closet.

Tidy up: You can't expect to have all the household chores done all the time. But you can decide to do one job once a day. Whether you do it in the evening or during the baby's afternoon nap, having the house somewhat neat can be a balm for a parent's soul. ■

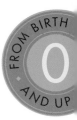

RIPPLING RIBBONS

VISIONS OF LOVELINESS

LONG BEFORE YOUR BABY is eagerly tearing paper off packages, ribbons will capture her curiosity and attention. Using masking tape, attach six-inch lengths of brightly colored ribbon to a piece of cardboard, or tie them securely to a wooden spoon. Lay your baby on the floor or changing table, or in an infant car seat. Then gently wave the ribbons around her face and hands. When she starts kicking her feet and jerking her arms, you'll know she's having fun with the colors, textures, and movement.

SKILL SPOTLIGHT

At this age, *watching the ribbons dance up and down and from side to side helps your baby develop her visual tracking skills. When she is older and starts swiping at objects, this activity lets her practice her eye-hand coordination and grasping skills, and lets her see the relationship between cause (I hit the ribbon) and effect (The ribbon swings and bounces).*

✔ **Eye-Hand Coordination**

✔ **Tactile Stimulation**

✔ **Visual Development**

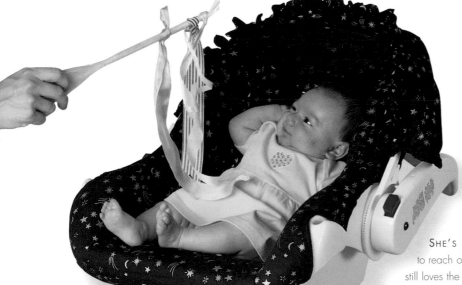

SHE'S NOT QUITE OLD ENOUGH to reach out and grasp yet, but she still loves the movement.

37

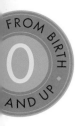

SOUND SPOTS

WHERE'S MOMMY'S VOICE?

SKILLSPOTLIGHT

Listening and looking *for your voice helps your baby develop both his visual tracking and auditory location skills. Equally important is your introduction of the idea that his family provides smiles, laughter, and praise. By the time he's six months old, he, too, will be smiling and laughing, and by the time he's one year old, he'll be trying to get you to turn your head toward him when he makes funny sounds.*

BABIES ARE BORN with an innate fascination with human voices, but they're not born with an immediate ability to locate the source of a sound in a room. To help your baby fine-tune his senses, try this: Place him in a car seat or infant chair in the middle of a room. Walk back and forth in front of him as you sing songs, make funny noises, or talk to him. Then try walking to the opposite side of the room and back again, letting him follow the sound of your voice. Although he won't turn his head at the sound of your voice, he'll hear the difference in sound as you move back and forth.

Listening	✔
Social Development	✔
Visual Development	✔

IF YOUR BABY ENJOYS THIS ACTIVITY, also try Noisemakers, page 44.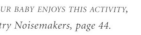

Most parents get a kick *out of claiming that their infant's personality—be it calm, restless, sweet, or belligerent—was foretold by his activity in the womb. But do such links between prenatal behavior and post-natal personality have any merit? In fact, researchers at Johns Hopkins University have found that several factors, including heart rate and movement in the womb, really can help predict what an infant's temperament will be during his first few months. According to the study, more active fetuses generally turn into more lively and unpredictable infants.*

FINDING MOMMY'S VOICE will eventually evolve into fun games of peekaboo and hide-and-go-seek.

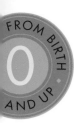

EYES ON TRACK

SPOT THE TOY

SKILLSPOTLIGHT

What's that sound? *What's that movement? As your baby moves her head from side to side, she learns to locate the source of noises and keep track of an object's whereabouts. At around three months, she'll swipe at the toy, and at about four months she'll grab at it.*

| Listening | ✔ |
| Visual Tracking | ✔ |

◀ *IF YOUR BABY ENJOYS THIS ACTIVITY, also try Rippling Ribbons, page 37.*

EVEN AS NEWBORNS, babies display interest in sights and sounds. Try moving a brightly colored squeaking toy back and forth slowly in front of your baby's eyes. When she's focused on the toy, move it to the left and to the right. Don't go too fast or far afield, though. If she loses sight of the toy, she'll figure it simply doesn't exist, and she'll lose interest in the game altogether.

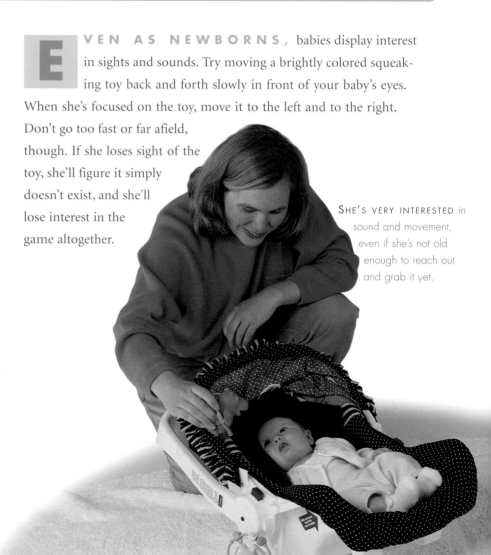

SHE'S VERY INTERESTED in sound and movement, even if she's not old enough to reach out and grab it yet.

ROCK THE BABY

BALANCE ON A BOLSTER

WHEN WE THINK OF ROCKING, we usually think of a baby on her back in a cradle or in our arms in a rocking chair. But one very soothing motion for an infant is to be gently rocked from side to side on her tummy. Roll up a towel or two together. Lay your baby on her stomach over the roll so that it supports her head, chest, stomach, and thighs. Turn her head to one side. Then very gently rock her from side to side while singing a song such as "Rock the Baby" (see the lyrics at right). The rocking motion helps her develop a sense of balance, while lying on her tummy gives her a chance to try to lift her head from a belly-down position.

THE PRESSURE on her tummy can be soothing; the rocking motion helps her gain an elementary sense of balance.

Rock the Baby

 to the *tune* of **"London Bridge Is Falling Down"**

**Rock the baby
side to side,
side to side,
side to side.
Rock the baby
side to side,
just like this.**

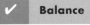

✔	**Balance**
✔	**Spatial Awareness**
✔	**Upper-Body Strength**

IF YOUR BABY ENJOYS THIS ACTIVITY, also try Beach-Ball Balance, page 42.

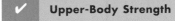

BEACH-BALL BALANCE

A ROCK AND ROLL GAME

SKILLSPOTLIGHT

Rolling back and forth *and from side to side stimulates baby's sense of balance. After the first month, most babies will also try to lift up their heads to see what's going on around them. That helps build upper-body strength. And the gentle pressure on the tummy can help babies with gas or colic.*

Balance	✔
Trust	✔
Upper-Body Strength	✔

◀ *IF YOUR BABY ENJOYS THIS ACTIVITY, also try Rock the Baby, page 41.*

YOUNG BABIES often don't like to lie on their tummies for very long. But most find it pretty interesting to lie on something big, soft, and round for a little while. Try placing your baby tummy-down on a slightly deflated beach ball. (But always be sure to support a newborn's head.) Turn her head to one side. Then, while securely holding her, rock her slowly forward and back or side to side on the ball. Sing or talk to her while you play; that will help keep her focused while the gentle rhythm and pressure soothe her tummy. Stop when she gets tired. When she's older and nearly able to sit up on her own, you can support her seated on top of the beach ball, and very gently bounce her up and down.

BRIGHT COLORS, a squishy surface, and a delightful rolling sensation make a winning combination.

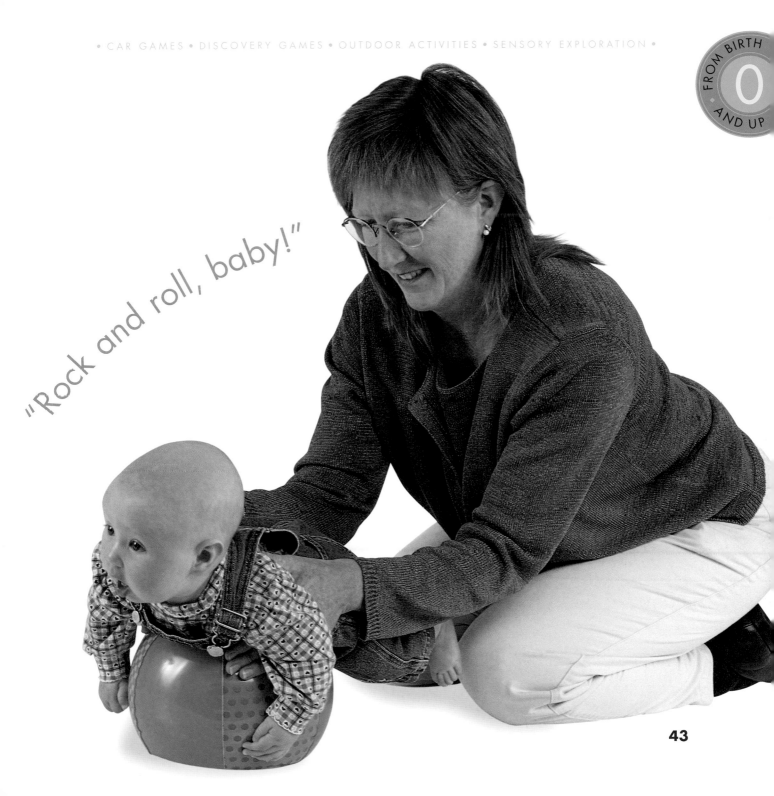

"Rock and roll, baby!"

43

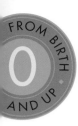

FROM BIRTH
0
AND UP

NOISEMAKERS

SOUND SENSATIONS

SKILLSPOTLIGHT

Hearing the various sounds
*from the dangling objects will
sharpen your baby's auditory
awareness and his visual discrimination skills. Seeing the objects
will help him focus. And in a few
months, when your baby is able to
swipe at objects, this activity can
encourage him to develop his
gross motor skills.*

Eye-Hand Coordination	✔
Listening	✔
Visual Development	✔

WHETHER THE SOUND is familiar, like that
of a musical mobile, or unfamiliar, like a new voice, noises
intrigue even the very youngest babies. Create a primitive
symphony of sound by stringing a number of noise-making objects—
jar lids, lightweight rattles, or plastic and wooden spoons—on
a rope or ribbon. Dangle and shake the noisemaker about
twelve inches in front of your baby. Or string
it across the crib and let him gaze up at it
as you shake the
rope or jiggle the
objects for him,
just don't leave
him alone with
this kind of toy.

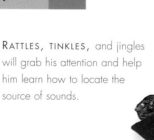

RATTLES, TINKLES, and jingles
will grab his attention and help
him learn how to locate the
source of sounds.

44

LITTLE BIRD WATCHERS

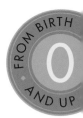

BABY'S FIRST NATURE CLASS

A **FLUTTER OF WINGS,** a flash of color, a sharp whistle or trill—such sights and sounds will fascinate almost any baby. The challenge, of course, is getting her close enough to actually see the birds. Try placing a bird feeder filled with seed just outside a window. As the birds begin to flock, hold your baby up so she can see them, or place her infant seat where she can watch them come and go. Soon she'll be crowing delightedly when she sees her feathered friends.

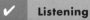

SHE LOVES TO WATCH these funny flying creatures flit about.

SKILLSPOTLIGHT

A newborn will have trouble *seeing the birds clearly, but she may detect a blur of color or motion. Over the next few months, watching birds will help her develop her visual tracking and focusing abilities. Her curiosity about the birds is a great example of her blossoming fascination with the world around her. A year from now—believe it or not—she'll be begging to help you fill the feeder!*

| ✔ | Listening |
| ✔ | Visual Development |

IF YOUR BABY ENJOYS THIS ACTIVITY, also try Rippling Ribbons, page 37.

45

BABYCYCLE

A BODY-AWARENESS ACTIVITY

SKILLSPOTLIGHT

By moving his legs *for him, you let your baby feel his little legs and feet moving in a new way— each side of the body working in reciprocal movement. You also mimic an action he'll be using later on as he learns to crawl.*

Body Awareness	✔
Gross Motor Skills	✔

◀ *IF YOUR BABY ENJOYS THIS ACTIVITY, also try Infant Massage, page 22.*

WHEN HE'S FIRST BORN, your baby has no idea that his body is actually separate from yours. But his expanding physical abilities will give rise to an increased interest in his own body parts that will last him well into toddlerhood. They also let him enjoy more physical, interactive games. In this simple exercise game, you very gently and very slowly move his legs in a bicycling motion, all the while talking and smiling at him to encourage him to wiggle his legs without your help. Before you know it he'll be grabbing his own little feet—and eventually pedaling all by himself!

IT FEELS GOOD to stretch and kick—especially when Mommy's guiding the movement.

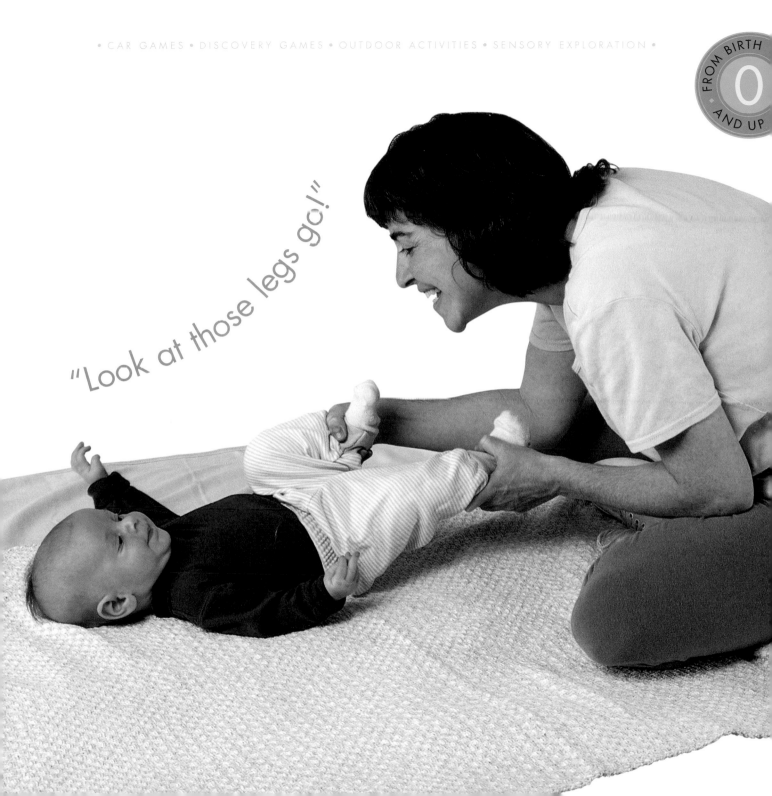

FROM BIRTH
0
AND UP

"Look at those legs go!"

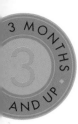
STRETCHING OUT

GENTLE GYM

I'm a Tiny Baby

to the *tune* of "Itsy-Bitsy Spider"

I'm a tiny baby
I'm soft and round and
small.
But when I'm busy stretching
I feel so big and tall.
My arms are getting long,
and my legs are getting
strong.
And the next thing you
know,
I'll be learning how to crawl.

| Body Awareness | ✔ |
| Tactile Stimulation | ✔ |

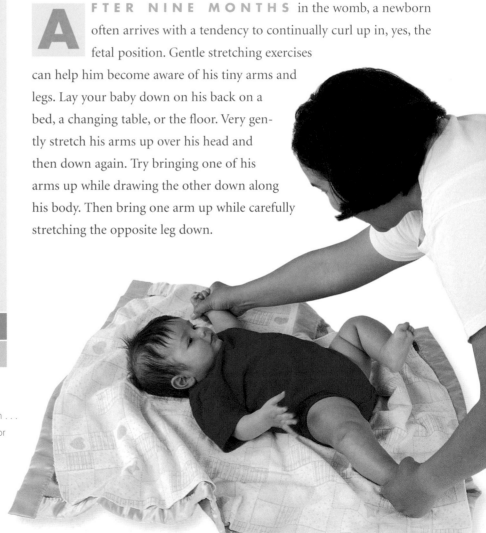

AFTER NINE MONTHS in the womb, a newborn often arrives with a tendency to continually curl up in, yes, the fetal position. Gentle stretching exercises can help him become aware of his tiny arms and legs. Lay your baby down on his back on a bed, a changing table, or the floor. Very gently stretch his arms up over his head and then down again. Try bringing one of his arms up while drawing the other down along his body. Then bring one arm up while carefully stretching the opposite leg down.

ONE ARM UP, one leg down . . . gentle stretching is relaxing for babies and parents alike.

SWAT THE TOY

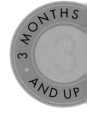

CATCH AS CATCH CAN

YOUR BABY may be able to see (at close range) as well as you can, but her ability to grasp objects is still not a match for yours. To help her, attach a small plush toy or teething ring to a brightly colored ribbon or plastic links. Dangle the toy in front of her and make it sway from side to side, encouraging her to reach across her body. Praise her efforts as she reaches out and swipes at—or even grabs— the toy. But never leave a baby alone with a long ribbon, as it poses a safety hazard.

WHEN YOUR BABY is grasping a pink plush puppy, she is exercising her ability to reach out and make contact with her world.

SKILLSPOTLIGHT

By three months, *most babies are using their heads and eyes together to track moving objects. That is, if an object moves to the left, the baby rotates her head to the left to follow the object, rather than just moving her eyes, as a newborn does. But she still needs to practice her grasping skills. Reaching for a moving object helps her fine-tune the coordination of both sides of her body.*

✓	**Eye-Hand Coordination**
✓	**Fine Motor Skills**
✓	**Visual Development**

IF YOUR BABY ENJOYS THIS ACTIVITY, also try Big Bouncing Ball, page 80.

49

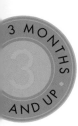

3 MONTHS AND UP

TARGET PRACTICE

A KICKING GAME

SKILLSPOTLIGHT

For babies, *eye-foot coordination is important. Eventually, using the feet in conjunction with the eyes will help him cruise the furniture and learn to walk.*

Body Awareness	✔
Eye-Foot Coordination	✔
Listening	✔

HE'S ALREADY DISCOVERED the joy of kicking his little legs. Give your baby's kicking a purpose by holding a target for him to try to hit. When he's on his back—on the changing table, a bed, or the floor—hold up a pillow, a plush toy, your hands, or a pie tin within easy reach of his little feet. If he doesn't understand the game, guide his feet to the target and praise him when he makes contact. Once he figures out what to do, he'll want to practice this one over and over.

HE SEES HIS FOOT make contact, he hears the resulting noise, and he feels the sole of his foot on the plate.

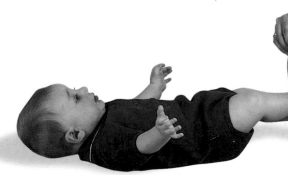

PEEKABOO GAMES

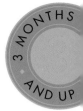

3 MONTHS AND UP

VARIATIONS ON A THEME

FIRST MOMMY'S THERE, then Mommy's gone, and then she's back again. Peekaboo is a perennial favorite with babies. Sometime around six or seven months, babies start to understand that objects continue to exist even when they are not present. Peekaboo is a great way to explore this concept with your little one. You can hold a blanket or diaper in front of your face while you say "Where's Mommy? Where's Mommy?" and then peek out from behind. Or put a light towel over your baby's face instead, then whisk it off, calling, "Peekaboo!" when her face emerges.

SKILLSPOTLIGHT

A newborn baby thinks *that when an object disappears, it no longer exists. When you appear and disappear behind the diaper, she begins to learn that even if you're momentarily hidden, you're still there. Grasping this concept— i.e., holding mental images—is a precursor to language development. When she gets old enough to put a blanket over her own face (albeit haphazardly), you'll see her kick and squirm with joy, as she's now in control of the disappearing act.*

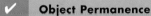
✔ **Object Permanence**

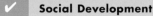
✔ **Social Development**

"PEEKABOO!" It's a relief and a revelation for her to realize you never really left at all.

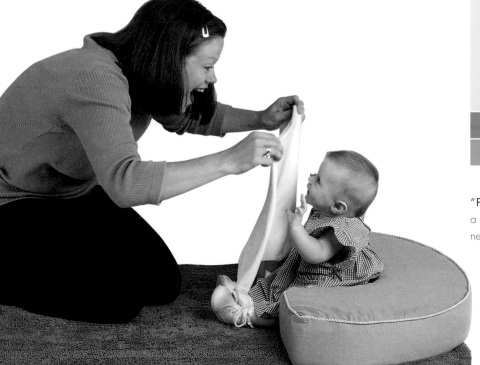

BABBLING WITH BABY

THE LITTLEST LANGUAGE LESSONS

SKILLSPOTLIGHT

Responding to your baby's *babbling supports his early efforts to communicate using sounds other than crying. Reinforcement of his vocalizations will show him that people value what he has to say, which will make it more rewarding for him to master language in the long run.*

Language Development	✔
Listening	✔
Social Development	✔

IF YOUR BABY ENJOYS THIS ACTIVITY, also try Fingerpuppet Fun, page 97. ▶

A THREE- TO SIX-MONTH-OLD BABY is often a delightfully social little being full of funny coos, gurgles, shouts, grunts, and irresistible smiles. Although he can't say real words yet (that won't come until he's nearing his first birthday), he utters those adorable sounds as a way of exploring the sounds he hears every day. He also learns from the responses you give to these vocalizations. Encourage his early efforts by holding a baby-babble conversation with him.

• When he says "aaah," listen, nod, and say "aaah" in return. When he says "goo!" you say "goo!" too.

• Once you're both warmed up, try changing his words slightly, by stretching them out ("bah!" becomes "baaaaaaah") or even adding to them ("ooh" becomes "oooh-wah!").

• Encouraging your baby to mimic you will inspire him to try ever more complex language patterns, which eventually will result in his attempting words and then phrases.

Note: This kind of baby talk is constructive only until a child begins talking. At that point, it's better to repeat words correctly than repeat his incorrect pronunciations, no matter how cute they are.

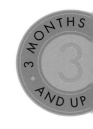

3 MONTHS
3
AND UP

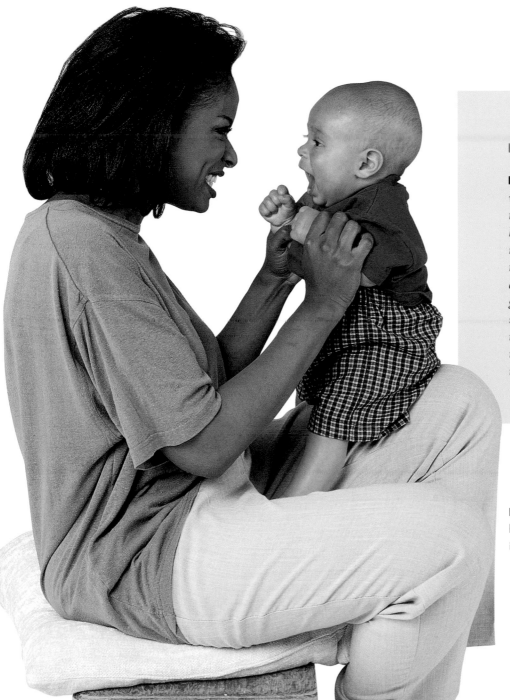

RESEARCH REPORT

For the first six months, *babies will babble whether you talk to them or not. But they'll learn how to talk more easily if you make a concerted effort to show them how language works. Indeed, all babies—no matter what language is spoken in their home—sound alike until they're about six months old. After that, they start repeating the sounds they hear most often around them.*

HE'LL SQUEAL AND SQUIRM when he realizes you're following his lead in this elementary conversation.

SLEEPING THROUGH THE NIGHT

BY THE TIME she's three or four months old, your baby will probably have developed some sort of sleep pattern. It may be a dream-come-true sleep pattern, or it may feel like your biggest life challenge—waking every hour on the hour at night, never napping for more than half an hour during the day, suddenly getting daytime (wake time) and nighttime (sleep time) reversed, or something in between.

Getting a baby to sleep on a "normal" schedule is actually a matter of common sense and logistics, with a little bravery and patience thrown in.

Develop a daytime routine: plan fairly regular times for outings, baths, play periods, and meals. External regularity will help her set her inner clock.

Develop a nighttime routine: a warm bath, cozy pajamas, a lullaby, and some books are classic ways of getting your baby to unwind. It's never too early to convince a baby that nighttime feedings are all business and kind of boring. Keep the lights low, don't talk to her very much, don't let her play with toys or watch television, and gently put her in her crib on her back as soon as she's done.

Once your baby is about six months old, she shouldn't really need to eat during the night. Some parents choose to use a modified "cry it out" program, letting her cry for a few minutes, then going in to reassure her, then letting her cry some more; some may continue to feed, cuddle, walk, or sing to their babies in hopes that eventually the child will sleep longer and longer on her own. Eventually, most babies will learn to put themselves to sleep, which is an important skill to have.

What's the best approach? It's a little bit different for every family. The magic formula is the method that you and your baby feel most comfortable with—and that's a personal decision. ■

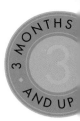

3 MONTHS AND UP

TUMMY BOLSTER

BUILDING UPPER-BODY STRENGTH

LEARNING HOW TO SIT requires far more than just keeping one's head up; it also calls on the muscles of the shoulders, torso, and upper and lower back. You can help your baby develop those muscles by bolstering him with a rolled-up towel, the ends secured with soft fabric hair bands. Slip the towel roll under his arms and chest while he lies on his tummy on the floor or carpet. The bolster helps him to raise his neck and shoulders up for longer periods and encourages him to use his arms for support. It also offers him an enticing view of the world around him.

SKILL SPOTLIGHT

Using a bolster *like this one helps your baby practice putting weight on his forearms, which helps him strengthen his arm and back muscles in preparation for sitting up and eventually crawling. And giving him a new position from which to view the world will stimulate his vision and inspire him to reach, roll, or even creep forward.*

✔	**Emotional Development**
✔	**Social Development**
✔	**Upper-Body Strength**

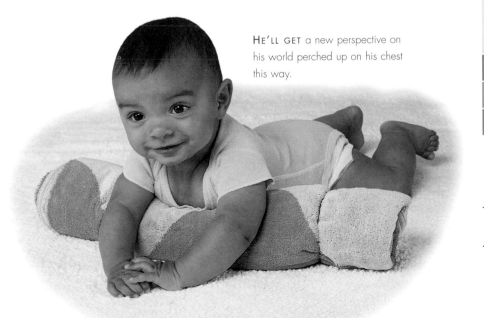

HE'LL GET a new perspective on his world perched up on his chest this way.

IF YOUR BABY ENJOYS THIS ACTIVITY, *also try Tummy Talk, page 60.*

55

FRIENDLY FACES

A BOOK OF MUG SHOTS

SKILLSPOTLIGHT

The combination *of your baby's visual abilities and desire for human interaction makes her highly sensitive to cues provided by facial expressions. A book full of different faces gives her many to contemplate. She may simply stare at them— glancing from their eyes to their mouths and back again. Or she may try to point or talk to the pictures.*

MAKING YOUR OWN

You can create a face book by gluing photos (either from magazines or from your own collection) on pieces of heavy cardboard. Preserve them with clear plastic contact paper or sheet protectors. Or simply place photos in a photo album.

BY THE AGE OF THREE MONTHS, your baby is so attuned to facial expressions that she responds to smiles or laughter. She can also tell the difference between her loved ones' faces and unfamiliar faces. That's why you get that special grin when your baby peers at you over someone else's shoulder and your friends just get a solemn gaze. It's also why her whole body wriggles when you peek at her over her crib rail in the morning; she recognizes your face, and she already loves it dearly.

Giving your baby a book with lots of faces— either one you buy or one you make—introduces your baby to a wide range of faces and the many emotions they express. You may even find that she develops favorites—perhaps the little boy gleefully holding a puppy, or the picture of Daddy looking sheepish in his fishing hat.

| Social Development | ✔ |
| Visual Discrimination | ✔ |

POINTING OUT THE PEOPLE in the pictures helps your baby begin to connect names with familiar faces.

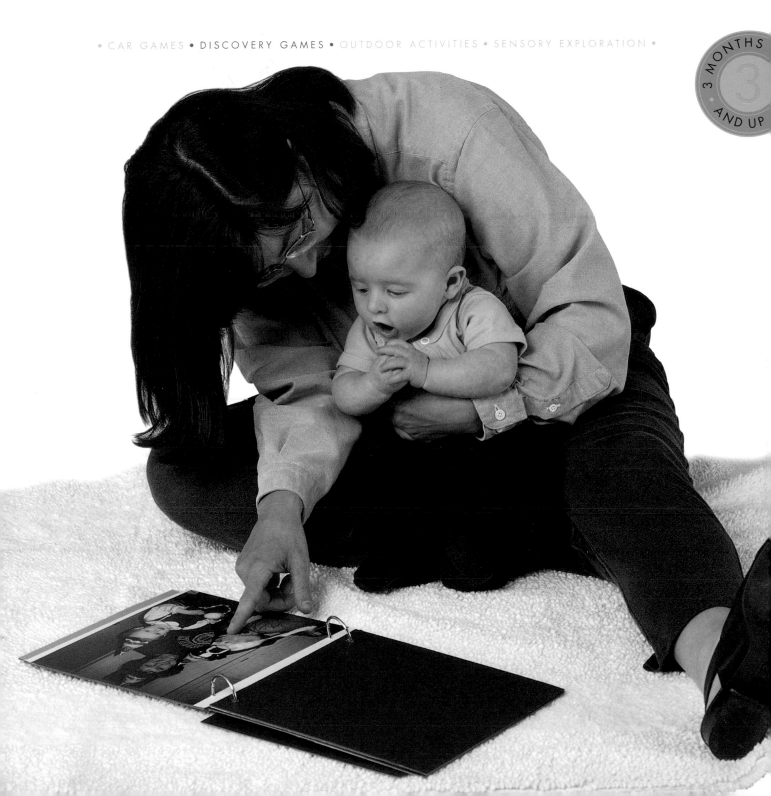

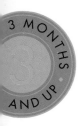

MIRROR PLAY

WHO'S THAT BABY?

SKILLSPOTLIGHT

Watching her own face *and interacting with her image in the mirror increases your baby's budding awareness of herself as a separate person. And if she lies on her stomach, it will help her strengthen the muscles needed for sitting and crawling.*

Upper-Body Strength	✔
Visual Stimulation	✔

◀ *IF YOUR BABY ENJOYS THIS ACTIVITY, also try Facial Expressions, page 24.*

A **THREE- OR FOUR-MONTH-OLD BABY** is just getting to the point where she can amuse herself for several minutes on end—an exciting breakthrough for baby and parents alike. You may hear her gurgling to her toes early in the morning, for instance; see her fiddling with her hands in front of her face; or catch her looking intently around a room. At around four months old, a baby can not only see but also track, which means that she can actually watch objects or people as they move around her. Now that your baby can lift her head while she's on her tummy, a mirror in her crib can provide a lot of fun. She doesn't yet understand that she's looking at herself in the mirror, and she won't until she's fifteen to eighteen months old. Still, she'll brighten and smile when she sees her own face—she's happy to be greeted by such an intriguing person!

YOUR BABY will be enchanted by her new playmate, even if she doesn't recognize it is her own image.

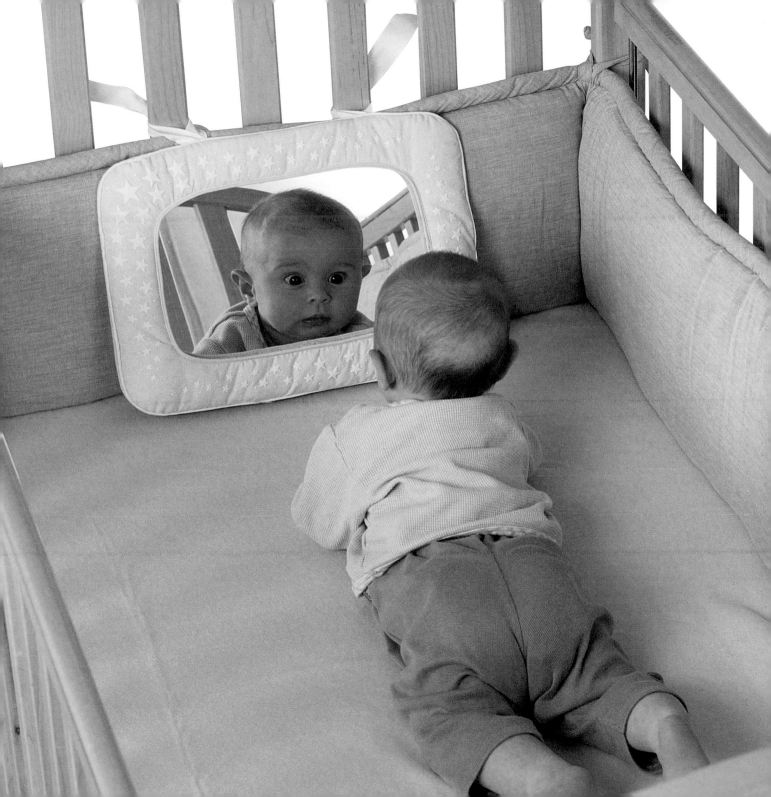

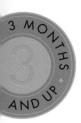

TUMMY TALK

STRENGTHENING THE NECK AND BACK

SKILLSPOTLIGHT

Every moment your baby spends on his tummy helps build up his strength. Your reassuring presence and pride in his accomplishments (however small) also help him learn that it's really OK to be on his stomach. When you roll him back over when he gets too uncomfortable (as indeed you should), he learns yet again that someone is paying attention to his cues and responding appropriately.

Emotional Development	✔
Social Development	✔
Upper-Body Strength	✔

AT THREE MONTHS, some babies may still cry in protest when placed on their tummies. But spending time in that position is crucial, as it helps them to strengthen the neck, shoulder, and back muscles in preparation for sitting and crawling.

• You shouldn't make your baby stay in a position he is not comfortable with, but you can persuade him to like it more by lying in front of him, placing a favorite toy in view, making eye contact, and socializing with him a bit.

• Encourage him if he starts improvising on the position. He may start "swimming" excitedly with his arms and legs, for instance. Or he may stiffen them in an "airplane" position and rock back and forth.

• Don't worry if he can only tolerate being on his belly for a minute or two. Follow his lead and quit when he's had enough. You can try again later. Plenty of babies are challenged by tummy time—and all of them learn to sit, crawl, and walk.

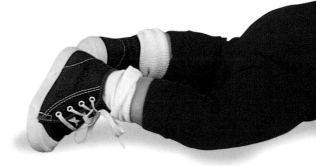

IF MOMMY'S DOING IT, then he may decide it's OK for him to try it awhile, too.

60

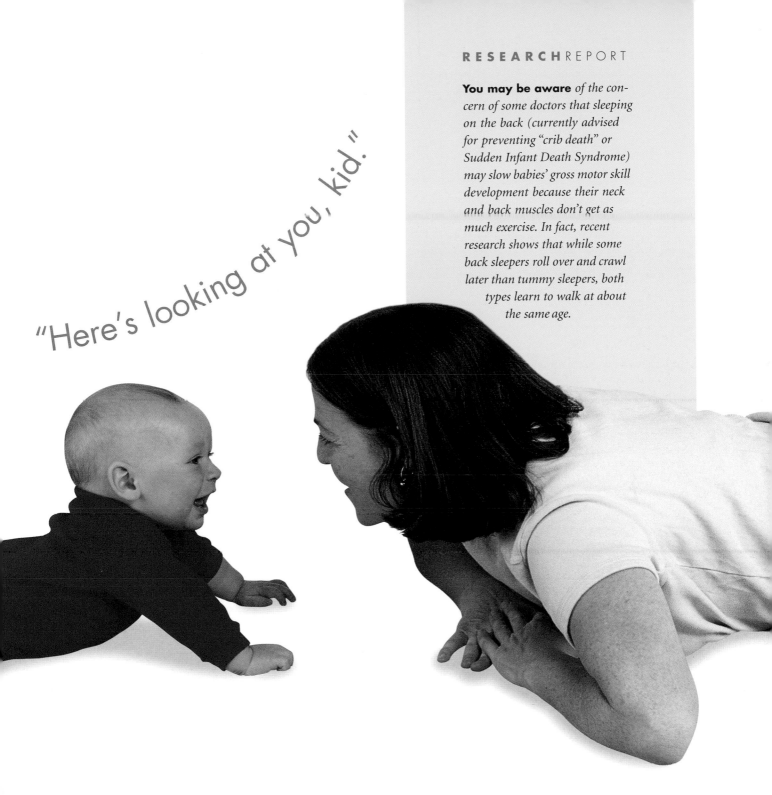

"Here's looking at you, kid."

RESEARCH REPORT

You may be aware of the concern of some doctors that sleeping on the back (currently advised for preventing "crib death" or Sudden Infant Death Syndrome) may slow babies' gross motor skill development because their neck and back muscles don't get as much exercise. In fact, recent research shows that while some back sleepers roll over and crawl later than tummy sleepers, both types learn to walk at about the same age.

GETTING OTHERS INVOLVED

I'S A FACT that in most families, Mommy takes on the lion's share of the care for young babies. Unfortunately, the more Mommy does it, the more she—and everyone else—starts feeling that she's the only one who knows how to do it right. Here are a few ways to help others get involved with your baby's care and play.

The other parent: If Mom stays at home and Dad goes to work, she changes ten times as many diapers as he does, prepares three times as many meals, and spends about eight times as long playing with the baby. If they're both working, statistics show, she's still spending more time with the baby. That can make her feel like she's the expert and him feel that he's all thumbs.

How do you let go? Tell your significant other what he needs to know for safety's sake (for example, the baby can now roll off the bed), and then walk away and let him figure it out. If he secures a diaper too loosely or puts the baby in a position she doesn't like, he'll soon discover his mistake.

Grandparents: They may have different or outdated ideas about child rearing, or have forgotten how to take care of a baby. But a grandparent's love is special and something your child shouldn't miss. Explaining what works and is safe for your baby will make everyone feel more comfortable. Let them know what your baby enjoys, and then let them indulge their love.

Baby-sitters: Regular baby-sitters will have a good idea of what toys your baby enjoys, what comforts her, and what trouble she's attracted to. Occasional baby-sitters need to have that information spelled out. Show all baby-sitters where extra bottles and clothing and the first-aid kit are kept. Leave emergency telephone numbers. Then leave! It's important for parents and babies alike to know that little ones are safe in the care of other adults. ∎

PINWHEEL MAGIC

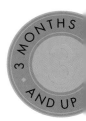

3 MONTHS AND UP

BLOWING IN THE WIND

BY FOUR MONTHS, your baby's vision has developed significantly, he can control his head, and he's starting to reach out to touch things. This means he's ready—and eager—to take in the wonders of the wide world. Try showing him the blur of beautiful colors that results when you blow on a pinwheel. He himself won't be able to blow on it until he's more than a year old, but he may enjoy watching you wave it in the air. (Most babies this age will try to grab at pinwheels. Don't let them, however, as the sharp edges could hurt them and small pieces could be swallowed.) You can also place the pinwheel outside in a planter box and seat your baby near it so that he can watch the colors go round.

SKILLSPOTLIGHT

A tantalizing pinwheel *will mesmerize most babies. A younger baby—around three months— will be fascinated by the blur of movement and may swipe vaguely at the pinwheel with closed fists. By six months, though, he'll be able to see and reach for the pinwheel. You can also sing a spinning pinwheel song to add to the fun.*

✔ **Social Development**

✔ **Visual Development**

GRANDPA'S colorful pinwheel will capture the baby's attention and possibly prompt a gleeful reaction.

63

TICK-TOCK

A CUCKOO GAME

Tick-Tock

Tick-tock, tick-tock,
swing baby from side to side

I'm a little cuckoo clock.
swing her from side to side

Tick-tock, tick-tock,
swing her from side to side

now I'm striking one o'clock.
lift baby up to the sky gently just once

Cuckoo! Cuckoo!

repeat verses with two and three o'clock, raising her up two and three times, respectively

WITH A SIMPLE CHANT, some soft swaying, and a gentle lift in the air, this activity is sure to please most babies. Hold your baby under her arms and keep her head upright. You can sit or stand with your baby either facing you or out into the room. Babies also like to watch each other doing this activity. So if your little one has a little playmate, let them face each other while the parents sing the song. When your baby gets too heavy for you to lift this way, you can turn the game into a lap ride by chanting the words as you rock back and forth and gently bounce her on your lap.

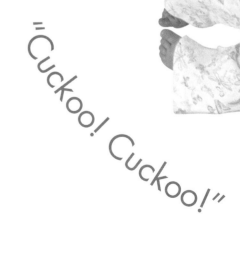

"Cuckoo! Cuckoo!"

Balance	✔
Body Awareness	✔
Listening	✔

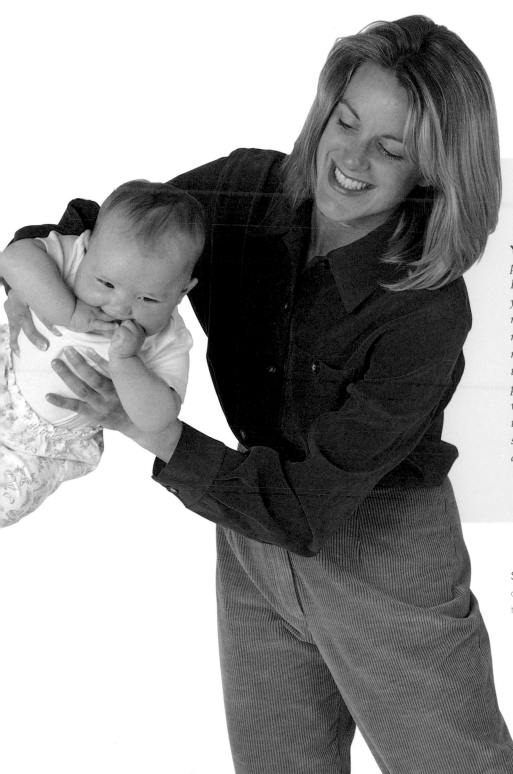

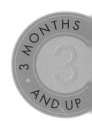

RESEARCH REPORT

You may think *your infant isn't paying attention to music yet. In fact, numerous studies in recent years have shown that babies can remember a melody and comprehend rhythm, and that music even sets off memories for them. In one study of three-month-old babies, researchers played a song while babies played with mobiles. When the babies heard that same song either one day or seven days later, they started inter- acting with their mobiles once again.*

SHE HAS NO IDEA what a clock is, but swinging from side to side is delightful just the same.

65

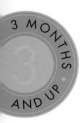
JUST OUT OF REACH

MOVEMENT MOTIVATION

SKILL SPOTLIGHT

Even before your baby can sit up on his own, he may be starting to roll from one side to the other. That means he's beginning to realize that he's a self-propelling creature. Enticing him with interesting-looking objects may encourage his emerging mobility. Accompanying the exercise with playful interactions helps build a close relationship between you and your child and sows the seeds for healthy self-esteem.

Gross Motor Skills	✔
Social Development	✔

YOU CAN ENCOURAGE your baby's early efforts to grab things and even to move his body by placing attractive objects (brightly colored balls, plush toys, favorite picture books, and, most especially, yourself) just beyond his reach. Encourage him to get to the objects in any way he can, whether by creeping forward on his tummy, rolling over on his side, or just plain s-t-r-e-t-c-h-i-n-g as far as he can go. Don't tease him, though. Instead, build success into the activity. If he starts to get frustrated, hand him the toy and praise his efforts.

STRETCHING, ROLLING, and "tummy time" build strength needed for crawling.

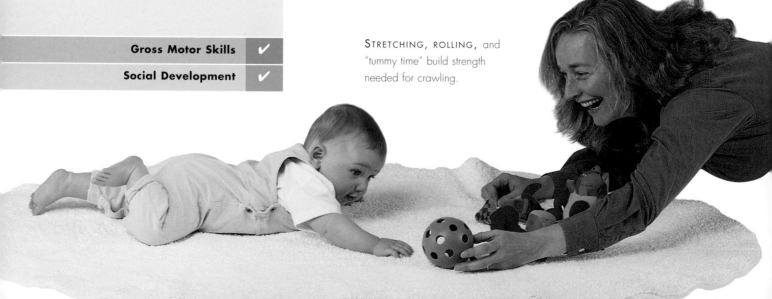

BELLY ROLL

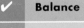

3 MONTHS AND UP

BODY AWARENESS FOR BEGINNERS

WHEN HE WAS FIRST BORN, your baby couldn't tell the difference between his being and your being, or where his body ended and yours began. You can boost his budding body awareness and stimulate his little body by gently rolling a small beach ball across his tummy and up and down his legs and arms. Does he want to grab it or kick it? Let him at it—it's excellent coordination practice. You can also try putting him on his tummy and rolling the ball down his back. Singing a song during this activity can add to the fun.

SKILL SPOTLIGHT

The gentle massage *from the ball provides tactile stimulation and helps your baby become aware of his own body. Grasping the ball helps him develop eye-hand coordination. Sitting upright and holding on to the ball with your support will help him learn balance.*

✔	**Balance**
✔	**Body Awareness**
✔	**Tactile Stimulation**

THE TICKLING PRESSURE OF a rolling beach ball helps him learn more about his body.

KITCHEN FUN

NOW YOU'RE COOKING

As he manipulates *cups and spoons by dropping them, picking them up, and placing them in his mouth, your baby learns about using his arms and hands. Exploring objects by mouth helps your baby learn about physical properties such as smooth, rough, cold, hard, light, and heavy. Your participation in such activities helps ensure your baby's success.*

Eye-Hand Coordination	✔
Fine Motor Skills	✔
Gross Motor Skills	✔

IF YOUR BABY ENJOYS THIS ACTIVITY, *also try Swat the Toy, page 49.*

JUST BECAUSE YOUR BABY can reach out and grasp something—a rattle, a stuffed animal, or a lock of your hair—doesn't mean he can control that object very well. Becoming truly dexterous requires fine control of the wrist, palm, and fingers, as well as the ability to judge distance and shapes. All that takes plenty of practice. Sets of plastic measuring cups and spoons are great toys at this stage because they're easy to grasp and have interesting surfaces. If your baby has learned to pick up things on his own, just place them around him on the floor. If his aim isn't yet perfected, place the spoons in his hand and encourage him to hold them. Don't be surprised or disappointed if the spoons immediately go in his mouth. Gumming objects is a healthy way for babies to learn about the world.

EXPLORING WITH SPOONS helps him understand how his hands, his arms, and various-sized objects actually work.

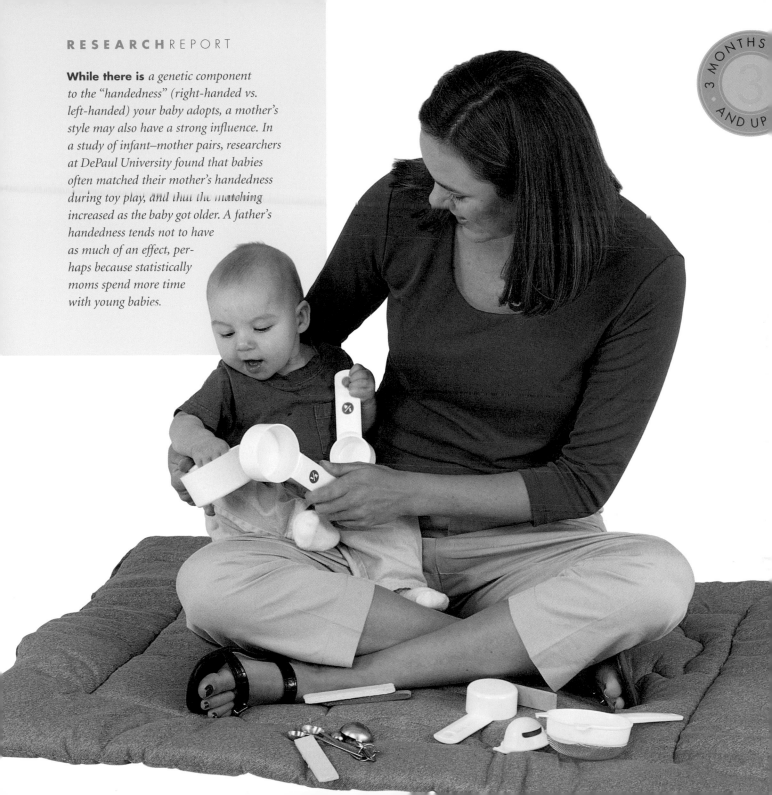

RESEARCH REPORT

While there is *a genetic component to the "handedness" (right-handed vs. left-handed) your baby adopts, a mother's style may also have a strong influence. In a study of infant–mother pairs, researchers at DePaul University found that babies often matched their mother's handedness during toy play, and that the matching increased as the baby got older. A father's handedness tends not to have as much of an effect, perhaps because statistically moms spend more time with young babies.*

KNEE RIDES

ADD A LITTLE BOUNCE to lap time by propping up your baby on your knee and gently rocking her back and forth while you sing a children's song. It's a good way for her to gain a sense of rhythm and challenge her sense of balance.

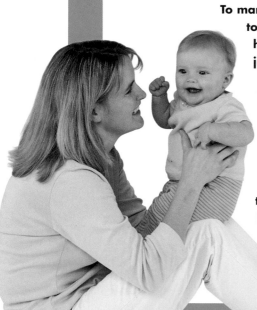

TO MARKET, TO MARKET

**To market, to market,
to buy a fat pig,
home again, home again,
jiggety jig.**

**To market, to market,
to buy a fat hog,
home again, home again,
jiggety jog.**

**To market, to market,
to buy a plum bun,
home again, home again,
marketing's done.**

TROT, TROT, TROT

Trot, trot to London,
rock baby side to side on lap
**trot, trot to Dover.
Look out, (baby's name),
or you might fall O-VER.**
tip baby to one side

Trot, trot to Boston,
rock baby side to side on lap
trot, trot to Lynn.
*support baby's waist and neck
with your hands*
**Look out, (baby's name),
or you might fall IN!**
*gently let the baby drop through
the space between your legs*

SKIP TO MY LOU

Skip, skip, skip to my Lou,
rock baby rhythmically from side to side
skip, skip, skip to my Lou,
skip, skip, skip to my Lou,
skip to my Lou, my darling.

Lost my partner, what'll I do?
rock baby back and forth
Lost my partner, what'll I do?
Lost my partner, what'll I do?
Skip to my Lou, my darling.

I'll find another one, prettier too,
raise baby up on knees, and down again
I'll find another one, prettier too,
I'll find another one, prettier too,
skip to my Lou, my darling.

Flies in the buttermilk, shoo fly shoo,
rock baby on knee, exaggerate "shoo" sound
flies in the buttermilk, shoo fly shoo,
flies in the buttermilk, shoo fly shoo,
skip to my Lou, my darling.

MY BONNIE

My Bonnie lies over the ocean,
rock baby to left
my Bonnie lies over the sea,
rock baby to right
my Bonnie lies over the ocean,
lean backwards
oh bring back my Bonnie to me.
pull baby tight to chest

Bring back, bring back,
rock baby back and forth
oh bring back my Bonnie
to me, to me.
Bring back, bring back,
rock baby back and forth
oh bring back
my Bonnie to me.
end with a big hug

FEW BABIES can resist a
silly song and a rhythmic
rock with a parent.

WAY HIGH

EARLY FLIGHT LESSONS

SKILLSPOTLIGHT

Although he's firmly held *by you, this "flying" activity helps him develop the large muscles in his back and shoulders, especially if he lifts his head up to look at the scenery. It also gives him a chance to develop a fledgling sense of balance. You won't let him go, of course, but he'll feel his center of gravity shifting as he "flies" up and down.*

Balance	✔
Upper-Body Strength	✔

◀ *IF YOUR BABY ENJOYS THIS ACTIVITY, also try Airplane Baby, page 32.*

YOUR UNCLE may have tossed you in the air when you were young—and you may have loved it—but such baby-as-beach-ball activities are no longer considered safe. You can still have fun "flying" with your baby, however—just be sure to keep a steady grip on his tiny torso and keep your movements gentle. Sit upright with your baby in front of you on the floor. Lift him up in the air, then roll onto your back, lifting him over your head. You can also place his tummy on your shins while you lie back and gently sway or lift your legs while holding his arms. Either way, he will enjoy the feeling of soaring through the air, even while you're safely supporting him. Sing a song like "I'm Flying High" (opposite) to add to his fun.

MOMMY'S STEADY HANDS, happy song, and smiling face make "rough-housing" safe and fun.

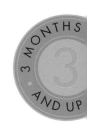

3 MONTHS
3
AND UP

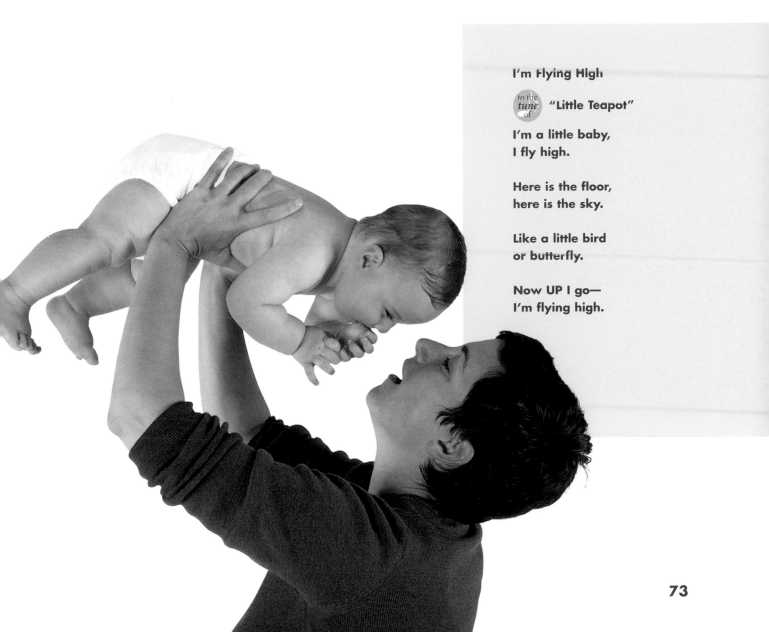

I'm Flying High

In the **tune** *of* **"Little Teapot"**

I'm a little baby,
I fly high.

Here is the floor,
here is the sky.

Like a little bird
or butterfly.

Now UP I go—
I'm flying high.

73

BABY'S FIRST BOOKS

READY FOR READING

SKILL SPOTLIGHT

The physical closeness *involved in reading envelops your baby with a sense of intimacy and well-being. Indeed, in time, a reading session can become a wonderful bedtime ritual and a nice way of calming a fretful, sick, or over-stimulated baby. And having the objects in the pictures named for him helps him develop a receptive vocabulary for language.*

Emotional Development	✔
Language Development	✔
Visual Development	✔

HE'S TOO YOUNG to understand a story line. He's probably too young even to turn the pages. But introducing your young baby to the pleasures of books is one of the best things you can do for him, as it builds a positive association with reading.

• Small, square board books are easiest at this age, as your baby can gum them, swat at them, and grab at them without damaging the pages. In the second half of this first year, when your baby learns to turn his own pages, look for plastic bath books or books with cloth pages, which will be easier for him to handle.

• Books with colorful pictures and a minimum of text are the best choices, as they introduce him to the magic of illustrated worlds without too much narration. Point out the objects in each picture—"See the duck?" "Where are the socks?" Someday soon he'll surprise you by pointing to such objects on his own.

• Most young babies won't sit still for a full narration and instead may enjoy simply exploring the pages. Other babies are lulled by the cadence of nursery rhymes and similar story lines. Your baby knows best what kind of storybook session he likes, so follow his lead.

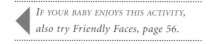

IF YOUR BABY ENJOYS THIS ACTIVITY, also try Friendly Faces, page 56.

He can hardly sit up *and he can't tell a chicken from a dump truck. So why read to a baby? Research shows that reading, even to young babies, helps them build their "receptive" vocabularies (the number of words they understand). In one study at Rhode Island Hospital, researchers compared the receptive vocabularies of two groups of eighteen-month-olds. One group had been read to often as babies; the other had not. The frequent-reading group's vocabulary had increased 40 percent since babyhood; the nonreading group's vocabulary had increased just 16 percent.*

EVEN THE YOUNGEST BABIES enjoy time spent snuggling, listening to words, and looking at colorful pictures.

3 MONTHS AND UP

75

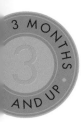

3 MONTHS AND UP

EYES, NOSE, MOUTH, TOES

A BODY EXERCISE

SKILL SPOTLIGHT

Your young baby *is not going to repeat any of these body-part names; that comes later on. But your touch provides tactile stimulation and helps her become more aware of her body's parameters and movements. Naming body parts often enough eventually will help her to recognize them and learn how to say them herself.*

Body Awareness	✔
Language Development	✔
Tactile Stimulation	✔

◄ *IF YOUR BABY ENJOYS THIS ACTIVITY, also try Babbling With Baby, page 52.*

HER KICKING FEET, waving hands, and general jiggling and giggling are all signs that your baby is beginning to understand that she can somewhat control the movements of her own body. Reinforce this dawning realization by pointing out the major body parts for her. Place her on a bed, carpet, or changing table. Touch her face and say "face." Then place her little hands on your face and repeat "face." Then do her eyes, nose, mouth, and chin, and her legs, tummy, feet, and toes, each time letting her feel both her own body and yours.

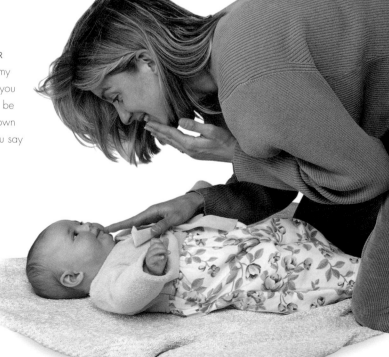

"THIS IS YOUR FACE, this is my face." Before you know it, she'll be touching her own face when you say the word.

WHAT'S SQUEAKING?

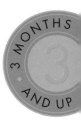

3 MONTHS AND UP

A HANDS-ON EXERCISE

BETWEEN THE THIRD and fourth months, most babies learn to reach for and grasp objects. This isn't an easy task; it requires your baby to have significant hand control. It's an exciting discovery, however, as he can now draw objects in the world toward himself rather than waiting for you to deliver them. To help him practice, hold two squeaky toys in front of him. Squeezing first one and then the other, encourage him to grab at the toys.

SKILL SPOTLIGHT

At first your baby *may just wave his hands and kick excitedly. But squeaky toys are enticing enough that he'll start swiping at them—which is good practice for his hand-eye coordination and shows him just how far his body reaches. If he makes contact with the toy, let him hold it; the sense of accomplishment and satisfaction he gets will be a reward that inspires him to try this activity again and again.*

| ✔ | **Eye-Hand Coordination** |
| ✔ | **Listening** |

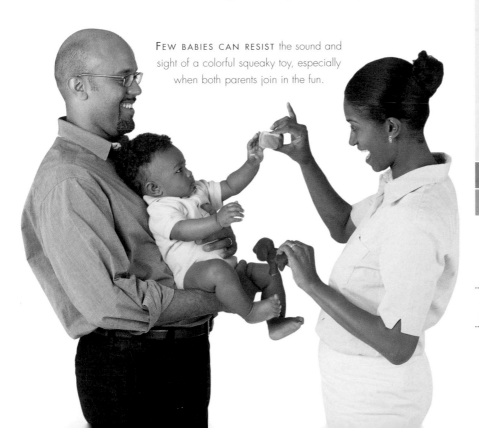

FEW BABIES CAN RESIST the sound and sight of a colorful squeaky toy, especially when both parents join in the fun.

IF YOUR BABY ENJOYS THIS ACTIVITY, also try Big Bouncing Ball, page 80.

BUBBLES FOR BABY

REACHING, TOUCHING, POPPING

SKILLSPOTLIGHT

Watching bubbles float *through the air helps your baby practice his visual skills such as eye tracking, distance, and depth perception. Trying to swat at them is excellent practice for his budding eye-hand coordination. And if he should actually catch one, he'll get a lesson in the relationship between cause (I touch the bubble) and effect (The bubble pops!).*

MAKING YOUR OWN

For the soap solution, mix 1 cup of water, 1 teaspoon of glycerin (available in pharmacies), and 2 tablespoons of dish-washing detergent. Make bubble wands from plastic lids with the center cut out. But be sure to keep these away from your baby.

Cause and Effect	✔
Eye-Hand Coordination	✔
Visual Development	✔

HAS IT BEEN DECADES since you last pondered the magic of iridescent bubbles floating in the air? Don't let that stop you from sharing this simple—and highly entertaining—activity with your baby.

• Buy a variety of bubble-blowing toys, and blow different-sized bubbles for your baby. If you aim large bubbles at a cloth, soft carpet, or bath water, the bubbles will stick longer, which will give five- and six-month-olds a chance to "catch" their first one. Or create a shower of small bubbles by blowing quickly through a wand or pipe. Tracking bubbles in midair hones your baby's developing visual skills.

• A cascade of bubbles makes a pleasant distraction during diaper-changing time. Blowing bubbles while he's bathing will make bath time fun (and the bathtub also helps contain the soapy residue that some bubbles leave on surfaces). Bubbles billowing outside are especially enchanting. Wave the wand way up high, or blow the bubbles low to the ground so they drift skyward on air currents.

IF YOUR BABY ENJOYS THIS ACTIVITY, also try Pinwheel Magic, page 63.

BUBBLES ARE FASCINATING
baubles—even for very young babies.

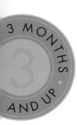

3 MONTHS
3
AND UP

BIG BOUNCING BALL

SWATTING PRACTICE

SKILLSPOTLIGHT

He can't grab objects *until he can literally learn to aim and fire those little hands and feet. That takes eye-hand and eye-foot coordination, as well as an understanding of just how far those arms and legs extend—all of which come from steady swatting and kicking practice.*

Eye-Foot Coordination	✔
Eye-Hand Coordination	✔
Tactile Stimulation	✔
Visual Development	✔

SOMETIMES IT'S THE SIMPLEST **TOYS** that give a baby the biggest kick for the longest amount of time. For instance, an old-fashioned, brightly colored punchball (available at toy stores) can engage a baby all through the first half of his first year—and even beyond. Newborns will gaze at the orb if it's hung from a ceiling or doorway. Three- to six-month-olds can swat it with their hands, kick it with their feet, and eventually try to get both arms around it. Can't find a punchball? Hang a beach ball instead. Whichever you choose, always supervise your baby with the ball.

HE'LL LOVE SWATTING
at this big, colorful ball.

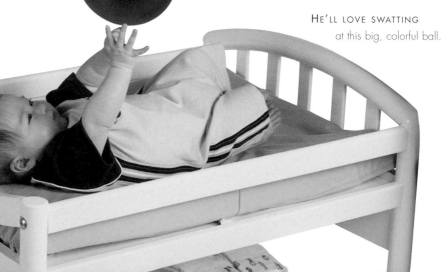

80

JACK-IN-THE-BOX

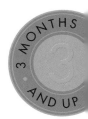

3 MONTHS AND UP

THE JOY OF SURPRISES

TAKE A GAME OF PEEKABOO, add a little music, throw in the surprise effect of having a toy clown pop out from a box, and you've got the perfect activity for a five- or six-month-old baby. Once she learns that a toy comes out every time, the anticipation will build until it's hard for her to contain her excitement. Soon she'll be helping you stuff the toy back in the box, and waiting expectantly for you to close the lid, turn the handle, and make the clown pop out again.

AFTER THE "POP," she'll help you stuff the clown back in its box.

SKILL SPOTLIGHT

The sound of a crank *going round and round, as well as the delicious "pop" of a toy springing from its box, provide auditory stimulation for your baby. Equally important, the repetition of the toy's appearance and disappearance reinforces her growing understanding of object permanence.*

✔	**Cause & Effect**
✔	**Listening**
✔	**Visual Stimulation**

 IF YOUR BABY ENJOYS THIS ACTIVITY, also try Peekaboo Games, page 51.

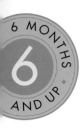
PUSHING GAME

LOWER-BODY EXERCISES

SKILLSPOTLIGHT

A baby's muscles develop *from the head and neck, shoulders, and arms; down the back; and finally to the hips, thighs, and calves. At this age your baby's upper body may be pretty well developed (that's why he can sit up), but his legs aren't quite sturdy enough for him to crawl. This exercise helps strengthen them and also gives him a taste of what it takes to get some forward motion.*

Balance	✔
Gross Motor Skills	✔
Upper-Body Strength	✔

◀ *IF YOUR BABY ENJOYS THIS ACTIVITY, also try Just Out of Reach, page 66.*

HE **THINKS HE CAN**, he thinks he can…he thinks he can move forward on his tummy, but he's not quite coordinated enough yet. Give him a boost by laying him on his front and letting him push against your hands or a rolled-up towel with his feet. Don't push, but support his feet with your hands as he inches forward each time. One minute of creeping practice now and again may be exhilarating; two minutes may be all he needs to get moving down the path toward greater mobility.

SOMETIMES A LITTLE SUPPORT from behind can help get your budding crawler moving.

SURPRISES INSIDE

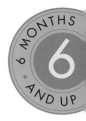

6 MONTHS AND UP
6

FINGER FUN AND PAPER MAGIC

HE'S RUMMAGING through the drawers, digging through the magazine rack, and pulling all his books off his shelf. His constant explorations are probably creating chaos in your home, but they're actually a sign of healthy infant development. Here's a way to put those little hands to good, nondestructive use: loosely wrap some of his toys in brightly colored paper, put them all in a big shopping bag, and let him dig through, unwrap, and rediscover his things. This is a great activity during car trips and airplane flights.

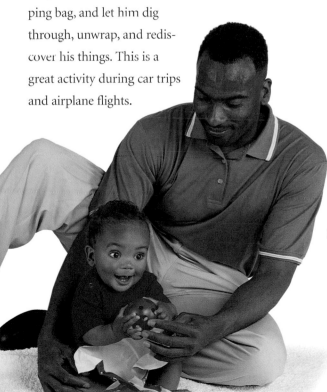

IT'S THE SAME BALL he's had for months, but it's a new surprise when he finds it inside brightly colored paper.

SKILL SPOTLIGHT

It takes fine motor skills *to figure out how to unwrap an object, and your baby will delight in the sound of crumpled paper. You may have to show him how to unwrap the objects at first, of course, but once he masters it, he'll soon understand that good things come in wrapped packages.*

✔	**Fine Motor Skills**
✔	**Problem Solving**
✔	**Tactile Stimulation**

IF YOUR BABY ENJOYS THIS ACTIVITY, also try Boxed Set, page 134.

SHAKE, RATTLE, AND ROLL

A RATTLE FOR BIG BABIES

SKILL SPOTLIGHT

Mastering the fun shaking *motion and creating the rattling sound will make your baby feel powerful and boost his awareness of cause and effect as he replicates the noise over and over again. It will also help him express his growing sense of rhythm and develop his gross motor skills.*

MAKING YOUR OWN

Plastic spice bottles work well for homemade maracas because they're small enough for your baby to wrap his hands around. Fill them with sand, dried beans, or pebbles; secure the tops firmly with duct tape or glue; and he's ready to shake!

BY SIX MONTHS, your baby has a pretty good sense that his hands are connected to his arms and has pretty good control of the movements of both his arms and hands. Now he wants to use his hands to explore his environment, whether by patting, stroking, or grabbing at nearly everything around him. As he discovers the properties of the objects he touches—their shape, weight, texture, and, of course, taste—he'll be particularly amazed by the various sounds they make. You can help his early experiments by providing a simple maraca made from a plastic bottle filled with something that will make noise. Show him how to shake it—but once he gets the idea, it may be hard to get him to stop!

Cause & Effect	✔
Gross Motor Skills	✔
Listening	✔

IF YOUR BABY ENJOYS THIS ACTIVITY, also try Music Maker, page 92.

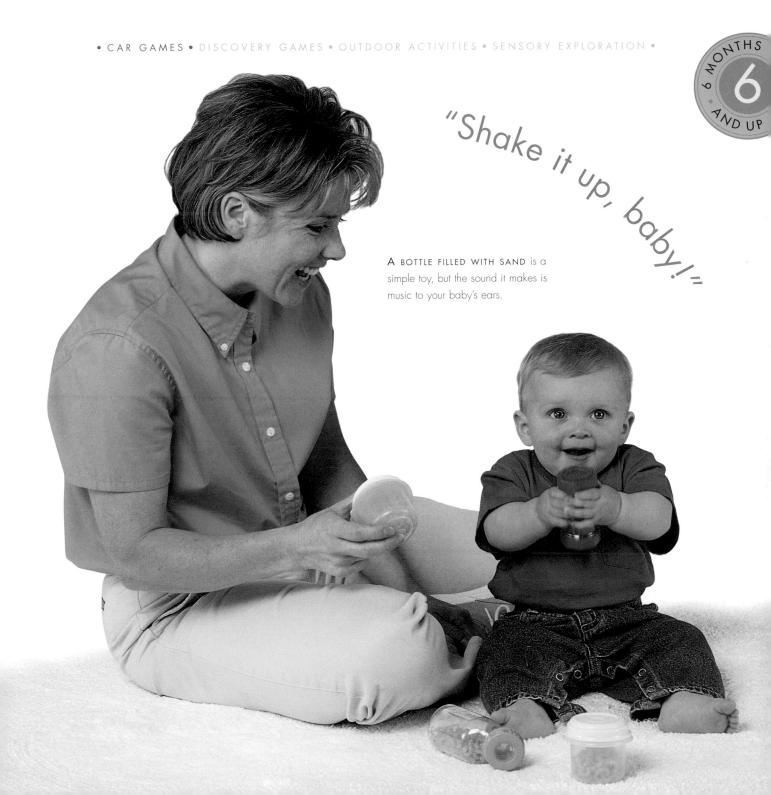

6 MONTHS AND UP

6

"Shake it up, baby!"

A BOTTLE FILLED WITH SAND is a simple toy, but the sound it makes is music to your baby's ears.

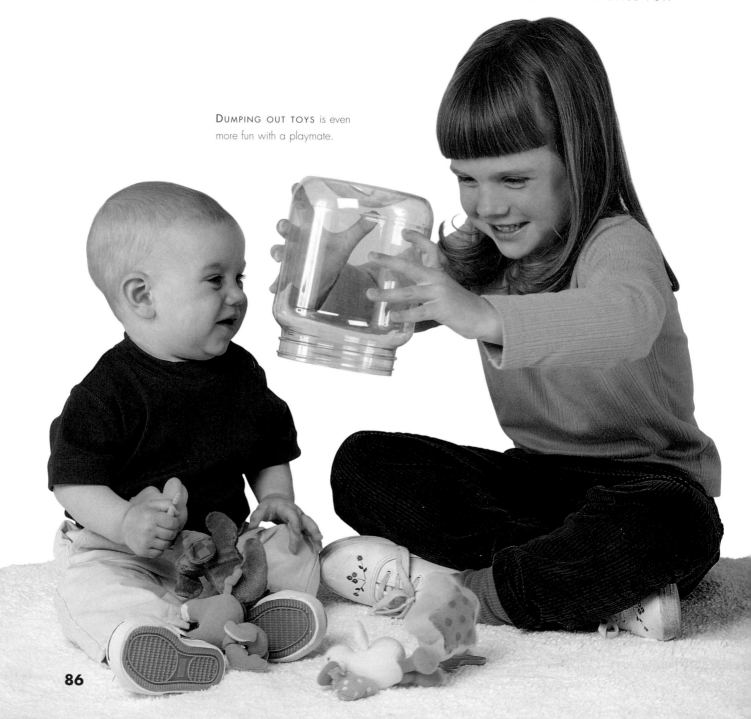

DUMPING OUT TOYS is even more fun with a playmate.

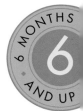

DUMPING DELIGHTS

A PUTTING-IN AND TAKING-OUT GAME

DUMPING THINGS out of containers and then putting them back in again is a favorite sport of babies who have learned to sit up and use their hands. Wherever he is in the house, your baby will probably find something to empty and fill. And while he will be happy to empty out the contents of your wastebaskets or cupboards all morning long, you can let him play a cleaner and more baby-friendly putting-in and taking-out game by giving him a wide-mouthed, gallon-sized plastic jar, a large plastic storage container, or even a large stainless steel bowl of his own. Fill the container with measuring cups, plastic bowls, blocks, small plush toys, plastic rings, and rattles. Then sit alongside him on the floor and help him fill and dump the container a few times. He will soon be busily doing the job on his own—over and over again.

SKILLSPOTLIGHT

Besides entertaining *your baby, dumping and filling containers teaches him about the relative sizes, shapes, and weights of various objects. It also introduces him to spatial concepts such as big and small, and empty and full. Dumping out and putting back exercises both fine and gross motor skills.*

✔	**Fine Motor Skills**
✔	**Gross Motor Skills**
✔	**Size and Shape Discrimination**
✔	**Spatial Awareness**

IF YOUR BABY ENJOYS THIS ACTIVITY, also try Baby's Cupboard, page 108. ▶

BABYPROOFING

WHETHER she's rolling, creeping, crawling, pulling up, or cruising at this stage, a mobile baby is quite capable of harming herself. Some kinds of babyproofing depend on your baby's particular interests (not all babies are fascinated with potted plants, for example). But some kinds need to be done regardless of your baby's current behavior, because the consequences can be dire.

Electrical outlets: Babies are very curious about tiny holes. Outlet covers are easy to install and can avert a possible disaster.

Cupboards: Any cupboard or drawer that contains sharp, poisonous, or breakable objects needs to have a babyproof lock. Better yet, move dangerous items out of your baby's reach.

Unstable furniture: If your baby bangs into or pulls up on a piece of unstable furniture, she could knock it over and injure herself. Bolt unstable furniture (such as bookshelves) to walls and keep heavy objects off furniture that wobbles when touched.

Choking hazards: Keep an eagle eye out for small objects that often fall on the floors of your home, such as buttons, needles, coins, pills, or earrings. Regular sweeping and vacuuming can help keep these hazards to a minimum.

Stairs: Install barriers at the top and bottom of each flight of stairs in your home.

Adult stuff: Be constantly on the lookout to make sure things such as knives, scissors, letter openers, razors, pens, power cords, and glasses stay out of your baby's reach.

Unfortunately, babyproofing is not a one-step operation. As your baby gets older, taller, more mobile, and bolder, you'll need to monitor what she can hit her head on, what she can reach, and what she can put her fingers into. ■

SWITCHING GAME

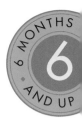

6 MONTHS
AND UP
6

TAKING TURNS WITH HANDS

BY NOW your baby has a good grasp of getting hold of objects—whether it's her favorite stuffed duck or a lock of your hair. But she may not be quite so adept at passing an object from one hand to another, which involves moving two hands at once. (Instead, she'll probably drop one object when offered another.) To help her practice using both hands, put a small toy in one. Let her play with it for a while, then hold another toy up toward that same hand. Encourage her to switch the first toy from one hand to the other, rather than simply dropping it. Her reward for accomplishing this tricky task? Getting to hold two toys at once!

SKILLSPOTLIGHT

Passing a toy *from one hand to another helps her learn to grasp and release simultaneously—not an easy task for a baby. It will also help her to cross over the vertical midline of her body with her hands, a precursor to crawling and walking.*

✔ **Bilateral Coordination**

✔ **Eye-Hand Coordination**

✔ **Fine Motor Skills**

✔ **Grasp and Release**

HOLDING TWO TOYS at once takes practice, but the result is twice as nice!

89

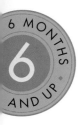
PLAY BALL

CRAWLING AND CATCHING FUN

SKILLSPOTLIGHT

Having a desirable object *move just beyond reach may inspire your baby to pursue the next mobility task, whether it's rolling, creeping, or crawling. Learning how to stop a moving object reinforces her developing sense of personal power as she exerts control over her environment. But don't expect her to roll or throw the ball back to you; those are skills she develops in her second year.*

Balance	✔
Eye-Hand Coordination	✔
Gross Motor Skills	✔
Spatial Awareness	✔

SHE'S NOT QUITE READY for a game of catch, but a game of fetch will please her no end. Roll a medium-sized whiffle ball, a blown-up beach ball, or a large cloth ball just beyond your baby so that she has to move to get it. Or try rolling it to her directly so that she can get used to stopping it with her hands. Here's a hint: letting a little air out of a big plastic ball or beach ball will make it easier for her to grab and handle.

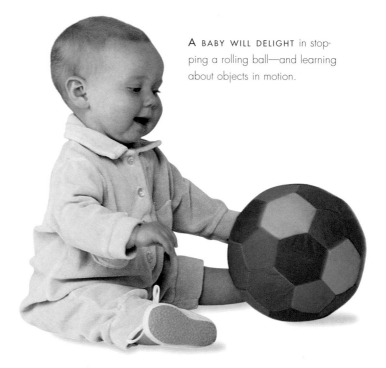

A BABY WILL DELIGHT in stopping a rolling ball—and learning about objects in motion.

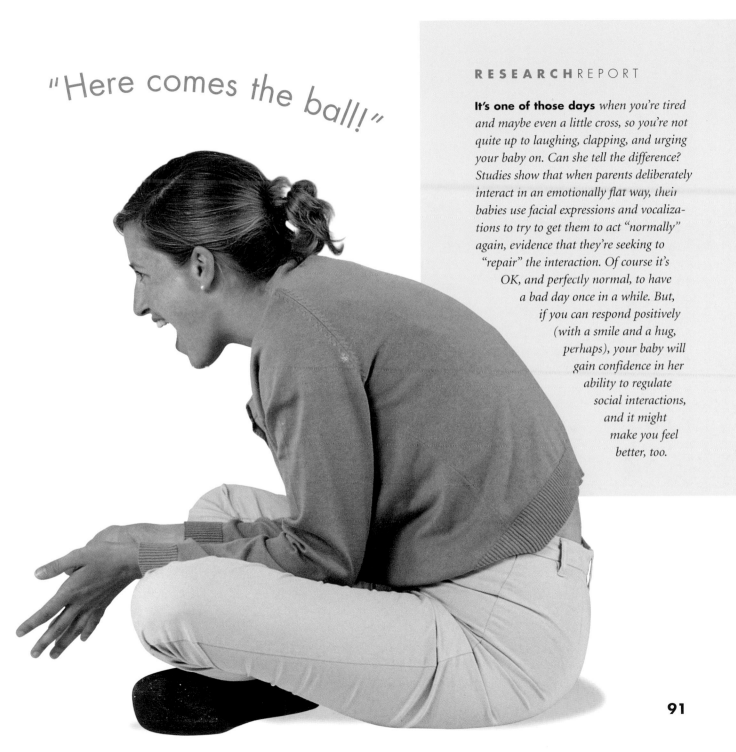

"Here comes the ball!"

91

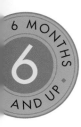
MUSIC MAKER

A SOUND BACKGROUND

SKILLSPOTLIGHT

Matching an external beat
isn't a part of her musical skill set yet, but understanding that music is participatory and fun helps both her musical and social development. This activity actually works on both her gross and fine motor skills and sets up a positive association with music.

Fine Motor Skills	✔
Gross Motor Skills	✔
Listening	✔
Rhythm Exploration	✔

◀ *IF YOUR BABY ENJOYS THIS ACTIVITY, also try Shake, Rattle, and Roll, page 84.*

IT'S NEVER TOO EARLY to expose your baby to music, but it's not until she's old enough to control objects (even somewhat) that she can become an active player. You can enhance her listening pleasure by giving her things to shake, rattle, and roll while she listens to music or you singing. Just gather together rattles, squeaky toys, and shakers. Show her how to use them, and then allow her to let loose.

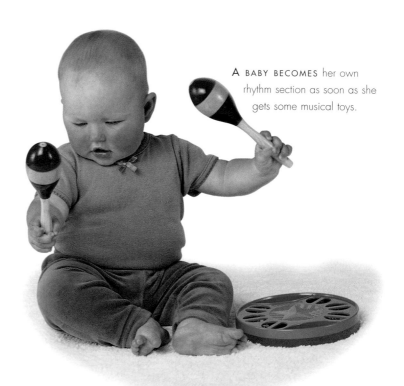

A BABY BECOMES her own rhythm section as soon as she gets some musical toys.

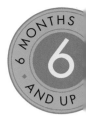

TOTALLY TUBULAR

A STACKING GAME

YOUR BABY may not have entered an ocean, a lake, or even a kiddie pool yet, but swim tubes provide plenty of fun on dry land, too. Sitters and crawlers alike enjoy using the tubes for sitting support. Or play a game of peekaboo in the rings. Just sit her down in one on a soft surface, stack the rest of them up to her chest, and lift them off while calling "Peekaboo!" Babies who are more mobile will take pleasure in creeping and crawling in and out of several tubes placed on the floor.

SKILLSPOTLIGHT

Playing peekaboo *with swim tubes lets babies experience a temporary visual separation from you, which will eventually help them understand that even if you leave, you haven't disappeared forever. Crawling in, out, and over the rings lets babies practice being mobile on an uneven surface, which helps them develop balance and coordination.*

✔	**Balance**
✔	**Gross Motor Skills**
✔	**Object Permanence**

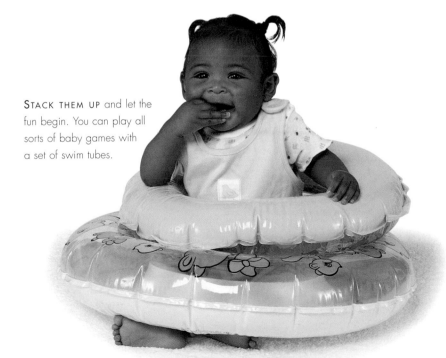

STACK THEM UP and let the fun begin. You can play all sorts of baby games with a set of swim tubes.

93

CLAPPING SONGS

AS YOUR BABY'S manual dexterity improves, she'll become fascinated with hand movements such as clapping, snapping, and waving. Amplify her delight by singing songs that incorporate simple gestures. While she won't be able to perform each movement right away, eventually she'll learn to clap or wave. Coax her by clapping or waving her hands for her, or clapping and waving yourself.

BINGO

There was a farmer had a dog
and Bingo was his name-o
B-I-N-G-O
B-I-N-G-O
B-I-N-G-O
and Bingo was his name-o.

There was a farmer had a dog
and Bingo was his name-o
clap-I-N-G-O
clap-I-N-G-O
clap-I-N-G-O
and Bingo was his name-o.
keep adding one clap and removing one letter

THIS OLD MAN

clap out rhythm throughout

**This old man, he played one,
he played knick knack on my thumb,
with a knick, knack, paddy whack,
give a dog a bone,
this old man went rolling home.**

**This old man, he played two,
he played knick knack on my shoe,
with a knick, knack, paddy whack,
give a dog a bone,
this old man went rolling home.**

*continue with additional verses:
three/knee, four/door, five/hive,
six/sticks, seven/up in heaven, eight/gate,
nine/spine, ten/once again*

WHETHER YOU'RE MAKING the
movement for her or she's making
elementary motions herself, putting
words, music, and gestures together
helps build your baby's vocabulary.

WORKING ON THE RAILROAD

**I've been working on the railroad
all the livelong day.**
make digging motions with hands

**I've been working on the railroad
just to pass the time away.
Can't you hear the whistle blowin'?**
pull an imaginary whistle string

Rise up so early in the morn.
raise hands into air

**Can't you hear the
captain shouting,**
clap

**"Dinah, blow
your horn."**

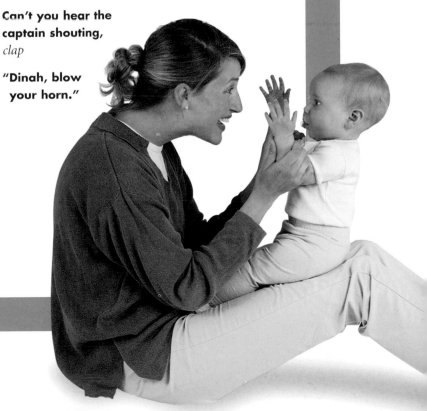

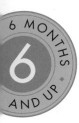

6 MONTHS
6
AND UP

LITTLE DRUMMER BABY

BANGING AWAY

SKILLSPOTLIGHT

At this age, *babies start to get a very elementary understanding of cause and effect. Hitting an object and having it make noise reinforces that concept while strengthening the baby's eye-hand coordination. And hearing the different sounds that various objects make helps him learn about the properties of those objects, which he'll later transfer to other situations.*

Cause & Effect	✔
Eye-Hand Coordination	✔
Listening	✔

◀ *IF YOUR BABY ENJOYS THIS ACTIVITY, also try Music Maker, page 92.*

BEING ABLE TO MANIPULATE OBJECTS is very gratifying for young babies who are working on fine motor control; being able to make noises with those objects is even more so. You can entertain your baby by setting pots, pans, and bowls near him and providing him with wooden spoons. Show your baby how to hit the "drums" to make a noise, then encourage him to try it himself. He may hit the pots accidentally, which will give him enough of a taste to start tapping them on purpose.

A RAT-A-TAT-TAT and a sis-boom-bang . . . this elementary drum set introduces him to the joys of noise, as well as to the idea that his actions influence his world.

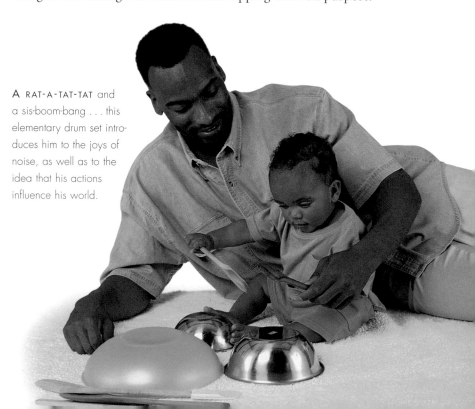

FINGERPUPPET FUN

MAGIC AT YOUR FINGERTIPS

MESMERIZED BY MOTION and enchanted by animal toys, babies are natural audiences for a miniature puppet show. Just slip on a fingerpuppet or two and let them bob, dance, kiss, tickle, sing, and talk to your littlest spectator. At this age, he's likely to reach out, grab a puppet, and start to mouth it. This is fine as long as the puppets have no small parts that can be pulled off and swallowed. He's equally likely to babble, gurgle, and blow raspberries at the animated actors. You can also find a song to go with your finger-puppets and make it a musical show!

SKILL SPOTLIGHT

Listening to the puppets *talk and sing will help him learn the art of conversation—that is, that first one person (or puppet, as the case may be) talks, and then the other person responds. Being tickled and nuzzled by his little friends provides both entertaining tactile stimulation and fun, posi-tive interaction with you.*

✔ **Social Development**

✔ **Tactile Stimulation**

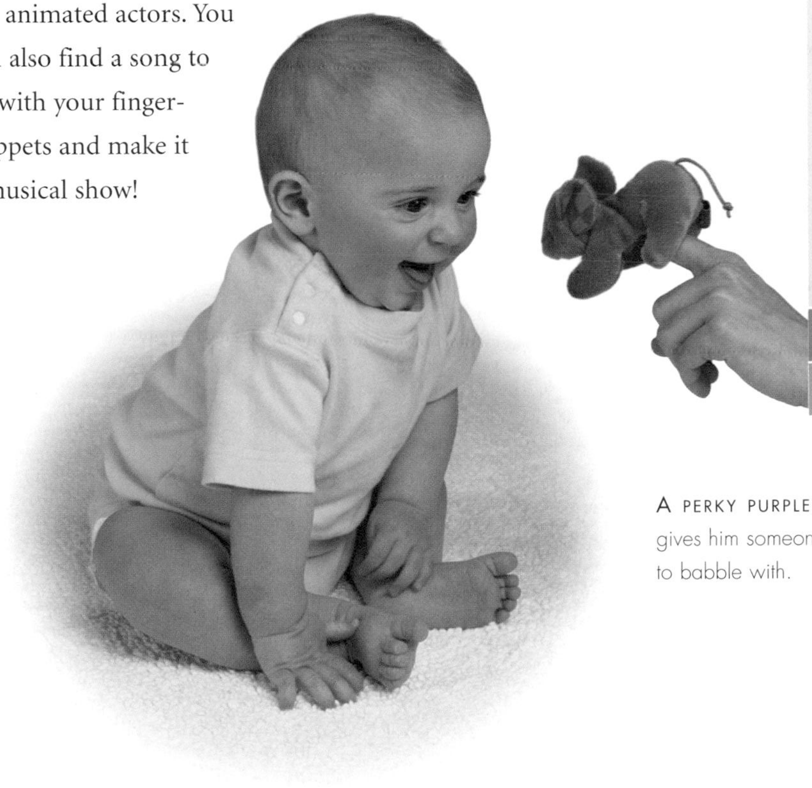

A PERKY PURPLE MOUSE
gives him someone new
to babble with.

97

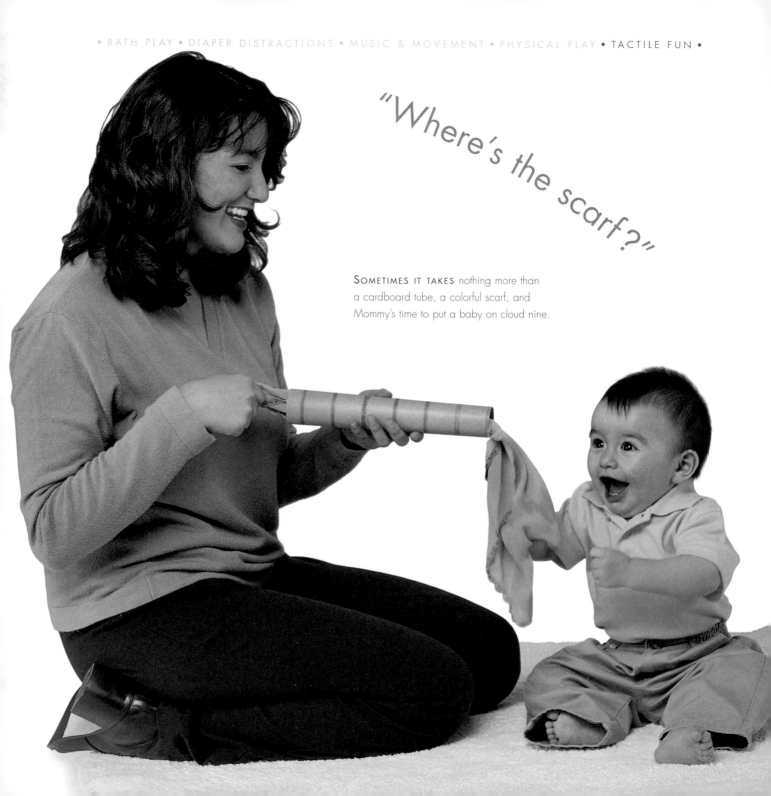

"Where's the scarf?"

SOMETIMES IT TAKES nothing more than a cardboard tube, a colorful scarf, and Mommy's time to put a baby on cloud nine.

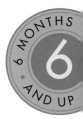

MAGIC SCARVES

A REAPPEARING ACT

IF YOU'RE LOOKING for a versatile toy that will last through several of your child's developmental stages, you need look no further than your own clothes closet. Silky scarves can delight and entertain him up through his preschool years. When he's still a baby, one of the best games you can play is to poke a brightly colored scarf through one end of a cardboard tube and let him pull it out the other side. You can play the game without the tube by hiding most of the scarf in your fist and letting him find and grab the end. Embellish the game by adding your own enticements—"Where's the scarf? Where did it go? Oh, there it is! Peekaboo!"—to help keep him engaged.

MAKING YOUR OWN

If you don't have any scarves, you can buy colorful squares of cloth at fabric or novelty stores. For a change, use an empty tissue box instead of the cardboard tube—show your baby how to stuff the scarf in and pull it out.

SKILL SPOTLIGHT

Grabbing the silky scarf and pulling it from the tube lets your baby work on his eye-hand coordination along with his fine motor skills. And seeing the scarf first disappear and then reappear at the other end will boost your baby's understanding of object permanence.

✔ **Eye-Hand Coordination**

✔ **Object Permanence**

✔ **Tactile Stimulation**

IF YOUR BABY ENJOYS THIS ACTIVITY, also try Busy Boxes, page 101.

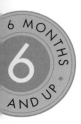
STOP THE TOP

FUN WITH SPINNING

SKILLSPOTLIGHT

Touching an object *that's just lying there, like a block, is one challenge. Tracking and touching an object that's moving is a completely different challenge—one that this activity lets your baby practice over and over again. In addition, seeing how a gentle touch can either stop the spinning top or send it careening across the floor teaches your baby valuable lessons about cause and effect.*

Cause & Effect	✔
Eye-Hand Coordination	✔
Spatial Awareness	✔

A **SPINNING TOP** is one of those old-fashioned toys that can delight all kinds of babies. Small babies obviously can't pump the handle up and down, but that doesn't mean they have to be passive observers. Instead, make the top spin in front of your baby. Then show him how to stop it by touching it with your hand. He'll soon start reaching out to control the whirling colors and whirring noises himself.

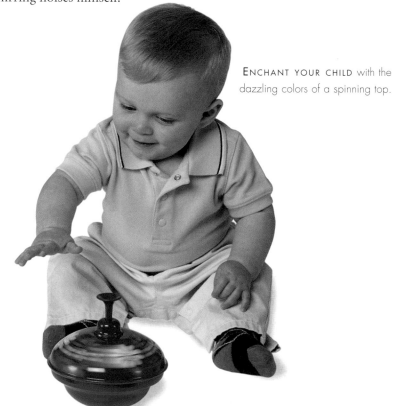

ENCHANT YOUR CHILD with the dazzling colors of a spinning top.

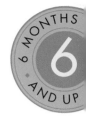

BUSY BOXES

LITTLE TASKS FOR LITTLE FINGERS

A **CTIVITY BOARDS** with cylinders that whirl, dials that spin, and buttons that squeak can provide hours of amusement for your baby's curious fingers. Just set up the board so she can reach all the stations, and show her how it works. Then let her try her own hand at it. At first, she may only be able to do the very simplest activities on the board, like swatting a rolling ball or sticking her finger in a hole on the dial. In the months to come, though, she'll learn to spin the dial and press the buttons.

YOU'LL PIQUE her curiosity and keep her fingers busy with one of these classic baby toys.

SKILL SPOTLIGHT

Even the simplest activities *help a baby develop finger dexterity and coordination, which leads to more advanced tasks in later months. Learning that touching different knobs creates different results helps her mentally classify those results, and also builds upon her sense of mastery.*

✔ **Cause & Effect**

✔ **Eye-Hand Coordination**

✔ **Fine Motor Skills**

IF YOUR BABY ENJOYS THIS ACTIVITY, also try Activity Book, page 128.

101

SEPARATION ANXIETY

JUST WHEN your baby is gaining a good deal of mobility and a tiny bit of independence, he suddenly wants to be joined to your hip once again. Your baby's new-found independence and his newly expressed separation anxiety are related. Now that he's mobile, he understands how easily the two of you can become separated.

Knowing that your presence means so much can feel flattering, but it can also fray your nerves. Here are some tips to get through this challenging period.

Respect him: Remember that your presence is still essential to your baby, and he can't help being distraught at the thought that you're not there.

Reassure him: Hold him, talk to him, sing to him, and, once he calms down, distract him by giving him a book or toy. Reassurance now will help him feel more secure later.

Protect him: Separation anxiety and stranger anxiety often arrive hand in hand. If strangers get too close, explain that your baby's not comfortable around new people and let him hide on your shoulder. Don't scold him for being shy; he can't help it. Given time, most babies will warm up to new people who are friendly and gentle in their approach.

Tell him the truth: It's tempting to try to slip out the back door when you have to leave him with a caregiver, but that won't help your baby. If he thinks that you really do suddenly disappear from time to time, he's more likely to panic if you step out of the room. Be cheerful and clear when you announce your departure, tell him you love him, and walk out the door. If he learns that he can trust you to be truthful and that you really will return, he'll feel more confident.

Remember, it's not forever: Infants, toddlers, and preschoolers all go through stages of separation anxiety. Given comfort, love, and encouragement, most children become quite independent over time. ∎

ROLY-POLY

PULL-UP PRACTICE

YOUR BABY has probably enjoyed rocking and even standing supported in your lap since she was just a few months old. Now that her muscles are getting stronger, she'll be even more motivated to stand on her own two feet with your assistance. Make practice fun by accompanying it with a merry movement chant. Start by laying your baby down on her back so that she's facing you with her legs out straight. Then gently help her to sit and stand as you engage in this roly-poly activity.

SHE'S STANDING, she's learning words, and, best of all, you and she are looking right at each other as you play.

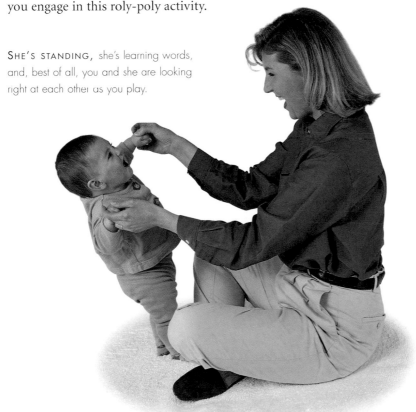

Roly-Poly

Roly-poly, roly-poly,
circle arms around one another
(repeat whenever singing roly-poly)
out, out, out.
move hands away from each other
Roly-poly, roly-poly,
in, in, in.
bring hands together
Roly-poly, roly-poly,
touch your nose.
touch baby's nose
Roly-poly, roly-poly,
touch your toes.
pull baby to seated position
Roly-poly, roly-poly,
up to sky.
pull baby up to standing
Roly-poly, roly-poly,
fly, fly, fly.
lift baby up into the air

✔	**Gross Motor Skills**
✔	**Language Development**
✔	**Lower-Body Strength**

103

LITTLE FOLKS' SONGS

SURE, children's television programs and videos provide lots of new songs for little kids. But sometimes it's the old songs that have the most charm, as they help knit the generations together. Engage your child by singing these songs with our suggested hand gestures, and invite the whole family to join in!

DAISY, DAISY

Daisy, Daisy,
give me your answer, do.
clap hands together

I'm half-crazy
over the love of you.
put hands on baby's cheeks

It won't be a fancy marriage—
I can't afford a carriage.
shrug shoulders with hands turned up

But you'll look sweet upon the seat
point at baby

of a bicycle built for two.
hug baby

IT'S RAINING, IT'S POURING

It's raining, it's pouring,
the old man is snoring.
He bumped his head,
and fell out of bed,
and couldn't get up
in the morning.

RAIN, RAIN, GO AWAY

Rain, rain, go away,
come again some other day.
Rain, rain, go away,
all the children want to play.

POLLY WOLLY DOODLE

**Oh I went down South for
to see my Sal,
sing Polly Wolly Doodle all the day.**
tickle baby under chin or ribs

**My Sal she is a spunky gal,
sing Polly Wolly Doodle all the day.**
tickle baby under chin or ribs

Fare thee well,
wave bye-bye

fare thee well,
wave bye-bye

fare thee well my fairy Faye.
wave bye-bye

For I'm going to Louisiana
run fingers up and down baby's body

**for to see my Susyanna,
sing Polly Wolly Doodle all the day.**
tickle baby under ribs

HEY DIDDLE DIDDLE

**Hey diddle diddle, the cat and
the fiddle,**
make fiddling motion with hands

the cow jumped over the moon.
sail hand through the air

**The little dog laughed to see
such sport**
put hands over eyes

**and the dish ran away
with the spoon.**
run fingers from baby's belly to chin

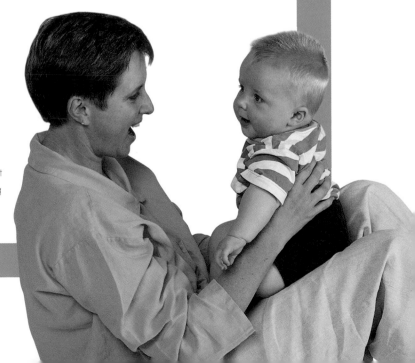

MOMMY'S LAP is the perfect place to perch while listening to favorite songs.

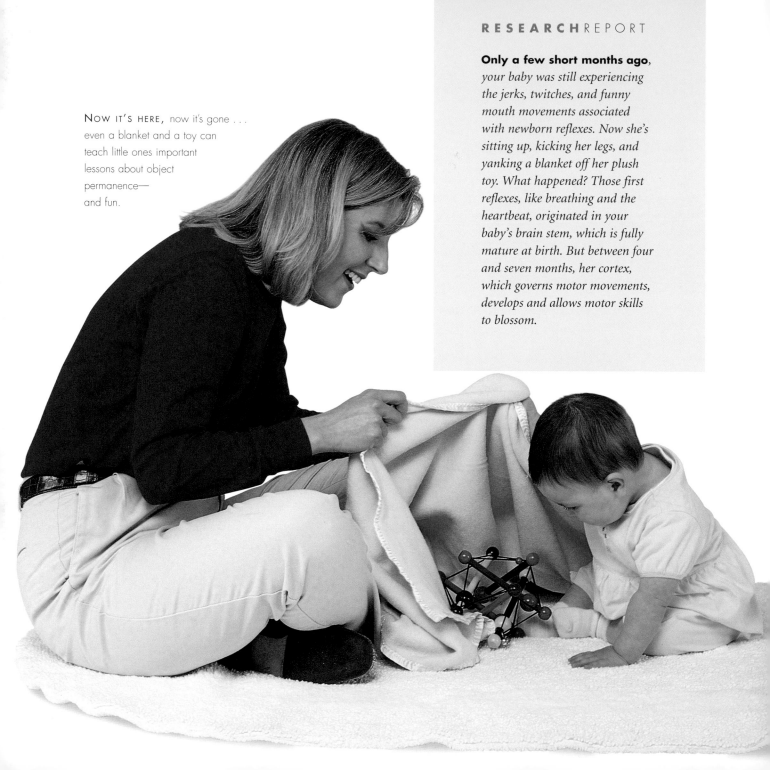

NOW IT'S HERE, now it's gone . . . even a blanket and a toy can teach little ones important lessons about object permanence— and fun.

RESEARCH REPORT

Only a few short months ago, *your baby was still experiencing the jerks, twitches, and funny mouth movements associated with newborn reflexes. Now she's sitting up, kicking her legs, and yanking a blanket off her plush toy. What happened? Those first reflexes, like breathing and the heartbeat, originated in your baby's brain stem, which is fully mature at birth. But between four and seven months, her cortex, which governs motor movements, develops and allows motor skills to blossom.*

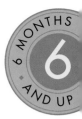

WHERE'S THE TOY?

MORE PEEKABOO PLAY

WHEN SHE WAS A NEWBORN, your baby was very much an "out of sight, out of mind" type of creature. That is, if you hid a toy from her, she figured it no longer existed. But now that she's reached the six-month threshold, she's on to better ideas. While she may not know exactly where the toy went or why it disappeared, she does understand that it still exists, somewhere, at least for a little while. You can bolster her understanding of this very basic fact by playing peekaboo games with toys.

• Partially hide a favorite plush toy or book under one of her blankets. Ask her repeatedly, "Where is it?" She may need some help finding it the first time, but once she realizes that the rest of the toy is connected to the part that's showing, she'll be diving under the blanket with joy.

• Soon you can begin hiding the toy completely. As long as your baby sees you hide it or notices the toy's outline beneath the blanket, she should be able to find it.

SKILLSPOTLIGHT

Learning that something *exists even when she can't see it helps your baby understand object permanence. This is key to her ability to tolerate separations from you, as well as to remember people, places, or objects she saw previously but that are currently out of sight. This ability is called "representational memory."*

| ✔ | **Fine Motor Skills** |
| ✔ | **Object Permanence** |

IF YOUR BABY ENJOYS THIS ACTIVITY, also try Peekaboo Games, page 51.

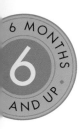
BABY'S CUPBOARD

EARLY EXPLORATIONS

SKILLSPOTLIGHT

Shelves filled *with tempting "toys" help your baby practice her "aim and fire" technique—that is, her ability to see an object, reach for it, and grab it. Having a variety of objects to manipulate lets your baby learn about physical properties such as size, shape, and weight. It also gives her a chance to explore and discover safe items on her own terms.*

Fine Motor Skills	✔
Gross Motor Skills	✔
Sensory Development	✔
Visual Discrimination	✔

NOW THAT YOUR BABY'S getting mobile, it's crucial that you babyproof any cupboards containing breakables, cleaning products, heavy pots and pans, or other materials that could harm her. But if she sees you taking things out of cupboards, it's guaranteed she'll want to do the same—grabbing games, like clearing shelves and emptying cupboards, are favorite pastimes of babies this age. You can keep your baby safe and satisfy her urge to explore and imitate by devoting a cupboard especially to her. An unlocked cabinet stocked with safe, appealing objects like towels, plastic bowls, measuring cups, muffin tins, and a few favorite toys will keep her happily occupied—and it will give you some time to focus on cooking, washing dishes, or even reading the newspaper!

◀ *IF YOUR BABY ENJOYS THIS ACTIVITY, also try Dumping Delights, page 86.*

BABY'S "WORKING" in the kitchen just like you, but she's not getting into trouble, or even making a mess!

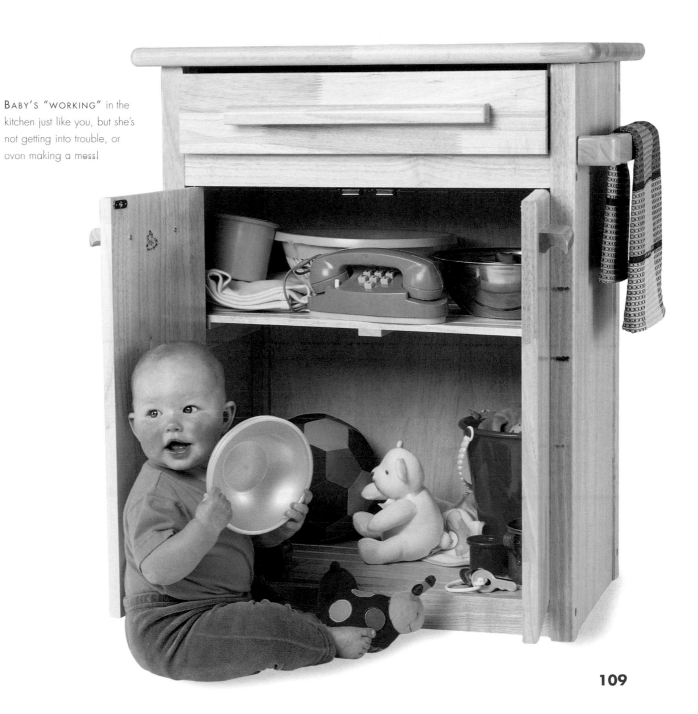

109

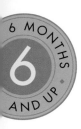

6 MONTHS
6
AND UP

I'M GONNA GET YOU

AN OLD-FASHIONED GAME OF CHASE

SKILLSPOTLIGHT

This is a game *for two to play, and it can help build your baby's social awareness as well as his sense of trust. Having an incentive to crawl also strengthens his balance and gross motor skills.*

Balance	✔
Gross Motor Skills	✔
Social Development	✔
Trust	✔

NO ONE REALLY KNOWS why babies love to be chased and surprised. Whatever the reason, even most early crawlers seem to think that having a beloved caretaker thundering along after them is very, very funny.

• Start crawling slowly after your baby, murmuring "I'm gonna get you …I'm gonna get you …I'm gonna get you!" Then gently grab your baby and say, "I got you!" You can lift him up in the air, kiss the nape of his neck, and give his ribs a little tickle, but keep the game gentle so you don't startle him—he's still a baby, after all.

• A good game of chase isn't just for crawlers; it will keep him on his toes as a toddler and eventually evolve into classic big-kid games like hide-and-seek and tag.

A GENTLE GAME OF CHASE teaches him that Mom can be fun and boisterous as well as cuddly and calm. This helps him understand the range of social behavior humans can show.

110

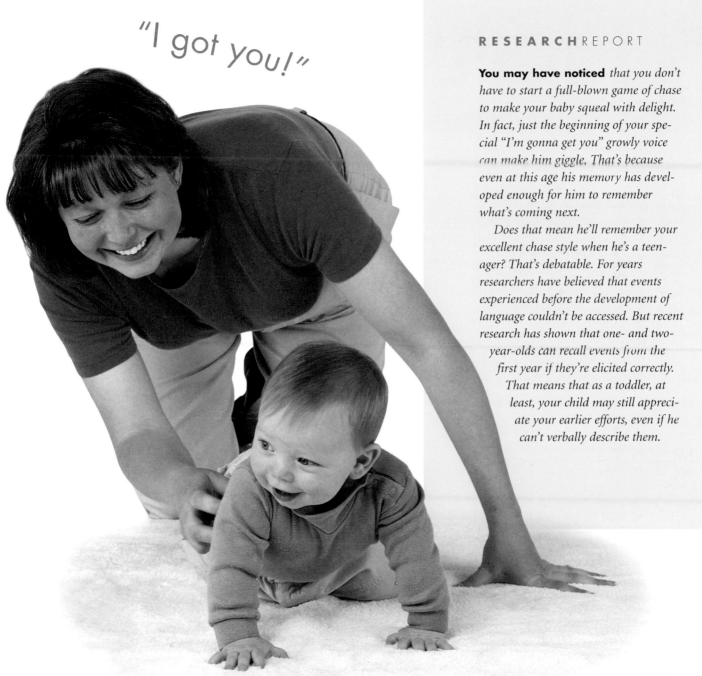

"I got you!"

RESEARCHREPORT

You may have noticed *that you don't have to start a full-blown game of chase to make your baby squeal with delight. In fact, just the beginning of your special "I'm gonna get you" growly voice can make him giggle. That's because even at this age his memory has developed enough for him to remember what's coming next.*

Does that mean he'll remember your excellent chase style when he's a teenager? That's debatable. For years researchers have believed that events experienced before the development of language couldn't be accessed. But recent research has shown that one- and two-year-olds can recall events from the first year if they're elicited correctly. That means that as a toddler, at least, your child may still appreciate your earlier efforts, even if he can't verbally describe them.

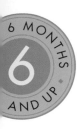

BOTTLE ROLL

GIVING CHASE

SKILLSPOTLIGHT

Encouraging your baby *to grab a rolling bottle will likely motivate him to crawl after it, thereby exercising his gross motor skills. If he prefers to just sit and roll the bottle back and forth, he'll still be working on his fine motor skills as well as his eye-hand coordination.*

Eye-Hand Coordination	✔
Fine Motor Skills	✔
Gross Motor Skills	✔

◀ *IF YOUR BABY ENJOYS THIS ACTIVITY, also try Play Ball, page 90.*

IT'S OK if your baby starts crawling later than the baby next door—they'll both be running and climbing with abandon in just a few short years. But if you'd like to coax a late or not very enthusiastic crawler into moving a bit more, a baby bottle filled with beans or grains can be an enticing lure. Just fill the bottle partially (so the contents can move) and roll it across the floor in front of your baby. Make sure the bottle top is safely secured. He still won't budge? Show him how to roll it back and forth himself, so he sees that it can provide plenty of sitting entertainment.

GO GET 'EM! He'll love to watch, listen to, and chase after these rolling bottles.

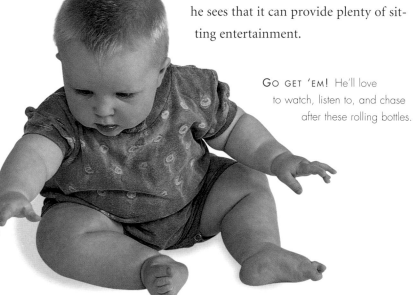

112

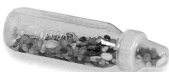

HOW PUZZLING!

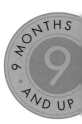

9 MONTHS AND UP · 9

FINDING THE RIGHT FIT

ASSEMBLING A JIGSAW PUZZLE is beyond your baby's reach, but she can easily grasp the concept behind the simple wooden puzzles made for older babies and toddlers. Those that feature simple shapes and large pieces with knobs are especially easy, as are those that have matching pictures underneath. There's a knack to getting even these big puzzle pieces in their places, however—you will probably need to guide the pieces as she moves them, so she can feel how they slip into place.

SKILLSPOTLIGHT

Playing with a puzzle—*even getting the pieces out—is great exercise for a baby's fine motor and spatial skills. And learning which piece goes where draws on both her visual memory and her understanding of shapes, sizes, and colors.*

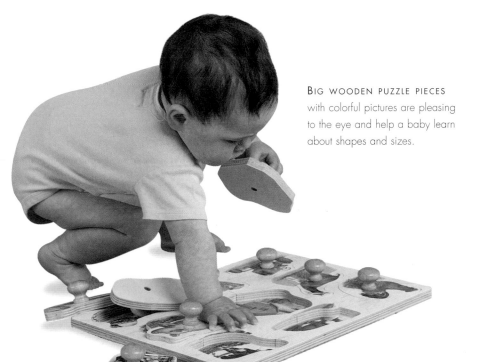

BIG WOODEN PUZZLE PIECES with colorful pictures are pleasing to the eye and help a baby learn about shapes and sizes.

✔	**Fine Motor Skills**
✔	**Problem Solving**
✔	**Size & Shape Discrimination**
✔	**Visual Discrimination**

IF YOUR BABY ENJOYS THIS ACTIVITY, also try Boxed Set, page 134.

113

SOUND STAGE

A LISTENING EXERCISE

SKILLSPOTLIGHT

Focused listening *builds the foundation for your child's language development. It allows him to locate and recognize sounds, and, when combined with other experiences and repetition, allows him to begin forming a repertoire of receptive language.*

Language Development	✔
Listening	✔
Sensory Development	✔
Social Skills	✔

NOT ALL OF YOUR TIME with your baby needs to be spent talking, playing, reading, or otherwise stimulating his little mind. Just sitting and observing the obvious can also build sensory and cognitive awareness. One listening exercise, for instance, is as simple as finding an area where your baby can hear a number of different sounds. It may be inside, where he can hear the dog's toenails clicking on the kitchen floor, the refrigerator running, the telephone ringing, or cars zooming by. Or it may be outside, where he can hear birds singing, leaves rustling, a wind chime jingling, or an airplane overhead. Call his attention to the sounds, point in the right direction, and tell him what they are. You can let him participate in the sounds by hitting the wind chimes, or show him how to imitate the sounds—the "tweet-tweet" of a bird, for instance, or the "vrooom" of a car driving by the house.

IF YOUR BABY ENJOYS THIS ACTIVITY, also try Let's Explore, page 118.

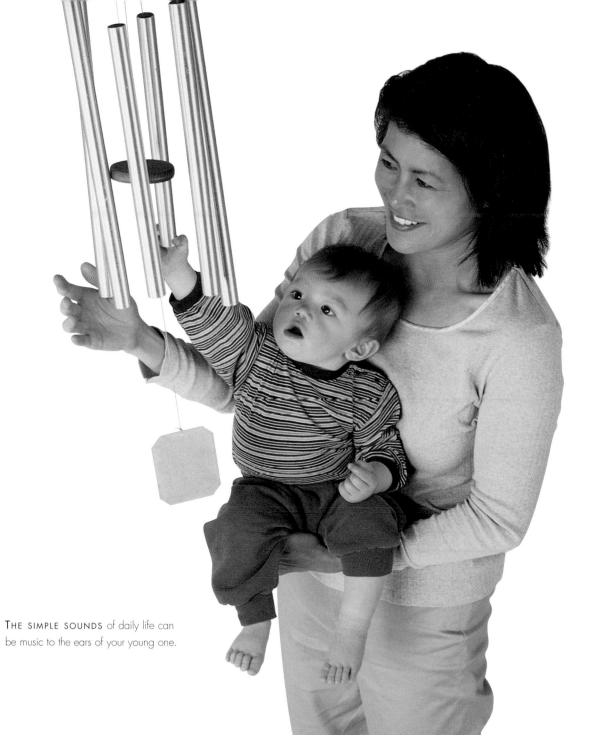

THE SIMPLE SOUNDS of daily life can
be music to the ears of your young one.

TRAVELING WITH BABY

BY THE TIME your child is nine months old, life at home has probably settled a bit. You've bonded with your baby, your home is somewhat childproof, and you know how to keep him entertained and safe throughout the day.

But once you leave the comforts of home, life with a baby this age can be unsettling. While a very young baby can sleep through plane changes and family reunions, an older baby has more distinct wants and needs and is less likely to go with the flow.

Does that mean you should avoid travel until your baby is an adolescent? Not at all. Families need to take vacations, and most relatives will relish a visit from you. The trick is to expect the best outcomes but plan for potential obstacles.

Remember his schedule: Planning your travel schedule around your baby's sleep times can help you avoid the stress of dealing with a tired baby once you reach your destination. Throughout your trip, remember that the more rested he is, the more fun your whole family will have.

Remember his important items: If your baby has a stuffed toy or blanket that he uses for comfort, be sure to bring it. Familiar things help to ease the transition to a new environment.

Remember his food: In a hotel or a friend's kitchen, it won't be as easy to whip up his favorite snack. Carry foods like crackers, dry cereal, and fruit, and do a quick shopping trip when you arrive so that you have the food you need on hand.

Remember to babyproof: You won't be able to relax if you're worried about his safety. If you pack a few outlet covers and cupboard locks, you won't need to worry.

Remember your needs: Travel is tiring even when you don't have a baby. Try to eat and sleep well and get some exercise. You can get precious time to yourself by asking a relative to watch your child or by hiring a recommended sitter. ■

RIDING HIGH

EXPLORING MOVEMENT

SOMETIMES it's hard to know just when to introduce certain toys, because it's hard to know how skilled a baby needs to be to use them. But even a baby who isn't yet walking can use a riding toy, provided her legs are long enough to reach the ground. At first you may have to push her a bit so she understands what this game is all about. But soon she'll be pushing herself along (although, as with crawling, she may go backward at first), and squealing delightedly as she rolls from room to room.

HER FIRST RIDING TOY acquaints her with the delights of independent mobility— and riding it is really good exercise!

SKILLSPOTLIGHT

Most babies won't figure out how to use their legs alternately on a riding toy until their second year. But as they move themselves forward and backward with both feet at once, they'll build strong gross motor skills and improve their balance.

✔	**Balance**
✔	**Gross Motor Skills**
✔	**Lower-Body Strength**

IF YOUR BABY ENJOYS THIS ACTIVITY, also try Push Me, Pull You, page 140.

117

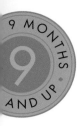

LET'S EXPLORE

BABY'S FIRST TOUR

SKILLSPOTLIGHT

It's easy for adults *to take the daily environment for granted. After all, we've been seeing and hearing it every day for years. But babies are greatly intrigued— and their brains stimulated—by new sights and sounds, and just about everything in your world is still new to them. Encouraging babies to explore the world with their senses, even if it's from the safety of your arms, helps teach them to be actively curious. Your narration also helps your baby build her vocabulary.*

Eye-Hand Coordination	✔
Listening	✔
Sensory Development	✔
Visual Development	✔

AT THIS AGE, your baby's curiosity about the world far exceeds her ability to explore it—even if she is already walking. Give her a lift toward making her first great discoveries by taking her around and describing the local sights.

• Inside the house, show her paintings, posters, books, knobs, and light switches. Let her work the light switch, pull a towel off the rack, or grab a toothbrush from its holder. Describe what she sees and touches—the nubby peel of an orange, for instance, or the soft towel in her hand.

• Take her outside and let her feel the bark of a tree, the leaves on a shrub, or the warmth of a stone in the sun. Lift her up to smell the blossoms on an apple tree or to meet a kitten by the window.

• Don't be surprised if something odd catches her fancy. Most children like animals, but during this stage they also have an interest in inanimate objects such as door hinges, stereo knobs, and push buttons, and are curious about how they work.

IF YOUR BABY ENJOYS THIS ACTIVITY, also try Sound Stage, page 114.

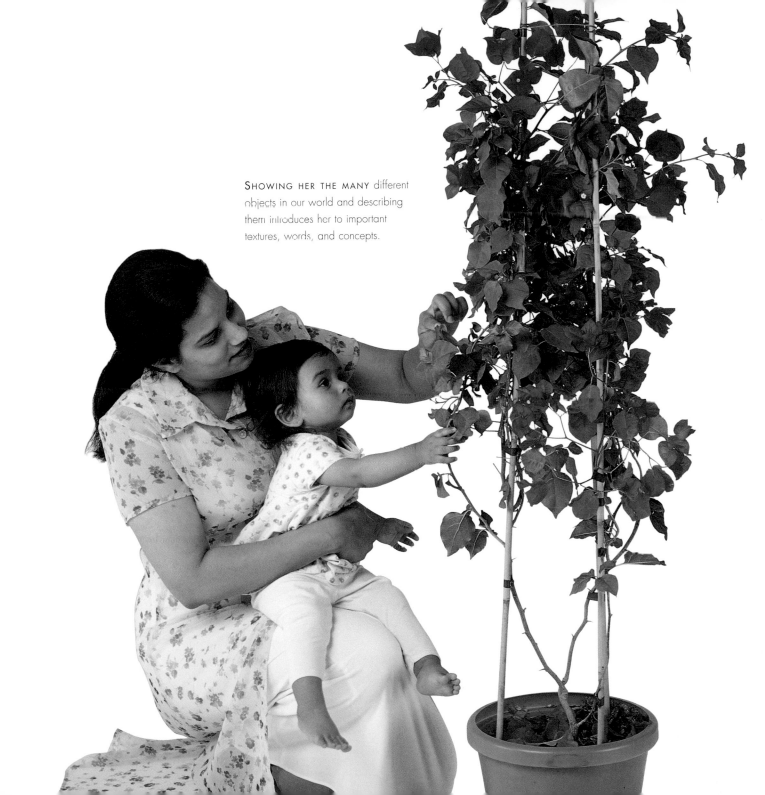

SHOWING HER THE MANY different objects in our world and describing them introduces her to important textures, words, and concepts.

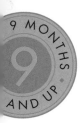
SEARCHLIGHT

CATCH THE SPOT

SKILLSPOTLIGHT

Whether your baby is crawling or walking, trying to catch the colored light improves his eye-hand coordination and agility. Walkers who chase after the beam of light also hone their balance and visual skills.

Balance	✔
Eye-Hand Coordination	✔
Gross Motor Skills	✔

INCREASED MOBILITY brings with it a whole new range of games that involve chasing and catching. Most of those games have you pursuing your baby. But he can play the pursuer when you show him how to "catch" a flashlight beam. Wrap and secure a layer of tissue paper around the end of a flashlight. Shine the colored light on the floor, on the wall, and on furniture, and encourage your baby to go get it.

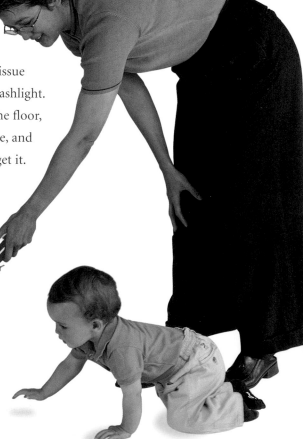

FOLLOWING THE CIRCLE of colorful light requires concentration and coordination.

120

OBSTACLE COURSE

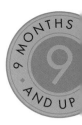

A MOBILE PURSUIT

WALKING ON A FLAT SURFACE is one challenge; crawling around or stepping over things while upright is another—and it's an important skill for a baby who's learning to maneuver through a sandbox, around pets, or over the roots of a tree. Help your baby learn to navigate around objects on the ground by setting up a series of small blocks, boxes, and plush toys. If she's walking, hold her hands and help her step over the objects. If she's crawling, encourage her to crawl around this makeshift obstacle course.

MASTERING the challenge of stepping over objects can boost her self-esteem and walking skills.

SKILLSPOTLIGHT

Whether your child is crawling or already tottering along without holding on, this game helps her learn how to keep her balance. It also helps her develop eye-foot coordination as she practices lifting her feet and putting them in a "safe" spot.

✔	**Balance**
✔	**Eye-Foot Coordination**
✔	**Gross Motor Skills**
✔	**Lower-Body Strength**

IF YOUR BABY ENJOYS THIS ACTIVITY, also try Upstairs, Downstairs, page 143. ▶

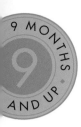
I CAN DO IT, TOO!

COPYCAT FUN

SKILLSPOTLIGHT

Learning how *to put a plush toy in a stroller, how to handle a broom, and how to stir with a plastic spoon helps your baby gain a better sense of spatial relations and develops her fine motor skills. Equally important is the opportunity to mimic what the big kids and adults in her world are doing.*

Fine Motor Skills	✔
Social Skills	✔
Spatial Awareness	✔

AT NINE MONTHS, your baby may already be imitating you by swiping at the floor when you're cleaning or by waving a wooden spoon at a bowl as you cook. Encourage her interest in the adult world by giving her baby-sized versions of brooms, mops, toolboxes, shopping carts, and strollers. If she's walking, you can show her how to take the stuffed dog for a stroller ride. She may not have great coordination at this age, but these are her very first explorations of what will become pretend play, a realm that will engage her increasingly in her toddler and preschool years.

NOTHING IS MORE compelling than doing what big brother does.

122

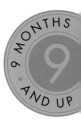

ZANY XYLOPHONES

SOUNDS OF MUSIC

YOUR BABY'S MUSICAL PURSUITS needn't be limited to baby stuff like rattles, bells, and windup toys. A xylophone designed for children under three years of age (available in music and toy stores) allows her to bang out a tune no matter where the mallet lands. It can also introduce her to the idea of musical scales if you show her how the notes go higher and lower when you play in different directions.

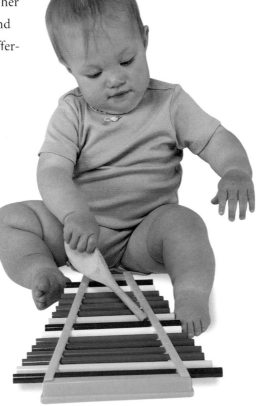

YOUR BABY WILL LOVE to discover that different colored xylophone bars make different sounds.

SKILL SPOTLIGHT

Learning how to hear *different notes, and eventually to associate them with different keys, helps your baby develop her listening skills. Gaining the skill to hit the bars one by one helps her develop eye-hand coordination and fine motor skills. And learning that she, too, can make music builds self-esteem.*

✔	**Eye-Hand Coordination**
✔	**Fine Motor Skills**
✔	**Listening**

◀ IF YOUR BABY ENJOYS THIS ACTIVITY, *also try Music Maker, page 92.*

123

POURING PRACTICE

FILLING FUN

SKILL SPOTLIGHT

When your baby *was younger, he didn't have the coordination to handle most objects. Now he's capable not only of lifting objects but also of tipping and twisting them. This game helps him work with his hands to develop fine motor skills. It also helps him practice his eye-hand coordination.*

Eye-Hand Coordination	✔
Fine Motor Skills	✔

EMPTYING AND FILLING one container is fun; emptying stuff from one container into another is twice as much fun. It's also an easy game to set up. Just gather some plastic cups, bowls, and buckets, plus spoons or small shovels. Then add either water (in a small basin or in the tub), sand (in the sandbox), or cornmeal (at the kitchen table or in a high chair). Show your baby how you fill the cup, spoon, shovel, or bowl with one of the substances. Watch as he enjoys fingering the sand or cornmeal or splashing the water—exploring the textures and how the items work together. Then show your baby how to pour the sand, cornmeal, or water out again. Before long he'll figure out how first to fill a container, then empty it into another.

IF YOUR BABY ENJOYS THIS ACTIVITY, also try Sand Skills, page 192.

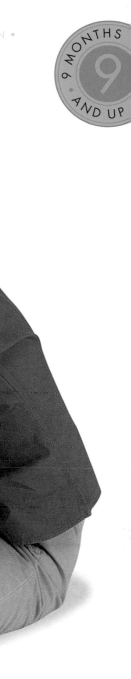

"There it goes!"

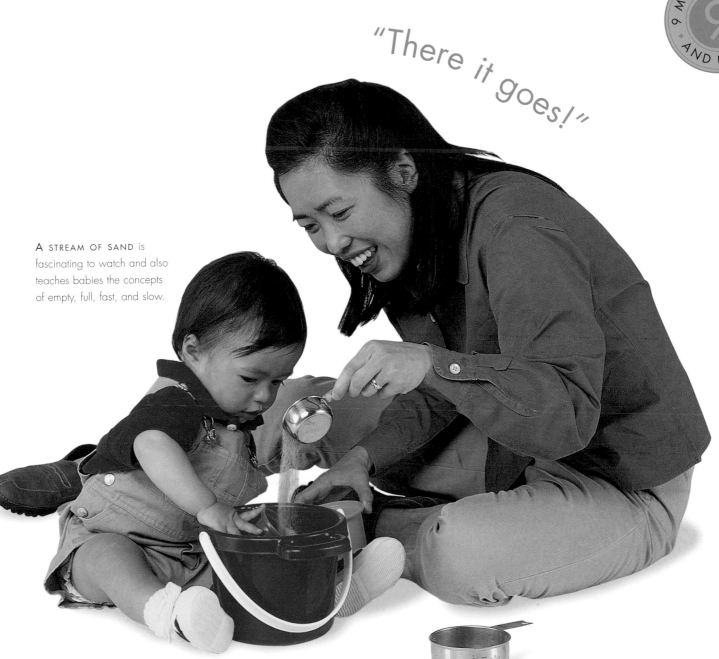

A STREAM OF SAND is fascinating to watch and also teaches babies the concepts of empty, full, fast, and slow.

ANIMAL SONGS

AT THIS AGE, most babies are beginning to notice the noises animals make and the ways they move. That means it's a good age to introduce songs with funny animal sounds. Your baby will be intrigued by the words and melodies that will later become part of his regular repertoire.

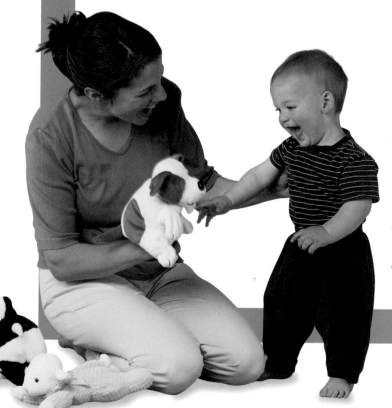

WHERE, OH WHERE

**Oh where, oh where
has my little dog gone?
Oh where, oh where can he be?
With his ears so short
and his tail so long,
oh where, oh where can he be?**

YOUR BABY WILL LOVE interacting with animal puppets as you sing silly animal songs.

SING A SONG OF SIXPENCE

Sing a song of sixpence,
a pocket full of rye,
four and twenty blackbirds,
baked in a pie.

When the pie was opened,
the birds began to sing.
Wasn't that a dainty dish
to set before the king?

MARY HAD A LITTLE LAMB

Mary had a little lamb,
little lamb, little lamb,
Mary had a little lamb
whose fleece was white as snow.

Everywhere that Mary went,
Mary went, Mary went,
everywhere that Mary went,
that lamb was sure to go.

OLD MACDONALD

Old MacDonald had a farm,
eee-i-eee-i-o.
And on his farm he had a dog,
eee-i-eee-i-o.
With a woof-woof here
and a woof-woof there,
here a woof, there a woof,
everywhere a woof-woof.
Old MacDonald had a farm,
eee-i-eee-i-o.

*continue the song, substituting other
animals and the sounds they make*

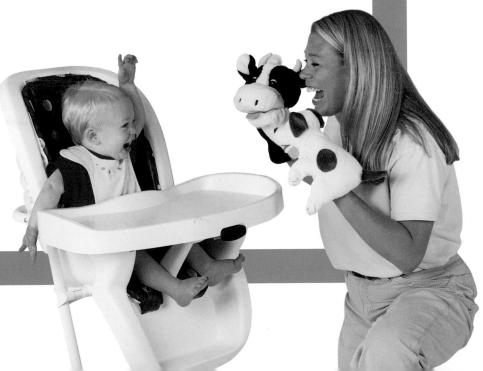

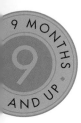
ACTIVITY BOOK

THINGS TO SEE AND DO

SKILLSPOTLIGHT

A book with cards *to open, textures to feel, and pictures to peruse boosts your baby's budding fine motor skills. Your narration as she looks at the book—"There's the kitty," "This is soft," or "Can you open this?"—helps her learn both words and concepts.*

Fine Motor Control	✔
Language Development	✔
Tactile Stimulation	✔

◀ *IF YOUR BABY ENJOYS THIS ACTIVITY, also try Friendly Faces, page 56.*

IS SHE TURNING book pages, fiddling with clothing labels, and pulling the ties off the tie rack? You can appeal to your baby's tinkering instinct by buying her an activity book or creating one from things found around your house. Just gather together pictures to look at (from magazines and postcards), textures to pat (cotton balls, fake fur, corduroy, crinkly tin foil, or bubble wrap), ribbons to tug, and old cards to open. You can securely glue them to pieces of cardboard and bind it all together with short pieces of ribbon.

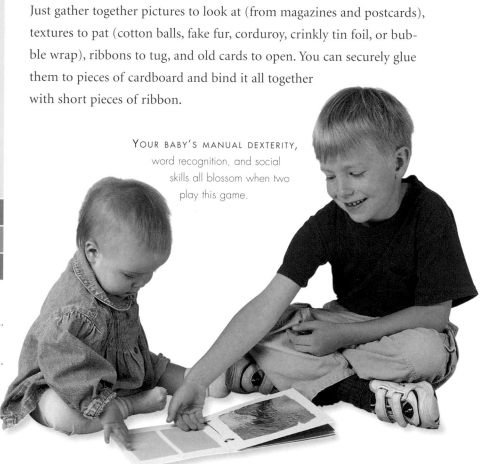

YOUR BABY'S MANUAL DEXTERITY, word recognition, and social skills all blossom when two play this game.

KNOCKDOWN

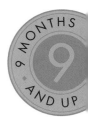

CREATING TOWERS

AS OLDER BABIES gain greater hand and arm coordination, they often take great joy in placing one object on top of another. You can nurture this budding talent by building towers of large blocks, books, cereal boxes, shoe boxes, or plastic bowls and cups for your baby. Remember there are two steps to this fun for your baby: watching you stack the objects and then knocking them down herself.

KNOCKING DOWN the tower is only part of the experience. She is also learning about sizes and shapes.

SKILLSPOTLIGHT

Playing with towers *of toys helps babies develop both gross and fine motor skills. Your baby also has the opportunity to explore spatial relationships and differences in size and shape.*

✔	**Fine Motor Skills**
✔	**Gross Motor Skills**
✔	**Size & Shape Discrimination**

IF YOUR BABY ENJOYS THIS ACTIVITY, also try Boxed Set, page 134.

129

BRIGHT COLORS, easy-to-handle rings, and some simple problems to solve keep babies motivated to stack the large rings again and again.

"Stack them up!"

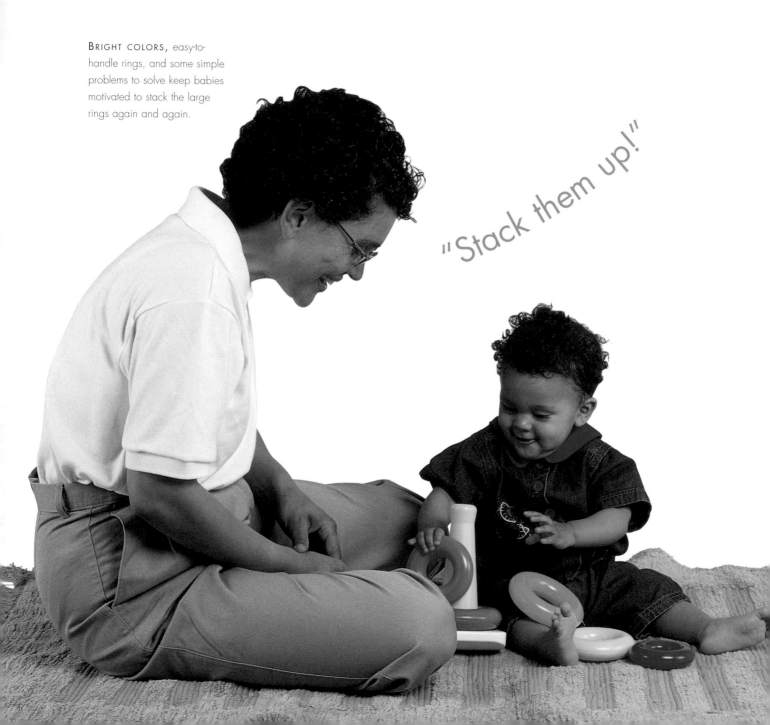

STACKING RINGS

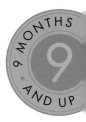

LEARNING ABOUT SIZE

SOME TOYS never go out of style. Good old-fashioned stacking rings are just as intriguing to babies today as they were to babies generations ago. You can buy sets made of wood or plastic, or make your own. A large set—made of bulky plastic rings, for instance—is usually easiest; older babies, with more advanced fine motor control, can tackle the sets with smaller poles.

• Start by showing your baby how to take the rings off—that's easier than fitting the rings over the pole. Don't be surprised if he just picks up the toy, turns it upside down, and dumps the rings all over the floor. He's showing you the most obvious solution to the problem!

• Learning to stack the rings according to size—with the large ring on the bottom and the small ring on top—comes much later in the second year. In the meantime, just let him practice getting the rings off and on the pole in any order.

◀ *IF YOUR BABY ENJOYS THIS ACTIVITY, also try Knockdown, page 129.*

MAKING YOUR OWN

As an alternative to a premade stacking ring, take the cardboard tube from a roll of paper towels and some Mason jar rings—or even rings cut from cardboard—and show your baby how to slide them on and off the tube.

SKILLSPOTLIGHT

Figuring out *how to get the colorful rings off—even if it's by dumping them all on the ground at once—helps your child build problem-solving skills. And learning how to place the rings over the pole helps him build both fine motor skills and an understanding of the concept of size.*

✔	**Eye-Hand Coordination**
✔	**Fine Motor Skills**
✔	**Problem Solving**
✔	**Size & Shape Discrimination**

131

PUBLIC ETIQUETTE

YOUR BABY won't always smile and coo in public—even the happiest baby falls prey to fussiness. And the public won't always be receptive to a fussy baby. But you and your baby have to travel in public, even if it's just for a quick trip to the post office. Your life will be far easier if you learn how to cope with potential conflicts early on.

Countdown to meltdowns: A sure way to create a frustrated, crying baby is to haul her from place to place when she's tired, hungry, or sick. Solution? Don't do it. Try to keep errands short; do them when your baby is rested and well fed; and bring a supply of books and toys for her to play with if you get stuck in a line or traffic jam.

Safeguard your privacy: Even mothers who felt perfectly comfortable nursing their newborn in public may feel a little bashful nursing an eleven-month-old in a shopping mall, especially if that eleven-month-old is walking and starting to talk. Strangers may give you funny looks for "still" nursing such a big baby. If this makes you uncomfortable and you find you have to breast-feed in public, try to find a private corner where you and your baby can be alone and have some quiet time together.

Protect against verbal assault: Blunt remarks about your baby can be annoying and hurtful. The best solution is for you to tactfully respond in a positive way. If someone at the grocery store declares that your baby boy is fat or mistakes him for a girl, you can reply with a very matter-of-fact "Yes, isn't he a gorgeous big boy?"

Part of the art of dealing with awkward situations in public is displaying model behavior for your baby. While he's not old enough to say "Please don't touch me" or "I'll outgrow my baby fat," he is old enough to perceive how you deal with potential conflicts. Staying calm, matter-of-fact, and loving will teach him to behave the same way. ■

UH-OH!

LEARNING ABOUT CAUSE AND EFFECT

IT'S A SIMPLE FACT that most older babies love to throw things from a higher perch—their highchair, Grandma's lap, etc. Grownups can make this habit into a fun game by engaging the child when she is doing so. Place plastic cups, rattles, large blocks, or small plush toys on the high-chair tray. Then sit on the floor next to the highchair and have the baby hand or toss the toys down to you. You can add to the fun by singing "uh-oh!" or "there it goes," or talking about how the toys go "down" and "up."

SKILLSPOTLIGHT

Dropping and watching *things fall helps a baby learn about cause and effect. At this stage, your baby is also just beginning to understand that through her actions she can exert control over others—something she will test more and more as she gets older.*

✔	**Cause & Effect**
✔	**Eye-Hand Coordination**
✔	**Grasp & Release**
✔	**Social Development**

YOU CAN TURN her natural instinct to throw things into a fun learning game.

133

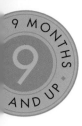

9 MONTHS
9
AND UP •

BOXED SET

OPENING, CLOSING, FILLING, AND EMPTYING

SKILL SPOTLIGHT

A box and a lid *provide an elementary puzzle for a baby, as she has to figure out how to get the lid off (easy) and how to put it back on (harder). This involves coordination and understanding the nature of both shapes and sizes. The activity also introduces her to the concepts of open, shut, full, empty, in, and out.*

Fine Motor Skills	✔
Problem Solving	✔
Size & Shape Discrimination	✔
Spatial Awareness	✔

A **BOX OF WIPES,** a bag of lentils, even the bowl of spaghetti left on the fridge's bottom shelf all fascinate your baby now. She wants to investigate everything in sight. You can safely keep her fingers busy by gathering a set of boxes with easy-to-manage tops (such as shoe boxes, empty diaper-wipe containers, and square gift boxes) and putting small toys and objects inside each.

• Put the same toys in the same boxes every time you play this game.
• Say the words "open" and "closed" as she plays with the boxes, as well as words like "in" and "out" as she plays with the toys.

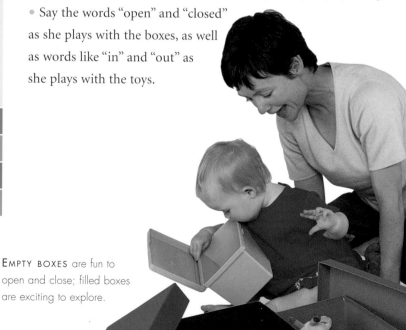

EMPTY BOXES are fun to open and close; filled boxes are exciting to explore.

134

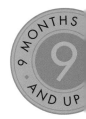

9 MONTHS
9
AND UP

BALL DROP

AN EYE-HAND COORDINATION EXERCISE

BALLS, BOWLS, and anything that bangs are big, big hits with older babies. How can you incorporate all those elements into one playtime? Just provide your baby with some lightweight balls (like whiffle or tennis balls) and a big metal bowl or plastic basket. Then show your baby how to drop the balls into the container. When the balls hit, they each make an interesting sound. Your baby will be intrigued by this activity and will gain an understanding of cause and effect.

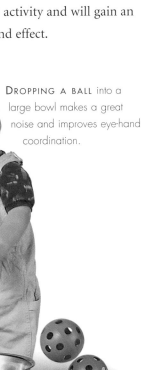

DROPPING A BALL into a large bowl makes a great noise and improves eye-hand coordination.

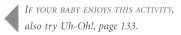

SKILL SPOTLIGHT

Grabbing a ball *comes pretty naturally to a baby after about the sixth month. Letting go of it again—as in a simple drop—is harder to learn, and intentionally throwing it is a future skill. This game lets your baby practice these first two skills while sharpening his eye-hand coordination.*

✔	**Eye-Hand Coordination**
✔	**Fine Motor Skills**
✔	**Grasp & Release**

◀ *IF YOUR BABY ENJOYS THIS ACTIVITY, also try Uh-Oh!, page 133.*

135

TUNNEL TIME

PLACES TO GO

SKILL SPOTLIGHT

Crawling through *small spaces helps your baby learn just how big her body is in relation to other objects, which helps her develop both spatial and body awareness. This game also helps develop visual skills such as depth perception and builds her self-confidence as she maneuvers through the tunnel without the benefit of peripheral vision.*

Body Awareness	✔
Gross Motor Skills	✔
Spatial Awareness	✔

◀ *IF YOUR BABY ENJOYS THIS ACTIVITY, also try Obstacle Course, page 121.*

EVER WONDER WHY your baby is so intent on wriggling under the bed, squeezing behind the couch, or curling up on the floor of your closet? A child this age is naturally intrigued with space—especially when it's just her size. You can cater to this fascination by providing a commercially made or cardboard tunnel for her to crawl through. Roll a ball down the tunnel and encourage her to go after it. Or put yourself, or small toys such as beanbags or plush toys, at the other end and coax her through.

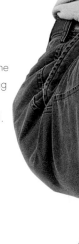

SHE'S BOTH LEARNING ABOUT the nature of small spaces and enjoying the thrill of discovery when she crawls through a baby-sized tunnel.

136

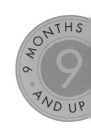

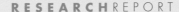

RESEARCH REPORT

Educators have long believed *that children exhibit distinct learning styles, or preferences, for taking in new information. Some kids need to physically explore something in order to understand it, while others need simply to see or hear it. Today some researchers believe that even infants show such preferences, as evidenced by their tendency to look at, listen to, or fiddle with objects very intently. Since babies need to develop all their senses, it's a good idea for parents to continue to offer their babies stimulating new environments to explore.*

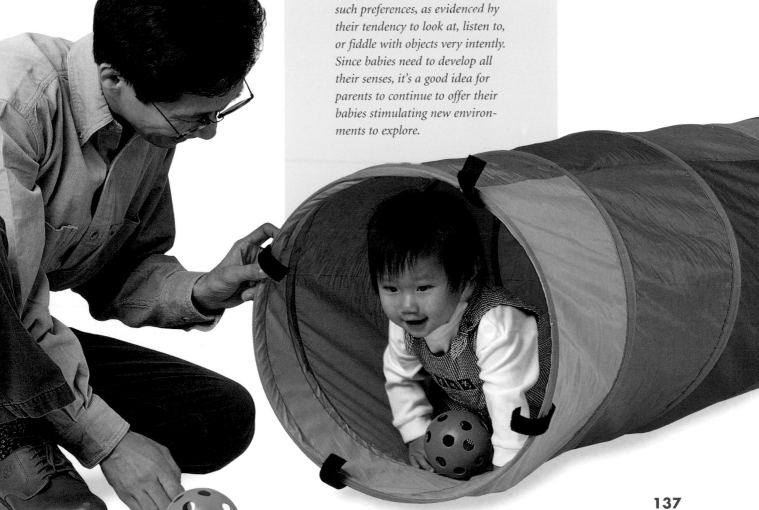

137

SING ABOUT ME

YOUR LITTLE ONE may not be able to say "mouth," "nose," "feet," or "toes," but he's probably already beginning to associate your spoken words with his body parts. You can boost his growing language and motor skills by teaching him these body songs. Gently move his arms and legs and use your hands and fingers to indicate the parts of his body.

PAT-A-CAKE

Pat-a-cake, pat-a-cake, baker's man,
clap hands together

bake me a cake as fast as you can.
clap hands

Pat it and prick it,
tap finger on one palm

and mark it with a B,
trace an imaginary B on one palm

and put it in the oven for Baby and me.
pretend to slide a cake into an oven

NOSE, NOSE, JOLLY RED NOSE

Nose, nose, jolly red nose—
tap your own nose

and who gave thee that jolly red nose?
point to baby's nose

Nutmeg and ginger, cinnamon and cloves—
wrinkle up your nose and pretend to sniff your palm

that's what gave me this jolly red nose.
tap baby's nose

138

HERE ARE THE TOES

 to the tune of **"Take Me Out to the Ball Game"**

Here are the toes of my (baby's name),
tap on baby's toes

**here are the toes of my (gal/guy),
and here are his feet and
his tiny knees—**
tap on baby's feet and knees

I can't help it—I'll give them a squeeze.
gently squeeze above baby's knees

**And he's got two arms
just for hugging,**
pat on baby's arms

and hands that clap and wave.
clap baby's hands for him

**But it's his eyes, nose,
mouth, and chin**
tap baby's facial features

that really draw me in!
lean in and kiss baby's face

HEY MR. KNICKERBOCKER

**Hey Mr. Knickerbocker,
boppity-bop,**
*standing with baby, rock
from side to side*

**I sure like the way you
walkity walk.**
lean baby forward and back

**I like the way you
walkity walk
with your feet,
ch-ch-ch-ch-ch-
ch-ch-ch-ch.**
walk forward

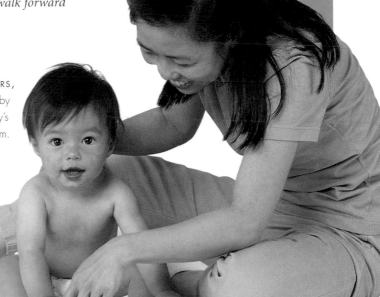

EYES, NOSE, FINGERS, and toes—your baby delights in Mommy's songs about him.

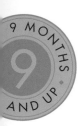
PUSH ME, PULL YOU

WALKING PRACTICE

SKILL SPOTLIGHT

The support provided *by a pushable object allows your baby to practice walking without holding on to furniture or your hands. By now, your baby has learned a little about how her body works— how she can work against gravity to keep herself upright as she moves forward. Walking and pushing helps her develop balance and gross motor skills.*

Balance	✔
Gross Motor Skills	✔
Lower-Body Strength	✔

IF YOUR BABY is walking, or even starting to toddle, she appreciates the support provided by a large object (like a push toy, stroller, or small chair) that she can push across the floor. A laundry basket filled with her toys also makes a great walking aid. You might help her at first by pulling from the other side—but then watch out! She will soon want to do it all by herself.

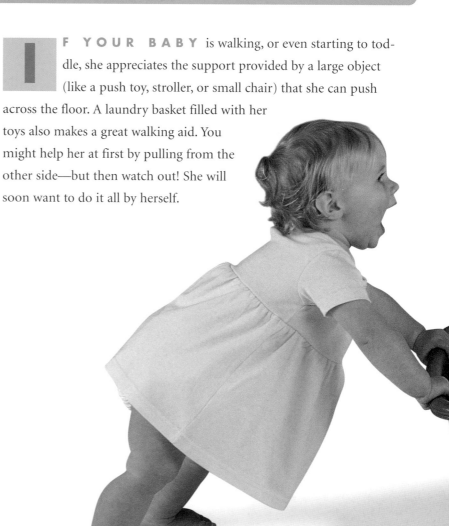

140

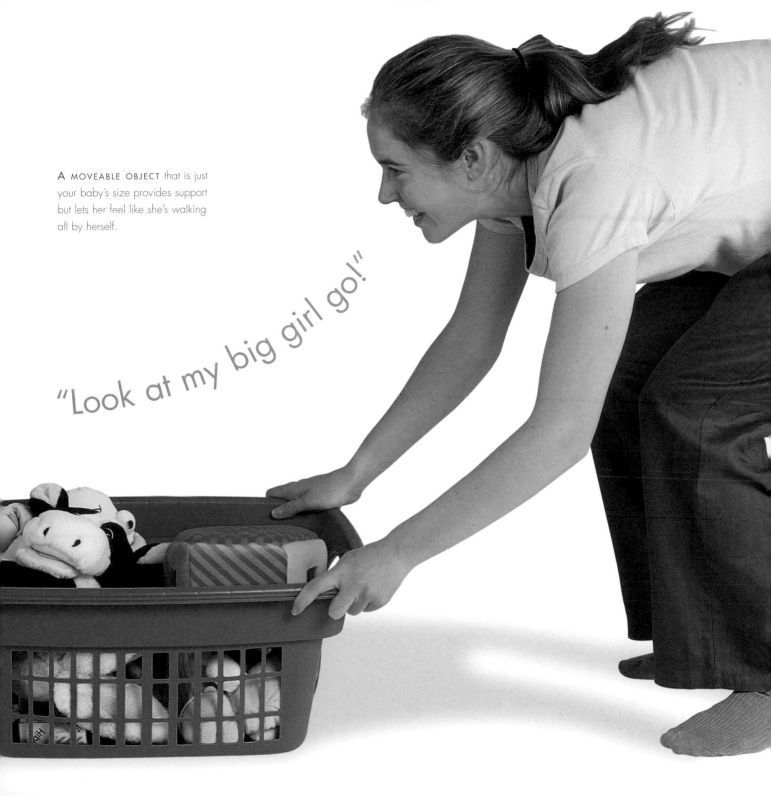

A MOVEABLE OBJECT that is just
your baby's size provides support
but lets her feel like she's walking
all by herself.

"Look at my big girl go!"

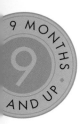
MONKEY SEE

Just Like Me

 to the *tune* of **"London Bridge Is Falling Down"**

Make your hands go
clap clap clap,
clap clap clap,
clap clap clap.
Make your hands go
clap clap clap,
just like me.

Make your head go
side to side,
side to side,
side to side.
Make your head go
side to side,
just like me.

Body Awareness ✔

Language Development ✔

142

IMITATING OLDER PEOPLE—whether siblings, parents, or next-door neighbors—is a prime source of learning for an older baby, and you can turn that imitation instinct into a game. Slap your knees, bang the floor or high-chair tray, put your hands over your eyes, open your mouth wide, or tip your head from side to side as you sing a song. She'll learn new words for her body and its movements, and also discover the joy of an interactive game.

CREATING NEW SOUNDS while directing arm and finger movements helps your child develop auditory memory and rhythm.

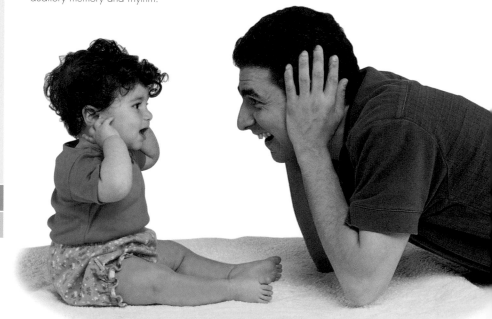

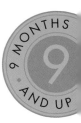

9 MONTHS AND UP
9

UPSTAIRS, DOWNSTAIRS

LEARNING STAIR SAFETY

ONCE YOUR BABY CAN CRAWL across the floor, he'll be eager to try crawling up the stairs, too. Going up is easy. It's getting down that's hard. Rather than banning him from the stairs, teach your baby how to descend safely by helping him turn around on his belly—feet first—and find the stairs with his feet. Guidance is important at first. Use consistent cue phrases such as "turn around" or "feet first" each time he approaches the stairs. And don't let him head for the stairs on his own.

LEARNING HOW to climb and descend stairs safely is a crucial skill for all budding toddlers as well as a fun activity.

SKILLSPOTLIGHT

Learning to reach his feet *into a space he cannot see and then find firm footing teaches your baby a lot about spatial relations and balance. Stair practice also helps your baby develop a better sense of height and depth, which makes him more cautious in his future climbing pursuits.*

✔	**Balance**
✔	**Gross Motor Skills**
✔	**Lower-Body Strength**
✔	**Spatial Awareness**

143

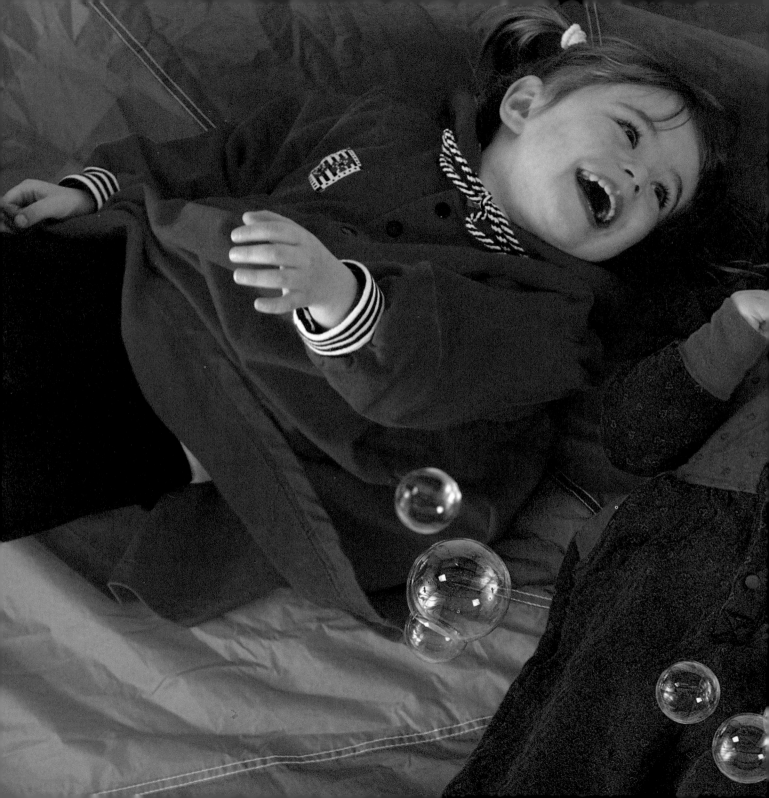

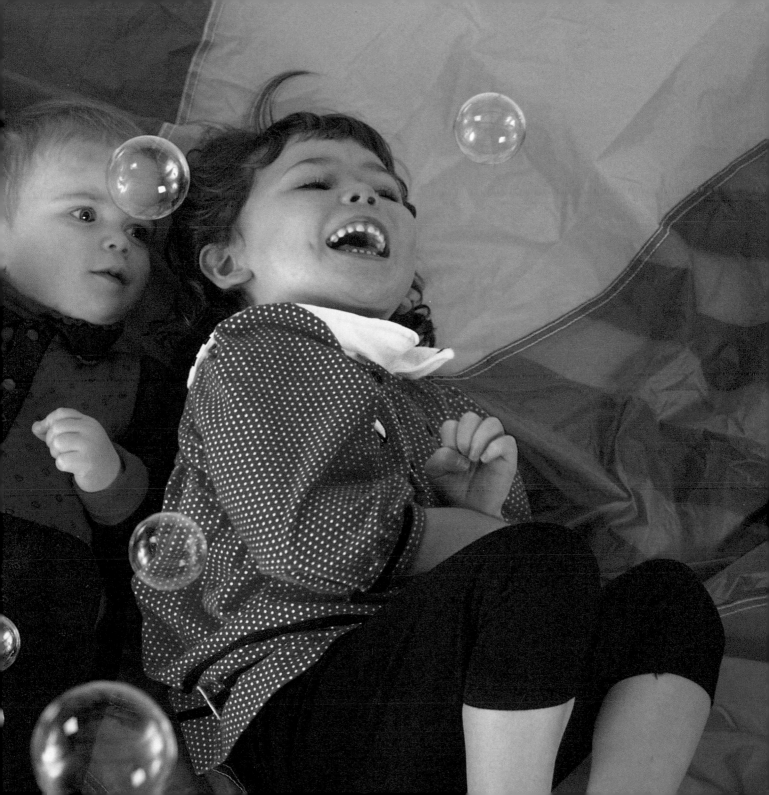

PLAYING WITH YOUR TODDLER

WHETHER THEIR expressions are marked by ear-to-ear grins or brow-furrowing intensity, toddlers at play are a wonder to behold. The concentration with which they examine—and whoops! occasionally disassemble—each new object, the enthusiasm they bring to each new endeavor, and the joy they radiate as they acquire each new skill

A STRING OF BUBBLES is a magical delight—and a dazzling demonstration of cause and effect.

demonstrate that for these young explorers, play is serious business. It's a way of learning about their world, other people, and themselves, of testing and pushing the limits of their abilities, of conquering everything from the physics of sand castles to the basic rules of social interaction.

These early years are ripe with unparalleled opportunities for you as a parent to unlock your child's potential. A toddler's brain is a work in progress profoundly influenced by her environment, and what she is now exposed to—or not exposed to—will have a lifelong impact. This might be a daunting prospect except for a few comforting facts. First, children are born primed to learn. Second, parents instinctively strive to provide the stimulation children need. And, most important, since play is a vehicle of learning for children, engaging in this task should be fun for parent and child alike.

THE BENEFITS OF PLAY

Because play comes so naturally to children and seems like nothing more than simple pleasure, it is easy to overlook the many far-reaching benefits that

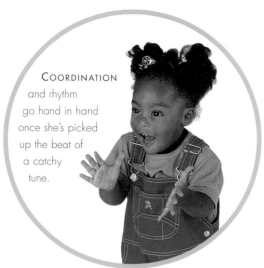

COORDINATION and rhythm go hand in hand once she's picked up the beat of a catchy tune.

engrossed in a variety of play activities teaches him how to concentrate and persevere.

Play also provides an invaluable window to your child's personality. By playing with him—or watching him play with others—you will soon learn how he reacts to obstacles, failures, and victories. You'll see his quirky sense of humor emerge and his social skills begin to develop over time. His manner of playing can reveal his emotions, aptitudes, and preferred learning styles—whether he's responding well

play contributes to your child's emotional, physical, and intellectual development. Through play, a toddler learns so many vital skills—how to communicate, count, and solve problems. He hones his gross motor skills by tossing balls or climbing up a slide, and polishes his fine motor skills by painting with brushes or drawing with crayons. His imagination soars as he pretends to converse on a toy telephone or dons a succession of silly hats in front of a mirror. His language skills improve as he listens to stories and strives to communicate his needs and preferences. Early play encounters with his peers, siblings, parents, and other adults teach him how to get along with others and to respect rules and boundaries. Becoming

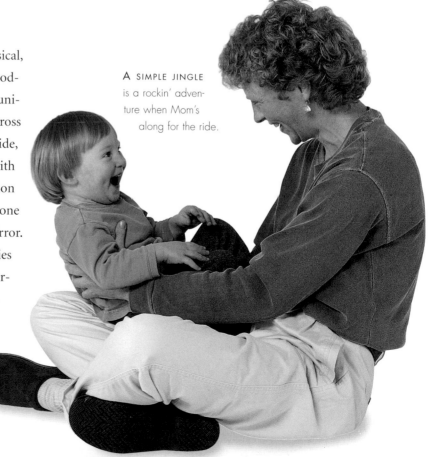

A SIMPLE JINGLE is a rockin' adventure when Mom's along for the ride.

to verbal instructions or visual images, for example, or if he retains information best after hands-on experiences.

Play also affords a wonderful opportunity for bonding with your toddler. When she is in a quiet mood, cuddling and looking at picture books or building an elaborate block tower creates a feeling of peaceful togetherness. When she's feeling a bit rowdier, a game of hide-and-seek or a beanbag toss imparts the notion that parents can be fun as well as sources of care and compassion. When you help her acquire new skills and praise her efforts, you convincingly demonstrate how you are always there to lend support and spur her progress—and countless studies demonstrate that children learn

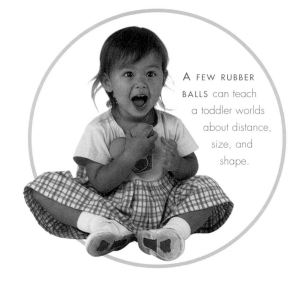

A FEW RUBBER BALLS can teach a toddler worlds about distance, size, and shape.

best in a loving, supportive environment. In so many ways, being your child's enthusiastic play partner creates a special closeness that will resonate throughout both of your lives.

ROLLING TO THE MUSIC lets toddlers (and moms) exercise their rambunctious sides.

DIFFERENT WAYS TO PLAY

This book is designed to help you make the most of the wonderful toddler years by providing a wealth of simple and diverse activities to enjoy with your child. You'll find rousing fingerplays to sing along to, art projects, bath-time activities, games with blankets and boxes and blocks, as well as many other imaginative suggestions. There are ways to introduce children to the joys of music, to encourage muscular coordination and strength, and to build budding vocabularies. The wide variety of activities touches upon every important component of a child's physical, mental, social, and emotional skills, and each has been carefully designed and selected for developmental appropriateness. Some are classics, some are Gymboree's own innovations, but all are designed to foster the type of loving, nurturing interaction that helps a toddler learn and forms a lasting bond between parent and child.

Although playing and learning are inextricably linked, the point of these activities is not to run your toddler through a rigid battery of exercises. Instead, this section's emphasis is on having fun first and foremost through activities that also happen to spur age-appropriate development in your child. These activities help build a solid foundation for all future learning. In other words, they help your toddler learn *how* to learn.

READY, SET, PLAY!

Far from being rigid, the instructions in this book are intended as guidelines for loosely structured play, open to modification as you respond to your own child's particular interests and inclinations. Get things going, then step back and allow your toddler the freedom to explore

and experiment as he wishes. This is key to encouraging him to work things out on his own, learn to problem-solve, think creatively, and achieve self-esteem and a sense of autonomy.

Setting up a well-designed, safe play environment also contributes to his growing sense of independence and provides stimulation: deck the walls in his room with shatterproof mirrors and colorful

BRING ON THE NONSENSE—no song is too silly as far as your giggly wiggle-worm is concerned.

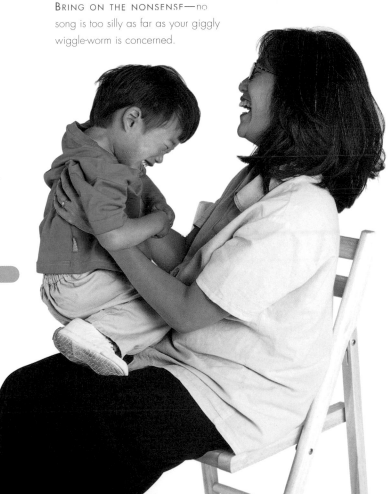

posters, and transform the ceiling into a starry sky or an undersea fantasy with glow-in-the-dark stickers. Arrange low bookcases or tables with a rotating assortment of toddler-friendly toys, books, and art supplies, providing bins for easy sorting and storage. Place a hamper within your child's reach, as well as a rack for hanging up clothes. Most important, don't think you need to stock up on a lot of expensive and elaborate playthings; classics such as puzzles, bubbles, puppets, blocks, tops, and balls remain versatile and engaging toddler toys.

As you become familiar with this book, feel free to return again and again to your child's favorite activities. Children benefit greatly from repetition. It allows them to test and refine what they have learned and it gives them a sense of accomplishment (for more on repetition, see page 176). And don't fret if your child doesn't seem to conform to the age bands listed—if your one-year-old, for instance, is having trouble handling the beach ball in Pass the Ball or, conversely, if your two-year-old quickly memorizes every song and fingerplay in the book. Keep in mind that each child develops at her own pace and in her own style (for more information on developmental differences, see page 160). The age bands are simply broad guidelines, and there are plenty of activities in this book to suit every child's unique needs and preferences.

So go ahead, put on your play clothes, warm up those vocal cords, and prepare to enter and enhance your toddler's world by trying the activities suggested in the following pages. They'll help you provide a richer, more stimulating environment for your child—and a treasury of happy memories for you, your child's first playmate.

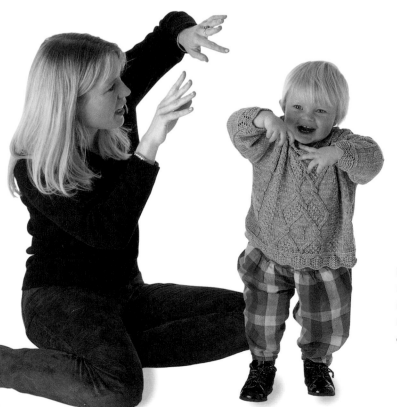

FINGERPLAYS
help your itsy-
bitsy spider flex
her verbal as well
as motor skills.

The following activities are grouped chronologically in six-month age ranges that match key stages in a child's development. These are general guidelines only, as there is a wide range of developmental differences among children.

12 MONTHS AND UP

Whether they're crawling, cruising, or walking, one-year-olds enjoy a newfound mobility that accompanies their enormous curiosity about the world. Their fine motor skills have developed to the point where they can assuredly pick up small objects and stack a few blocks. They love listening to their parents' voices, such as when reading a story or singing a song. They understand many words and respond to some simple commands, most also begin saying a few words of their own.

18 MONTHS AND UP

Children this age are determined to explore, handle, taste, and shake, rattle, and roll everything in sight. Their increasingly sophisticated gross motor skills allow them to walk, run, and climb, and their fine motor skills permit them to eat with a spoon and throw a ball. They enjoy games that engage their tactile senses and can express an appreciation of music by swaying. Their vocabulary averages more than a dozen words, and they can usually form simple two- and three-word phrases.

24 MONTHS AND UP

Children's strength, flexibility, and balance are stronger and surer now: they can unscrew the lid of a jar and perform other tasks that showcase their developing fine motor abilities. Their enthusiasm for music continues, and they are beginning to use their imaginations. Most enjoy the company of peers, although rather than engaging in joint activities they tend to play independently side by side. Two-year-olds might have more than two hundred words in their vocabulary, and they begin to speak in simple sentences.

30 MONTHS AND UP

Older toddlers delight in activities that refine and stretch their physical abilities, such as running, jumping, tricycle riding, and playing a simple game of catch. They continue to hone their fine motor skills, such as holding a crayon or paintbrush. Their attention spans increase, and they often show a passion for classifying activities and sorting games. Their fluency with language grows dramatically, and they catch on to the notion of abstractions, making for a rich repertoire of fantasy play.

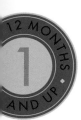

12 MONTHS
1
AND UP

PASS THE BALL

BALL PLAY FOR BEGINNERS

SKILLSPOTLIGHT

Learning to roll *or even stop a ball helps toddlers refine their gross motor skills and develop eye-hand (or eye-foot, as the case may be) coordination. Playing with balls helps them develop a sense of timing as they attempt to figure out how long it will take before the ball reaches them.*

FEW TODDLERS can actually catch a ball—that takes a good bit of coordination—but most love to push, kick, and grab this engaging toy. To start your toddler out on ball play, choose a flat, grassy spot outside or a cleared space inside, and sit just a couple of feet away from her. Gently roll the ball to your child and encourage her to roll it back in your direction. As she gets better at it, sit farther and farther away. Try softly bouncing the ball between the two of you, as well.

Body Awareness	✔
Coordination	✔
Gross Motor Skills	✔

A BALL THAT'S ABOUT THE SIZE of your child's head is just right; it's not so big that it will overwhelm her and not so small that she'll have trouble handling it.

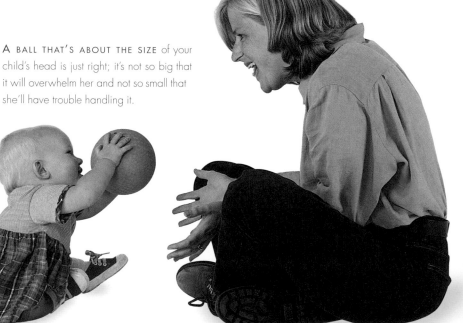

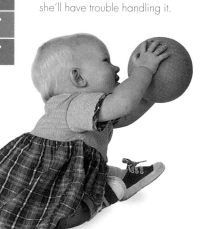

IF YOUR CHILD ENJOYS THIS ACTIVITY, also try Tube Tricks, page 218. ▶

THE FINGER BAND

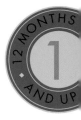

A SONG WITH IMAGINARY INSTRUMENTS

IT'S NEVER TOO EARLY to give your toddler music lessons, especially when the instruments are make-believe. As you sing "The Finger Band" (lyrics at right), pretend to play different instruments such as drums, a flute, cymbals, and a piano. Don't worry if your child has never heard a clarinet, much less seen a trombone—she will enjoy watching and imitating your hand movements. Make your gestures distinct and energetic. If at first she can't copy you, move her hands and fingers for her. As she gets more coordinated, march your legs up and down as you sing and play. Alternate between singing softly and loudly, explaining the difference as you do so.

PROP YOUR LITTLE MAJORETTE on your lap and introduce her to your finger band before launching into this musical parade.

 to the tune of **"The Mulberry Bush"**

**The finger band has come to town,
come to town, come to town,
the finger band has come to town,
so early in the morning.**
hold up and wiggle your fingers

**The finger band can play the drums,
play the drums, play the drums,
the finger band can play the drums,
so early in the morning.**
pantomime playing a drum

**The finger band can play the flute,
play the flute, play the flute,
the finger band can play the flute,
so early in the morning.**
pantomime playing a flute and continue with other instruments

✔ **Eye-Hand Coordination**

✔ **Language Development**

✔ **Listening Skills**

153

PARACHUTE PLAY

FUN WAYS TO BUILD BALANCING SKILLS

SKILL SPOTLIGHT

Parachute play *enhances your toddler's ability to balance—a skill that translates to freedom and independence, because it's a precursor to walking, running, and more complex physical actions such as skipping or even doing a somersault. Parachutes are also intrinsically interesting items to use because of their slick feel and bold colors; reinforce your child's color-recognition skills by naming the colors as you play.*

Balance	✔
Tactile Stimulation	✔
Visual Discrimination	✔

YOUR TODDLER will cheer as you treat him to a slip-and-slide parachute ride, and in the process you'll safely challenge his ability to balance while in motion. On a carpeted floor, seat or lay him on a colorful mini-parachute, blanket, or sheet, then gently and gradually pull him around, taking care to avoid any furniture and sharp corners as you explore the great indoors.

• Recruit another adult to help you hold the blanket or parachute over your child's head. If your child can stand with ease, test his balance by slowly raising and lowering the parachute while he stands underneath it and admires the colors or pattern. Do this carefully; even a lightweight parachute can topple an unsteady toddler.

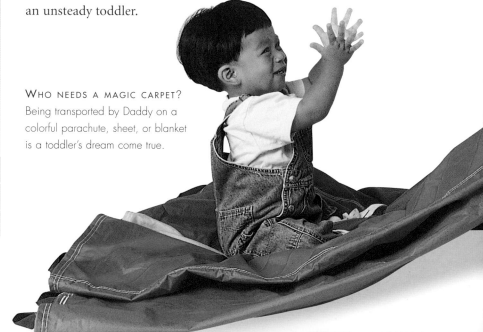

WHO NEEDS A MAGIC CARPET? Being transported by Daddy on a colorful parachute, sheet, or blanket is a toddler's dream come true.

154

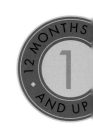

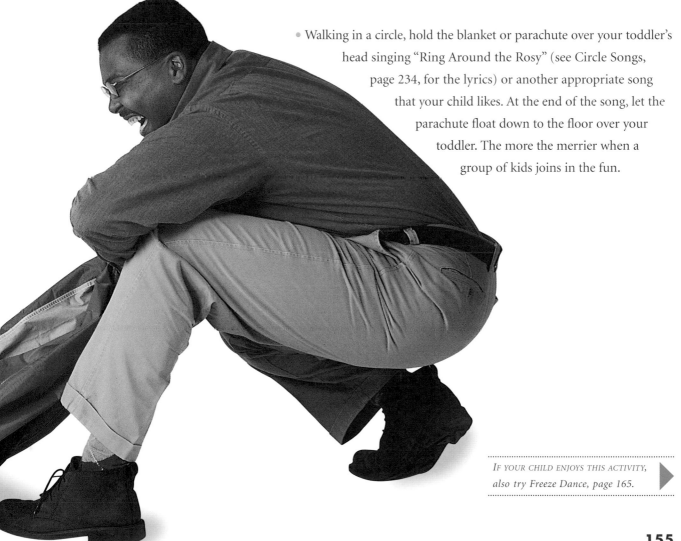

• Walking in a circle, hold the blanket or parachute over your toddler's head singing "Ring Around the Rosy" (see Circle Songs, page 234, for the lyrics) or another appropriate song that your child likes. At the end of the song, let the parachute float down to the floor over your toddler. The more the merrier when a group of kids joins in the fun.

IF YOUR CHILD ENJOYS THIS ACTIVITY, also try Freeze Dance, page 165.

BUBBLE BUSTERS

A POP-THE-BUBBLE GAME OF CHASE

SKILL SPOTLIGHT

Chasing, catching, and popping bubbles contributes to eye-hand coordination, sensory stimulation, body awareness, and gross motor skills. And if your toddler tries to blow bubbles herself, she'll learn about cause and effect. Your bubble buster is also discovering that when she touches an apparently solid object, it sometimes pops—her first lesson in physics!

Eye-Hand Coordination	✔
Gross Motor Skills	✔
Language Development	✔
Tactile Stimulation	✔

MAKING YOUR OWN

For the soap solution, mix 1 cup of water, 1 tablespoon of glycerin (available in most pharmacies), and 2 tablespoons of dishwashing detergent. Fashion bubble wands from pipe cleaners, plastic bag ties, even plastic cups with the bottom cut out.

IF THERE IS A MAGIC EQUATION for entrancing a toddler, it must be the combination of a simple soap solution and a bubble wand. Blowing, chasing, and popping bubbles is an excellent opportunity to encourage movement, stimulate eye-hand coordination, and introduce the concepts of big and small, high and low. Experiment with an assortment of bubble wands in varying sizes. Don't be surprised if your toddler enjoys this activity so much that "bubble" becomes one of her favorite words!

• Use a large wand to make big bubbles and cheer her as she chases and pops them, then repeat the activity with a smaller wand. Blow forcefully when you're creating a shower of tiny bubbles and softly when you're making a huge bubble. Blow the bubbles up high and down low, saying "high" or "low" as they float away.

• When you blow bubbles outdoors, explain that the wind that rustles the leaves and blows her hair also carries the bubbles away. Encourage your toddler to pop the bubbles with her fingers or stomp on them with her feet. Walk backward as you blow on the bubble wand so she'll chase you to catch the bubbles.

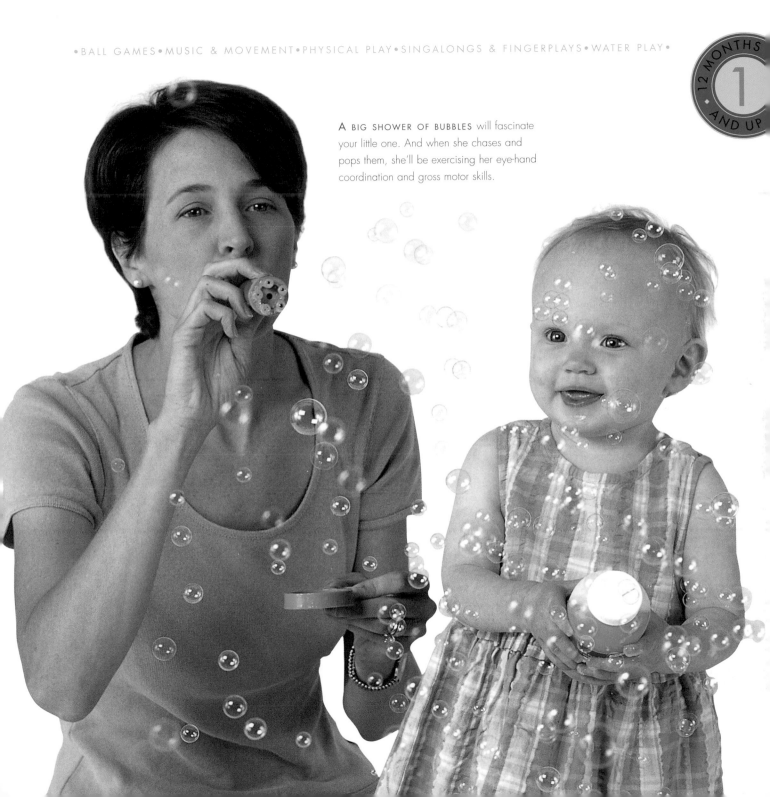

A BIG SHOWER OF BUBBLES will fascinate your little one. And when she chases and pops them, she'll be exercising her eye-hand coordination and gross motor skills.

CLAP, CLAP, CLAP

A MOVE-YOUR-BODY SONG

SKILL SPOTLIGHT

Learning the words *for body parts, and learning to control those hands, arms, and feet, is serious business for kids this age. While your toddler may already be pointing to her body parts when you name them, this song gives her a chance to practice isolating and moving her hands, feet, arms, and lips.*

Body Awareness	✔
Gross Motor Skills	✔
Listening Skills	✔
Social Skills	✔

IF YOUR CHILD ENJOYS THIS ACTIVITY, also try Just Like Me, page 181.

IF YOU'RE FAMILIAR with the ever-popular song "The Wheels on the Bus" (see page 168), you can add a new twist to the tune with these lyrics (right). "Clap, Clap, Clap" coaxes your little one to coordinate body movements with words. Associating words and actions with a melody and a beat will enhance her understanding of rhythm, because she'll be able to feel it and mimic it with her body.

• Young toddlers are eager to learn the words for body parts, so be sure to emphasize those words in the song—"hands," "arms," "mouth"—by enunciating them or singing them more loudly. Make big motions at first to underscore the meaning of the words.

• Try variations: ask your child to tap her knees, shake her hips, or nod her head.

• After she's learned the song, make a few "mistakes"—clap your hands when you're supposed to be tapping your foot. Her laughter shows she already has a sense of humor.

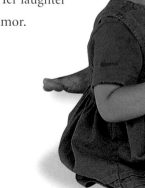

YOUR TODDLER WILL ENJOY imitating you as you clap your hands and tap your foot in this music game.

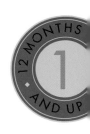

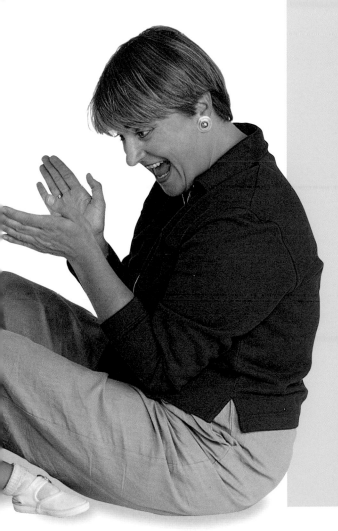

 to the *tune* of **"The Wheels on the Bus"**

**You take your little hands
and go clap, clap, clap,**
clap your hands
**clap, clap, clap,
clap, clap, clap.
You take your little hands
and go clap, clap, clap,
clap your little hands.**

**You take your little foot
and go tap, tap, tap,**
tap your foot
**tap, tap, tap,
tap, tap, tap.
You take your little foot
and go tap, tap, tap,
tap your little foot.**

**You take your little arms
and go hug, hug, hug,**
hug each other
**hug, hug, hug,
hug, hug, hug.**

**You take your little arms
and go hug, hug, hug,
hug your mom and dad.**

**You take your little mouth
and go kiss, kiss, kiss,**
pucker your lips
**kiss, kiss, kiss,
kiss, kiss, kiss.
You take your little mouth
and go kiss, kiss, kiss,
kiss your mom and dad.**

**You take your little hand
and wave bye, bye, bye,**
wave good-bye
**bye, bye, bye,
bye, bye, bye.
You take your little hand
and wave bye, bye, bye,
wave your little hand.**

159

AT THEIR OWN PACE

BABIES SIT UP at six months. They utter their first "dada" at nine. They crawl at seven months and walk at age one. When parents are confronted by the firm developmental timetables sometimes espoused in popular child-care books, they often are pleased if their children achieve a milestone a few weeks or months ahead of schedule—and panicked if their offspring are late. But while pediatricians used to treat these timetables as if they were carved in granite, most practitioners today agree that there is a much wider developmental range in perfectly healthy children.

A child may first roll over, for example, at any time from two to six months of age. Children can vary the age at which they start talking by a year or more, and future soccer stars may take their first steps as early as seven months and as late as eighteen. Although children generally follow the prescribed developmental sequence, some will skip a milestone completely—they might never learn to crawl, for example. Instead, when their muscle tone and coordination skills are ready, they just get up and start walking.

All of these developmental milestones are a matter of complex neural and muscular maturation, which is affected by both inherited and environmental factors—a child may walk late in life, for example, if the family has a history of late walkers. Often a child lags in one area while accelerating in another. In rare instances, a delayed milestone can signal significant problems, but in the vast majority of cases it's just a matter of a child developing at her own rate. As educational psychologist Jane Healy observes in her book *Your Child's Growing Mind:* "A child who is lagging slightly in development is on the same track as the others. His train simply goes at a slower pace, although it stands every chance of reaching the same destination." ■

ITSY-BITSY SPIDER

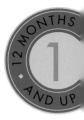

12 MONTHS AND UP
1

A FAVORITE FIRST FINGERPLAY

IN THIS POPULAR SONG, you can portray the trials of the hapless itsy-bitsy spider with fun-to-mimic hand motions. By repeating the song and the gestures you are not only entertaining your toddler, you're also stimulating her listening and language skills. Add tactile stimulation by crawling the spider up her tummy, "pouring" the rain down over her shoulders, and crossing her arms above her head to make the sun. When she seems proficient, try singing the song and cuing her to perform the finger movements—eventually she may surprise you with a solo rendition.

**The itsy-bitsy spider
went up the water spout,**
walk your fingers up in the air

**down came the rain and
washed the spider out.**
*wiggle your fingers downward
to make rain*

**Out came the sun and
dried up all the rain,**
*form a circle with your
fingers above your head*

**and the itsy-bitsy spider
went up the spout again.**
walk your fingers up again

✔	**Fine Motor Skills**
✔	**Listening Skills**
✔	**Tactile Stimulation**

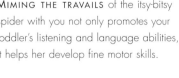

MIMING THE TRAVAILS of the itsy-bitsy spider with you not only promotes your toddler's listening and language abilities, it helps her develop fine motor skills.

161

THE PILLOW COURSE

FIRST STEPS ON A PATH OF PILLOWS

SKILL SPOTLIGHT

Movement and exploration *are near and dear to a toddler's heart, so an opportunity to move around in an interesting environment is bound to be met with joy. This activity is also an excellent way for your toddler to build his motor skills by challenging large muscle groups and to increase both his balance and coordination as he faces physical obstacles.*

Balance	✔
Body Awareness	✔
Eye-Foot Coordination	✔
Gross Motor Skills	✔

CREATE A SAFE OBSTACLE COURSE in your living room by laying out a simple zigzagging path of pillows and cushions.

• Encourage your child to complete the course by crawling or walking along the path. It will be a bumpy, lumpy route, so even if he's already walking be sure to hold on to his hands as he begins the journey. Once he becomes more sure-footed, let him take some steps on the pillows by himself, but stay nearby just in case he starts to topple. Remove your toddler's shoes and socks to help him keep his balance.

• Vary the height of the path by stacking a couple of pillows. To make the course more challenging, run it under a table so he has to crawl underneath, or position pillows around the room so he must maneuver around soft furniture (avoid furniture with sharp edges).

• Use cushions and pillows of varying sizes, colors, and textures to keep the course interesting. Don't be surprised if your young athlete stops occasionally to feel the obstacles with his hands or feet. Allow him to explore, then gently encourage him to keep going.

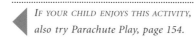
IF YOUR CHILD ENJOYS THIS ACTIVITY, also try Parachute Play, page 154.

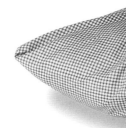

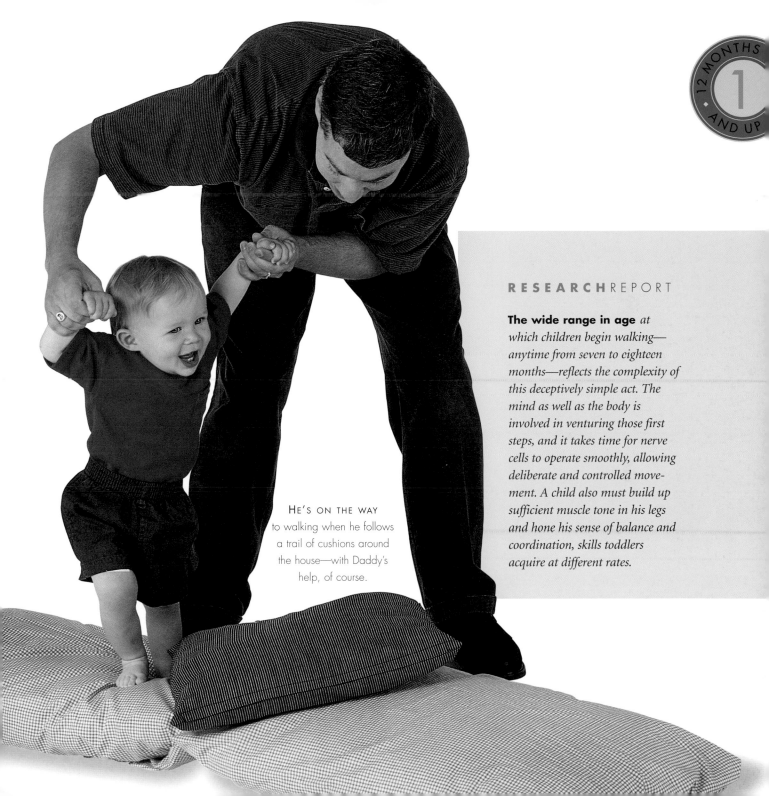

RESEARCHREPORT

The wide range in age *at which children begin walking— anytime from seven to eighteen months—reflects the complexity of this deceptively simple act. The mind as well as the body is involved in venturing those first steps, and it takes time for nerve cells to operate smoothly, allowing deliberate and controlled move- ment. A child also must build up sufficient muscle tone in his legs and hone his sense of balance and coordination, skills toddlers acquire at different rates.*

HE'S ON THE WAY to walking when he follows a trail of cushions around the house—with Daddy's help, of course.

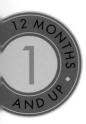

12 MONTHS AND UP

HATS ON!

EXPERIMENTING WITH DIFFERENT HEADGEAR

SKILLSPOTLIGHT

Talking to your toddler *about the hats the two of you are wearing helps expose him to new words that will someday become a part of his vocabulary. And seeing you in different hats teaches him that you're still Mommy even if you look a little different. When your child is a bit older, he'll start to enjoy role-playing with the hats, a game that will stretch his capacity for imaginative play.*

Concept Development	✔
Language Development	✔
Social Skills	✔

YOUR TODDLER WILL MARVEL at your elaborate headdress and smile when you make him a fire chief—especially if you mimic special sound effects, such as an engine siren, to go with each hat.

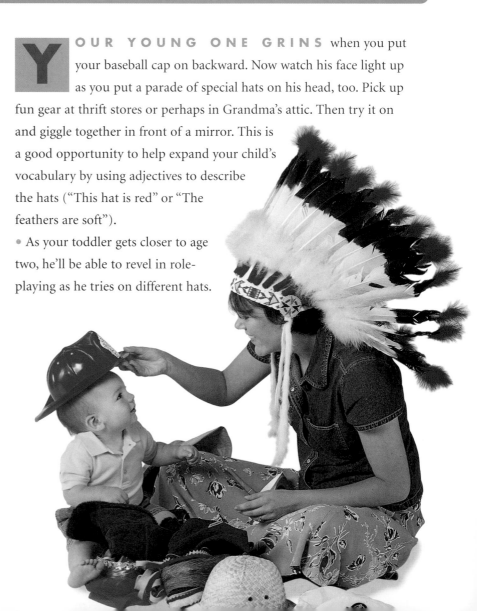

YOUR YOUNG ONE GRINS when you put your baseball cap on backward. Now watch his face light up as you put a parade of special hats on his head, too. Pick up fun gear at thrift stores or perhaps in Grandma's attic. Then try it on and giggle together in front of a mirror. This is a good opportunity to help expand your child's vocabulary by using adjectives to describe the hats ("This hat is red" or "The feathers are soft").

• As your toddler gets closer to age two, he'll be able to revel in role-playing as he tries on different hats.

FREEZE DANCE

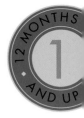

12 MONTHS
1
AND UP

STOP-AND-GO MUSICAL FUN

PLAY MUSIC and put a friend or older child in charge of the volume control while you take your young dancer for a twirl. Hold your toddler in your arms; when the music starts, exaggerate your dance moves by swaying from side to side and dipping her on occasion. When the music stops, hold your stance; begin dancing when the music starts again, then freeze each time it halts. Older toddlers may be able to dance—and stop—on their own, but most are just as happy to "freeze" in your embrace.

SKILLSPOTLIGHT

By taking a ride *in your arms as you dance the night away, your toddler experiences the rhythm of music, a crucial first step in developing both language and music skills. And when you freeze in mid-action, she learns to balance herself in your arms. Suddenly turning the music on and off gives your toddler something she dearly loves—a surprise—and cultivates listening skills as well.*

✔	**Balance**
✔	**Listening Skills**
✔	**Social Skills**

SWINGING TO THE BEAT is a surefire way to thrill her—especially when you surprise her with sudden pauses in your boogie.

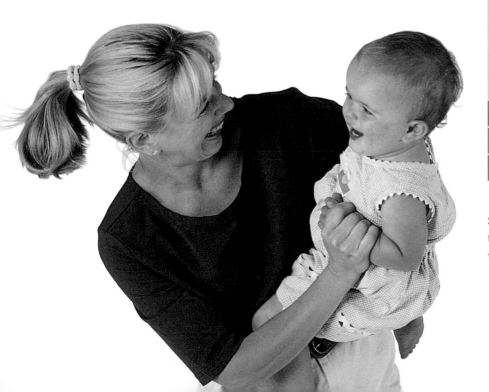

165

TWINKLE, TWINKLE

SOME SONGS ENDURE generation after generation, giving parents and grandparents a chance to share their old favorites with young children. But old favorites can be changed in new and surprising ways, so as you sing these suggested variations of "Twinkle, Twinkle Little Star," try to come up with some simple—or silly—improvisations of your own.

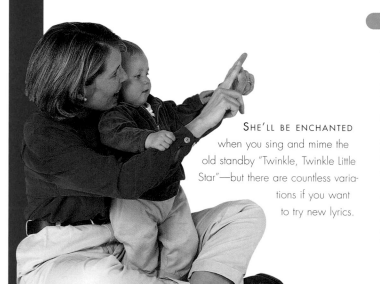

SHE'LL BE ENCHANTED when you sing and mime the old standby "Twinkle, Twinkle Little Star"—but there are countless variations if you want to try new lyrics.

TWINKLE, TWINKLE LITTLE STAR

Twinkle, twinkle little star,
hold hands up, opening and closing fists
how I wonder what you are!

Up above the world so high,
point upward
like a diamond in the sky.
create a diamond with thumbs and forefingers

Twinkle, twinkle little star,
open and close fists
how I wonder what you are!

THE APPLE TREE

 to the *tune* of "Twinkle, Twinkle Little Star"

Way up high in the apple tree
stretch arms up high
two little apples
looking down at me.
make circles around eyes with thumbs
and forefingers

I shook that tree
just as hard as I could,
shake an imaginary tree with
both hands
down came the apples
float fingers down
and mmm they were good!
rub tummy and smile

I shook that tree
just as hard as I could,
shake an imaginary tree with
both hands
down came the apples
float fingers down
and mmm they were good!
rub tummy and smile

THE SKY SO BLUE

 to the *tune* of "Twinkle, Twinkle Little Star"

Way up in the sky so blue
reach up to the sky with both hands
two little clouds said "peekaboo."
play peekaboo with hands

The wind blew the clouds
just as hard as it could,
rub hands together and shiver
down came the raindrops
flutter fingers down
and oooh. . . they felt good!

The wind blew the clouds
just as hard as it could,
rub hands together
and shiver
down came the raindrops
flutter fingers down
and oooh. . . they felt good!

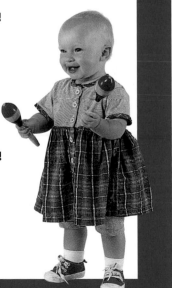

167

THE WHEELS ON THE BUS

A MUSICAL TRANSPORTATION TOUR

SKILL SPOTLIGHT

The catchy tune *and easy-to-follow gestures make this sing-along a skill-building activity for all toddlers. Repeating the song stimulates your toddler's auditory development, while the hand movements help him conceptualize what the words mean. As his motor skills and memory improve, he will readily imitate most of the hand gestures and even begin to anticipate many of them.*

Body Awareness	✔
Concept Development	✔
Coordination	✔
Language Development	✔
Listening Skills	✔

168

THIS SONG is an all-time toddler classic. You can perform it in many ways, but it's easiest with your child seated facing you or on your lap facing away from you. If he's propped up on your lap, gently guide his hands through the movements.

• Begin by showing him the different motions as you sing, then encourage him to join in.

• Don't be afraid to improvise your own verses and corresponding hand movements if the spirit moves you—your toddler will love it!

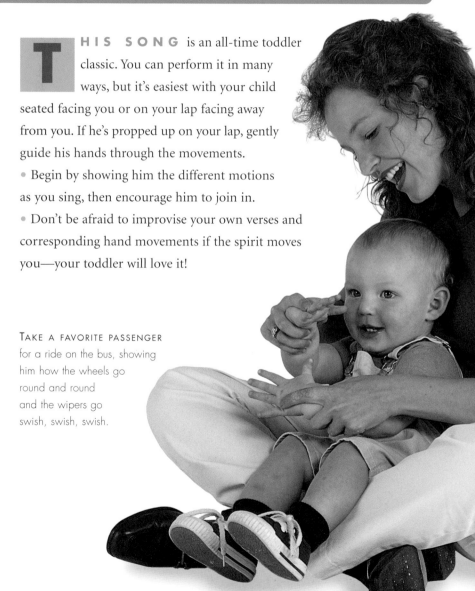

TAKE A FAVORITE PASSENGER for a ride on the bus, showing him how the wheels go round and round and the wipers go swish, swish, swish.

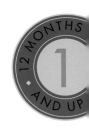

12 MONTHS
1
AND UP

The wheels on the bus go round and round,
roll forearms forward in a circular motion

round and round,
continue to roll arms

round and round.
roll arms

The wheels on the bus go round and round,
roll arms

all through the town.
draw a circle in the air

The horn on the bus goes beep, beep, beep,
press imaginary horn with hand

beep, beep, beep,
press horn with hand

beep, beep, beep.
press horn with hand

The horn on the bus goes beep, beep, beep,
press horn with hand

all through the town.
draw a circle in the air

continue with:

The wipers on the bus go swish, swish, swish . . .
sway forearms back and forth

The driver on the bus says "Move on back" . . .
point over your shoulder with your thumb

The lights on the bus go blink, blink, blink . . .
open and close fists

The baby on the bus goes waah, waah, waah . . .
make cradling motion with your arms

The parents on the bus say "I love you" . . .
hug your child

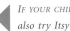

IF YOUR CHILD ENJOYS THIS ACTIVITY, also try Itsy-Bitsy Spider, page 161.

169

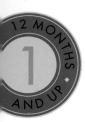
BAND ON THE RUN

MUSIC FROM THE KITCHEN CABINET

SKILLSPOTLIGHT

One way toddlers learn *cause and effect is by making sounds with a variety of objects. As a child bangs on a bowl, he learns that he is capable of creating sounds by himself. As he practices, he improves his coordination and his understanding of rhythm, and as he experiments with the various "instruments" in his cabinet, he learns that he can create a myriad of interesting (and loud!) sounds.*

Cause & Effect	✔
Coordination	✔
Listening Skills	✔
Rhythm Exploration	✔

CLEAR OUT A KITCHEN CUPBOARD (near the floor) for your child and fill it with sturdy wooden spoons, metal bowls of different sizes, lightweight pans (cake pans and small frying pans work well), wooden salad bowls, metal lids of various sizes, and plastic measuring cups. The greater the variety of "instruments," the greater the variety of sounds you and your toddler will be able to make, so be creative as you stock the cupboard. If you have toy instruments on hand, add them to the mix.

• With older toddlers, create a stop-and-go band. Have your child bang on the "instruments" while listening to you—the bandleader—give directions to stop the music and start it again.

• As your young musician plays, encourage him to experiment with sound by banging in different ways: with enthusiasm, gently, slowly, fast. Demonstrate to show him the difference.

• Play music (tunes with a strong beat are best) and encourage him to add his own percussion sounds.

EVERYTHING BUT THE KITCHEN SINK—and that would probably work as well—is a potential instrument for a budding musician.

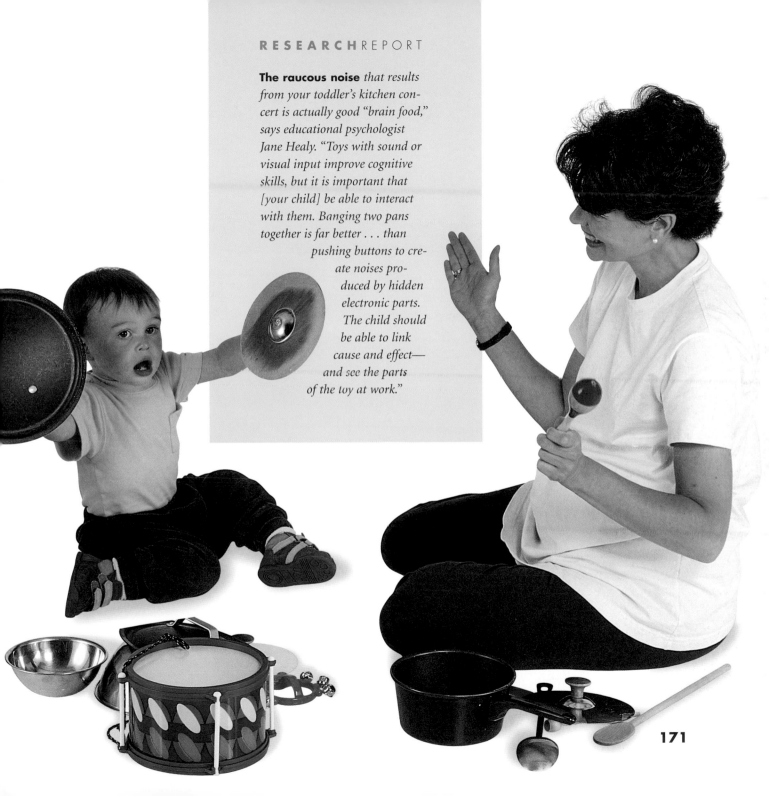

The raucous noise that results from your toddler's kitchen concert is actually good "brain food," says educational psychologist Jane Healy. "Toys with sound or visual input improve cognitive skills, but it is important that [your child] be able to interact with them. Banging two pans together is far better . . . than pushing buttons to create noises produced by hidden electronic parts. The child should be able to link cause and effect— and see the parts of the toy at work."

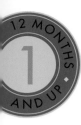

12 MONTHS AND UP

PEEKABOO BOXES

PUTTING NAMES TO FAMILIAR FACES

SKILLSPOTLIGHT

This activity refines *your child's visual memory and fine motor skills. Most significantly, matching a word with its visual representation helps build the language skills he'll need later, when he begins reading and writing. As your child's vocabulary expands, surprise him now and then by pasting new pictures inside the boxes.*

Fine Motor Skills	✔
Language Development	✔
Social Skills	✔
Visual Memory	✔

COLLECT AN ASSORTMENT of cigar boxes, shoe boxes, or gift boxes. Cut out pictures of family members or easily recognizable objects (such as household items, animals, or toys) and paste one inside the lid of each box. Open the boxes and discuss the images inside. As your child's confidence grows, ask him to open the boxes and name the pictures. Once he masters this (around two years of age), test his memory: ask him which box contains the picture of Daddy, a horse, or a ball.

FINDING A PHOTO of Mommy, Daddy, or the family dog under the lid of a box is a great way to boost your little one's sense of discovery while enhancing his visual memory.

FUNNY FEET

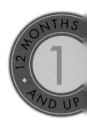

EXPLORING TEXTURE WITH YOUR TOES

EVEN A CHILD who has been toddling for several months is still getting used to the sensations involved in walking. Take advantage of her curiosity by removing her shoes and leading her outside across a variety of textures, such as warm sand, smooth pebbles, cool concrete, wet grass, and gooey mud. As she gets older, ask her what she feels as she's walking. If she doesn't know the words yet, suggest some: "warm," "prickly," "soft." If you're worried about dirty feet, finish off by stomping in a basin of warm, soapy water.

YOUR TODDLER WILL DELIGHT in the feel of different textures, such as soft grass, on her sensitive soles. Kick off your shoes and join in the fun!

SKILLSPOTLIGHT

Walking barefoot *is easier for your young toddler than walking with shoes because she can use her toes to help with balance. And while the sensations of walking on unusual surfaces may make her giggle, she'll start to grasp the properties associated with different materials, as well as a few words to describe them.*

✔ **Body Awareness**

✔ **Language Development**

✔ **Sensory Exploration**

✔ **Tactile Discrimination**

173

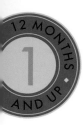

PICTURE THIS

GROWING A BOOKWORM

SKILLSPOTLIGHT

Reading is an important tool *for learning language. Toddlers learn most of the rules of grammar simply by hearing you and others speak. And recent studies show that the size of a toddler's vocabulary depends on how much speech she hears in a meaningful context. So the more you read to your child, the easier it will be for her to develop strong language skills.*

Language Development	✔
Listening Skills	✔
Visual Discrimination	✔
Visual Memory	✔

SHE MAY NOT BE ABLE to talk and she may not understand all your words, but even a young toddler loves to "read books" with a parent or grandparent. The rhythm of the words engages her; the pictures teach her about her world.

• Choose books with clear pictures of familiar objects and point them out to your child as you read. It will help her learn the words for everyday things, such as "chair," "house," and "car."

• Select books made of cloth, plastic, or heavy cardboard. They can withstand toddlers' eager jaws and paws more readily than paper. And small books with padded covers are easier for little hands to handle.

• Edit out long narratives and hard words. Instead, abridge the plot and spend time talking about the illustrations or photographs. That will keep her interested and help her develop observational skills.

• Emphasize the rhymes and funny words that engage her.

• Tailor your reading session to her attention span. Let her wander off to play with her toys when she wants to. Ending the session while it's still fun will ensure that you're building a positive association with reading that will last a lifetime.

EVEN A CHILD who is too young to understand the plot will delight in the colorful pictures, the simple rhymes, and the cadence of Grandma's voice.

174

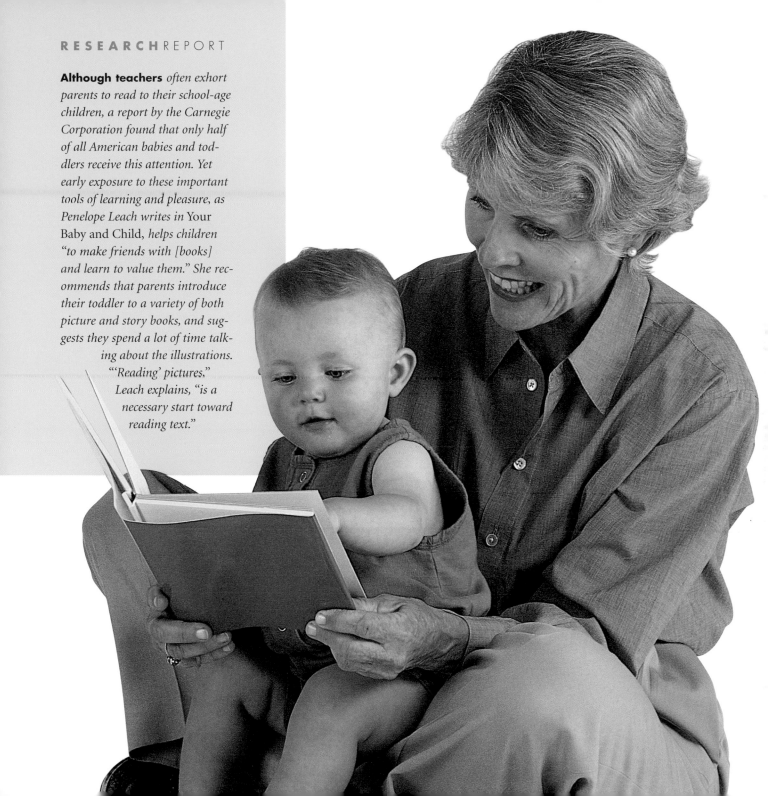

Although teachers *often exhort parents to read to their school-age children, a report by the Carnegie Corporation found that only half of all American babies and toddlers receive this attention. Yet early exposure to these important tools of learning and pleasure, as Penelope Leach writes in* Your Baby and Child, *helps children* "to make friends with [books] and learn to value them." *She recommends that parents introduce their toddler to a variety of both picture and story books, and suggests they spend a lot of time talking about the illustrations.* "'Reading' pictures," *Leach explains,* "is a necessary start toward reading text."

REPETITION IN PLAY

THINK YOU'LL GO nuts if you have to spend another minute rolling a ball back and forth with your toddler? Bored with reading his favorite book over and over again? Or maybe you're just worried that your child needs more variety in his play and you feel you should try to keep him from returning again and again to a few preferred activities.

Although it may try your patience, never underestimate the value of repetition when it comes to a child's development. As educational psychologist Jane Healy says in her book *Your Child's Growing Mind,* "An activity must be repeated many times to firm up neural networks for proficiency." In other words, by repeating the same story to your child every evening you are helping to stimulate the brain cells that allow your child to make the association between words and the objects they represent. And when it comes to rolling that ball, you'll soon see how his eye-hand coordination improves. A simple activity such as this helps prime him for more complex tasks in coming years, whether it's understanding the nuances in James Joyce's *Ulysses* or playing little-league baseball.

Besides, kids don't get bored as easily as adults do. As neurologist Ann Barnet notes in *The Youngest Minds,* "Nursery rhymes and simple games enthrall small children precisely because they become familiar." Mastering a new skill gives them a lot of confidence and even whets their appetites for future challenges.

This isn't to say that parents can't overdo it by spending too much time interacting on one activity with their child—even young minds and bodies can get overtaxed. So be sure to take your cues from your child: watch for signs of frustration or restlessness, but if he's enjoying an activity, let him do it . . . over and over and over again. ■

FUN-FILLED JARS

12 MONTHS AND UP
1

FINDING OUT WHAT'S INSIDE

COLLECT A FEW LARGE, clear plastic jars with easy-to-remove lids. Place a favorite toy or colorful scarf inside each jar and close the lid. Ask your child to take off the lid and pull out the toy or scarf. (You might need to start this activity with loose lids so her not-so-nimble fingers can remove the toys more easily.) Your toddler will be eager to remove the toys again and again. When you're filling the jars, select toys that are more than 1¼ inches (4.5 cm) in diameter (so there won't be a choking hazard).

A TOY INSIDE a jar provides plenty of incentive to lift off the lid.

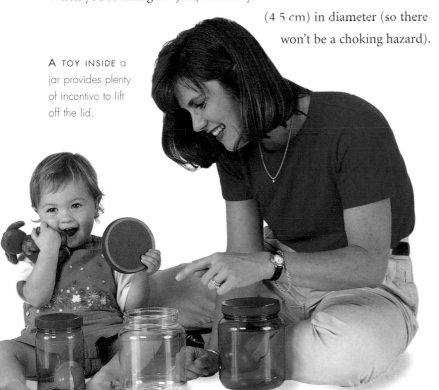

SKILLSPOTLIGHT

Learning to remove a lid, *even if it's already unscrewed, helps your toddler develop coordination and fine motor skills. And just attempting to unscrew a lid enhances these skills as well. In this activity, success is immediately rewarded, ensuring that your toddler will want to try removing the lids again and again.*

✔ **Fine Motor Skills**

✔ **Language Development**

✔ **Social Skills**

IF YOUR CHILD ENJOYS THIS ACTIVITY, also try Cereal Challenge, page 202.

177

SILLY LAP SONGS

SITTING ON A PARENT'S LAP is not a passive activity for a busy toddler. Although your lap is a safe haven for your child—a place to relax and cuddle between activities—it's also associated with such pleasures as reading, rocking, and singing the following songs—and pretending to be an airplane, a pony, or even a funny frog.

THE AIRPLANE SONG

 to the *tune* of **"Row, Row, Row, Your Boat"**

Fly, fly, fly your plane,
fly your plane up high.
Merrily, merrily, merrily, merrily,
high up in the sky!

hold your child firmly with both hands and raise him overhead

MAKE YOUR TODDLER feel secure as he soars like a plane by looking at him, smiling, and having as much fun as he is.

DOWN BY THE BANKS

Down by the banks of the hanky panky,
where the bullfrogs jump
from bank to banky.
They went oops, opps, belly flops.
One missed the lily pad
and went . . . kerplop!

*bounce your child on your lap as you teach
her this song; holding her securely, let her slip
partway between your legs on "kerplop"*

TROT LITTLE PONY

 "Hush Little Baby"

Trot little pony, trot to town,
trot little pony, don't slow down.
Don't spill the buttermilk,
don't spill the eggs,
trot little pony, trot to town.

*holding your toddler securely on
your lap, gently bounce her up
and down*

WHEN WE ALL ROLL OVER

 "Have You Ever Seen a Lassie"

When we all roll over,
roll over, roll over,
when we all roll over,
how happy we'll be!

Roll this way, and that way,
and this way, and that way,
when we all roll over,
how happy we'll be!

*bounce your toddler on your
lap as you sing, or, lying on
your back, place him facedown
on your stomach and rock him
gently from side to side*

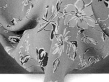

179

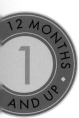
I HAVE A LITTLE DUCK

MAKING WAVES WITH A SONG

 to the tune of **"The Wheels on the Bus"**

**I have a little duck that says
quack, quack, quack,
quack, quack, quack,
quack, quack, quack,
I have a little duck that says
quack, quack, quack,
all day long.**
"quack" your hands to the beat

**I have a little duck that goes
splash, splash, splash . . .**
splash the water gently

**I have a little duck that goes
swim, swim, swim . . .**
skim your hands on the surface

Cause & Effect	✔
Language Development	✔
Listening Skills	✔
Rhythm Exploration	✔
Sensory Exploration	✔

SHARE THIS FAMILIAR TUNE with your child as you play in the baby pool or bathtub—and use a family of rubber ducks as colorful props. Your toddler won't need much encouragement to splash, so be sure you are both ready to get wet. In the first verse, "quack" your hands (place your palms together as if you're miming a duck bill) in the water. Little will your toddler know that in the midst of all the hilarity, you are stimulating her auditory memory and enhancing her sense of rhythm.

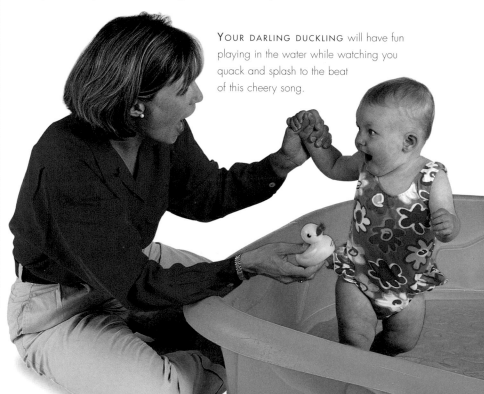

YOUR DARLING DUCKLING will have fun playing in the water while watching you quack and splash to the beat of this cheery song.

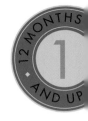

JUST LIKE ME

A FOLLOW-THE-LEADER SONG

MAKE THE MOST of your toddler's natural instinct to mimic with this lively activity. Give yourself plenty of room and either sit with your child on your lap or stand facing him. Emphasize the name of each body part as you sing and point it out on your toddler's body as you make the movements. If your child is hesitant, gently help him raise and lower his arms, shoulders, and legs. Between repetitions of the song, ask him to point to his own arms or legs. Once he's following you like a pro, try adding some movements of your own invention.

 to the *tune* of **"London Bridge Is Falling Down"**

**Make your arms go up and down,
up and down, up and down,
make your arms go up and down,
just like me.**

Continue with:
**Move your hands up and down . . .
Move your shoulders up and down . . .
Flap your elbows up and down . . .
Make your legs go up and down . . .
Move your feet up and down . . .
Move your body up and down . . .**

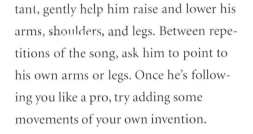

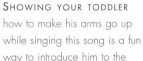

SHOWING YOUR TODDLER how to make his arms go up while singing this song is a fun way to introduce him to the names of his body parts.

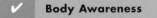

✔	**Body Awareness**
✔	**Concept Development**
✔	**Coordination**
✔	**Creative Movement**
✔	**Listening Skills**

181

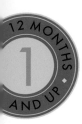
A STAR IS BORN

TALKING ON TAPE

SKILLSPOTLIGHT

As you may have noticed, *your toddler is quite focused on herself at this stage—and with all things belonging to her. Just as a mirror intrigues her because she can see herself, a tape recording lets her revel in the sound of her voice. This helps her develop her listening skills, which are crucial to language development.*

Language Development	✔
Listening Skills	✔
Social Skills	✔

YOU'VE SEEN HOW your little one perks up at the sound of other children's voices. And you've noticed how she responds to seeing her face in the mirror. Now imagine her delight upon hearing a "reflection" of her own voice! Recording your child's voice gives her a whole new sense of herself and gives your entire family an audio baby journal to cherish for years to come.

• Record your toddler's sounds—laughing at Daddy's funny faces, babbling to herself as she plays, talking on a toy phone (see Ring-a-Ling, page 237), or shrieking with glee in the tub.

• Try recording a session the next time you read to your toddler. Later, she can listen to your story-time voice and her own commentary.

• You can use a cassette recorder with a built-in microphone, but a separate microphone that can be plugged into the recorder will provide a sharper sound.

• When your young crooner is older, around age two or three, encourage her to sing songs on tape—alone or with you or her friends.

IF YOUR CHILD ENJOYS THIS ACTIVITY, also try Mirror, Mirror, page 184. ▶

ONCE YOUR STARLET understands the purpose of the microphone, she'll reach for it and talk into it enthusiastically, which allows her to experience herself in a whole different way.

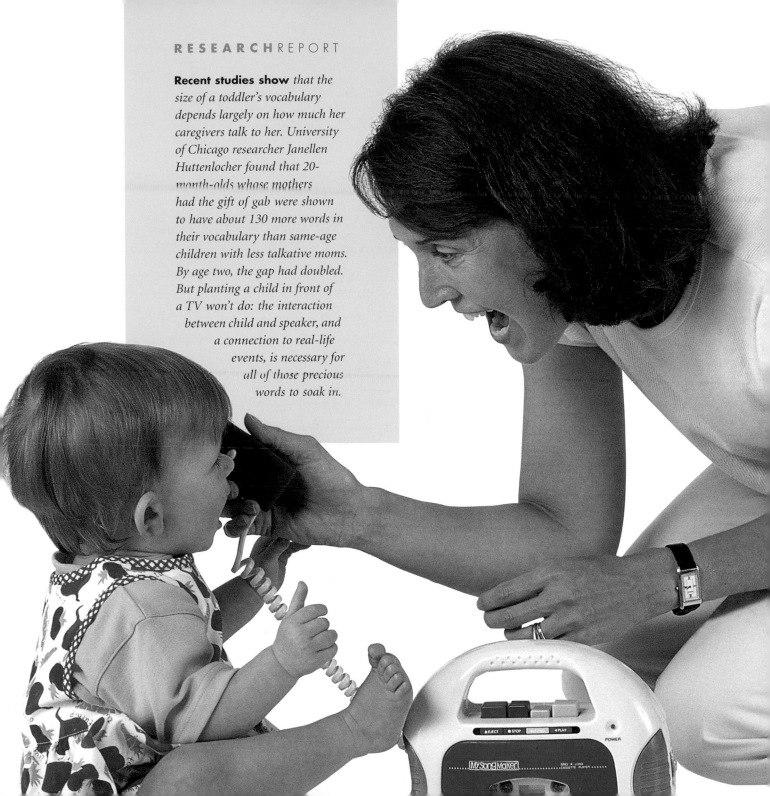

Recent studies show *that the size of a toddler's vocabulary depends largely on how much her caregivers talk to her. University of Chicago researcher Janellen Huttenlocher found that 20-month-olds whose mothers had the gift of gab were shown to have about 130 more words in their vocabulary than same-age children with less talkative moms. By age two, the gap had doubled. But planting a child in front of a TV won't do: the interaction between child and speaker, and a connection to real-life events, is necessary for all of those precious words to soak in.*

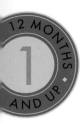
MIRROR, MIRROR

GETTING TO KNOW ME

SKILLSPOTLIGHT

A sense of herself as a person
(hence her intrigue with the notions of I and mine versus you and yours) is key to your toddler's development. Playing with mirrors helps her develop this concept of self as separate from others. Toddlers are also intrigued with their bodies; labeling the parts of her body in front of the mirror helps her understand the names of those parts and encourages her to further explore her own identity.

Body Awareness	✔
Language Development	✔
Self-Concept	✔
Social Skills	✔
Visual Discrimination	✔

184

YOUR CHILD has no doubt been fascinated with her own image since she was a wee baby. But mirror fun really begins in toddlerhood, because now she understands that the image is of herself—and understanding herself and all her body parts are her primary interests.

Sit or stand together in front of a mirror and make faces—happy, sad, and goofy. With an older toddler, encourage her to follow suit. Then point out her arms, legs, eyes, nose, and other body parts. Point out your own, as well.

Ask her who's the baby and who's the mommy—pretty soon she'll surprise you by pointing to the right image.

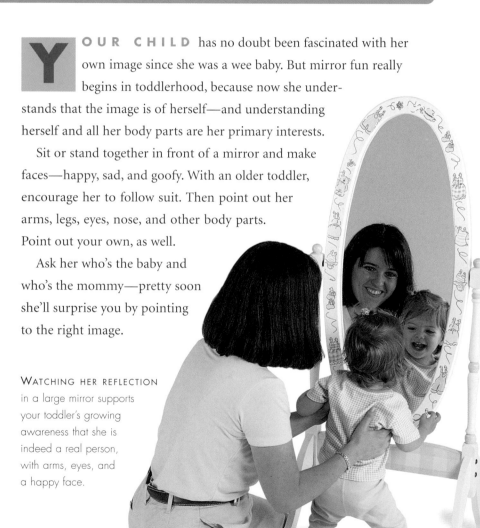

WATCHING HER REFLECTION in a large mirror supports your toddler's growing awareness that she is indeed a real person, with arms, eyes, and a happy face.

HEY MR. KNICKERBOCKER

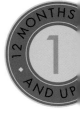

12 MONTHS AND UP **1**

PLAYING IN A ONE-KID BAND

SEAT YOUR TODDLER on your lap or on the floor in front of you for this favorite chant with silly sound effects. Create a slow beat by alternately slapping your hands on the floor and then clapping them together. Encourage your child to clap with you once you begin the chant. Repeat the chant's first two lines before you make a new motion and sound. When your toddler attempts to control his body to make a specific type of sound—such as stomping his feet or clicking his teeth—he improves both his language and motor skills.

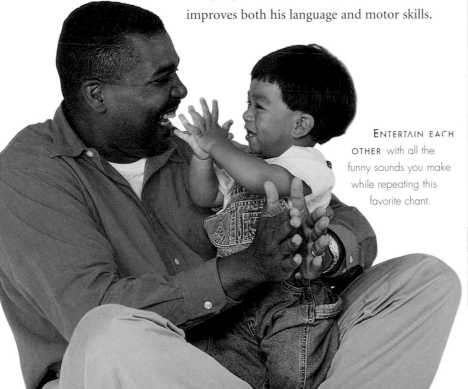

ENTERTAIN EACH OTHER with all the funny sounds you make while repeating this favorite chant.

Hey Mr. Knickerbocker, boppity, bop!
pat your hands flat on the floor once, clap, then repeat

I like the way you boppity, bop!
continue alternately patting and clapping to establish a beat

Listen to the sound we make with our hands.
rub palms to make a chafing sound

Listen to the sound we make with our feet.
stomp feet loudly on floor to the beat

Listen to the sound we make with our knees.
tap fingers softly on knees to the beat

Listen to the sound we make with our teeth.
click teeth together

continue with other body parts

✔ **Fine Motor Skills**

✔ **Gross Motor Skills**

✔ **Listening Skills**

185

PAPER-BAG BLOCKS

STACKING BIG BLOCKS

SKILL SPOTLIGHT

Children enhance *their fine motor skills and their ability to discriminate among shapes and sizes when they explore and play with blocks. Most kids also love to practice stacking the blocks—then knocking them down, of course. That provides a good lesson in balance, as well as in cause and effect. And if your child builds a little fort or cave, having a private space that's just his size can bolster his emerging sense of identity.*

Cause & Effect	✔
Fine Motor Skills	✔
Problem Solving	✔
Size & Shape Discrimination	✔
Spatial Awareness	✔

AT THIS AGE, his hands may be too small to skillfully maneuver heavy wooden blocks. But you can make large, lightweight blocks from paper bags and milk cartons that are both easy to handle and soft on impact.

• To make large blocks, fill a paper grocery bag to the brim with crumpled newspaper. Fold and tape the sides of the open end as if you were wrapping a present. Help your child decorate the oversize blocks using non-permanent markers, crayons, wrapping paper, or stickers.

• For smaller blocks, thoroughly rinse and dry empty milk cartons. Open the tops and vertically cut through the corner creases to create flaps. Tape the flaps shut and cover the cartons with colored construction paper or even contact paper with a brick motif (to create a "brick" house).

• Now let your kinder-contractor begin to build. Encourage him to stack the blocks as high as he can or to use them to create little forts. A couch or a table and sheets can provide additional walls and a roof.

• Also show him how to stack the small blocks on top of the big blocks to build a toddler-size tower. When it's time to disassemble the stack, take turns removing one block at a time, and count the blocks out loud as you remove them. Then create new structures with your little builder.

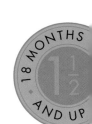

"Stack them high!"

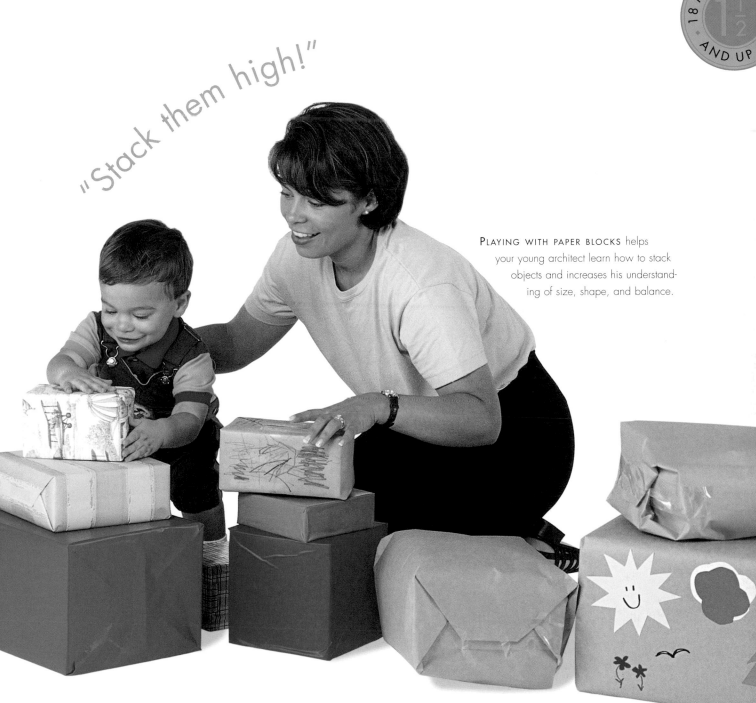

PLAYING WITH PAPER BLOCKS helps your young architect learn how to stack objects and increases his understanding of size, shape, and balance.

SIZE WISE

SORTING OUT NESTING CUPS

SKILLSPOTLIGHT

A nesting game *keeps toddler minds and hands busy as they learn to recognize differences in size. It also helps children learn to solve problems ("How do I get these to all fit together?") and enhances eye-hand coordination and fine motor skills. The give-and-take between parent and child is important, too: your toddler is learning to listen and let you show her how to do things.*

Eye-Hand Coordination	✔
Fine Motor Skills	✔
Problem Solving	✔
Size & Shape Discrimination	✔

YOUNG TODDLERS derive endless pleasure from taking objects out of a container and then trying to put them back again. Increase the complexity and fun of this type of activity by introducing your child to nesting objects, which require her to fit things together in a particular order.

• You can buy nesting containers at toy stores. Or use measuring spoons, mixing bowls, or cardboard boxes of different sizes for the same effect.

• Some toddlers do not yet have the manual dexterity to get the objects to nest or to pull them apart again. Start out slowly by introducing your child to this activity with only two or three nesting cups that vary dramatically in size. Demonstrate how the items fit within each other. You may need to show her several times, but eventually she'll be able to help you; then she'll figure out how to nest the objects on her own.

• Gradually add to the number of nesting objects once she has mastered fitting the first few cups or bowls together.

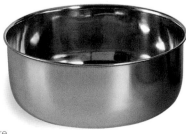

NESTING BOWLS TOGETHER teaches your toddler some important lessons about size differences while satisfying her curiosity about your shiny kitchenware.

188

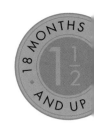

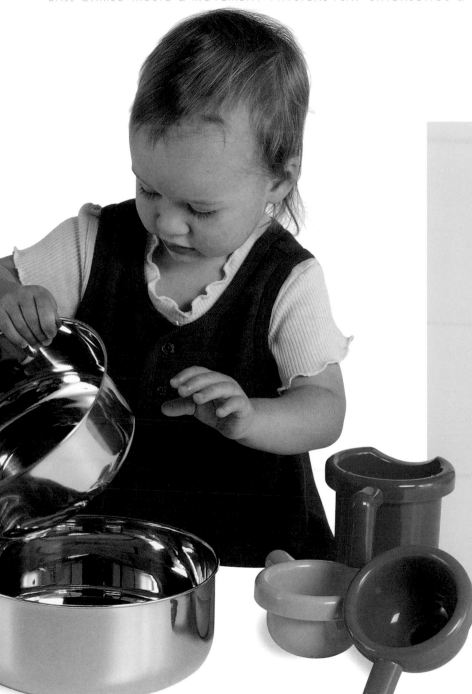

RESEARCH REPORT

A toddler's ability *to sift through a jumble of cups and bowls and sort them into piles by size or shape demonstrates the dawning of logical reasoning. As exciting as it is to see a child master the simple but important concepts of same and different, it's obviously still a long journey to the type of sophisticated thinking associated with higher forms of logic. Jonas Langer, a psychologist at the University of California at Berkeley, notes that a child's logical powers make a big jump in complexity between the ages of four and eight, but she isn't able to truly comprehend notions of abstract symbolism until she reaches age eleven or so.*

189

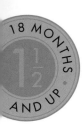

HIDE YOUR EYES

 to the *tune* of **"The Farmer in the Dell"**

**Can you hide your eyes,
can you hide your eyes?
Yes you can, you surely can,
you can hide your eyes.**
cover your eyes with your hands

**Can you hide your nose,
can you hide your nose?
Yes you can, you surely can,
you can hide your nose.**
cover your nose with your hands

**Can you hide your feet,
can you hide your feet?
Yes you can, you surely can,
you can hide your feet.**
cover your feet with your hands

*continue with chin, knees, toes,
elbows, ears, and so on*

Body Awareness	✔
Creative Movement	✔
Language Development	✔

T HIS SINGALONG takes a toddler favorite—the peekaboo game—and applies it to several parts of your child's body. In turn, this helps her learn the words for many of her body parts as well as how to sing along with others.

• Kick off the "Can You Hide Your Eyes?" song with the names of some easy body parts, such as eyes, nose, feet, and toes. Then graduate to less familiar words, like elbows, knees, chin, and neck.

• Make a few mistakes once in a while to see if she catches them—cover your knees when you say "toes," for instance, or cover her knees instead of yours. She'll be amused by these silly contradictions.

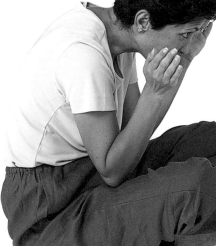

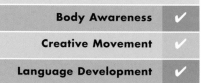

YOUR CHILD GETS TO PLAY peekaboo while singing when you add these new lyrics to an old, familiar tune.

190

SHAKE IT UP, BABY!

18 MONTHS
1½
AND UP

EXPERIMENTING WITH SOUND

INTRODUCE YOUR CURIOUS CHILD to new sounds and rhythms by supplying her with maracas or other percussion instruments (available in most toy stores). Or create your own musicmakers by filling a few plastic bottles with rice, dried beans, or pennies. Close the lids tightly and seal them with packaging tape to avoid any spillage (items under 1¾ inches, or 4.5 cm, in diameter are choking hazards). Begin by shaking each instrument, then pass it to your toddler, commenting on the unique sound it makes. Play a selection of familiar songs with different tempos and encourage her to make music and move her body to the beat.

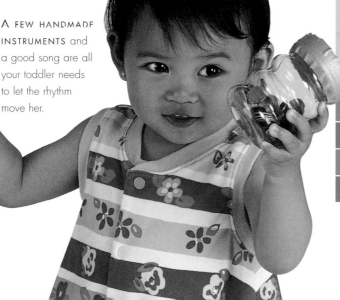

A FEW HANDMADE INSTRUMENTS and a good song are all your toddler needs to let the rhythm move her.

SKILLSPOTLIGHT

Playing with musicmakers *stimulates auditory reflexes and nurtures a child's innate sense of rhythm, both of which are fundamental to language development. Identifying various kinds of sounds helps train the ear to recognize pitch and volume, while dancing and shaking or playing the instruments will encourage creative expression. If you make your own maracas, provide your child with additional tactile stimulation by allowing her to feel the rice, beans, or pennies before you put them in the bottles (but make sure she doesn't try to eat them).*

✔ **Creative Movement**

✔ **Listening Skills**

✔ **Rhythm Exploration**

✔ **Sensory Exploration**

191

SAND SKILLS

MAKING DESIGNS IN THE DIRT

SKILL SPOTLIGHT

Sand is wonderful *for artistic explorations because it allows a toddler to safely wallow in the medium from head to toe. Grasping and releasing the sand and using tools to manipulate it also exercise his fine motor skills and stimulate his sense of touch.*

Creative Expression	✔
Fine Motor Skills	✔
Tactile Stimulation	✔

Z EN MASTERS DO IT. Bulldozers do it. And toddlers can do it, too. Whether you're at the beach, on a playground, or in a backyard sandbox, making designs in the sand is absorbing, creative, and entertaining. It also provides a great way to combine artistic endeavors with healthy outdoor play.

• Gather a variety of tot-size tools, including sand toys (plastic buckets, shovels, and molds), kitchen utensils (spatulas, wooden spoons, and plastic containers), and garden tools (watering cans and miniature rakes).

• Pour water over the sand to make a more pliable palette.

• Show your child how to use the tools to make designs. He can draw a rake through the sand, for instance, to create straight or wavy rows of lines. Or press a pie pan into the sand to make a big circle. Use empty yogurt containers and wet sand to add towers and turrets.

• Show your toddler how he can erase his creations by simply running his hands over the sand or by dumping a bucket of water on top of his mini masterpieces. Then let him wipe out and recreate his sand structures and patterns as many times as he likes.

IF YOUR CHILD ENJOYS THIS ACTIVITY, also try Nature Art, page 206. ▶

MOST TODDLERS ARE THRILLED to play in a pile of sand; you can add to their fun by showing them how to make designs with sand toys and kitchen utensils.

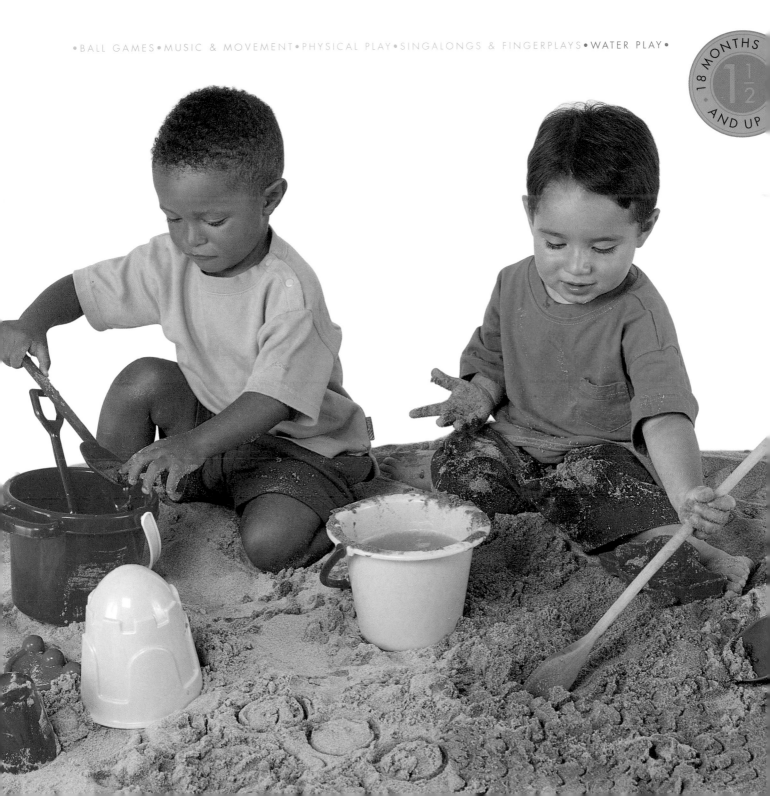

PHOTO FUN

PUTTING NAMES TO FACES

SKILL SPOTLIGHT

Your toddler picks up *the rules of grammar by hearing your speech patterns. But she can't learn who Auntie is or what an ostrich looks like just by listening. She needs a picture to put a face to a name. This activity aids in expanding her vocabulary, which in turn helps her organize and share her memories.*

Language Development	✔
Visual Discrimination	✔
Visual Memory	✔

MAKING YOUR OWN

Tape or glue photos to playing cards or index cards. For extra protection from enthusiastic little hands, laminate the cards at a copy or framing shop. To hang, use tape or large magnets; avoid thumbtacks and small magnets.

IT MAY SEEM like your toddler has nothing but a Be Here Now (or Give It to Me Now) perspective on life. But she's been able to store and retrieve memories since she was about six months old. Now she's driven to remember and practice saying the names of people and objects around her. This flash-card activity is a means of memorizing while having some fun.

• Tape or glue photos of family members and friends to index cards (this will enable your child to pick them up more easily). Point to someone in a picture and say the person's name. Pretty soon she'll be calling out their names even before you do.

• Glue these photos to a piece of construction paper and laminate it for a personalized place mat.

• Using photos cut out of magazines, make cards depicting appealing things that aren't already in her daily life, such as an anteater, giraffe, or helicopter. Hang the cards at eye level (on the refrigerator, for example) and point them out to her often.

• Attach stories to the images so your toddler will have an easier time remembering them. You can say "We made cookies with Grandma, didn't we?" or "Rob has a big dog at his house, doesn't he?" This helps her learn how to tell stories, and it shows her that people are interested in them. It also helps her mentally process familiar events.

194

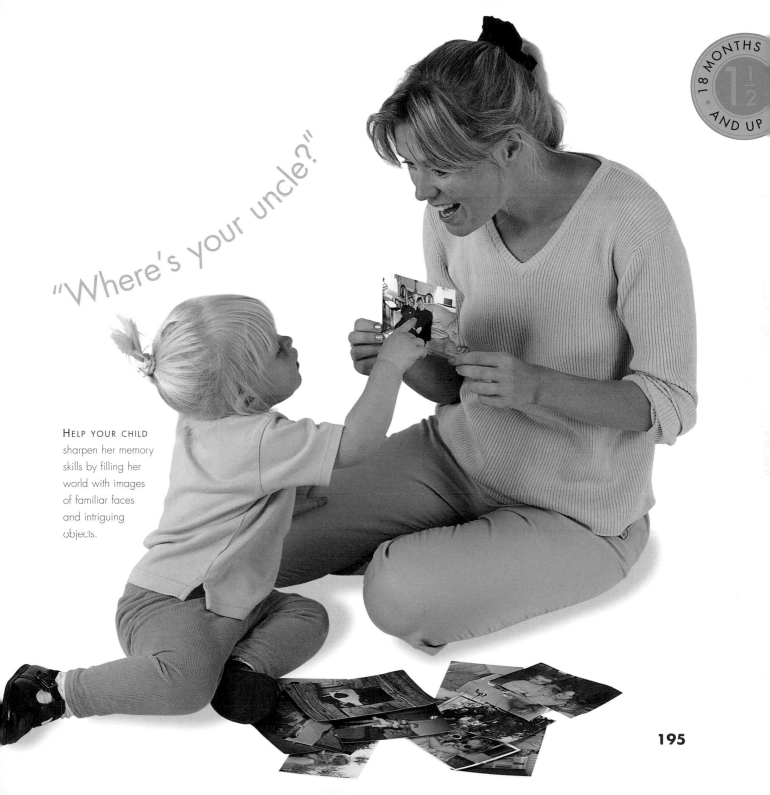

"Where's your uncle?"

HELP YOUR CHILD sharpen her memory skills by filling her world with images of familiar faces and intriguing objects.

195

THE MAGIC OF MUSIC

THE PASSION for music is a universal human trait, a gift parents from every culture instinctively bestow on their children. We coo lullabies as babies drift off to sleep, clap as toddlers make their first wobbly forays onto the living-room dance floor, and play endless games of patty-cake with our youngsters. Which is a good thing: recent studies, such as the one outlining the much-publicized Mozart effect detailed on page 233, suggest that exposure to music has far-reaching intellectual benefits that go beyond imparting a sense of melody and rhythm.

Mark Tramo, a neuroscientist at Harvard Medical School, explains that the same mental pathways used to process music also seem to serve as conduits for language, math, and abstract reasoning. "This means that exercising the brain through music strengthens other cognitive skills," Dr. Tramo concludes. The governor of Georgia, among many others, found this evidence so compelling he decided to send every baby born in Georgia home from the hospital with a recording of classical music.

This book includes simple and enjoyable suggestions for filling your child's world with the sound of music, from the tape-recorded parent-and-child duets on page 182 to the percussion games on page 210. Many of the activities link movement with music, which helps your toddler assimilate language and rhythm, develop coordination, and heighten body awareness. Complement these exercises by listening to a variety of music—while driving, eating, or doing chores, for example—and you'll further enhance her auditory senses and broaden her musical horizons. Don't feel you have to play classical music: introduce your child to the tunes you enjoy, and your pleasure will only make her more receptive to the value and power of all music. ■

196

TAMBOURINE TIME

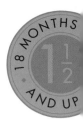

18 MONTHS
1½
AND UP

MAKING MERRY MUSIC

THE TAMBOURINE IS MUSIC to your toddler's ears, arms, fingers, toes, and just about any other body part. Give him a tambourine and encourage him to shake it and tap it to the beat of his favorite songs—or to accompany you if you play an instrument. Move around as you play. Experiment with tambourines of different sizes: how do the sounds of large and small ones compare? How does the sound change when you shake the tambourine hard, then tap it gently? The two of you can delight in each other's musical discoveries.

SKILL SPOTLIGHT

Simple musical instruments *offer toddlers a rich variety of activities that both stimulate and fine-tune auditory and tactile senses. As children play and listen, they begin to discriminate among different rhythms and types of sounds. And a tambourine, which can be either tapped or shaken, reinforces what toddlers are already discovering: that the world is full of unique and varied sounds —sounds they not only can recognize but can produce themselves.*

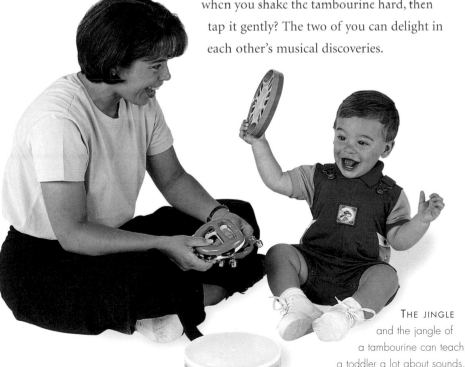

✔	**Eye-Hand Coordination**
✔	**Listening Skills**
✔	**Rhythm Exploration**
✔	**Social Skills**

THE JINGLE and the jangle of a tambourine can teach a toddler a lot about sounds.

197

CRAYON CREATIONS

ARTWORK ON A GRAND SCALE

SKILL SPOTLIGHT

Grasping and using a crayon *builds fine motor skills and eye-hand coordination. It also can help a child learn to identify colors. More important, letting him express himself by choosing his colors and scribbling in whatever way he pleases allows him to give color and shape to his budding sense of identity. Discussing what the two of you are doing as you draw helps cement concepts in his memory and develop his communication skills.*

Concept Development	✓
Fine Motor Skills	✓
Social Skills	✓
Visual Memory	✓

EVEN CHILDREN as young as eighteen months are thrilled to put crayon and pen to paper. It can be hard for them to aim, however, and difficult to understand that the crayons or markers need to stay inside the paper's edges (and not on the table or floor). Rather than fence him in with standard letter-size paper, let your child spread his artistic wings to create mural-size artwork.

• Clear a large area on the floor and tape down poster-size sheets of paper. Sit next to your toddler, hand him some non-permanent markers or crayons, and encourage him to scribble on the paper. You may have to show him how at first, but once he gets going, he won't want to stop.

• Talk about what you're doing as you draw. When he picks up a crayon, tell him what color it is. Encourage him to use different colors and praise whatever marks he makes on the paper.

• With an older child, ask him to describe what he is drawing. If he's drawing a circle or square, for example, identify the shape and explain that it's round like a ball or square like a box. Control your desire to help him make perfect shapes. His drawings may look like only a bunch of squiggly lines to you, but they're masterpieces to him.

IF YOUR CHILD ENJOYS THIS ACTIVITY, also try Play With Clay, page 254.

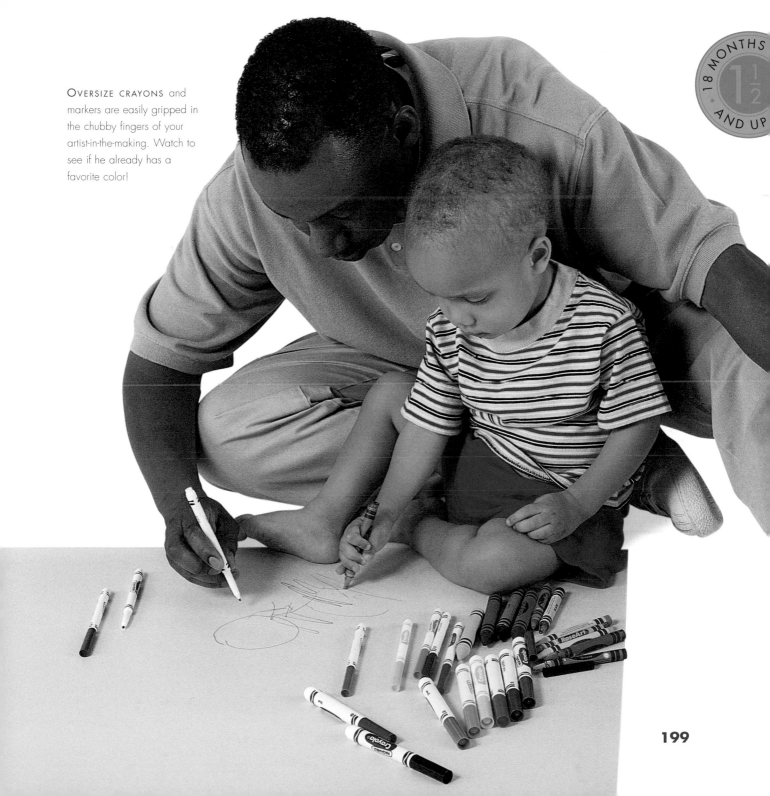

OVERSIZE CRAYONS and markers are easily gripped in the chubby fingers of your artist-in-the-making. Watch to see if he already has a favorite color!

COUNT WITH ME

YOUR TODDLER is always happy to bounce on your knee and hear you sing, but songs and chants that emphasize counting add educational fun. While your child will love just to listen to you, she'll also begin to recognize numbers. Repetition reinforces the learning, so sing an encore or two.

FIVE LITTLE RAINDROPS

Five little raindrops falling from a cloud,
wiggle fingers on one hand downward
the first one said,
**   "My, the thunder's loud."**
hold up one finger; cover ears

The second one said,
"It's so cold tonight."
hold up two fingers; shiver and hug body

The third one said,
"Oh, the lightning's so bright."
hold up three fingers; cover eyes

The fourth one said,
"Listen to the wind blow."
hold up four fingers; cup hand at ear

The fifth one said,
"Look, I'm turning into snow."
hold up five fingers; float fingers down

So down they tumbled through the cold winter's night,
roll arms downward in front of body
and turned all the earth to a frosty, snowy white.

COUNTING RAINDROPS, caterpillars, and crayons is a fun way to introduce your child to the concept of numbers.

THE CATERPILLAR

One little caterpillar crawled on my shoe.
wiggle finger like a worm on a shoe

Along came another and then there were two.
show two fingers

Two little caterpillars crawled on my knee.
wiggle two fingers on knee

Along came another and then there were three.
show three fingers

Three little caterpillars crawled on the floor.
walk three fingers across the floor

Along came another and then there were four.
show four fingers

Four little caterpillars all crawled away.
walk four fingers across the floor

They will all turn into butterflies one fine day!
flap your arms like a butterfly

TEN LITTLE CRAYONS

 to the tune of **"Ten Little Indians"**

One little, two little, three little crayons,
four little, five little, six little crayons,
seven little, eight little, nine little crayons,
ten little crayons in a box.
hold up one finger for each crayon as you count them

Take out a red one and draw a big circle.
draw a circle with your finger

Take out a blue one and draw a straight line.
draw a straight line

Take out a yellow one and draw a little triangle.
draw a triangle

Then put them back in the box!
pretend to replace them in the crayon box

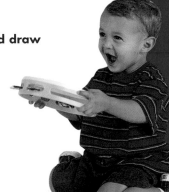

201

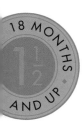

CEREAL CHALLENGE

GETTING TO THE CONTENTS

SKILLSPOTLIGHT

This is a deceptively simple *activity that promotes problem-solving techniques and demonstrates the concepts behind in and out as well as the principle of cause and effect. Once your child has mastered this challenge, raise the stakes with this visual memory game: take three small plastic containers such as bottles and hide a cereal bit in one of them. Mix them up, then urge her to find the one with the cereal (also see Magic Cups, page 247).*

Cause & Effect	✔
Concept Development	✔
Fine Motor Skills	✔
Problem Solving	✔

FIND A CLEAN, unbreakable small-mouthed bottle (a baby bottle or water bottle works well). Drop some of your toddler's favorite cereal or snack into it. Show your toddler the cereal in the open bottle and ask her to get it out. Allow her to experiment, but if she becomes overly frustrated, demonstrate how to tip the bottle over. Increase the challenge by lightly screwing on the top or asking her to drop the cereal back into the bottle. To further fine-tune her motor skills, try this with a variety of containers that have different types of lids.

BOTTOMS UP! There's nothing like a snack to motivate your budding genius—just watch how quickly she catches on.

202

SHAPE TO FIT

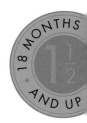

PUZZLING OUT A SOLUTION

WHICH SHAPES GO WHERE? Toddlers love a mystery, and this is one they can solve with some help from you. Use a shape-sorter toy or cut out three or four shapes on the top and sides of some sturdy cardboard boxes. (Make sure the shapes are about the same size so the triangle won't fit into the hole for the circle, for instance.) Ask your toddler to drop the shapes into the matching holes. Demonstrate the activity to get your child started, then let your young detective work on this visual mystery at her own pace.

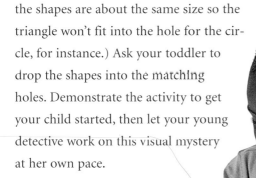

MATCHING UP SHAPES teaches more than geometry; a child also learns how to solve new challenges.

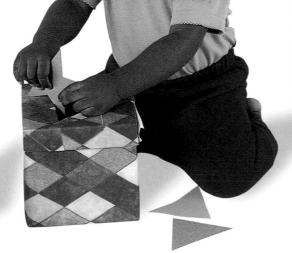

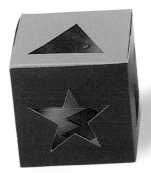

SKILLSPOTLIGHT

The ability to classify *as well as discriminate among sizes and shapes is a fundamental skill that not only helps toddlers make sense of the world but prepares them for activities they'll encounter in play groups, camps, and preschool. Sorting, grasping, and fitting shapes promotes the development of fine motor skills and eye-hand coordination, which will in turn aid toddlers as they practice using forks and spoons, manipulating toys, and coloring. It may take some time before your child is able to easily discriminate among shapes, but most children this age enjoy practicing.*

✔	**Classifying Skills**
✔	**Eye-Hand Coordination**
✔	**Fine Motor Skills**
✔	**Size & Shape Discrimination**

203

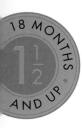

POINT OUT THE PARTS

TALKING ABOUT THE BODY

SKILLSPOTLIGHT

Identifying and repeating *the names of specific body parts plays a role in language development; not only is your child learning to match your real nose to the word "nose," she's also feeling what a nose is by touching it or sniffing with it. The resulting physical sensations increase her awareness of her body and her body parts.*

Body Awareness	✔
Concept Development	✔
Language Development	✔
Listening Skills	✔

LABELING BODY PARTS is an important first step in your child's sense of herself as a separate person. This simple activity aids the process of self-discovery, which begins at the end of the first year of life and blossoms in the second. Learning and saying the names of body parts sharpens your toddler's verbal skills and memory, and increases her awareness of her body.

• To start, sit facing your child and touch her nose. Then take her finger in your hand and guide it to your nose. Say "nose" several times as you tap her finger on your nose. Then ask her to point to her own nose. Continue with other body parts, such as head, arm, leg, and foot. It may take her awhile to distinguish between "Mommy's nose" and "baby's nose"—that's natural. But eventually this will become a favorite game of hers and one that gives her a sense of accomplishment.

• If she has the verbal skills to say some of the names, ask her to repeat them as you point to them. Or initiate a movement game that shows her how to shake her head, stomp her foot, and wiggle her toes.

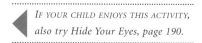

IF YOUR CHILD ENJOYS THIS ACTIVITY, also try Hide Your Eyes, page 190.

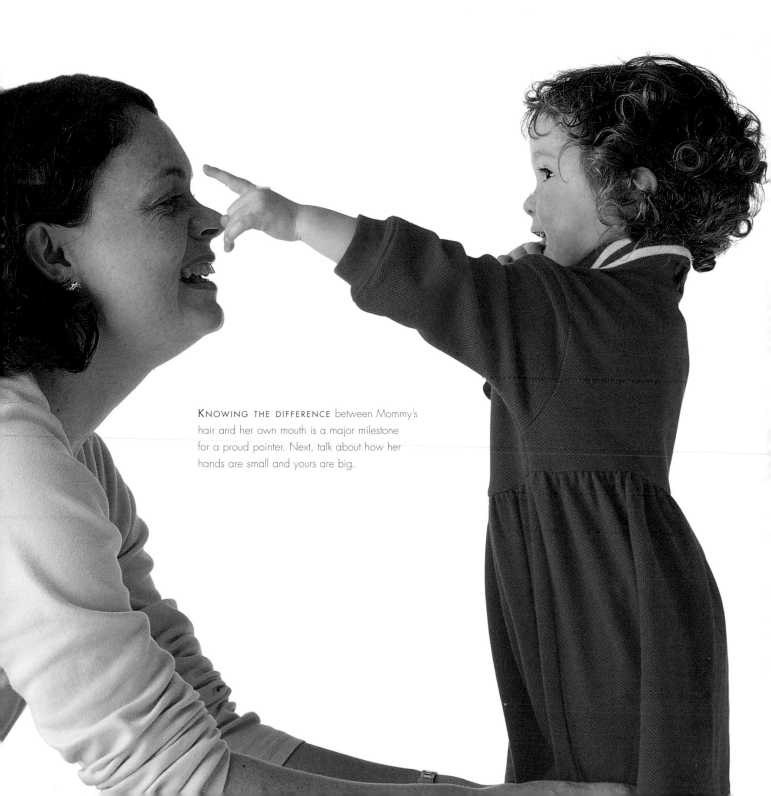

KNOWING THE DIFFERENCE between Mommy's hair and her own mouth is a major milestone for a proud pointer. Next, talk about how her hands are small and yours are big.

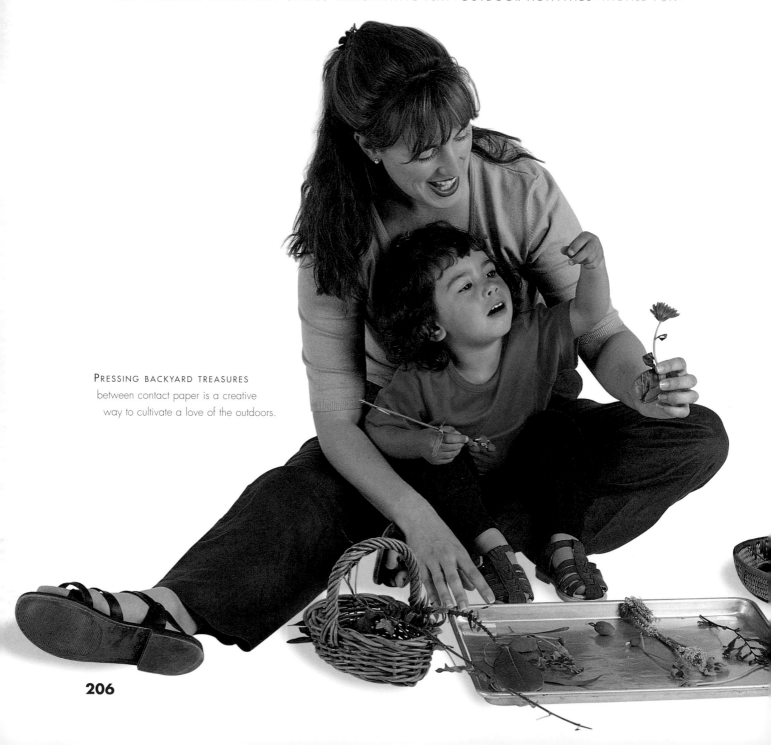

PRESSING BACKYARD TREASURES
between contact paper is a creative
way to cultivate a love of the outdoors.

NATURE ART

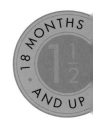

18 MONTHS 1½ AND UP

TODDLERS LOVE THE OUTDOORS, love to collect things, and love to dabble in the arts—as you've no doubt noticed with your child's oatmeal finger paintings at breakfast time or perhaps her crayon murals. Nurture this trio of passions by helping your toddler create a collage of natural elements.

• Take her on a walk in your backyard, a park, or the woods and collect small leaves, flowers, grass, sticks, feathers, and whatever else she finds that appeals to her (and is safe to handle).

• Use the outing as a time to expose your child to some new words and concepts by talking about what you find ("See this feather? That's from a blue jay." "Look, the flowers are turned toward the sun.").

• Once you're home, place a piece of clear contact paper, sticky side up, on top of a cookie sheet with a rim. Tape each corner of the contact paper to the cookie sheet to keep the paper from sticking to your hands.

• Help your child arrange her outdoor treasures on the contact paper.

• Place another piece of transparent contact paper, sticky side down, over the first one to help preserve your toddler's work of art.

• Hang the collage in a window, on the refrigerator, even in your child's room . . . anywhere she can proudly showcase her creation.

SKILLSPOTLIGHT

Letting your child choose *her own objects (a red flower versus a yellow one, for instance) and arrange them herself helps her identify and express her personal preferences. Talking to her about nature as you explore the outdoors encourages her to notice and describe the world. And the task of applying objects to paper—especially a sticky contact sheet—helps enhance her fine motor skills.*

✔ **Creative Expression**

✔ **Eye-Hand Coordination**

✔ **Fine Motor Skills**

✔ **Language Development**

207

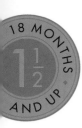

18 MONTHS
1½
AND UP

WATER THE PLANTS

A MUSICAL MIME

 to the *tune* of **"The Mulberry Bush"**

This is the way we water the plants,
put one hand on hip and bend the other like a curved spout
water the plants,
water the plants.

This is the way we water the plants whenever they get dry.

We water the plants so they will grow,
crouch down on the floor, then slowly stand up
they will grow,
they will grow.

We water the plants so they will grow way up to the sky.
raise your hands skyward

Balance	✔
Coordination	✔

THIS GARDENING SONG will teach your tyke a fundamental lesson about nature: that plants need water to grow! Show your child how to tip way over as he "pours" the water from his "spout." That's good balance practice. If he likes rowdier play, pick him up and tip him over instead. Reinforce the gardening lesson by asking him to help you water real plants, either inside or outside. He'll enjoy both participating in your chores (see Copycat, page 290) and nurturing living things.

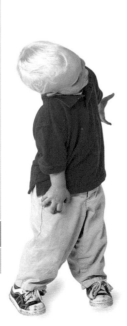
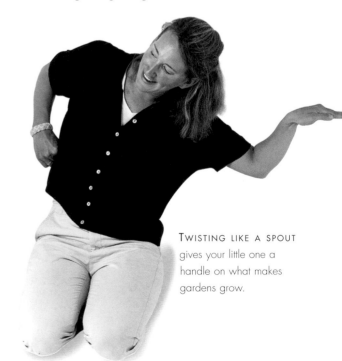

TWISTING LIKE A SPOUT gives your little one a handle on what makes gardens grow.

SURPRISE!

18 MONTHS
1½
AND UP

UNWRAPPING TOY TREASURES

FOR TODDLERS, the wrapping paper on a present is at least as fun as the gift itself. They love the brightly colored paper, the noise it makes when they crinkle it, and the challenge of discovering what's inside. Your child can enjoy this activity any day of the year if you gather several of his favorite toys and wrap them loosely in colorful paper (no tape) while he watches.

Show him one package at a time, asking, "What's inside the paper?" Let him remove the wrapping—but lend a helping hand if he gets frustrated. Wad up the paper while commenting on the sound it makes and how it feels.

THE ACT OF UNWRAPPING stimulates the senses and helps develop coordination.

SKILLSPOTLIGHT

Unwrapping an object *requires solving problems and having nimble fingers. Playing with different patterns and textures stimulates a child's visual, tactile, and auditory senses, especially when the paper crinkles or pops as he handles it.*

✔ **Coordination**

✔ **Problem Solving**

✔ **Sensory Exploration**

✔ **Tactile Discrimination**

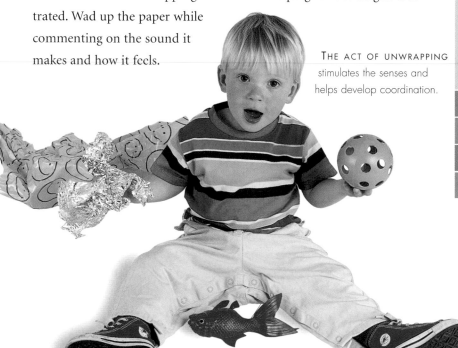

209

RHYTHM TIME

FUN WITH A DRUM

SKILLSPOTLIGHT

Your child is born with an innate sense of rhythm. But learning to pound out a beat—especially while practicing with you—lets her see how it fits into music, dance, and other rhythmic activities. Drumming also enhances her eye-hand coordination, and learning to vary the pace and volume fine-tunes her muscle control.

Cause & Effect	✔	
Creative Expression	✔	
Listening Skills	✔	
Rhythm Exploration	✔	

MAKING YOUR OWN

Creating a drum is as simple as turning over a saucepan or wooden bowl. Try metal, plastic, and wooden spoons for varying sound effects; use different-size containers to create varying pitches (the smaller they are, the higher the pitch).

YOUR CHILD ALREADY KNOWS how to make plenty of noise by banging her spoon on the table, clapping her hands, and pounding on the door she wants opened. You can direct this energy toward more musical pursuits—as well as encourage her sense of rhythm—by showing her how to bang out a beat with a drum.

• Buy a drum and mallet, or make your own. Sit down with your child and show her how to hit the drum with either a mallet or her hand. Demonstrate how to hit the drum softly, then loudly. Vary the pace of the drumming so she experiences fast beats as well as slow ones.

• Put on some lively music and demonstrate how to drum to the beat. Don't expect her to follow the music exactly—that will come when she's older. Sway back and forth, tap your foot, clap your hands, and toss your head from side to side to show her other ways of expressing rhythm. Or get your own drum and pound out a noisy duet.

◀ IF YOUR CHILD ENJOYS THIS ACTIVITY, also try Shake It Up, Baby!, page 191.

SHOW YOUR LITTLE DRUMMER GIRL
the different sounds she can make, then
let her march to her own beat.

"Bang, bang the drum!"

TODDLER PARADE

MAKING A SPECIAL DAY WITH EVERYDAY TOYS

SKILL SPOTLIGHT

This is the very beginning *of fantasy play: they are pretending to be a member of the parade and they're mentally converting their toys (and you) into appropriate props. Walking or marching to music can help them learn rhythm. And they'll develop new levels of coordination by figuring out how to pull their pretend-parade behind them.*

Creative Expression	✔
Fine Motor Skills	✔
Gross Motor Skills	✔

EVERYONE LOVES A PARADE— but you don't have to wait for a holiday or struggle with crowds to let your toddler participate in one. Instead, create a pint-size parade in your own home, complete with music, celebrities (albeit fuzzy ones), and an emcee. Make your child the grand marshal of the event.

• Help her collect her wheeled toys in the "staging grounds" (for example, your living room). Tie the toys together with short lengths of string so she can pull the makeshift contraption behind her. If you have a toy wagon, prop stuffed animals inside to serve as famous folk. To get really fancy, decorate the "floats" with streamers and ribbons. You could even make confetti!

NOTHING CAN RAIN on their personal parade when they have their rolling elephants, horses, and lion marching right along behind them.

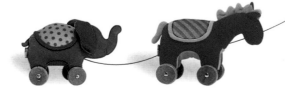

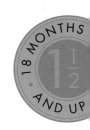

• When your toddler gets a little older, play lively marching music, outfit yourself with a drum (a spoon and a pot will do) or a fake baton, and parade around with your child in tow. She probably won't be able to march and pull her toys at the same time, so pull the floats for her while she practices stepping high and swinging her little arms.

RESEARCH REPORT

In studies conducted *in the United States and Britain, psychologists Anthony Pellegrini and Peter K. Smith showed that children instinctively seem to understand the importance of play and freedom of movement. When their free play was restricted for a period of time, the "deprivation led to increased levels of play when opportunities for play were resumed," the psychologists concluded. In other words, when finally let loose, the kids tried to make up for lost playtime.*

◀ *IF YOUR CHILD ENJOYS THIS ACTIVITY, also try Band on the Run, page 170.*

213

PLAYING WITH SIBLINGS

WHEN PLAYING one-on-one with a toddler, you can easily adapt to your child's needs and desires. But when a sibling is introduced into the group, the dynamics change dramatically, calling for a parent to exercise a bit more imagination and diplomacy.

Several factors complicate the situation: toddlers aren't always keen on sharing their parents' attention, even with a beloved brother or sister. If there's more than a two-year gap in ages, just finding an activity that suits both children can be a challenge. Then there are different play styles to consider: one child may be the quiet type who prefers to play alone with blocks, while his dynamo of a sister likes nothing more than to help him build block towers—before knocking them down. No wonder a session of family fun can leave you feeling more like a referee in a particularly fierce World Wrestling Federation match than a play partner.

Still, there are many ways to ensure smoother, more enjoyable play sessions. Taking into account the children's ages and personalities, devise activities that will be fun for both and accommodate different play styles. Art projects such as drawing with sidewalk chalk or painting, for instance, can be enjoyed by toddlers and young school-age children alike. Going to a playground outfitted with a variety of equipment allows children to play together for a while, and then pursue individual interests. And don't forget to stock up on duplicate toys and supplies when possible; having two sets of watercolors and two rainbow-colored balls has saved many a parent from sibling meltdown. It's also important to dole out attention in fairly equal measures. While it's natural to pay more attention to the younger child, as she might need more help, remember to offer words of praise or encouragement to the older sibling. ■

214

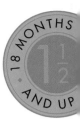

18 MONTHS
1½
AND UP

BABY BASKETBALL

SLAM-DUNKING A FAVORITE GAME

GATHER A FEW medium-size balls and place them in a large container such as a laundry basket, cardboard box, or plastic bowl. Show your child how to empty the balls onto the floor, then demonstrate how to drop the balls one by one into the basket. Initially, your toddler may enjoy simply putting the balls in the basket and taking them back out. When he's ready, have him stand back and try throwing the balls into the basket. Increase the challenge by placing a few containers around the room, then urge your athlete to aim toward a different one each time.

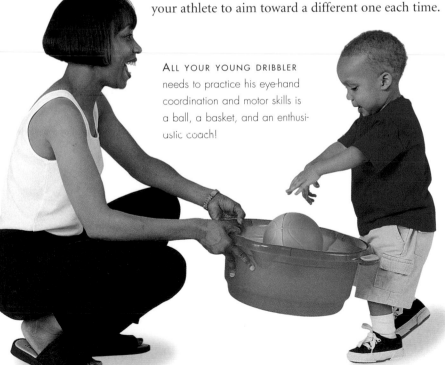

ALL YOUR YOUNG DRIBBLER needs to practice his eye-hand coordination and motor skills is a ball, a basket, and an enthusiastic coach!

SKILLSPOTLIGHT

When your child *practices aiming, he improves his eye-hand coordination and gross motor skills. And if you count the balls out loud as your toddler throws them into the containers, you'll help lay the foundation for understanding numbers. Whether your child is tossing the ball into a basket or at you, actively participate by gently throwing the ball back to him. Encourage him to take another (more difficult) fundamental step: learning to catch.*

✔	**Eye-Hand Coordination**
✔	**Gross Motor Skills**
✔	**Social Skills**

THE NOBLE DUKE OF YORK

A CLASSIC SONG AND MIME

SKILL SPOTLIGHT

Your toddler *is beginning to form a clearer sense of himself as an object in space. This song game—while fun to play with a parent—helps him learn the meanings of spatial words, such as "up," "down," and "over." And while your child may not be quite old enough to tell right from left, he'll get the idea, at least, that those words refer to something other than straight ahead.*

Concept Development	✔
Language Development	✔
Spatial Awareness	✔

IF YOUR CHILD ENJOYS THIS ACTIVITY, also try The Choo-Choo Train, page 220.

216

YOUR CHILD'S UNDERSTANDING of the concepts of space and movement increases slowly but surely in the toddler years. If your child loved lap songs as a baby, he'll get a big kick out of this more advanced version, which teaches him just some of the ways he can move about in the world.

• As with all song games, enunciating the sounds clearly and emphasizing the corresponding movements help teach your toddler the meaning of the most important words. Those emphases also create a song with more drama and vigor, which makes it more exciting for the two of you.

• As your toddler gets older, he can sing this song standing on the floor instead of sitting on your knees. Try marching during the first stanza, then stretching up and crouching down in the second stanza. With the third stanza, have him drop to the floor and lie on his back, then gently push his legs left, right, and up in the air.

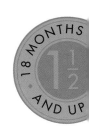

18 MONTHS 1½ AND UP

THIS FUN TUNE—bolstered by Mommy's bouncy movements—helps your little duke learn about moving up and down.

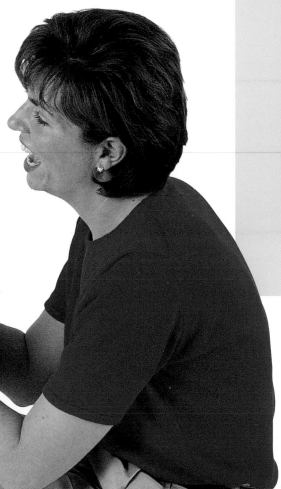

The noble Duke of York, he had ten thousand men,
bounce child on your knees, facing outward
he marched them up to the top of the hill,
march your legs upward with child still on knees
and he marched them down again.
march your legs downward with child still on knees

And when you're up, you're up.
raise both legs
And when you're down, you're down.
drop both legs

And when you're only halfway up,
raise both legs halfway up and pause
you're neither up nor down.
move legs up and down quickly

He rolled them over left,
lean to the left
he rolled them over right,
lean to the right
he rolled them over upside down,
lie backward with child lying on top of you
oh, what a funny sight!
return to original position

217

TUBE TRICKS

WHERE DOES THE BALL GO?

SKILLSPOTLIGHT

Balls and disappearing acts, *as well as repetition, fascinate children at this age. But it's not all fun and games here. Dropping balls into a tube and then catching or chasing them exercises your toddler's fine motor skills and eye-hand coordination. And fitting different-size balls into the tube helps her sort shapes in her mind. Taking turns at either end of the tube promotes sharing.*

Cause & Effect	✔
Fine Motor Skills	✔
Size & Shape Discrimination	✔

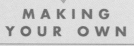

MAKING YOUR OWN

You can find tubes of all sizes at hardware stores, hobby stores, art galleries, photo shops, and the post office. Any soft balls that fit in the tube will work: tennis balls, racquet balls, or balls made of cloth, soft rubber, or foam.

I N ONE END and out the other. It seems simple to us, but to a toddler it's like playing hide-and-seek with a ball, which is sure to puzzle and thrill her. Even when she's mastered the mystery ("Where did the ball go? There it is!"), she'll want to play this game again and again.

• Start with a wide plastic or cardboard tube and a supply of tennis, racquet, or other soft balls. Put the balls in one end of the tube, tilt the tube so they roll down inside it, and have her retrieve them from the other end. Repeat several times. Then have her put the balls in and you catch them.

• Increase the complexity by using balls of different sizes. Which ones fit in the tube? Which ones don't? Be sure to choose balls that are at least 1¾ inches (4.5 cm) in diameter so they do not pose a choking hazard.

• You can turn this activity into a coordination exercise by asking her to catch a ball as it's falling out of the tube. She waits at the bottom end of the tube, and as the ball pops out, she tries to grab it. The smaller the ball, the greater the challenge.

◄ *IF YOUR CHILD ENJOYS THIS ACTIVITY, also try Baby Basketball, page 215.*

218

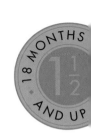

18 MONTHS 1½ AND UP

A **CLEAR TUBE** lets her watch the blue balls roll all the way from top to bottom; an opaque tube will add an element of surprise to the game.

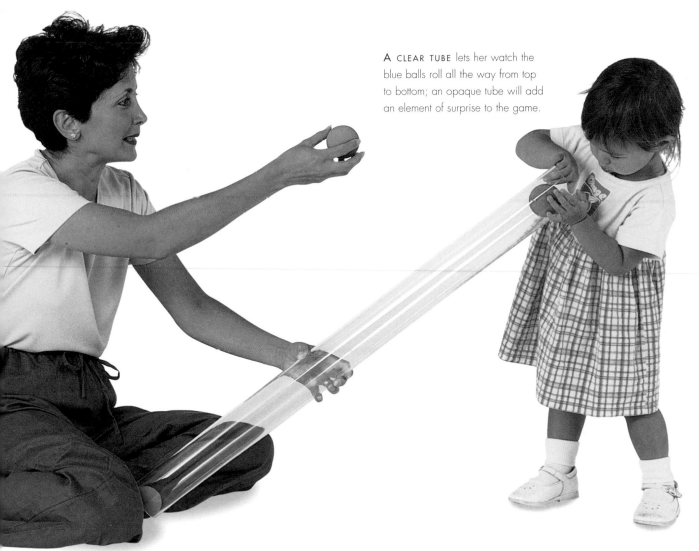

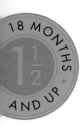

18 MONTHS
1½
AND UP

THE CHOO-CHOO TRAIN

AN EXCURSION IN RHYME

sit facing your child and hold both of her hands

Here comes the choo-choo train, coming down the track. First it's going forward, then it's going back.
pull one hand toward you while pushing the other toward your child; continue to alternate

Now the bell is ringing: ding, ding, ding!
ring imaginary bell

Now the whistle blows: whoo, whoo, whoo!
pull imaginary whistle cord

What a lot of noise it makes
cover both of your ears
everywhere it goes!

| Language Development | ✔ |
| Rhythm Exploration | ✔ |

TODDLERS DON'T NEED a melody to sense rhythm: they can feel beats with simple chants. When you add appealing rhymes, fun movements, an ever-friendly train theme, and an enthusiastic parent, you've got an activity that will keep your little one chugging merrily along.

• While you chant "Here Comes the Choo-Choo Train," play up the rhythm so your toddler can hear it and mimic it with her body. Ham up the movements, too. Emphasizing the gestures will help your eager engineer understand the meaning of the accompanying words.

THIS CHANTING game teaches your little conductor to feel a beat and understand the basics of forward and backward motion.

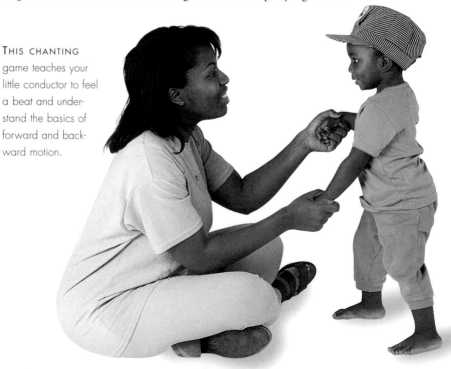

220

TANTALIZING TEXTURES

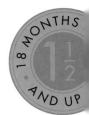

18 MONTHS 1½ AND UP

A BOOK OF SENSATIONS

HE'S ALREADY DETERMINED to get his hands on everything in (and out of) sight, including dollops of jam, dead bugs, and months-old cereal bits. Let his fingers experience the world safely by introducing him to a book filled with tactile adventures. You can buy a texture book or make your own.

• To create the book, collect a variety of materials, such as cloth, burlap, foil, wax paper, and bubble wrap. Glue a large square of each material onto cardboard or construction paper. Then tie or tape the sheets together.

• When you explore the book with your toddler, describe the different sensations you both are feeling.

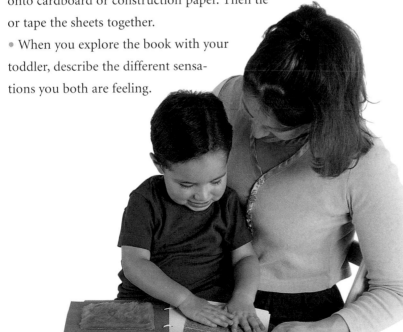

SKILL SPOTLIGHT

A texture book *lets your toddler discover a variety of different materials and helps him learn concepts such as rough, smooth, bumpy, and even squishy. The book can also give your child the chance to express his preferences: Does he like the scratchy feel of burlap? Or does he prefer the crinkliness of the foil?*

✔	**Language Development**
✔	**Tactile Discrimination**
✔	**Tactile Stimulation**

BOOK PAGES made of unusual textures, such as fine sandpaper or fake fur, let your child explore the world from the safety of your lap.

221

MAGNET MAGIC

PLAYING WITH TOYS THAT STICK

SKILLSPOTLIGHT

Grasping and moving *magnets helps build fine motor skills—the ones he'll need for drawing, completing puzzles, fastening little buttons, and, eventually, writing. Discussing these intriguing magnets helps him learn to distinguish among colors and sizes and helps expand his vocabulary, while making a magnet "disappear" exercises his visual memory.*

Counting Concepts	✔
Fine Motor Skills	✔
Size & Shape Discrimination	✔
Visual Memory	✔

MAKING YOUR OWN

Create personalized magnets by gluing or taping photos of family members onto inexpensive, flat magnets. Or attach photos, drawings, or magazine pictures of your child's favorite animals. Photo stores carry magnetized photo frames, as well.

MANY CHILDREN display their manual dexterity by pulling magnets off the refrigerator—and then crowing delightedly over their finds. You can make magnets even more fun by using them for a variety of games that engage your child's eyes and memory, as well as his curious fingers.

• Gather several colorful magnets and place them on a metal cookie sheet (note: magnets won't adhere to aluminum sheets). Use magnets with images of objects, such as animals, flowers, food, storybook characters, numbers, and vehicles. Avoid magnets that are smaller than 1¾ inches (4.5 cm) in diameter because they pose a choking hazard. And choose magnets with well-defined edges so your child can pick them up easily.

• Ask your toddler to take the magnets off the sheet—then ask him to put them back on. Talk to him about the colors, sizes, and characters he sees on the magnets. Encourage him to move them around to create his own design. With an older toddler, remove a magnet from the sheet and ask him to guess which one is missing.

IF YOUR CHILD ENJOYS THIS ACTIVITY, also try Tantalizing Textures, page 221.

222

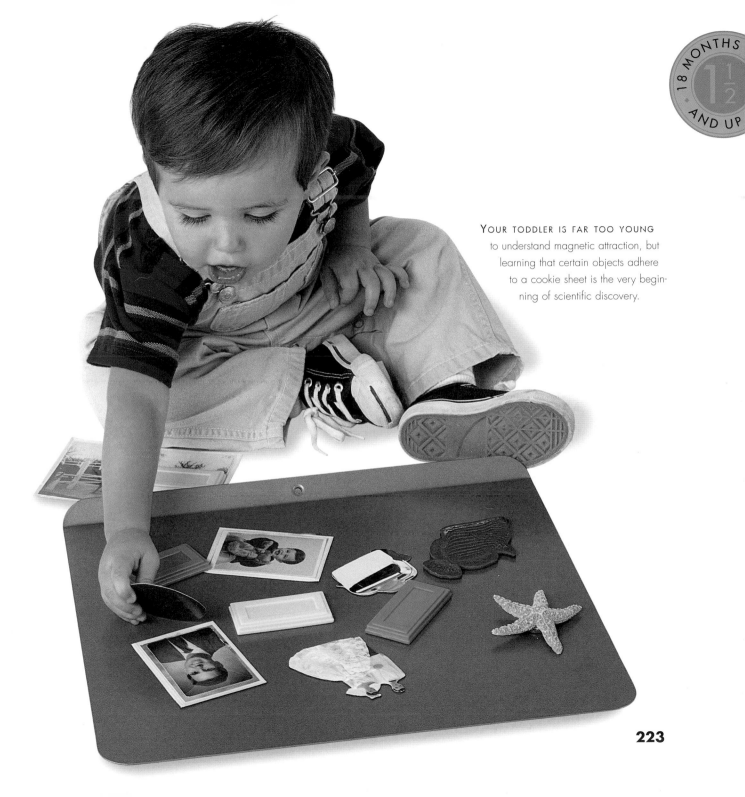

YOUR TODDLER IS FAR TOO YOUNG to understand magnetic attraction, but learning that certain objects adhere to a cookie sheet is the very beginning of scientific discovery.

223

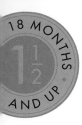

OPEN SHUT THEM!

A TICKLING RHYME AND CHANT

Open shut them,
open and close fists
open shut them,
give a little clap, clap, clap!
clap three times

Open shut them,
open and close fists
open shut them,
put them in your lap, lap, lap!
pat lap three times

Creep them, crawl them,
slowly creep them,
right up to your chin, chin, chin!
walk fingers from chest to chin,
tickling your child along the way

Open wide your little mouth,
touch lips with a finger
but do not let them in!
quickly run fingers down to lap,
tickling your child along the way

Creative Expression	✔
Fine Motor Skills	✔
Language Development	✔

TODDLERS HAVE A GREAT LOVE for their own little bodies—and the names of their own little body parts. They also enjoy tickle and surprise games. This chant gives your child a chance to show off her knowledge of her body and at the same time play a creepy-crawly tickle game.
• Start out by demonstrating the chant's gestures on yourself and see if she can follow along. If she seems confused, do the fingerplay on her instead—until she is ready to copy you.

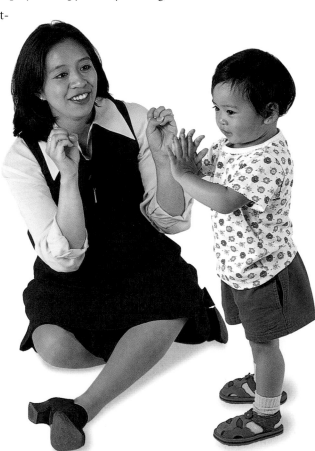

YOUR CHILD will enjoy playing the creepy-crawly game with her fingers—especially when Mommy is an active participant.

224

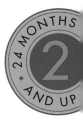

24 MONTHS
2
AND UP

BEACH-BALL CATCH

A TOSS-AND-CATCH BALL GAME

MOST TODDLERS are able to throw a ball before they can catch one. But they love trying to wrap their little arms around airborne balls, and with a healthy dose of patience and practice you can help your child learn the basics of catching. Start by rolling a ball to her and asking her to roll it back to you (see Pass the Ball, page 152). When she's ready to attempt catching, use a slightly deflated beach ball (it's easier for small hands to grasp).

• Kneel or sit a couple of feet apart and ask her to throw the beach ball to you. Demonstrate how to catch, then toss the ball to her and ask her to catch it. Once she accomplishes this (it will take a lot of practice), increase the distance between you, little by little.

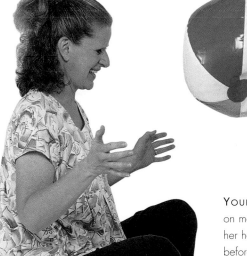

YOUR CHILD will catch on more quickly if you show her how to grab the ball before you toss it her way.

SKILL SPOTLIGHT

Playing a game *of catch with a toddler is a fun and simple exercise in socialization that builds gross motor skills and eye-hand coordination. Successful catches demand quick reflexes and good spatial awareness, which may take awhile for your toddler to achieve. By enthusiastically supporting your child in her attempts to catch, you are teaching her to appreciate being part of a game in a noncompetitive way.*

✔	**Eye-Hand Coordination**
✔	**Gross Motor Skills**
✔	**Social Skills**

225

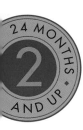
BALANCING ACT

STANDING TALL ON A BALANCE BEAM

SKILLSPOTLIGHT

Just like logs and low walls, *balance beams present an irresistible challenge to curious young children. As she perfects her walk along the beam, her ability to balance increases, and she develops crucial eye-foot coordination—skills that will help her as she moves from walking to running, jumping, hopping, skipping, and—who knows?—maybe even perfecting a gymnastic dismount.*

Balance	✔
Eye-Foot Coordination	✔
Spatial Awareness	✔

IF YOUR CHILD ENJOYS THIS ACTIVITY, also try Footstep Fun, page 241. ▶

ATTEMPTING TO BALANCE on narrow walkways is a natural and universal activity for young children, so you probably won't have to do much to encourage your child to try. You can find beams low enough to walk on safely at gyms, parks, and playgrounds. Demonstrate how to walk across, then hold your child's hand as she tries to walk slowly on the beam.

• If your toddler is reluctant at first, place a toy at the other end of the beam and encourage your young gymnast to hold your hand and walk across to retrieve it. Be sure she practices this balancing act above a soft or cushioned surface.

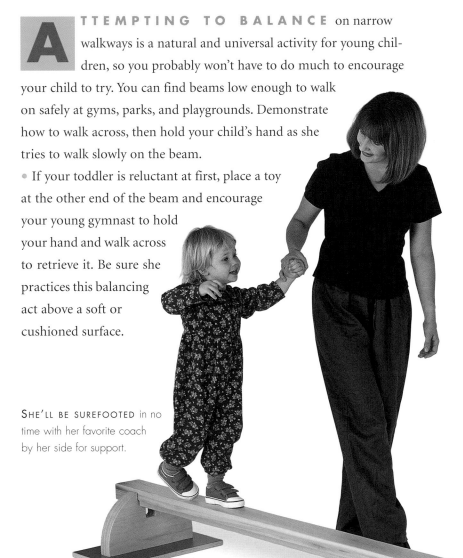

SHE'LL BE SUREFOOTED in no time with her favorite coach by her side for support.

PUPPET PLAY

AN OLD-FASHIONED STAGE SHOW

CHILDREN ADORE PUPPETS because they're toys that seem to magically come to life. They'll love them even more when you put on a live, slapstick show. You can buy puppets—or just use brightly colored felt-tipped pens to draw a face on a sock or a bag. You can even tape ears or horns on your home-made puppet and glue "hair" made of yarn to its top.

• Make a stage by draping a blanket over the back of a chair or a safety gate   or position yourself behind a sofa. With one or two puppets, tell your child stories and sing songs. Use a different voice for each puppet.

• Ask your child questions with the puppets and encourage him to converse. Question him about his favorite foods, his special toys, or his mommy and daddy. And ask him to show the puppet his nose and toes—toddlers love to point these things out.

SKILLSPOTLIGHT

By the age of two, *your child is attributing all sorts of human traits to his toys; he considers them his best friends. By making puppet toys act more like humans, you stimulate his imagination. And by telling stories and conversing with him, you accelerate his back-and-forth conversational skills.*

✔	**Imagination**
✔	**Language Development**
✔	**Social Skills**

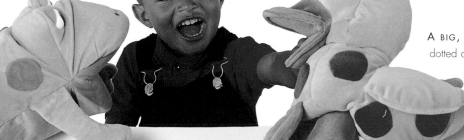

A BIG, FAT FROG and a polka-dotted duck can share some pretty funny stories with their little human friend.

227

TRAIN TRIPS

AN IMAGINARY LOCOMOTIVE

SKILLSPOTLIGHT

In this activity, *your little engineer enhances her upper body muscle coordination and learns to move with the rhythm of a chant. Puffing along as your pint-size passenger, she develops whole body coordination as well as balance—after all, it's hard to stay seated on Mommy when you're busy giggling like crazy. Role-playing also greases the gears of the imagination.*

YOU CAN HARNESS your child's abundant steam power by taking her on an imaginary train trip. Announce your destination ("First stop, Mommy's lap!"), pretend to pull the whistle ("Whoo whoo!"), then invite her to sit on your lap. As you chant "chug-a-chug-a-choo-choo," push her hands in a circle (like the rolling train wheels) or help her blow the whistle. Alternatively, you can both "chug" around the house ("Next stop, your bedroom!") with your child as the engine and you as the caboose.

• Pretend to navigate around curves by bending both of your bodies from side to side. Go through "tunnels" (don't forget to duck your heads!) and stop from time to time to let passengers off at the "depot."

• Sing a favorite train song or chant (see The Choo-Choo Train, page 220) while you chug around the house together.

• To help a toddler appreciate trains and enjoy this activity even more, take her to a real train station—or even the subway—and show your young conductor what it's like to ride the rails.

Coordination	✔
Gross Motor Skills	✔
Imagination	✔
Social Skills	✔

IF YOUR CHILD ENJOYS THIS ACTIVITY, *also try Drive the Fire Truck, page 250.*

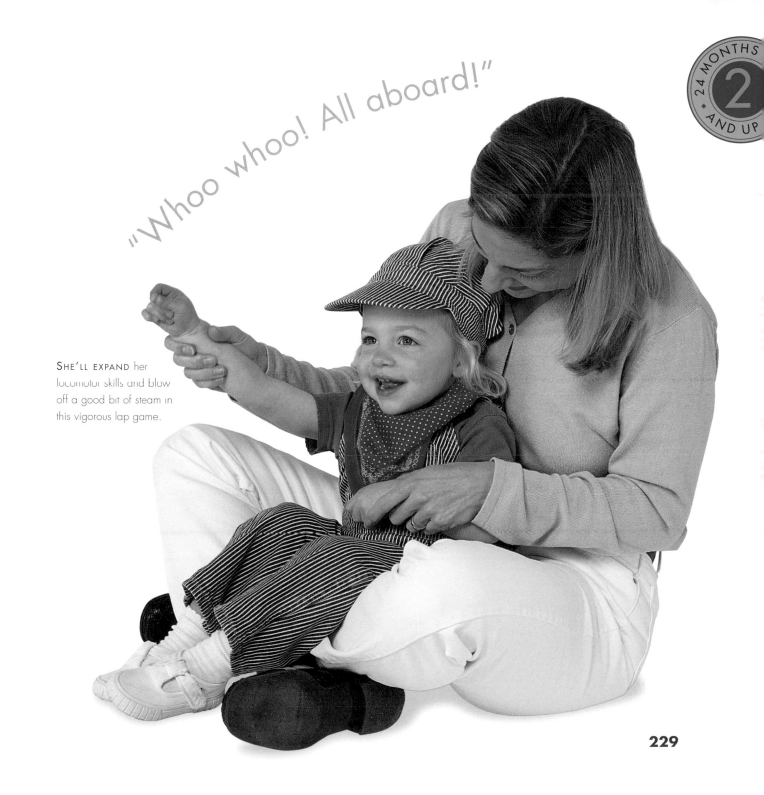

"Whoo whoo! All aboard!"

SHE'LL EXPAND her locomotor skills and blow off a good bit of steam in this vigorous lap game.

THE "NO" STAGE

A BIG SHOCK to first-time parents is the transformation of their easygoing, compliant infants into mercurial toddlers whose favorite word seems to be no—as in "no bananas," "no bath," and "no songs," even though they never seemed to mind these things before. As Dr. Benjamin Spock wrote in *Baby and Child Care*, "When you suggest something that doesn't appeal to them, they feel they must assert themselves. . . . Psychologists call it 'negativism.'" While admitting that this spell of negativism can test the resources of even the most patient parents, Spock also noted that this stage is an important signal that children are maturing into independent human beings who can think for themselves.

Being calm, cooperative, and reasonable with your toddler is one of the most effective ways to teach him to be a calm, cooperative, and reasonable person himself—but it will take time. Until he learns more self-control, you can expect temper tantrums when he doesn't get his way. It's best to ignore such behavior—if you can—to convey that he can't get what he wants in this unseemly manner. In *Raising Good Children*, developmental psychologist Thomas Lickona advises parents to keep toddlers happily busy, offer diversions when they get restless, and allow lots of free play in safe settings. He also recommends counting, such as saying, "Let's see if you can get in your chair by the time I count to ten." Another strategy is to present a child with alternatives. If he insists on wearing clothes that aren't appropriate for the weather, you could pick out two suitable outfits and say, "Which would you like to wear today?" Such maneuvers might seem transparent to adults, but they are wonderfully effective in making a headstrong toddler feel a measure of the control and freedom he so desires. ■

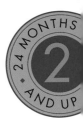

24 MONTHS
2
AND UP

PONY RIDES

TAKING A LIVING-ROOM TROT

SHE'S FASCINATED by pictures of horses, but a wee bit wary of the real thing. Give her a leg up on balance skills by playing the pony part yourself. Get down on your hands and knees and let your child ride on your back or shoulders. Make sure she hangs on tight, and be ready to grab a leg if she starts sliding.

• If you want to add music to this activity, sing "Trot Little Pony" (see Silly Lap Songs, page 178, for the lyrics) or another of your toddler's favorite songs as you crawl around the room. To help her learn to adjust her balance, lower your upper body to the floor, raise it (not too high!), or wiggle from side to side.

GIDDYAP DADDY! You can start your little cowgirl's riding lessons early by doing some of the legwork in your living room.

SKILLSPOTLIGHT

Sure, a two-year-old *can walk pretty well. But that doesn't mean her balance is fully developed. As you crawl and wiggle your way through the house, your child is learning how to find and keep her center of gravity. She'll also be stretching her imagination by pretending she's riding a pretty pony —or perhaps a dashing steed.*

✔	**Balance**
✔	**Gross Motor Skills**
✔	**Imagination**

231

HEAD TO TOES

GENTLE GYM

touch the body part with both hands as you sing its name

Head, shoulders, knees, and toes.

Knees and toes!

Head, shoulders, knees, and toes.

Knees and toes!

Eyes and ears and mouth and nose, head, shoulders, knees, and toes.

Knees and toes!

Body Awareness	✔
Gross Motor Skills	✔
Listening Skills	✔
Rhythm Exploration	✔
Visual Memory	✔

YOU MAY REMEMBER this song from your own childhood, when you sang it at camp, in school, or with your friends or parents. It's also a great tune for helping toddlers learn—and remember—the names of body parts.

• Sing "Head, Shoulders, Knees, and Toes" to your child and place both hands on your body parts as you call out the name of each part.

• Keep singing the song over and over, increasing the tempo each time. You'll probably both get mixed up and a bit breathless toward the end— but that's part of the fun!

• Is your toddler having trouble keeping up? Try touching her body as you sing to help her learn how the words and motions fit together.

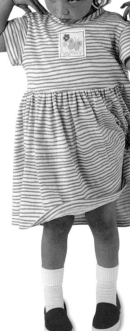

IF YOUR CHILD ENJOYS THIS ACTIVITY, *also try Circle Songs, page 234.* ▶

232

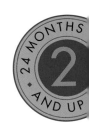

24 MONTHS
2
AND UP

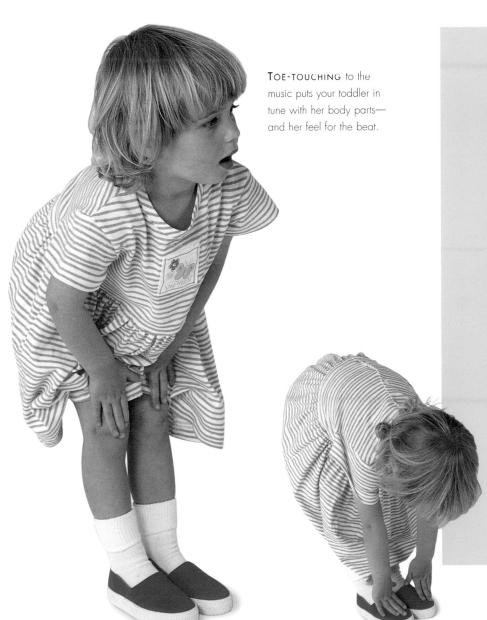

TOE-TOUCHING to the music puts your toddler in tune with her body parts—and her feel for the beat.

RESEARCHREPORT

Not only does music soothe *the savage breast, it seems to perk up the mind as well. Physicist Gordon Shaw and psychologist Frances Rauscher made worldwide headlines in 1993 with a research project showing that college students who listened to Mozart's Sonata for Two Pianos in D Major for ten minutes before a test of their spatial-temporal reasoning ability averaged an eight- or nine-point jump in scores. This finding, along with other studies, so impressed Florida legislators that they enacted the "Beethoven's babies law" in 1998, which requires state-funded day care centers to play classical music for thirty minutes every day. While "Head, Shoulders, Knees, and Toes" is a far cry from Mozart, Rauscher believes any complex music (be it classical, jazz, or rock) might enhance brain development.*

CIRCLE SONGS

THESE PERENNIAL FAVORITES are a perfect choice when your toddler has the urge to move all around. Best of all, there's a camaraderie and joy that comes with circling, singing, and holding hands—whether with Mommy and Daddy or a few cherished friends.

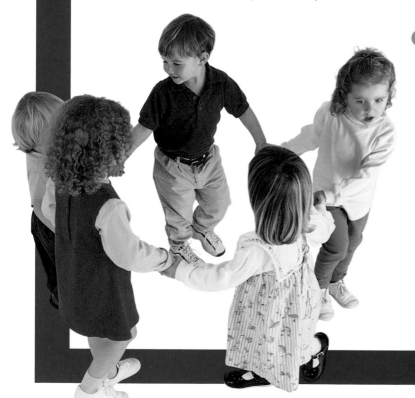

RING AROUND THE ROSY

Ring around the rosy,
hold hands and walk in a circle
pocket full of posies,
ashes, ashes,
we all fall down!
fall to the ground

The cows are in the pasture,
remain seated in the circle
eating buttercups,
pretend to eat
thunder, lightning,
pound hands on the floor
we all stand up!
stand up quickly

234

THE MULBERRY BUSH

Here we go round the mulberry bush,
hold hands and walk in a circle
the mulberry bush,
the mulberry bush.
Here we go round the mulberry bush,
so early in the morning.

This is the way we clap our hands,
clap hands while standing in a circle
clap our hands,
clap our hands.
This is the way we clap our hands,
so early in the morning.

This is the way we stamp our feet . . .
This is the way we turn around . . .
This is the way we twist and shout . . .
This is the way we reach and stretch . . .
This is the way we run and run . . .
This is the way we sit right down . . .
This is the way we wash our face . . .

LOOBY LOO

Here we go looby loo,
hold hands and walk in a circle
here we go looby light,
here we go looby loo,
all on a Saturday night.
jump up with arms extended skyward

POP GOES THE WEASEL

All around the cobbler's bench,
hold hands and run in a circle
the monkey chased the weasel,
the monkey thought
it was all in fun,
POP goes the weasel!
*jump up, then fall
to the ground*

UP, DOWN, ALL AROUND:
Circle songs give your toddler a
dizzying array of tunes to move to
and supportive hands to hold.

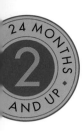

SCARF TRICKS

CATCHING THE FLUTTERING FABRIC

SKILLSPOTLIGHT

A two-year-old is biologically driven to practice gross motor movements of all kinds, such as running, kicking, jumping, and rolling. This activity gives her a new object with which to practice throwing and catching: a silky, fluttering scarf that is as engaging to watch as it is to touch.

Eye-Foot Coordination	✔
Eye-Hand Coordination	✔
Gross Motor Skills	✔

SHE MAY HAVE almost mastered catching a rolling ball, a wobbling plastic lid, or the family cat. Here's something altogether different to challenge her eye-hand coordination. Gather some brightly colored, lightweight scarves. Scrunch up a few of them simultaneously in your hand and throw them high in the air, then ask your child to try to catch them as they float and flutter toward the ground. After a few rounds, let her throw some of the scarves while you take a turn at nabbing them midair. As she gets older, encourage her to spin around or clap her hands before catching the scarves.

PLUCKING A RAINBOW of color from the air is as visually stimulating as it is physically challenging—and fun!

RING-A-LING

FUN WITH PHONES

TODDLERS ARE DRAWN to telephones like bears are drawn to honey. But rather than shooing your two-year-old from your carefully programmed cordless telephone, give her a phone of her own. You can use a castoff from your basement, or buy a toy phone (some even have push buttons that beep).

Encourage her to use it by holding the receiver to her ear and asking simple questions, such as "What's your name?" "What are you doing today?" and "May I talk to your daddy, please?"

"THIS IS CHRISTINA. Can you visit today?" A pretend phone call with Grandpa or Auntie helps your budding socialite learn the give-and-take of conversation.

SKILLSPOTLIGHT

Learning to hold *a conversation, even if it's an imaginary one, helps children exercise their emerging language and social skills. This activity is also a useful way to introduce basic phone etiquette ("Who's calling, please?" or "I'm fine, thank you") before your toddler starts picking up your phone and talking to your callers.*

✔	**Creative Expression**
✔	**Language Development**
✔	**Self-Concept**
✔	**Social Skills**

IF YOUR CHILD ENJOYS THIS ACTIVITY, also try Doll Talk, page 258.

237

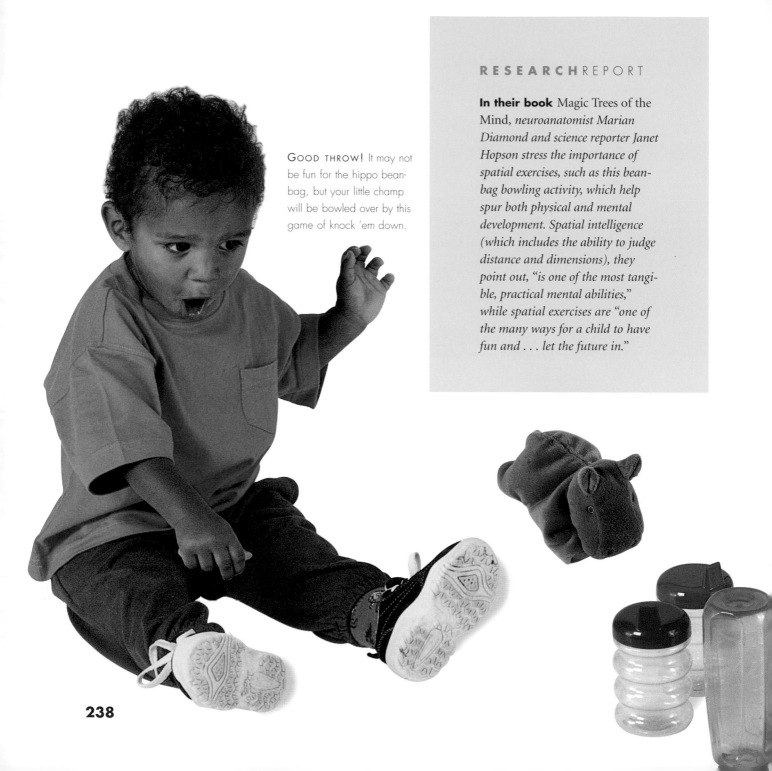

GOOD THROW! It may not be fun for the hippo bean-bag, but your little champ will be bowled over by this game of knock 'em down.

238

BEANBAG BOWLING

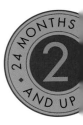

24 MONTHS
2
AND UP

LEARNING HOW TO THROW

WHETHER IT'S PUSHING his fork off his highchair tray or pulling your CDs off the shelves, your toddler delights in putting objects in motion—just to see what will happen (and often to see how you'll react). This is a natural way for toddlers to learn about cause and effect. It's also a good way for them to learn about concepts like gravity and force (not that they need to learn those words—at least not yet). If you're concerned with concepts such as object fragility, however, channel your child's curiosity about crashes into a game the two of you can play.

• Stack several tall, lightweight plastic bottles, cups, or empty cans. Show your child how to throw a beanbag animal to knock them down. (It will be easier for him to do this from a seated position.) Then take turns tossing the beanbags—but don't bother keeping score.

• Vary the activity by using different-size balls or even pincushions—without pins, of course—instead of beanbags. Also try seating your child at varying distances from the stack. He'll soon discover that he needs to throw with more force when he's farther away from his target.

• Once your baby bowler improves his game, ask him to toss the beanbags while standing. And to make the activity more fun for you, encourage him to collect the "pins" he has now learned to blast into all corners of the room!

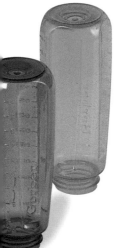

SKILL SPOTLIGHT

Throwing beanbag toys or balls at targets helps toddlers develop their eye-hand coordination and adds to their understanding of cause and effect. This activity also helps your child learn to take turns, a skill he'll work on throughout his early years. Taking turns will be crucial to later social interactions, such as at school, when children need to share to get along with others.

✔	**Balance**
✔	**Cause & Effect**
✔	**Eye-Hand Coordination**
✔	**Gross Motor Skills**

239

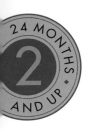

WHO ARE WE?

PLAYING DRESS-UP

SKILLSPOTLIGHT

Most two-year-olds *have strong preferences when it comes to their clothing. And many are determined to dress themselves no matter how long it takes. This activity gives them the license to choose their clothes—and the luxury of dressing themselves at their leisure. Role-playing activities also act as dress rehearsals for social interactions later in life.*

Creative Expression	✔
Imagination	✔
Role-Playing	✔
Social Skills	✔

A PRINCESS, A COWBOY, a movie star . . . children love the costume dramas that dressing up inspires.

SHE STARTED TOYING with your scarves, hats, and soft sweaters when she first learned to grab; she headed for your closets as soon as she could crawl. Now it's time to let her go wild with her own wardrobe. Keep a variety of dress-up items on hand (garage sales and thrift stores are great, often inexpensive sources) and let your child don what she may to be whoever she pleases. Participate in the fun by asking her who she is that day, and invite some of her pals to join in on the act.

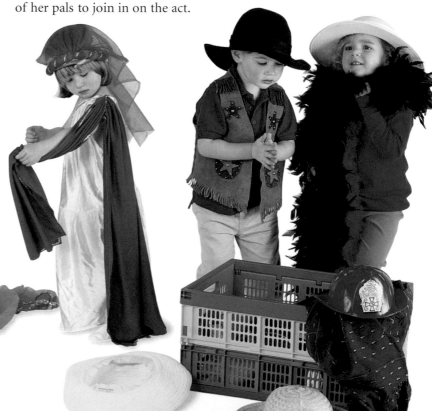

FOOTSTEP FUN

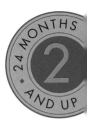

FOLLOWING THE FEET

EVER SINCE your toddler was a baby, he's been fascinated by his own feet, whether it's the taste of his toes or the look of his first walking shoes. Let him get a whole new view of his feet—as well as strong motor skills practice—by teaching him to follow his own footsteps. Trace the outline of the soles of his shoes onto colored pieces of paper. Cut out the foot shapes and glue them onto cardboard squares. Place the squares on the floor to form a path, then encourage your trailblazer to place his feet inside each of the silhouettes.

BY ASKING YOUR LITTLE ONE to follow a path of colorful footprints, you provide stepping stones to greater coordination.

SKILLSPOTLIGHT

Following a trail *of any sort requires good balance and coordination. Changing the shape of the path or the distance between the squares, or asking your toddler to jump on and off the path, further challenges that balancing act. Calling out "red," "blue," and "green" as he steps on those colors also helps him expand his vocabulary.*

✔	**Balance**
✔	**Coordination**
✔	**Eye-Foot Coordination**
✔	**Gross Motor Skills**

IF YOUR CHILD ENJOYS THIS ACTIVITY, *also try Balancing Act, page 226.*

241

BATH TIME FOR BABY

LESSONS IN TENDER, LOVING CARE

SKILLSPOTLIGHT

Two-year-olds are old enough to play "pretend" and to want some measure of control over their world. This activity lets your child be the parent to her "baby" and also allows her to be the little boss—a great way to practice her social skills and exercise her imagination. Learning to hold a soapy doll and wash its tiny body parts also promotes the development of fine motor skills.

Body Awareness	✔
Fine Motor Skills	✔
Imagination	✔
Role-Playing	✔
Social Skills	✔

YOUR LITTLE ONE may already be playing "Mommy" or "Daddy" with her dolls and stuffed animals by rocking them, feeding them, and putting them to bed (see Doll Talk, page 258). She'll love giving her baby dolls baths, too; it's a chance for her to be the caretaker at bath time, to learn about keeping the body clean, and to shower her little friends with love.

• Set up a doll's bathtub by filling a basin—or a baby bathtub if you still have one—with warm, soapy water. Provide towels, washcloths, soap, and bath toys to make it even more realistic.

• Encourage your toddler to test the water's temperature ("Is it too hot for your doll? Is it too cold?") and to be gentle while washing the doll.

• Point out many of the doll's body parts ("That's her nose! And those are her toes!"). This gives your toddler more practice in labeling her own body parts, a favorite activity at this age.

• Pretend the doll is dirty and encourage her to clean behind the doll's ears, between the toes, and in all the other areas that need washing.

• When the doll is clean, let your toddler dry it with a towel. Then remind her to clean one more thing: her dolly's teeth!

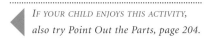

IF YOUR CHILD ENJOYS THIS ACTIVITY, also try Point Out the Parts, page 204.

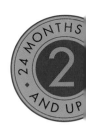

24 MONTHS AND UP

2

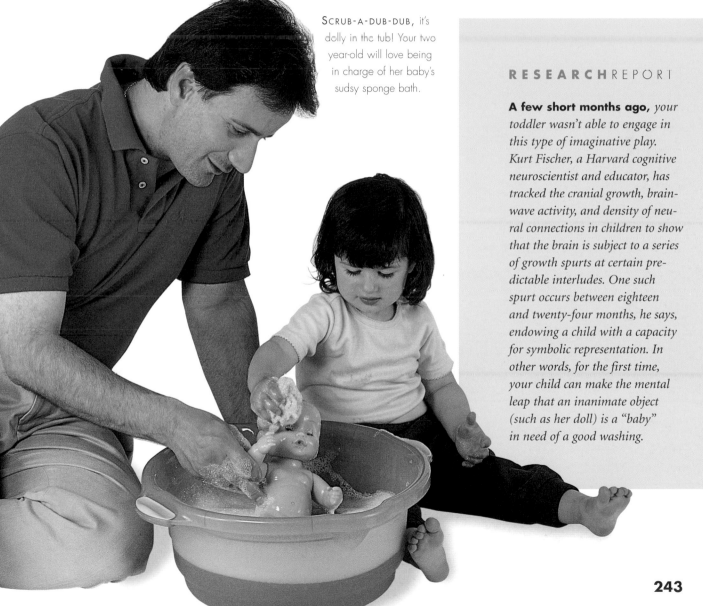

SCRUB-A-DUB-DUB, it's dolly in the tub! Your two year-old will love being in charge of her baby's sudsy sponge bath.

RESEARCH REPORT

A few short months ago, *your toddler wasn't able to engage in this type of imaginative play. Kurt Fischer, a Harvard cognitive neuroscientist and educator, has tracked the cranial growth, brain-wave activity, and density of neural connections in children to show that the brain is subject to a series of growth spurts at certain predictable interludes. One such spurt occurs between eighteen and twenty-four months, he says, endowing a child with a capacity for symbolic representation. In other words, for the first time, your child can make the mental leap that an inanimate object (such as her doll) is a "baby" in need of a good washing.*

243

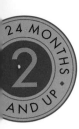

CARE FOR THE ANIMALS

LEARNING TO NURTURE OTHER CREATURES

SKILLSPOTLIGHT

This game of pretend *teaches your child empathy and lets her practice nurturing others. It also helps enhance her awareness of the animal world: birds have wings, tigers have paws, and elephants have trunks. Talking to your child about the ways animals get sick ("The horse ate too much sugar and got a tummy ache") expands her knowledge of them.*

Concept Development	✔
Creative Expression	✔
Fine Motor Skills	✔
Imagination	✔
Role-Playing	✔

SHE LOVES HER ANIMALS (real and stuffed) and she's keen on bandages and the notions of "boo-boo" and "sick." That means she's more than ready to open up a veterinary practice in her own home. It's all pretend, of course, but she'll enjoy learning how to care for her little friends.

• Help your toddler gather her favorite stuffed and plastic animals for this activity. (Make sure the toys are more than 1¾ inches [4.5 cm] in diameter so they won't pose a choking hazard.)

• Provide small boxes or berry baskets for her to use as cages or carriers. She can use napkins or small scarves as blankets.

• Talk to her about the ways in which animals get hurt: how they cut their paws, get bugs in their ears, break their wings, or get stomachaches.

• Help her care for her sick animals by washing and bandaging their wounds, wrapping their broken limbs with gauze, and giving them a clean, quiet place to sleep (plus lots of pats and kind words). A toy doctor's kit will provide helpful instruments for conducting a thorough exam and treatment of her ailing friends, too.

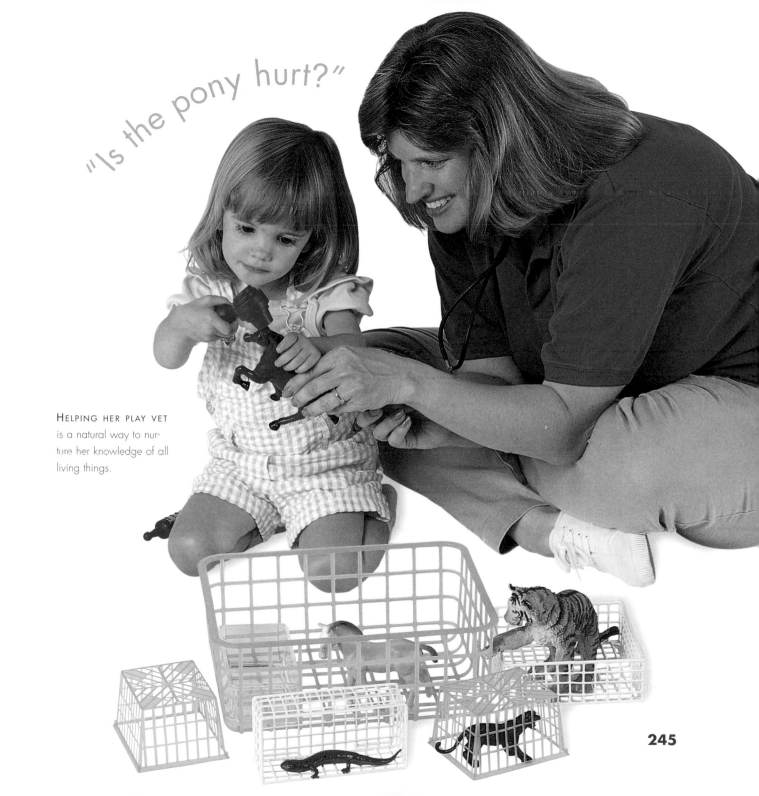

"Is the pony hurt?"

HELPING HER PLAY VET is a natural way to nurture her knowledge of all living things.

THE MANY FORMS OF PLAY

WHILE THIS BOOK emphasizes the playful interactions between a parent and child, it's also important to understand how a toddler will play with peers.

One-year-olds are primarily involved in solitary play, busy as they are exploring a world that is totally new to them. They are curious about other children, however, and often will imitate their actions or the noises they make. As they get a little older, toddlers begin engaging in parallel play—that is, two or more youngsters playing with similar toys or activities side by side but without much interaction, such as building block towers individually. Around age two, as child psychologist Penelope Leach notes in *Your Baby and Child,* "Toddlers increasingly need the companionship of other children." Most adore taking part in play groups, but their ability to share toys or to indulge in mannerly back-and-forth exchanges is still a little precarious. As they approach their third birthday, true cooperative play begins to emerge— two toddlers will build a single block tower together, for example— although there are still likely to be standoffs over treasured playthings or the attention of beloved adults.

These early play encounters plant the seeds for acquiring important attributes such as empathy, self-control, sharing, fairness, and self-esteem, and they help cultivate much-needed tools for dealing with different social situations. As Dr. Benjamin Spock explained in *Baby and Child Care,* "In play, children . . . learn how to get along with other children and adults of different personalities, how to enjoy give-and-take, how to solve conflicts." These are valuable lessons indeed, and ones that parents can foster by providing plenty of opportunities for play with other children. ■

MAGIC CUPS

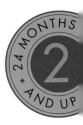

24 MONTHS
2
AND UP

A CHALLENGING MEMORY GAME

THIS TODDLER ACTIVITY is a step up from peekaboo, but operates on the same principle. First it's here, then it's gone, then it's back again—but only if your toddler remembers where it was! To start the game, hide a small toy under one of three cups while your child is watching. Then move the cups around and ask her to guess which one conceals the toy.

• If you've seen street entertainers play this game, you know it can be confusing, even for adults. So don't move the cups too quickly or else she won't be able to keep track of her toy.

SKILLSPOTLIGHT

When your toddler was a baby, you could cover up a toy and she would forget it ever existed. Now she understands that the covered object is still there—this is called object permanence—and she's delighted to find it. By asking her to concentrate on one cup as it moves, you encourage her to recall the toy and you help sharpen her visual memory.

✔ **Problem Solving**

✔ **Visual Memory**

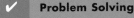
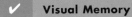
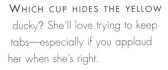

WHICH CUP HIDES THE YELLOW ducky? She'll love trying to keep tabs—especially if you applaud her when she's right.

247

BEEP, BEEP

PLAYING WITH TRUCKS AND CARS

SKILLSPOTLIGHT

Playing with toy cars *is a great way for your toddler to exercise her imagination, and it gives her a chance to imitate a mundane part of your adult world: driving the car. (Don't worry; it's interesting to her!) It also lets her develop the fine motor skills of pushing and pulling and teaches her to discern noises in her everyday world.*

Creative Expression	✔
Fine Motor Skills	✔
Imagination	✔
Language Development	✔

MOST TWO-YEAR-OLDS are fascinated with all things vehicular, ranging from their own strollers to the cars, trucks, and buses on the street to the choo-choo trains they see in picture books. They're especially excited by watching trains and cars enter tunnels and cross bridges. Enhance their wonder (and let them feel like they're finally behind the wheel of one of these grown-up contraptions) by giving them a chance to play with toy trucks, cars, and tunnels.

• Choose a large, colorful toy vehicle, rather than a miniature one, so she can control it more easily.

• Show her how to push the truck along the floor. Teach her all of the noises it makes, including the "beep, beep" of the horn, the "scre-e-e-e-ch" of the tires, and the "vrooom" of the engine. Point out those same sounds to her when you're driving in a real automobile.

248

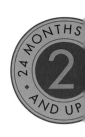

• Cut holes in both ends of a big cardboard box to make a tunnel and show her how to push the truck through it. Talk about the different parts of the truck (steering wheel, tires) and explain why she might need to "turn on" the headlights when she drives into the dark tunnel. Also see if she can guess which part of the truck will come out of the tunnel first—the front or the back.

STEER HER ENERGY into a little creative car play, and watch those motor skills grow.

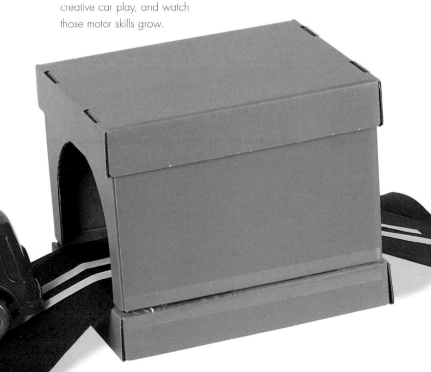

RESEARCH REPORT

A toddler's *apparently boundless enthusiasm for play reflects the fact that she is in a unique and wondrous period of development. A child's brain at age two years consumes twice as much metabolic energy as an adult's, and it possesses twice as many synapses (the connections between nerve cells that convey the electrical impulses needed for all the body's functions, including cognition). "Children are biologically primed for learning during this time," state neurologist Ann Barnet and her co-author and husband, Richard, in their book* The Youngest Minds. *This golden window of opportunity lasts only until age ten or so, when the brain starts to lose the synaptic connections that haven't yet been put to use.*

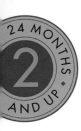

24 MONTHS
2
AND UP

DRIVE THE FIRE TRUCK

A FAVORITE MOVEMENT SONG

to the *tune* of **"Ten Little Indians"**

Hurry, hurry,
drive the fire truck,
make driving motions
hurry, hurry,
drive the fire truck,
hurry, hurry,
drive the fire truck,
ding, ding, ding, ding, ding!
swing hand as if ringing a bell

Hurry, hurry,
climb the ladder,
pretend to climb a ladder
hurry, hurry,
climb the ladder,
hurry, hurry,
climb the ladder,
ding, ding, ding, ding, ding!

Hurry, hurry,
squirt the water,
make squirting motions
hurry, hurry,
squirt the water,
hurry, hurry,
squirt the water,
ding, ding, ding, ding, ding!

Language Development	✔
Role-Playing	✔

RING THE BELL! Sound the alarm! This fast-paced song lets your truck-loving tyke pretend to drive the biggest, brightest rig around—a fire truck—while letting him play one of the most exciting roles in town. Face your child while you teach him the hand gestures, or have him stand with his back to you and help him do them himself. If he is ready to act out the role of a firefighter, find a heavy-duty cardboard box, paint it bright red, and push him around in it as you sing "Hurry, Hurry, Drive the Fire Truck" and he makes the motions.

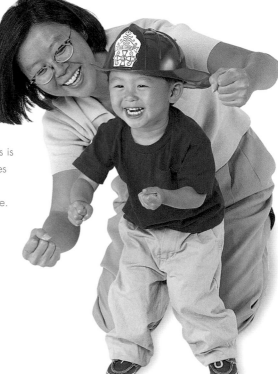

YOUR LITTLE FIRE CHIEF will think this is the hottest game of all when he realizes he gets to drive the truck and put out the imaginary fire with his pretend hose.

PURSE TREASURES

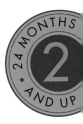

24 MONTHS
2
AND UP

EXPLORING GOODIES IN THE BAG

GRANTED, A TODDLER'S boundless curiosity about the treasures in your purse or briefcase is adorable. But it can lead to chaos (like lost credit cards) and even danger (opened pillboxes and pointy pencils). Safely encourage her explorations by giving her a purse of her very own. Fill it with harmless objects such as those she might find in your bag: a comb, keys, mirror, notepad—even a wallet. Encourage her to find things without looking ("Can you feel the keys in there?"), or ask her to name each item as she pulls it out.

SKILLSPOTLIGHT

You can enrich *your child's understanding of all the items in her purse by explaining the use of each object as she pulls it out ("I'm glad you found the car keys. Now we can drive to the grocery store." Or, "Would you like to comb your hair with that?"). Frequently changing the objects in the purse further challenges your child's identifying skills.*

✔	**Concept Development**
✔	**Language Development**
✔	**Listening Skills**
✔	**Tactile Discrimination**

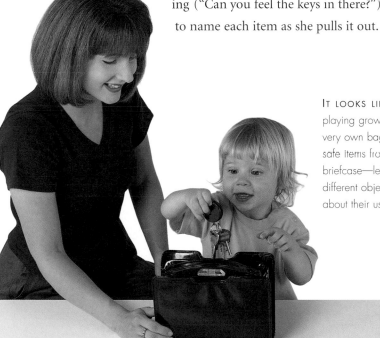

IT LOOKS LIKE she's just playing grown-up. But her very own bag—filled with safe items from a parent's briefcase—lets her explore different objects and learn about their uses.

TOUCH AND TELL

WHAT'S IN THE PILLOWCASE?

SKILLSPOTLIGHT

Learning to describe *the objects in his world helps your child feel some measure of control over them. It also helps him develop his language skills. And adding a tactile component to his developing visual memory helps him understand objects in a three-dimensional way.*

Concept Development	✔
Language Development	✔
Listening Skills	✔
Problem Solving	✔
Tactile Discrimination	✔

YOUR TODDLER is getting into just about everything now, mostly because he's compelled to explore how everything feels, tastes, sounds, looks, and moves. Help him investigate and identify the sensations of different shapes and textures with this variation of the classic show-and-tell game.

• Place a familiar object such as his toy truck, ball, doll, or favorite spoon or cup inside a pillowcase or canvas bag.

• Ask your child to reach into the pillowcase (no peeking!) and feel the object. Then ask him to guess what it is. (He may need to guess more than once.) If he doesn't guess the right answer, tell him what it is before he grows too frustrated.

• Pull out the object and talk to him about its tactile characteristics. Introduce the concepts of hard and soft, fuzzy and smooth.

• Put another toy inside and repeat the exercise. Encourage him to use the words you've introduced as he's guessing what the toy is.

• To vary the game, let him hide a toy in the pillowcase so you can play detective. Also try putting an object inside and asking your young sleuth to guess what it is by feeling it from *outside* the pillowcase.

IF YOUR CHILD ENJOYS THIS ACTIVITY, also try Mystery Sounds, page 257. ▶

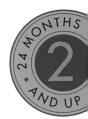

24 MONTHS
2
AND UP

"Look! It's my cup!"

HE'LL GET A FEEL for textures and learn to name those sensations in this hands-on guessing game.

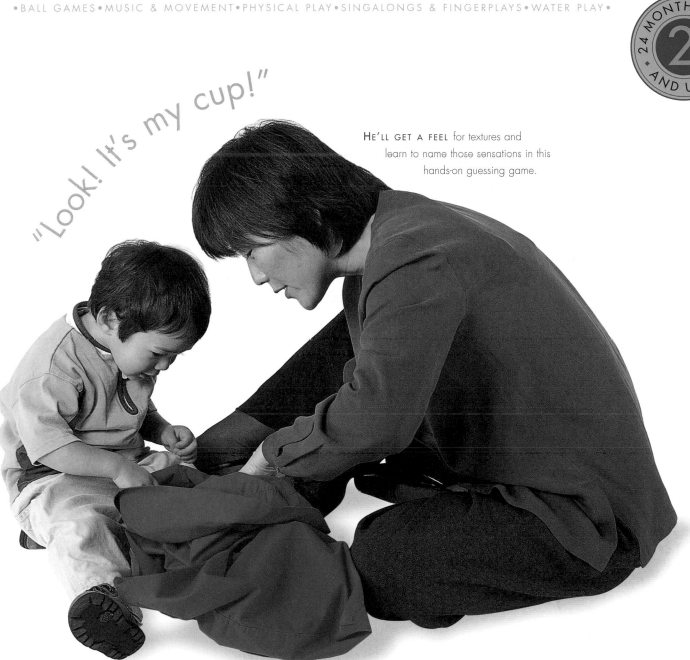

253

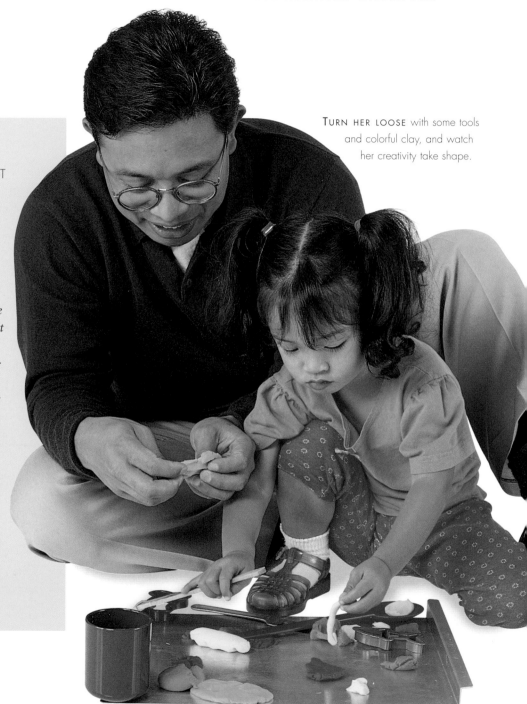

TURN HER LOOSE with some tools and colorful clay, and watch her creativity take shape.

RESEARCH REPORT

Squishing and shaping
modeling clay does more than encourage the budding artist in your child. By allowing her to handle these and other tactile delights, you're helping her develop "knowledge of how the world works and proficiency at using different materials," states Esther Thelen, a psychologist at Indiana University in Bloomington. Educational psychologist Jane Healy is another believer in the benefits of clay, sand, finger paint, and mud, which she says help refine a child's tactile ability. She also offers this advice to fastidious parents: "If you tend to be fanatic about cleanliness, close your eyes and imagine little [neural] dendrites branching inside that muddy head."

254

PLAY WITH CLAY

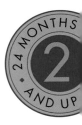

24 MONTHS
2
AND UP

MAKING SHAPES AND SCULPTURES

YOU MAY HAVE FOND MEMORIES of molding clay into silly shapes, and now your two-year is ready to dive into the colorful stuff. Purchase non-toxic modeling clay in any toy store or make a few colorful batches yourself (see the recipe for clay at right). Provide ample working space and a few safe tools, such as a rolling pin, a potato masher, and cookie cutters. Then let the sculpting begin.

• Most young children prefer to experiment with mushing the clay into abstract shapes. Guide her in manipulating the clay by rolling it into a ball and letting her smash it. Or make a long roll that she can tear into pieces and press back together.

• Show your child how simple shapes such as circles, squares, and triangles fit together to make recognizable objects like faces, hats, or trees.

• To store the clay, gather several airtight containers and mark each lid with the same color as the clay it contains. When she's done playing with the clay, ask her to put it in its appropriate container.

MAKING YOUR OWN

Mix 1 cup flour, 1 cup salt, 1 tablespoon cream of tartar, 1 cup water, and 1 tablespoon vegetable oil. Simmer in a pot until clay begins to pull away from the pot's sides. When cool, add 5 drops of food coloring, and knead until smooth.

SKILLSPOTLIGHT

Playing with modeling clay *allows your child to experience shapes and textures in three dimensions. In addition, manipulating the clay stimulates the senses and builds fine motor skills. Help increase your child's vocabulary by teaching her the words for colors, shapes, and textures.*

✔	**Cause & Effect**
✔	**Creative Expression**
✔	**Fine Motor Skills**
✔	**Language Development**
✔	**Sensory Exploration**

◄ *IF YOUR CHILD ENJOYS THIS ACTIVITY, also try Sand Skills, page 192.*

255

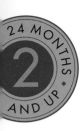

IF THE SHOE FITS

SORTING SHOES OF SEVERAL SIZES

SKILLSPOTLIGHT

This easy-to-assemble *project allows toddlers to practice their early sorting skills and make discoveries about size and materials. As you talk together, your toddler's use of language expands; when you ask him to guess or make assumptions about the different shoes and their uses, you encourage the development of his problem-solving abilities.*

Classifying Skills	✔
Language Development	✔

IF YOUR CHILD ENJOYS THIS ACTIVITY, also try Car Capers, page 280. ▶

MANY CLASSIFYING ACTIVITIES are too frustrating for younger toddlers, but by age two to two-and-a-half, most children are eager to perform a fairly simple sorting task—especially if it involves playing with Mommy's or Daddy's shoes. Put two or three pairs of shoes on a table, separating each shoe from its mate. Choose shoes of distinct sizes and types, such as adult boots, baby shoes, and your fuzzy slippers. Ask your child which shoes match. As he searches for the mate, talk about the types of shoes, whom they fit, and what they're used for. Some toddlers find it easier to sort if they have shoe boxes to put the pairs into.

WHICH SHOES BELONG together? Toddlers can try to successfully combine pairs of family footwear in a challenging game of mix-and-match.

256

MYSTERY SOUNDS

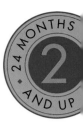

FINDING THE HIDDEN NOISE

WHAT'S THAT SOUND? Where is it coming from? Those are the questions to pose to young detectives in this game of auditory hide-and-seek. Use a long-playing musical toy or other noisemaking item (such as a kitchen timer, clock, or metronome) and hide it on a low shelf or table—or behind a cupboard door. Search together with your child to locate the source of the sound and retrieve the object. As you hunt, ask your toddler to try to guess what toy or object is making the mysterious sound.

SKILLSPOTLIGHT

Young children love *guessing games, and this one helps fine-tune auditory skills. Locating an object by listening to a sound teaches your toddler to find an answer through the process of elimination—and it reinforces the notion that a thoughtful guess is part of the learning process.*

USING HER EARS to find the source of a sound may become a young sleuth's favorite guessing game.

✔ **Listening Skills**

✔ **Problem Solving**

IF YOUR CHILD ENJOYS THIS ACTIVITY, also try Mighty Megaphones, page 283.

257

DOLL TALK

LEARNING TO NURTURE

SKILLSPOTLIGHT

Toddlers learn *to be kind to others—whether they are animals or people—often by watching their parents' behavior. Participating in your child's doll (or animal) play gives you the opportunity to model appropriate words and gestures. It also gives her a chance to feel confident about her emerging feelings of gentleness and love.*

Creative Expression	✔
Fine Motor Skills	✔
Imagination	✔
Listening Skills	✔
Social Skills	✔

SEEING A TODDLER'S TENDERNESS toward the dolls, teddies, and other cuddlies in her world is truly touching. Her enthusiasm, however, may sometimes make her a bit too rough—especially with animals or other children. You can help refine her nurturing abilities by interacting with your child as she plays with her pretend friends.

• Give your child a favorite doll or stuffed animal to hold. Suggest that she gently brush the doll's hair or rock it in her arms. Or help her learn to pat animals by showing her how on a plush toy.

• Tell her that the doll or teddy bear is cold, and ask her to comfort it by putting shoes and socks and warm clothes on the doll (she may need help with snaps and buttons) or by covering a plush toy with a blanket.

• Then suggest that she feed her doll or pet because it hasn't eaten all day and must be quite hungry. She can offer it pretend food, or give her a spoon and a small dish of cereal or raisins, which are easy to clean up.

• Join your child in singing a favorite lullaby to her charge while helping her rock it to sleep, then ask her to gently tuck it into bed.

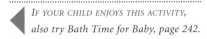

IF YOUR CHILD ENJOYS THIS ACTIVITY, also try Bath Time for Baby, page 242.

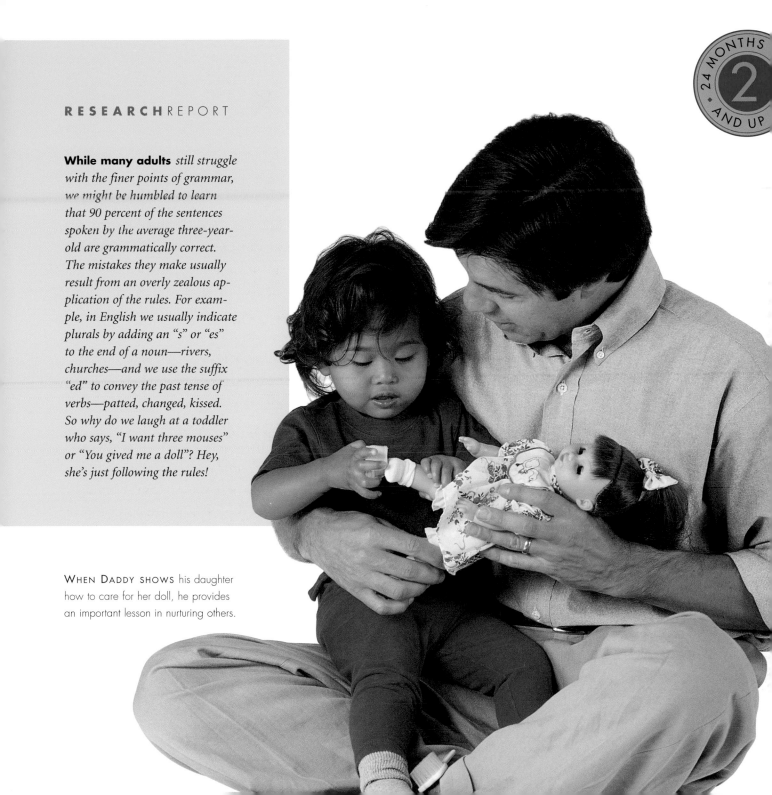

RESEARCH REPORT

While many adults *still struggle with the finer points of grammar, we might be humbled to learn that 90 percent of the sentences spoken by the average three-year-old are grammatically correct. The mistakes they make usually result from an overly zealous application of the rules. For example, in English we usually indicate plurals by adding an "s" or "es" to the end of a noun—rivers, churches—and we use the suffix "ed" to convey the past tense of verbs—patted, changed, kissed. So why do we laugh at a toddler who says, "I want three mouses" or "You gave me a doll"? Hey, she's just following the rules!*

WHEN DADDY SHOWS his daughter how to care for her doll, he provides an important lesson in nurturing others.

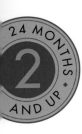

COLOR CLUSTERS

A SORTING, SPINNING, AND COUNTING ACTIVITY

SKILLSPOTLIGHT

This elementary abacus *enhances your toddler's ability to categorize objects by helping him identify different colors and sizes. It also provides a great opportunity to introduce your child to comparison words, such as big, bigger, and biggest.*

COLORFUL, REVOLVING BALLS on a rope are sure to catch toddlers' eyes, as they love both bright colors and spinning motions. But besides being fun, this activity can teach your little one some pretty big concepts. To start, thread a thin rope through a group of colored balls with holes (available at many toy stores) and tie the rope firmly between two chairs. Show your toddler how to spin the balls and slide them from one end of the rope to the other. Then ask him to spin only a particular color or only the large balls.

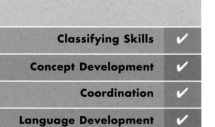

MAKING THE BRIGHT BALLS spin quickly is fun, but so is learning to identify blue and red, large and small, and more and less.

Classifying Skills	✔
Concept Development	✔
Coordination	✔
Language Development	✔

WATER TARGETS

30 MONTHS
2½
AND UP

MAKING A SPLASH LANDING

WATER, BALLS, THROWING, SPLASHING — the elements in this activity may get you and your toddler a bit wet, but she'll enjoy it so much you won't mind. Find two or three big plastic bowls or pots and fill them halfway with water. Gather an assortment of small balls, preferably ones that float (plastic or tennis balls work well). Ask your child to throw the balls into the water targets. Count how many balls she can land inside each bowl and be sure to applaud every attempt, even when she misses. As she gets better at this activity, increase the challenge by having her stand farther away from the bowls.

YOUR LITTLE PITCHER makes a big splash when she gets the ball in—and she fine-tunes her coordination skills as she aims for her water targets.

SKILLSPOTLIGHT

This water game *helps build your toddler's eye-hand coordination and gross motor skills. The activity is also a fun way to introduce your toddler to counting ("That's one in, two in. Look! Three balls in the water!").*

✔	**Coordination**
✔	**Counting Concepts**
✔	**Eye-Hand Coordination**
✔	**Gross Motor Skills**

IF YOUR CHILD ENJOYS THIS ACTIVITY, also try Up It Goes!, page 266.

261

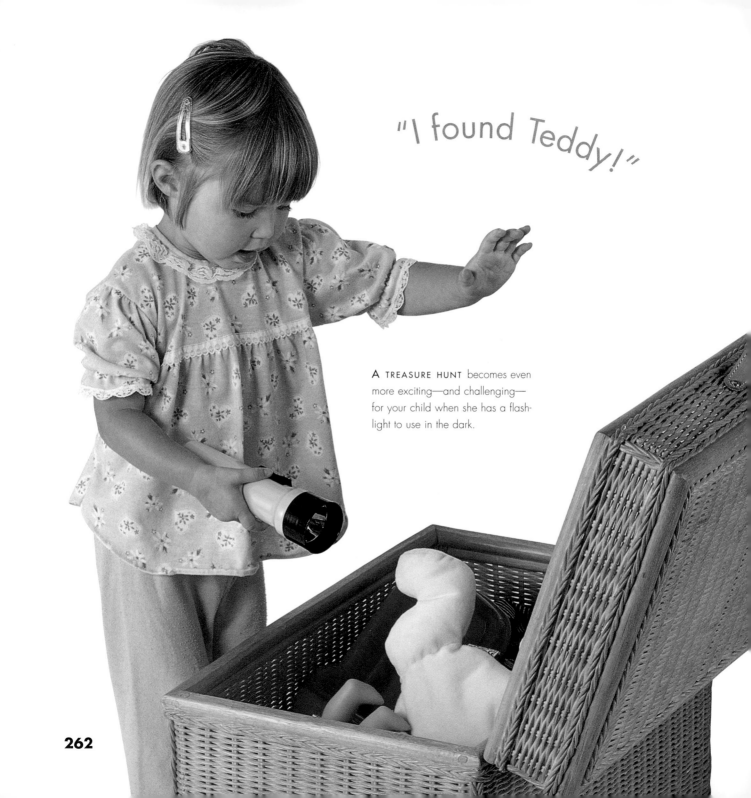

"I found Teddy!"

A TREASURE HUNT becomes even more exciting—and challenging—for your child when she has a flashlight to use in the dark.

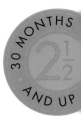

FLASHLIGHT FUN

FINDING HIDDEN TOYS IN THE DARK

WIELDING A FLASHLIGHT sparks wonder in most toddlers: the tool gives them control over the dark and changes the look of everything around them.

• Start this activity in the evening by hiding one of your child's favorite items, such as a doll, a book, or her beloved teddy bear. Limit the hunting area to one or two rooms so it won't be too difficult for her to find the hidden treasure.

• Tell your toddler what to look for, turn off (or just dim) the lights, and hand her a lightweight flashlight. (You may have to show her how to use it at first.) Be sure to equip yourself with a flashlight too, so you can join in the fun.

• Keep the game lively and silly by providing her with several clues: "You're getting warmer, warmer, warmer! Oops! Now you're cooling down." If she starts to get a little frustrated, use the beam of your own flashlight to help guide her to the hiding place.

• This is an ideal activity for a toddler to play with an older sibling or a group of kids, because you can hide several objects at one time—some in harder places than others—and it's a great spectacle to watch the children waving their bright beams of light at one another.

IF YOUR CHILD ENJOYS THIS ACTIVITY, also try Purse Treasures, page 251.

SKILL SPOTLIGHT

Searching for an object *presents a problem that your child has to concentrate on in order to solve. The first step for her, of course, is to listen to your description of the hidden object, which involves comprehension skills. Then she has to think about places that aren't immediately visible to her—a type of abstract thinking that is a big step for a young child. This nighttime game may also allay fears and negative feelings that children often have about darkness.*

✔	**Listening Skills**
✔	**Problem Solving**
✔	**Social Skills**
✔	**Visual Memory**

NATURE VS. NURTURE

DO WE COME into this world imprinted with immutable abilities, foibles, and personality traits? Or are we born blank slates, waiting for the environment to etch its effect on our psyches? For many scientists, the new influx of brain research has settled the age-old question of nature versus nurture once and for all. The verdict? It's a draw.

For decades, behavioral studies have suggested that some traits, such as aggressiveness, shyness, and a willingness to take risks, have a genetic origin. But just when Mother Nature seemed to be the winner in the ancient debate, neurologists demonstrated how unfinished the human brain is at birth and how environmental factors exert powerful influences on a person's disposition—even altering the shape of the brain in some cases. Scientists in the 1990s have reconciled these two competing forces by concluding that while people are indeed born with certain tendencies and abilities, the degree to which those traits are manifested depends a great deal on what people are exposed to, especially during early childhood. As neurologist Ann Barnet states in her book *The Youngest Minds,* "Current estimates made by behavioral geneticists for the relative influence of heritable factors and environment are about 50-50."

This split has important implications for parents. For one thing, it means that if a child is innately inclined to some particular behavior, parents can work with her to overcome that tendency—helping her become more outgoing if she's shy, for example, or instilling a little impulse control if she's inclined to take too many risks. Conversely, it also suggests that even if a child is born with certain gifts, such as outstanding musical or artistic ability, those talents might never be realized if there's no opportunity for them to flourish. ■

264

HEY MR. JUMPING JACK

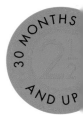

WIGGLE AND SHAKE TO A BEAT

GET YOUR LITTLE ONE giggling and wiggling to this upbeat chant that encourages rhythm and movement. Hold your child on your lap, facing you, and then tap out a rhythm with your feet as you say the words. When Mr. Jumping Jack jumps high, lift your toddler up high; when he jumps low, give him just a little lift. For the second verse, wiggle your child gently as you lift him high and low (hard shaking is dangerous). Add your own verses and movements—clapping, flapping, and waving, for example. And when your toddler is steady on his feet, let him jump and wiggle on his own as you chant and clap.

SECURE in Mommy's arms, your toddler will laugh out loud as he soars up and down to the words of this cheery chant.

Hey Mr. Jumping Jack,
a funny old man,
he jumps and he jumps
whenever he can.
He jumps way up high,
he jumps way down low,
and he jumps and he jumps
wherever he goes.

Come on and jump!

Hey Mr. Jumping Jack,
a funny old man,
he wiggles and he wiggles
whenever he can.
He wiggles way up high,
he wiggles way down low,
and he wiggles and he wiggles
wherever he goes.

Come on and wiggle!

| ✔ | **Listening Skills** |
| ✔ | **Rhythm Exploration** |

IF YOUR CHILD ENJOYS THIS ACTIVITY,
also try Teddy Bear Tunes, page 270.

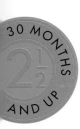

30 MONTHS
2½
AND UP

UP IT GOES!

A BALL-AND-PARACHUTE GAME

SKILL SPOTLIGHT

This game challenges *your toddler's coordination and visual acuity. To toss the ball straight up, she has to try to raise the blanket in sync with you. To catch it squarely on the blanket, she needs to keep her eye on the ball as it comes back down. This activity takes planning and some sense of cooperation with her partner— and she may need to practice it several times before she catches on.*

Cause & Effect	✔
Eye-Foot Coordination	✔
Eye-Hand Coordination	✔

◀ *IF YOUR CHILD ENJOYS THIS ACTIVITY, also try Beach-Ball Catch, page 225.*

SUMMER OR WINTER, indoors or out, a beach ball—or another very lightweight ball—makes for all kinds of merriment when there's a toddler around. To play this game, you and your child hold opposite ends of a blanket or parachute. Place a beach ball in the center and toss it up in the air, catching it in the parachute as it comes down again. Start with gentle tosses so the ball doesn't go too high. As your toddler's coordination improves, bounce the ball higher and higher.

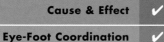

SHE FOLLOWS the bouncing ball in this delightful game that exercises her ability to coordinate muscle movements with motion.

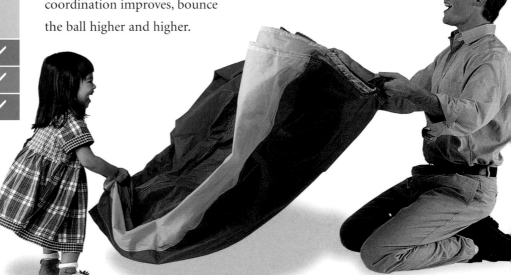

PAPER PUZZLE

FITTING THE BIG PIECES TOGETHER

IF YOUR CHILD is already happily playing with wooden puzzles and shape sorters, it might be a prime time to enhance his ability to understand and organize shapes spatially by creating an elementary puzzle for him. Find an engaging, colorful picture of something your toddler might like—an animal, a truck, a baby, or a favorite food, for instance. (Magazines are rich sources for large photographs.) Then glue the image onto a letter-size piece of paper or cardboard. Cut the picture into four large sections. Now help him rearrange the pieces to put the picture back together again. When he's figured that out, you can make the puzzle more difficult by cutting it into smaller pieces.

PUTTING TWO AND TWO together to make a butterfly is just the kind of puzzle your toddler is now ready to tackle.

SKILL SPOTLIGHT

This activity allows *your toddler to exercise his understanding of spatial relations. It also lets him create—and recreate—a picture that he likes (a test of his visual memory skills), which will give him the confidence to eventually try more difficult puzzles.*

✔	**Concept Development**
✔	**Problem Solving**
✔	**Size & Shape Discrimination**
✔	**Visual Discrimination**
✔	**Visual Memory**

267

COMMON SCENTS

AN ODYSSEY OF ODORS

SHE SMILES WHEN EATING a cookie and purses her little lips at the sight of broccoli, so you know she has a discriminating palate. But how's her sense of smell? Help her learn to match aroma to food with this simple sniffing game.

• Gather several strongly scented foods that your child already knows, such as chocolate-chip cookies, oranges, and onions.

• Blindfold her with a handkerchief or scarf (or just cover her eyes with your hand). Then ask her to take a big sniff (no peeking!) and guess what the smells are. After she guesses, let her taste the food to better match different smells with different tastes.

• As she masters this activity, choose foods with more subtle aromas. For example, see if she can distinguish between a peach and an apple, a cookie and a cake, or a lemon and an orange.

• You can do this with outside smells, too. Test her olfactory memory on flowers, pine needles, damp dirt, and common herbs.

• Or ask your toddler to identify smells she might encounter in the neighborhood, such as fresh bread in a bakery, barbecued chicken in a restaurant, or summer fruits at a sidewalk stand.

IF YOUR CHILD ENJOYS THIS ACTIVITY, also try Touch and Tell, page 252.

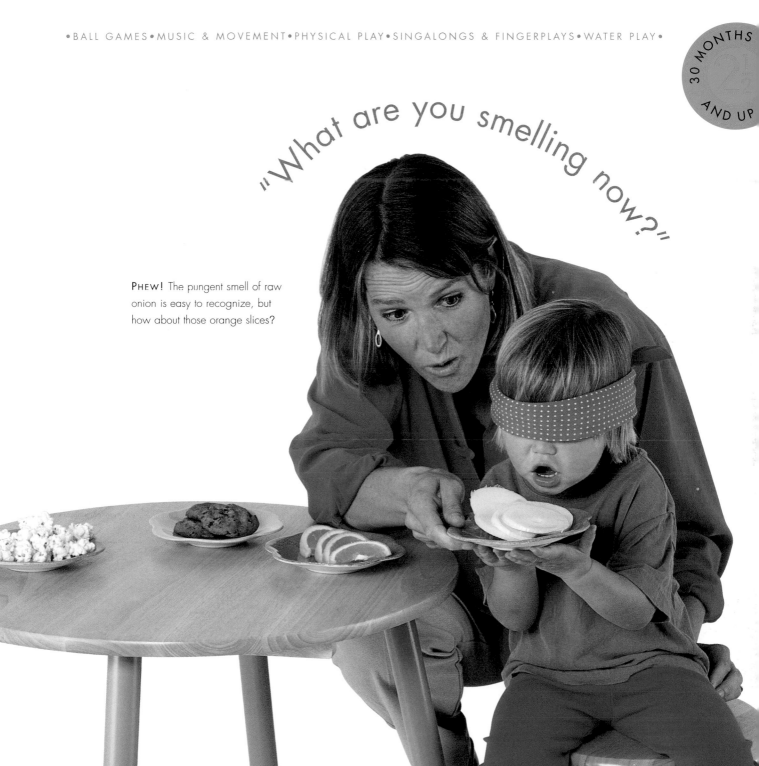

30 MONTHS AND UP

"What are you smelling now?"

PHEW! The pungent smell of raw onion is easy to recognize, but how about those orange slices?

TEDDY BEAR TUNES

TODDLERS LOVE teddy bears—and the rhythm and repetition of these teddy tunes give them a timeless appeal. With your child on your knee, bounce her gently to the beat of these songs while encouraging her to sing along—or join her (and her plush toys) in acting out the appropriate gestures.

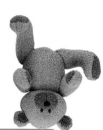

THE BEAR

to the tune of **"For He's a Jolly Good Fellow"**

**The bear went over the mountain,
the bear went over the mountain,
the bear went over the mountain,
to see what she could see.**

**To see what she could see,
To see what she could see.**

**The bear went over the mountain,
the bear went over the mountain,
the bear went over the mountain,
to see what she could see.**

TEDDY BEAR, TEDDY BEAR

Teddy bear, teddy bear, turn around.
*turn around in circles with your child
as you teach her this chant*

**Teddy bear, teddy bear,
touch the ground.**
touch the floor

**Teddy bear, teddy bear,
show your shoe.**
bring one foot forward

**Teddy bear, teddy bear,
crawl right through.**
let your child crawl between your legs

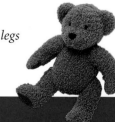

MARCHING BEARS

 to the *tune* of **"The Saints Go Marching In"**

**Oh when the bears
go marching in,
oh when the bears go marching in,
oh, how I want to be a big teddy,
when the bears go marching in.**
march in place with your child

**Oh when the bears
go jumping in,
oh when the bears go jumping in,
oh, how I want to be a big teddy,
when the bears go jumping in.**
jump up and down

**Oh when the bears
go wiggling in . . .**
wiggle your body

**Oh when the bears
go tiptoeing in . . .**
tiptoe around the room

**Oh when the bears
go hopping in . . .**
hop up and down

BEARS ARE SLEEPING

 to the *tune* of **"Frère Jacques"**

**Bears are sleeping,
bears are sleeping,
in their caves, in their caves.
Waiting for the springtime,
waiting for the springtime.
Shh! Shh! Shh!
Shh! Shh! Shh!**

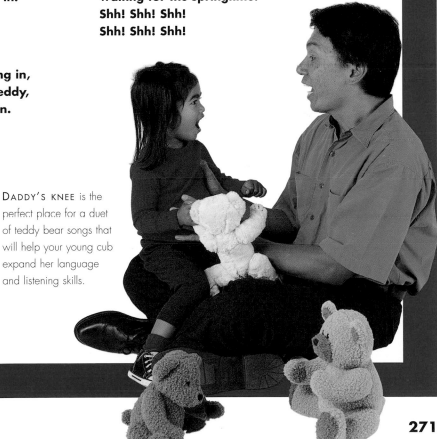

DADDY'S KNEE is the perfect place for a duet of teddy bear songs that will help your young cub expand her language and listening skills.

271

ON TARGET!

LANDING ON THE MARK

SKILL SPOTLIGHT

The act of jumping *works muscles on both sides of the body, thereby increasing bilateral coordination. This provides a good counterpoint to activities, such as rolling a ball, that work only one side of the body. Jumping also improves eye-foot coordination and balance in an older toddler: she needs to put her feet where she's looking and then she has to try to stay upright after landing.*

Balance	✔
Eye-Foot Coordination	✔
Gross Motor Skills	✔
Spatial Awareness	✔

JUMPING IS A BIG ACCOMPLISHMENT for toddlers, one that takes coordination, strength, and a dash of courage. It's also a skill that thrills: just observe the joy on your puddle jumper's face after leaping into a big pool of rainwater. You can help improve her form and aim and boost her confidence by setting up jumping target practice using a stable stool, block, or another safe launching pad that won't slide out from beneath her.

• Use a large piece of construction paper or a colored paper plate as a target, and adhere it to the ground with strong packaging tape so it won't slip when she lands. Encourage your child to jump directly onto the target—this will likely take some practice. Applaud every attempt.

• As your toddler's abilities increase, make the target smaller. Or ask her to jump from a greater (though still safe) height.

• Some children may be nervous about bounding into space this way. Soothe her fears by showing her how to jump—or hold her hand as she makes the leap. Once she becomes confident in her jumping abilities, she'll want to aim for the target again and again.

IF YOUR CHILD ENJOYS THIS ACTIVITY, *also try Turn Around, page 277.*

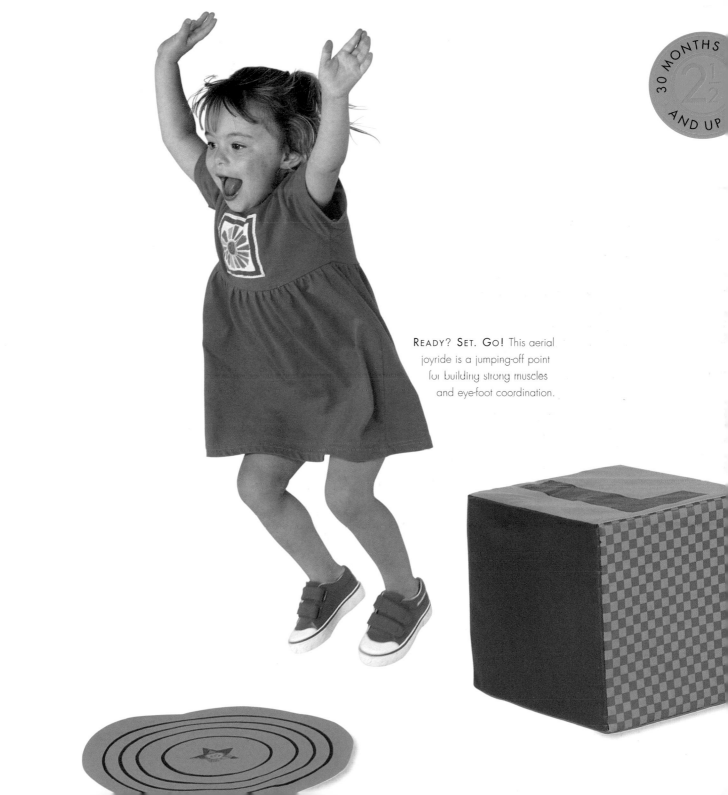

READY? SET. GO! This aerial joyride is a jumping-off point for building strong muscles and eye-foot coordination.

RESEARCH REPORT

Enriching experiences *such as assembling a collage provide children with creative stimulation that is vital to their development. Researchers at Baylor College of Medicine in Houston, Texas, found that children deprived of playthings and playmates (as well as nurturing caregivers) have brains 20 to 30 percent smaller than normal. To provide the proper stimulation, parents needn't stock up on all sorts of techno-gadgets and expensive toys; an extensive study conducted at the University of Alabama found that the basics, such as art supplies, blocks, and puzzles, were still the best at promoting cognitive and physical development.*

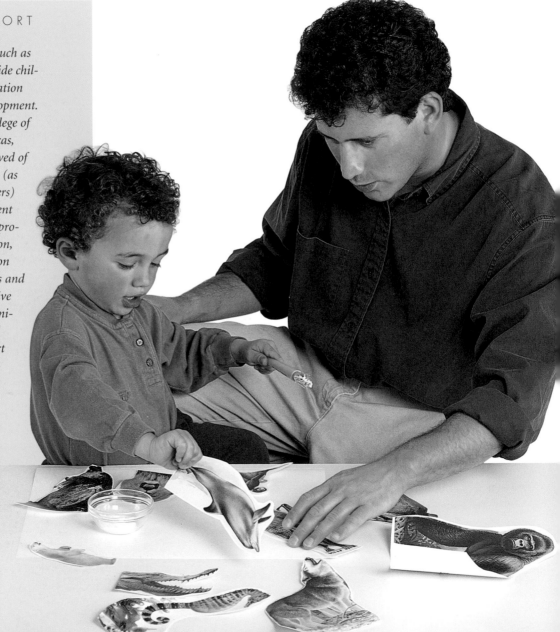

274

COLORFUL COLLAGES

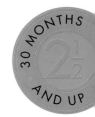

30 MONTHS
2½
AND UP

COLLECTING INTRIGUING IMAGES

EVEN AT THIS EARLY AGE, your child has distinct likes and dislikes. He may be fascinated by music, for instance, or animals, or occupations such as gardening and cooking. Encourage him to enjoy his natural interests by helping him create a fun collage made from related pictures.

• Collect colorful pictures of his current passion from magazines, newspapers, or even junk mail, and place them in a big basket or bowl.

• Invite your toddler to look through them and talk about the pictures as he picks them up. Ask him to name the objects he sees (for example, a violin, a whale, a flower, a blueberry muffin).

• Ask him to pick out his favorite pictures. Place them on a large sheet of heavyweight paper, such as construction paper.

• Using children's (nontoxic) glue, show him how to put glue onto the back of a picture, then press it down onto the paper to make a collage.

• Once you both have completed the collage, hang it someplace visible, such as in his bedroom, on the refrigerator, or even in the front hallway. Children's art should be seen—not hidden!

SKILL SPOTLIGHT

Letting your child *select his own pictures for a collage gives him a chance to practice expressing his preferences. Encouraging him to discuss the images is a way to help build his vocabulary. And teaching him to handle glue and sticky pieces of paper aids him in developing his fine motor skills.*

✔ **Creative Expression**

✔ **Fine Motor Skills**

✔ **Language Development**

✔ **Visual Discrimination**

"I LIKE DOLPHINS because they live in the ocean." Learn more about your child while creating a work of art that reflects his personality and preferences.

IF YOUR CHILD ENJOYS THIS ACTIVITY, also try Paper Puzzle, page 267.

275

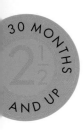

BEAUTIFUL BOX

DECORATING A TOY CHEST

SKILLSPOTLIGHT

This project nurtures *a toddler's creative spirit while encouraging her to express herself on something other than flat paper. By combining drawing, painting, coloring, and collage, it introduces her to several different artistic media. This activity also polishes fine motor skills and can help develop communication skills, especially if parents engage their children in a discussion as they're decorating the box together.*

Creative Expression	✔
Fine Motor Skills	✔
Social Skills	✔

◀ *IF YOUR CHILD ENJOYS THIS ACTIVITY, also try Play With Clay, page 254.*

TAKE YOUR TODDLER'S natural (albeit elementary) artistic abilities to a new dimension by helping her decorate a box for her toy treasures. Use a plain or colored cardboard box (or cover a printed box with white paper). Give your child non-permanent markers and crayons for drawing lines and circles on the box; help her glue glitter, ribbons, or paper cutouts on it as well. You can start with a theme (such as the sea) and encourage her to elaborate on that topic with stickers of waves, fish, boats, and beach balls. When she's done, write her name on her special box.

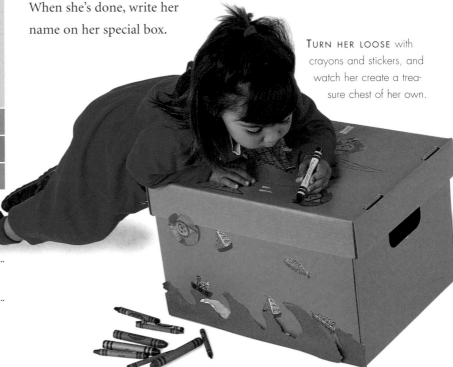

TURN HER LOOSE with crayons and stickers, and watch her create a treasure chest of her own.

276

TURN AROUND

30 MONTHS
2½
AND UP

A SING-WHILE-YOU-SPIN SONG

THIS MOVE-YOUR-BODY SONG is a fun way to combine singing with some vigorous exercise. Sing "Turn Around" a few times, following the instructions in the lyrics, and exaggerate your actions—for example, leap high in the air when you sing, "Up we go!" Your little jumping bean will love imitating you; at the same time he'll develop better body control and gross motor skills. Acting out the lyrics also improves your child's comprehension of up and down and high and low.

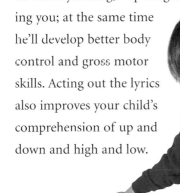

MOVING TO THE MUSIC helps his body confidence grow by leaps and bounds.

 to the *tune* of **"Frère Jacques"**

Perform the actions as indicated by the lyrics; do them slowly until your child understands all the movements.

**Turn around,
turn around,
touch your toes,
touch your toes.**

**Do a little jumping,
do a little jumping.**

Squat real low.

Up we go!

✔ **Balance**

✔ **Coordination**

✔ **Gross Motor Skills**

IF YOUR CHILD ENJOYS THIS ACTIVITY, also try Head to Toes, page 232.

277

MINI MIMES

ACTING OUT A TEA PARTY

SHE WANTS TO DO just about everything you do, right? Let her participate in grown-up activities by miming all sorts of fun things along with you.

• Try having a tea party—with no tea set. Act out pouring the tea, passing the plate of cookies, and drinking and eating. Be sure to say "Please," "Thank you," and "Mmm . . . this is delicious!" That helps her to learn good manners, and the conversation brings the party to life.

• Bake a cake together without any pans or ingredients. Crack the pretend eggs, mix in the flour, and pour the batter into a pan. Dust the flour off your hands when you're all done—and then treat yourselves to a big piece of scrumptious cake.

• Other activities to act out include flying an airplane, cleaning up the house, or galloping around on a horse.

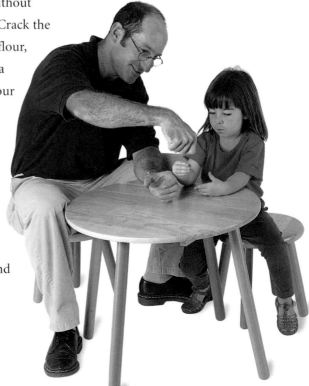

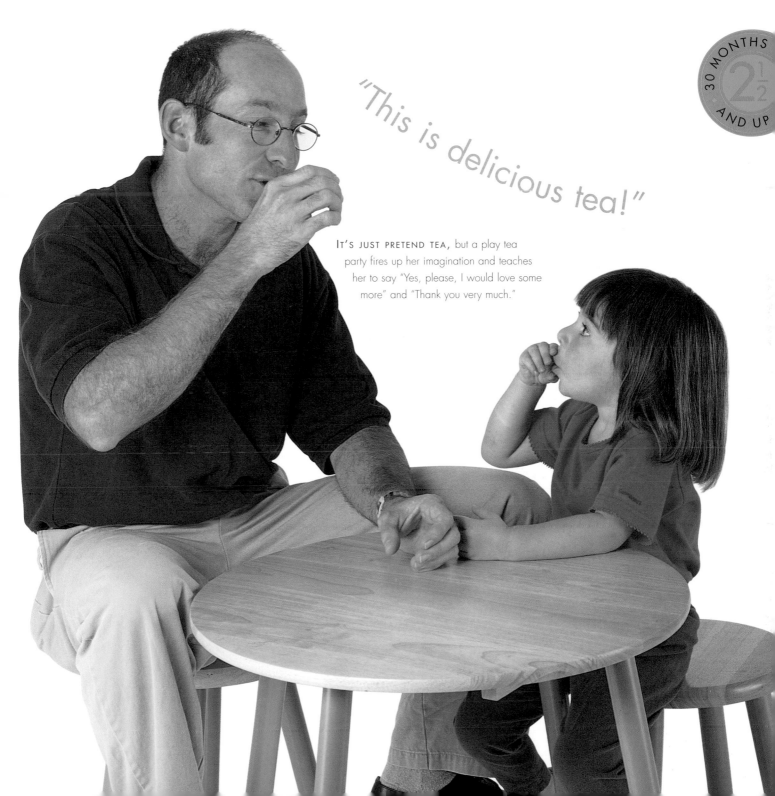

"This is delicious tea!"

IT'S JUST PRETEND TEA, but a play tea party fires up her imagination and teaches her to say "Yes, please, I would love some more" and "Thank you very much."

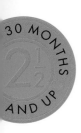

CAR CAPERS

A MATCHING-COLORS GAME

SKILLSPOTLIGHT

Successfully matching colors
helps train a toddler's eye to com-
pare and contrast different
objects. It also engages his mind
by making him link up two very
different items that share one
common characteristic (in this
case, color). And repeating the
names of the colors aloud as he
matches the car to the paper helps
strengthen his vocabulary.

Classifying Skills	✔
Concept Development	✔
Problem Solving	✔
Visual Discrimination	✔

MOST TWO-YEAR-OLDS are fascinated by colors and are compelled to identify them. This activity takes advantage of your child's interest in colors while strengthening his ability to recognize them. Find some paper that matches the colors of the cars or trucks and other vehicles in his toy collection. Call out the color of the paper as you lay it on the floor. Park a car of the same color on each piece of paper (red car on red paper, yellow truck on yellow paper, for example). Then mix them up and ask your child to "drive" the vehicles onto their correct, color-coded parking spots.

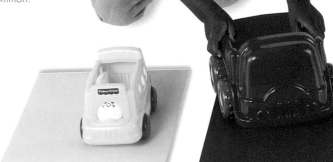

FINDING THE RIGHT parking place helps him begin to recognize what two different objects have in common.

IF YOUR CHILD ENJOYS THIS ACTIVITY, also try Leaf Lineup, page 289. ▶

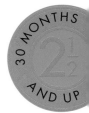

FUNNY FACES

TALKING ABOUT FEELINGS

YOUR TODDLER is just beginning to understand the concept of emotions—that he feels happy sometimes and perhaps angry or sad at other times. Wooden spoon puppets can help him identify and express his feelings in appropriate ways. Draw a happy face, a sad face, and a mad face on three wooden spoons. You can also dress them up with construction paper: add "hair," a "mustache," or a bow tie. Have the spoons express their "feelings" to your child or to each other. The happy-face spoon can say, "Oh boy! I'm going to the zoo today!" And the mad face can say, "No! I don't want to wear my coat!" Encourage your child to express his emotions, too.

SKILLSPOTLIGHT

Up until a few months ago, *your child probably had only one way of expressing "difficult" feelings: crying. Now he's getting old enough to say when he's happy, sad, or mad. Spoon puppets can model such conversations for him. Notice how he's getting rather demanding these days? Let the happy-face spoon show him how to politely ask for a glass of water instead of insisting on one.*

✔	**Concept Development**
✔	**Creative Expression**
✔	**Language Development**
✔	**Social Skills**

IT'S OFTEN EASIER for children to express themselves through play—so let your toddler practice talking about feelings with spoon puppets.

TODDLER TALK

JUST AS CHILDREN seem to come into this world hard-wired to learn language, parents instinctively do much to promote this vital skill. In countless cultures around the world, for example, they naturally speak to their babies and toddlers in a high-pitched, repetitive, singsong voice that linguists have dubbed "parentese." It is now universally accepted that this melodic, pared-down speech speeds up a child's ability to connect words with the objects they represent and offers the simplified syntax and repetition she needs to learn many of the rules of grammar.

Parents can do several other things to help. As the Research Report on page 183 highlights, the simple act of talking to your child—a lot—even before she is capable of talking back is critical to building her vocabulary. "Tell your baby and toddler everything you can think of," advise Dr. Marian Diamond and Janet Hopson in *Magic Trees of the Mind*. "Bathe your child with spoken language." Having a toddler point to the pictures in a book, echo some of your words, or add sound effects keeps her engaged and helps stretch her attention span.

Introducing new words in a real-life, emotional context also is important—a child picks up the meaning of "later" and "now" much more quickly when the words are linked to the time that she's going to get a favorite snack or go to the park. Feeding her boundless interest in knowing the names of everything she sees in the house, passes in the car, or spots in the local market is key to fulfilling her labeling instinct, which is going full throttle as she approaches her second birthday. Finally, keep in mind the benefits of hands-on parenting: cuddling a child as you talk or read together adds a dimension of loving, physical contact that also seems to hasten language acquisition. ■

282

MIGHTY MEGAPHONES

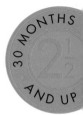

FUN WITH BOOMING VOICES

SHE'S SPEAKING quite well now, and her vocalizations often range from a murmur (when she's "reading" to her teddy bear) to a shriek (when it's time to leave the playground). You can expand her verbal and auditory skills even further with a paper megaphone. Just roll up a big sheet of thick paper and show her how talking into the small end of the cone can change the tone, direction, and volume of her voice. Take turns talking loudly and softly with the megaphone, or use it for amplifying songs and silly sounds.

NOW HEAR THIS: She'll love expanding her vocal range with this improvised amplifier.

SKILLSPOTLIGHT

Children naturally explore *their senses during play, but this activity encourages a focused exploration of listening and making sounds. Toddlers are also natural performers (hence the physical frenzy that often greets guests). Improvising with this megaphone helps turn up the volume on their creativity.*

✔ **Cause & Effect**

✔ **Creative Expression**

✔ **Listening Skills**

✔ **Sensory Exploration**

283

RIBBON RINGS

FANCY DANCING WITH FLYING STREAMERS

SKILL SPOTLIGHT

When you add *ribbon rings to a toddler's dance session, she'll become more aware of how she's moving her arms and body to make the ribbons float in different ways. This helps her develop gross motor skills and coordination. The rings also encourage rhythm exploration as well as creativity.*

Body Awareness	✔
Coordination	✔
Creative Movement	✔
Gross Motor Skills	✔
Rhythm Exploration	✔

284

SHE ALREADY LOVES to dance, but adding rings of colorful, floating ribbon will make her spinning and twirling all the more magical—and fun.

• Purchase a pair of ribbon rings (sold at specialty toy stores) or make your own by buying a dozen fabric ribbons or cutting fabric or old sheets into strips that are between 12 and 25 inches (30 to 64 cm) in length. Securely tie one end of each of the ribbons or strips around small embroidery rings or canning rims.

• Talk to your child about the different colors of the ribbons and ask her to show you which one is her favorite.

• Show her how to incorporate the rings into her dance routine: wave them up and down and swing them from side to side.

• Play dancing music you both enjoy, and join your toddler as she swings to the beat and makes the ribbons float and twirl.

• Put the rings on the floor and dance around them, or pass the rings back and forth as you sashay past each other. Encourage her to improvise with her pretty new props.

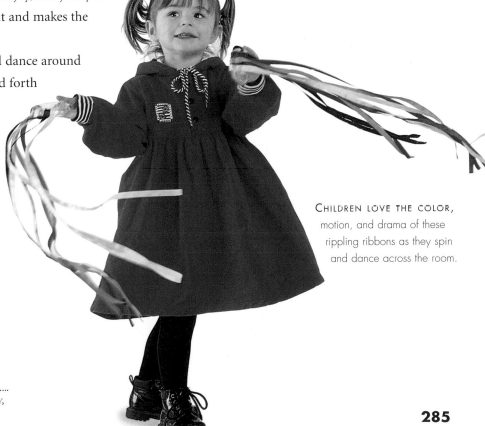

CHILDREN LOVE THE COLOR, motion, and drama of these rippling ribbons as they spin and dance across the room.

◀ *IF YOUR CHILD ENJOYS THIS ACTIVITY, also try Scarf Tricks, page 236.*

MAGNIFY MATTERS

GETTING A BUG'S-EYE VIEW OF THE WORLD

SKILLSPOTLIGHT

Using a magnifying glass *is a superb way to help a child appreciate nature. When a leaf isn't just a leaf but a complex maze of intersecting lines, or when a tiny bug suddenly has eyes, legs, and a mouth, your toddler learns that nature is rich and complex. Helping her describe what she sees builds her vocabulary, too.*

Concept Development	✔
Language Development	✔
Size & Shape Discrimination	✔
Tactile Stimulation	✔
Visual Discrimination	✔

AN ORDINARY ROCK and pinecone become intriguing landscapes of texture when your child has the chance to examine them up close and personal.

ENHANCE YOUR CHILD'S curiosity about her world—and her understanding of it—with a magnifying glass. She'll marvel at how grains of sand look like multicolored boulders and how flat green leaves are etched with tiny lines.

• Start your exploration by taking your child on a walk outdoors. Show her how to hold the magnifying glass up to different objects—such as leaves, rocks, grass, flowers, sand, even bugs—and look through it. Encourage her to touch the objects under scrutiny and help her find the appropriate words to describe them.

• Talk about concepts of size ("That pebble was little until we looked at it with the magnifying glass. Now it looks really big!"). Be sure to

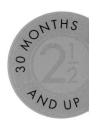

exercise extreme caution on sunny days; when the sun's rays are shining through the magnifying glass they can burn skin or even start a fire.

• Take her for a walk indoors, too. Tell her to get an up-close view of a blanket, her toast, a houseplant, her stuffed animals, or the hair on your pet. Ask her to describe what she sees, suggesting words if she doesn't have the vocabulary.

• Also use the magnifying glass to build body awareness. Let her explore her toes, fingerprints—and even your eyes and tongue.

287

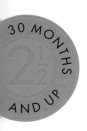

COUNT AND SEEK

FINDING THE MATCHING OBJECTS

SKILLSPOTLIGHT

Finding the objects *will boost your child's self-esteem (so don't hide the objects too well). Counting aloud as he finds them will help him learn both the sequence of numbers and an elementary concept of addition. The challenge of finding an object that he saw just a few moments ago also helps build visual memory.*

Counting Concepts	✔
Visual Discrimination	✔
Visual Memory	✔

IF YOUR CHILD ENJOYS THIS ACTIVITY, also try Flashlight Fun, page 262.

YOUNG CHILDREN of all ages love finding a hidden object—whether it's a baby's rattle, Mommy's face, or a cookie hidden in Daddy's pocket. Asking a child to find more than one object adds counting practice to the fun. Simply collect three or more similar items such as cups, shoes, wooden spoons, or colored balls. Show them to your toddler, hide them around the house (leaving a part of the "hidden" objects exposed so your child can find them more readily), then ask him to search for them. Count out loud and applaud every time he finds one. To make the game harder, hide more matching objects.

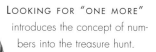

LOOKING FOR "ONE MORE" introduces the concept of numbers into the treasure hunt.

288

LEAF LINEUP

SORTING BY SIZE

YOUR CHILD IS QUITE INTENT on identifying his possessions ("That's my spoon!") and sorting them into various categories ("These are my hats. These are my shoes."). Take advantage of his dual love of possessions and sorting by creating a leaf collection. Gather small, medium, and large leaves. Tape one example of each size onto the sides of paper bags or small boxes. Place the rest of the leaves in a pile. Ask your child to sort the leaves into the correct bag or box according to size. While he sorts, talk to him about the leaves—where they came from, for instance, and their colors. Having a hard time finding leaves? Cut out some leaf shapes from colored construction paper.

SKILLSPOTLIGHT

Categorizing things *is immensely interesting for toddlers because it's a way of organizing and even controlling the world around them. This activity lets them learn the concepts of big and small and practice identifying which objects are which size. Talking about leaves also teaches children the words for colors and sizes and gives them a brief nature lesson.*

✔	**Classifying Skills**
✔	**Concept Development**
✔	**Language Development**
✔	**Size & Shape Discrimination**

WHAT GOES WHERE? Sorting a leaf collection is a great way to expand his understanding of big, medium, and small.

289

DUST BUSTING IS a chore toddlers adore, so let your little helper make this task more fun for you—and let her know that her work is appreciated.

RESEARCH REPORT

Many parents *are surprised at the gusto a young child will bring to everyday activities such as sweeping the floor or sponging off a counter. Yet almost a century ago, an Italian physician and educator named Maria Montessori trumpeted the value of meaningful chores—among many other revolutionary notions about early childhood. She said such chores help promote a child's sense of responsibility and self-esteem, and allow her to feel like she's contributing to the family or classroom. Today at the thousands of schools worldwide where teaching is based on Montessori's theories, classrooms are stocked with low-standing sinks, pint-size brooms and mops, and other cleaning supplies, and even the youngest preschoolers are expected to help.*

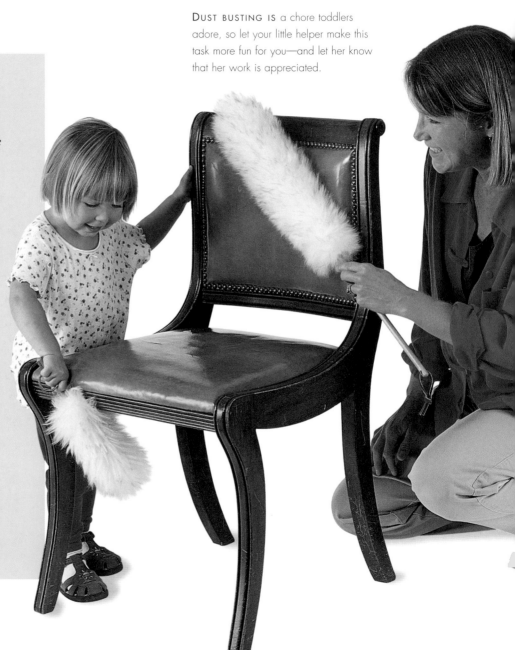

COPYCAT

IMITATING THE ADULT WORLD

SHE'S CARRYING YOUR HANDBAG and talking to the pets the same way you do. Sometimes it's delightful and sometimes it's embarrassing: do you really say, "Get down!" in that tone of voice? Now make imitation a joint activity—and get some chores done in the process.

• Encourage your child to "help" you rake leaves, dust, sweep, build a birdhouse, or fix a broken step. You can give her tot-size tools or safe adult ones, or just let her perform her tasks with make-believe supplies. She'll love giving you a helping hand.

• If you have a family pet, ask your toddler to help you feed, groom, exercise, or play with it. Not only will she learn new skills, she'll also learn to nurture the animal just as you nurture her.

• A garden is an ideal place for a child to lend a hand. Demonstrate how to plant seeds, then let her try. When the planting is long forgotten and the first shoots come up, you can surprise your young gardener by showing her the fruits of her labor.

• Adding music to your projects is a great way to enhance any task—especially if you whistle (or sing) while you work.

◀ *IF YOUR CHILD ENJOYS THIS ACTIVITY, also try Mini Mimes, page 278.*

SKILL SPOTLIGHT

Children learn *by observing others —especially their parents. This wonderfully interactive activity is a good way to show your child day-to-day chores (although she's not ready to be assigned large tasks yet). It also boosts her confidence as she pretends to accomplish what Mommy and Daddy do. Imitating your voice and gestures builds auditory and visual skills; doing it to music helps her explore rhythm.*

✔	**Coordination**
✔	**Gross Motor Skills**
✔	**Listening Skills**
✔	**Role-Playing**
✔	**Social Skills**

GLOSSARY

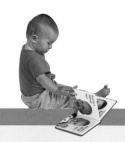 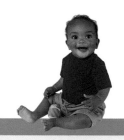

ABSTRACT THOUGHT

The ability to imagine and discuss people, ideas, and objects when they are not physically present. Pretending, notions of time, finding a lost object, and making plans to visit a friend all require some degree of abstract thought.

AUDITORY DEVELOPMENT

The auditory system's maturation, which is necessary for spoken language development.

BALANCE

The ability to assume and maintain body positions against the force of gravity. A sense of balance is crucial for learning how to roll over, sit, crawl, stand, walk, and run.

BILATERAL COORDINATION

The ability to use both sides of the body simultaneously, whether or not the movements are symmetrical. A child needs bilateral coordination to crawl, walk, swim, catch, climb, and jump.

BODY AWARENESS

An understanding of what limbs, joints, and muscles feel like and the ability to locate one's body parts.

CAUSE & EFFECT

How one action affects another. Experience with cause and effect helps a child learn how her actions create a result.

CLASSIFYING SKILLS

The ability to group objects according to a common characteristic, such as size, shape, or color.

COGNITION

Mental or intellectual abilities, including the ability to solve problems and remembering routines, people, and object placement.

COGNITIVE DEVELOPMENT

A child's growing understanding and knowledge, and her developing ability to think and reason.

CONCEPT AWARENESS

An understanding of specific concepts, such as open/closed and big/little, gained through play, exploration, movement, and experience.

COORDINATION

The ability to integrate all of the senses to produce a movement response that is smooth, efficient, and skillful, such as reaching for and grasping an object.

COUNTING CONCEPTS

The ability to recite numbers in the correct order and to recognize one-to-one correspondence.

CREATIVE EXPRESSION

Using voice, movement, or art (such as painting or drawing) to communicate feelings and ideas.

CREATIVE MOVEMENT

Using bodily motion (such as imitating animals or dancing) to communicate feelings and ideas.

DENDRITES

Branching neurons that carry nerve impulses within the brain. Researchers believe mental stimulation increases the size and complexity of dendrite networks, which consequently improves cognition.

EYE-FOOT COORDINATION

Gauging distance and depth with the eyes and processing that information to coordinate when and where to place the feet. Eye-foot coordination is required, for example, when kicking a target or walking on an uneven path.

EYE-HAND COORDINATION

Directing the position and motion of the hands in response to visual information, such as reaching out and grasping an offered toy.

FINE MOTOR SKILLS

Control of the small muscles, especially those in the hands, to execute small movements, such as picking up a raisin or plucking a blade of grass. This progresses to using tools such as spoons, pencils, or scissors.

GRASP AND RELEASE

The ability to purposefully reach out and retrieve an object and let it go.

GROSS MOTOR SKILLS

Control of the large muscles, such as those in the arms and legs. Gross motor activities include crawling, walking, and running.

IMAGINATION

The ability to form mental images of what is not present. Imagination involves the act of creating new ideas by combining past experiences. It also involves abstract thought. Imagination enables a child to practice roles, predict outcomes of his behavior, and create new scenarios.

LANGUAGE DEVELOPMENT

The complex process of acquiring language skills, including understanding human speech, producing sounds and spoken language, and eventually learning how to read and write.

LISTENING SKILLS

The ability to discern various sounds, including music, rhythm, and pitch, as well as the intonations of spoken language.

LOGICAL REASONING

The ability to make decisions or take actions based on an understood progression of facts or physical characteristics. Sorting, nesting, and stacking objects all depend on logical reasoning. A toddler's understanding that she needs to drag a chair over to the desk in order to reach the computer also shows logical reasoning.

LOWER-BODY STRENGTH

The development of muscles in the legs and lower trunk, which is crucial to crawling, walking, and eventually running and climbing.

NEURONS

Long nerve cells that carry electrical impulses throughout the body. Different kinds of nerve cells enable us to move our body, think, use our senses, and experience emotions.

OBJECT PERMANENCE

The concept that an object that is no longer visible still exists.

PROBLEM SOLVING

The ability to work out a solution to a mental or physical puzzle. A child solves a problem when he figures out how to fit a piece into a puzzle, stack nesting boxes, or open a package.

REFLEXES

Automatic responses to stimuli and events (for example, putting your hand up to stop a ball from hitting you).

RHYTHM EXPLORATION

The act of exploring the rhythms and underlying beat of music through movement.

GLOSSARY

ROLE-PLAYING
Mimicking the actions of others and eventually using imagination to pretend to be someone or something else.

SELF-CONCEPT
A child's understanding that he is an individual person separate from his parents.

SENSORY EXPLORATION
Using the senses—hearing, sight, smell, taste, and touch—to learn about the world.

SHAPE RECOGNITION
The ability to identify specific forms, such as circles and triangles. Shape recognition eventually helps a child learn to read and write.

SIZE & SHAPE DISCRIMINATION
The ability to identify objects of different dimensions and their relationship to each other, such as nesting boxes or pieces in a puzzle.

SOCIAL DEVELOPMENT
A child's growing understanding of her interactions with people and her influence on her world.

SOCIAL SKILLS
Interacting and relating to other people, including recognizing other people's emotions through their tone, actions, or facial expressions.

SPATIAL AWARENESS
Knowing where one's own body is in relation to other people and objects. A child uses spatial awareness to crawl under a bed, walk between two objects, and generally move through space.

SYNAPSES
The tiny gaps between neurons through which electrical impulses jump, thus allowing nerve cells to communicate with one another.

TACTILE DISCRIMINATION
The ability to determine differences in shape or texture by touch. Being able to discern textures helps children explore and understand their environment and recognize objects.

TACTILE STIMULATION
Input to receptors that respond to pressure, temperature, and the movement of hairs on the skin. Tactile stimulation enables a child to feel comfortable with new experiences such as first foods and unexpected touch.

UPPER-BODY STRENGTH
The development of muscles in the neck, shoulders, arms, and upper trunk, which is crucial to crawling, sitting, pulling up, and walking.

VISUAL DEVELOPMENT
The maturation of a child's eyes and eyesight.

VISUAL DISCRIMINATION
The ability to focus on and distinguish objects within a visual field. A toddler uses visual discrimination to find a bird in a picture, a desired toy in a basket, or locate a parent in a crowd.

VISUAL MEMORY
The ability to recall objects, faces, and images. Visual memory allows a child to remember a sequence of objects or pictures. It also serves as a foundation for learning to read.

VISUAL TRACKING
The ability to follow the movement of an item by moving the eyes and rotating the head.

SKILLS INDEX

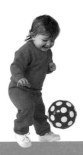
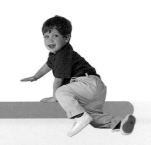

SKILLS INDEX

SKILLS INDEX

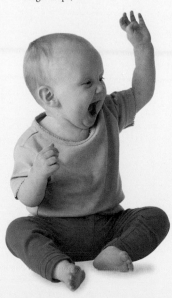
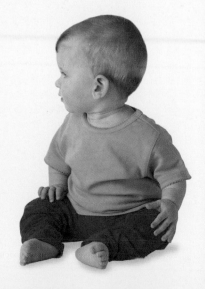

INDEX

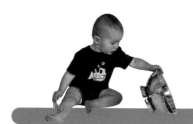
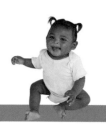

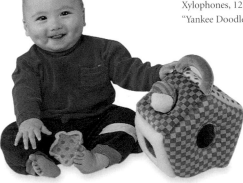

ACKNOWLEDGMENTS

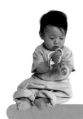
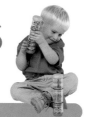

A VERY SPECIAL THANKS to all the children, parents, and grandparents featured in this book:

Tyler & Ashlynn Adams
Robin & Jessica Alvarado
Eric Anderson
José & Anna Arcellana
Lisa & Summer Atwood
Greg, Denise, & Aiden
  Ausley
Debbie & Karly Baker
Madeleine Barnum
Maiya Barsky
Leticia & Mikailah Bassard
Dana, Nicholas & Robbie
  Bisconti
Whitney Boswell
Annamaria & Sean Mireles
  Boulton
Catherine & Lizzie Boyle
Brynn & Riley Breuner
Jackson Breuner-Brooks
Danielle Bromley & Tyler
  Primas
Chizzie & Patrick Brown
Ashley Bryant
Madison Carbone
Millie Cervantes & Norma
  Foreman
Kailah Chavis
Christian Chubbs
Tami & Averie Clifton
Katherine & Parker Cobbs
Kelly, Mark, & Rebecca Cole
Jamila Coleman
Kevin & Sofia Colosimo
Kim & Katherine Daifotis

Bolaji, Kyle, & Miles Davis
Jane, Lauren, & Robert Davis
John & Jessica Davis
Keeson Davis
Justice Domingo
Elaine Doucet & Benjamin
  Martinez
Kimberly & Jacob Dreyer
Margaret & Lauren Dunlap
Stacy, Sydney, & Sophie
  Dunne
Tiffany & Simon Eng
Edgar & Melanie Estonina
Masooda & Sabrina Faizi
Christina Fallone
Kristen & Kaitlin Fenn &
  Susan Carlson
Quinn Folks
Shannon & Clayton Fritschi
Terri & Jacob Giamartino
Kristen Gilbert & Phenix
  Dewhurst
Wendi & Joshua Gilbert
Patricia & Nathan Gilmore
Galen Gold
Sharon & Annabel Gonzalez
Alexa Grau
Carrie Green-Zinn &
  Zaria Zinn
Jade & Jordan Greene
Candace Groskreutz &
  Matthew & Clare Colt
Annette, Katie, & Connor
  Hagan

Walter, Ester, & Whitney
  Hale
Danny & Yasmine Hamady
Drew Harris
Arthur & Reed Haubenstock
Ashley & Alyssa Hightower
Cameron & Bix Hirigoyen
Laurasia Holzman-Smith
Justin Hull
Margy Hutchinson & Isaiah
  Hammer
Rochelle Jackson
Ryan Jahabli-Danekas
Stephanie Joe & Alexander &
  Isabelle Weiskopf
David Johnson
Lynne Jowett & Eloise Shaw
Elana Kalish
Gilda & Megan Kan
David & Giselle Kaneda
Ashley Kang
Esther Aliah Karpilow
Isabella Kearney
Thomas Keller
Denise, Chloe, & Ian Kidder
Caecilia Kim & Addison
  Brenneman
Jeff, Jennifer, Sydney,
  & Gunner Kinsey
Sonya Kosty-Bolt & Owen
  Bolt
Dan & Martin Krause
Isabelle Jubilee Kremer
Olivier & Raphael Laude

Mark & Samantha Leeper
Mary & Simon Lindsay
Darien & Nicholas Lum
Peg Mallery & Elliot Dean
Alicia & Devon Mandell
Lily Marcheschi
Kim & Miles Martinez
Beth & Alison Mason
Lisa & Zachary Mayor
Nathaniel McCarthy
Ryan McCarty
Meredith & Sam McClintock
Susan McKeever & Sophia
  Rosney
Jennifer, Jim, & Abigail
  McManus
Alex Mellin
Maya & Jakob Michon
Sarah Miller & Elizabeth
  Schai
Justin Miloslavich
Kimberly Minasian &
  Isabelle Schulenburg
Lou, Terri, & Lou Molinaro
Mikayla Mooney
Nikolaus Moore
Theresa & Gabriel Moran
Mary, Jeff, & Amanda Rose
  Morelli
Tom, Genevieve, & Graham
  Morgan
Madeleine Myall
Chantál & Kalle Myllymäki
Betsy & Megumi Nakamura

Abby Newbold
Carly Olson
Sue, Katie, & Christine Partington
Terry, Kim, & Hunter Patterson
Elizabeth & Hayden Payne
Abigail Peach
Lori Pettegrew & Andrew Pike
Henrietta & Katie Plessas
Santiago Ponce
Bronwyn & Griffin Posynick
Jim & Kira Pusch
Shanti Rachlis
Ann Marie Ramirez & Damien Splan
Miles Reavis
Wayne & Thomas Riley
Kali Roberts
Aliyah Ross
Blake Rotter
Lori, Mark, & Zayle Rudiger
Renée Rylander & Ryan Ditmanson
Christine & Matthew Salah
Leigh & Kai Sata
Eloisa Tejero & Isabella Shin
Joseph Shin
Haley Shipway
Kathryn Siegler
Michelle Sinclair & Nicolas Amerkhanian
David Sparks
Colleen & Maxwell Smith

Nicole & Marlo Smith
Julia Stark
Jackie & Jaylyn Stemple
Denise & Adam Stenberg
Brisa & Diva Stevens
Quincy Stivers
JoAnne Skinner Stott & Sonja Stott
Lori & Karl Strand
James & Jayson Summers
Sandi, Kimberly, & Jacquelyn Svoboda
Michelle & Tatum Tai
Dylan Thompson
Rico & Deena Tolefree
Alisa & David Tomlinson
Kathi & Lauren Torres
Lila & April Torres
Mahsati & Kiana Tsao
Annalisa & John "Jack" VanAken
Paula Venables
Jim Vettel & Peyton Raab
Sebastian & Julian von Nagel
Gabriel Wanderley
Jenifer Warren & Grace Bailey
Patty & Shawn Weichel
Molly & Jamie Wendt
Kathleen & Meredith Whalen
Pernille & Sebastian Wilkenschildt
Daisy & Karinna Wong

Emma Wong
Sara Wong & Dean & Jack Fukushima
Catherine Wood
Tina & Anna Wood
Ajani Wright
Amy & Marissa Wright
Preeti & Shama Zalavadia
Allison, Jill, & Nicole Zanolli

Karen Zimmerman & Jarred Edgerly
Lisa Zuniga & Maria Carlsen

Mirror on page 184 courtesy of Mudpie in San Francisco. Crayola and serpentine design are registered trademarks of Binney & Smith and are used with permission.

ABOUT GYMBOREE

For more than a quarter century, Gymboree has helped parents and children discover the many pleasures and benefits of play. Based on established principles of early childhood education and administered by trained teachers, The Gymboree Learning Program emphasizes the wonder of play in a nurturing, noncompetitive environment. Gymboree has contributed to the international awareness of the importance of play and runs its interactive parent-child programs in twenty-nine countries.

OUR CONSULTING EDITORS

Dr. Wendy S. Masi is a developmental psychologist specializing in early childhood. She has designed and implemented programs for preschools, families with young children, and early childhood professionals for more than twenty-five years. The mother of four children, Dr. Masi is dean of the Mailman Segal Institute for Early Childhood Studies at Nova Southeastern University in Fort Lauderdale, Florida.

Dr. Roni Cohen Leiderman is a developmental psychologist specializing in emotional development, positive discipline, and play. For more than twenty-five years, she has worked with children, families, and professionals. She is associate dean of the Mailman Segal Institute for Early Childhood Studies at Nova Southeastern University and the mother of two children.

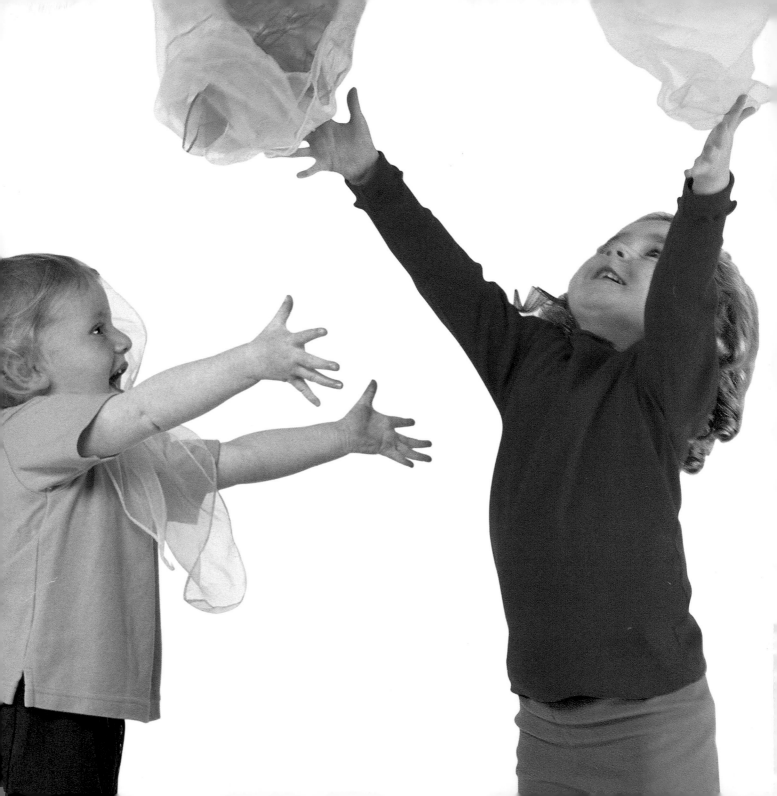

THE
ATLAS
OF
WILD
PLACES

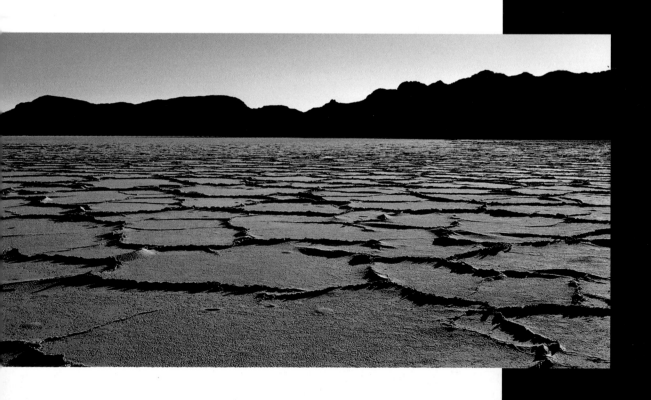

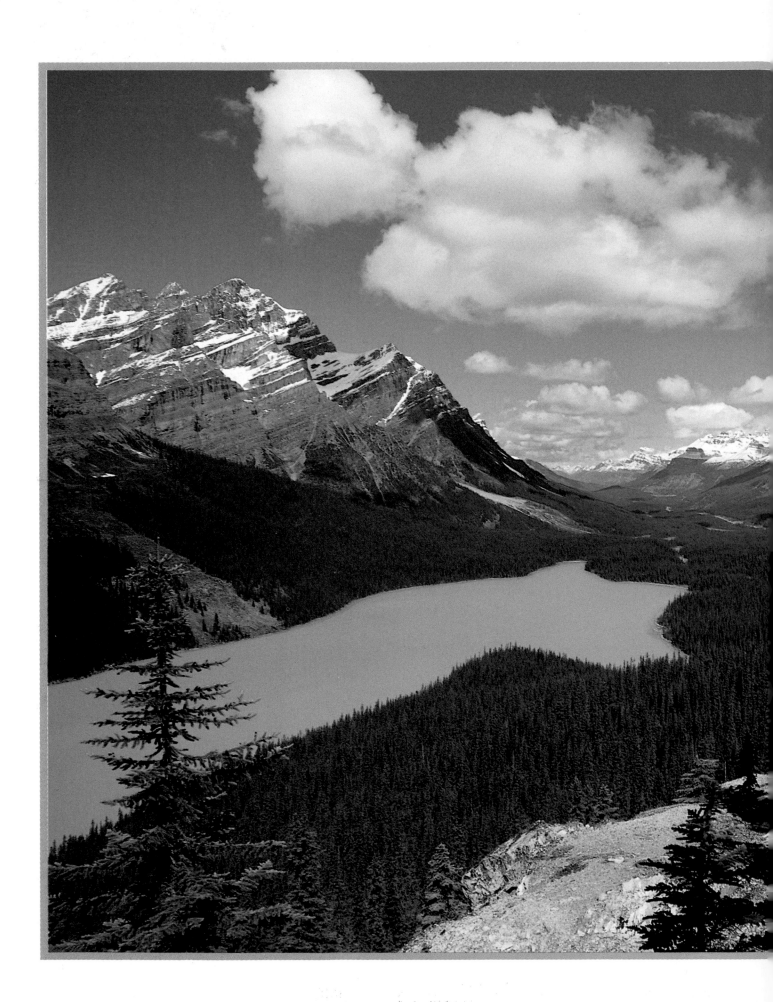

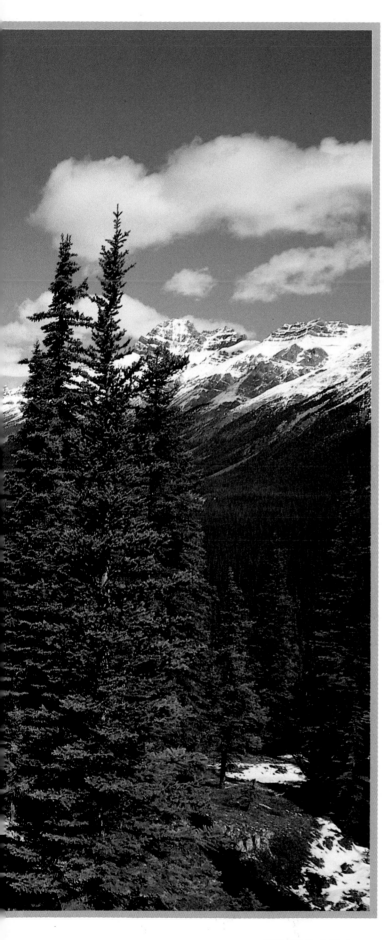

THE

ATLAS

OF

WILD

PLACES

*In search
of the
Earth's
last
wildernesses*

ROGER FEW

Facts On File®

A Marshall Edition
This book was conceived, edited,
and designed by Marshall Editions,
170 Piccadilly, London W1V 9DD

Facts On File, Inc.
460 Park Avenue South
New York NY 10016

Library of Congress Cataloging-in-Publication Data

Few, Roger.
    The atlas of wild places : in search of the
earth's last wildernesses / Roger Few.
        p.   cm.
    Includes index.
    ISBN 0-8160-3168-1
    1. Natural history.   2. Biotic communities.
    3. Wilderness areas.
I. Title
QH45.5.F48 1994

Facts On File books are available at special
discounts when purchased in bulk quantities for
businesses, associations, institutions or sales
promotions. Please call our Special Sales
Department in New York at 212/683-2244 or
800/322-8755.

Contributors
Roger Few Pages 6–7, 10–29, 66–97,
98–131, 156–187, 188–199
Duncan Brewer Pages 132–155, 226–236
Sophie Campbell Pages 200–225
Ed Zahniser Pages 30–65

Editor   **Jinny Johnson**
Art director   **Dave Goodman**
Picture editor   **Zilda Tandy**
Research   **Jon Richards**

Printed in Spain by Printer Industria Grafica

10 9 8 7 6 5 4 3 2 1

This book is printed on acid-free paper

Page 1
A huge salt flat on the Bolivian Altiplano
Page 2
Peyto Lake in Banff National Park

CONTENTS

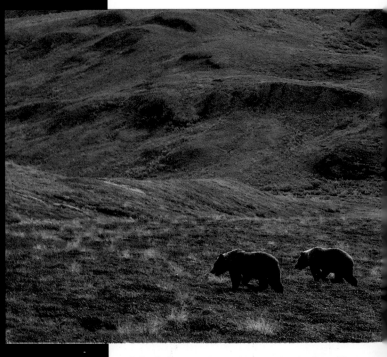

Grizzly bears roam the tundra in Denali National Park.

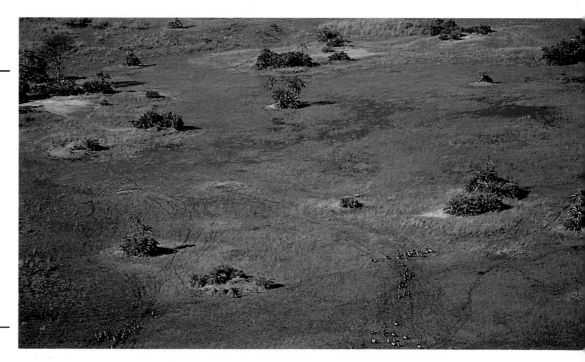

Herds of lechwe antelope graze on the Okavango Delta.

PREFACE

"Landscapes that have never been tamed by human activity – where nature still prevails"

The notion of "wilderness" invokes feelings that are a mixture of fear and fascination. The word suggests something outside the familiar, ordered world – an environment utterly exposed to the elements, where true darkness still reigns at night and where savage creatures lurk. And yet part of us craves more knowledge of that other world. It is a part of us that feels trapped by the very buildings, roads, powerlines, factories and fields that give us comfort. Even if we cannot experience that world directly, we can savor it through the printed word, through photographs and film, and wonder at these landscapes that have never been tamed by human activity.

The places featured in this book share that essential wilderness quality, but otherwise they differ immensely. Compare the luxuriant forests of Tasmania with the barren, icebound Antarctic Peninsula, where only a few minuscule plants exist. Contrast the flat terrain of the Coto Doñana with the towering peaks of the Pamirs, and the intense aridity of the Skeleton Coast with the water-soaked Okefenokee Swamp. Some wild places, like the great stony wastes of the Gobi Desert, are vast. Others, such as Itatiaia National Park, are merely islands in surrounding seas of cultivation. And while clement summer weather and magnificent scenery lure many tourists to the Banff and Jasper National Parks, far fewer visitors brave the interior of the dusty, bleak and inhospitable Patagonian Plain.

These wildernesses, with their varied appeal, reflect with great intensity the world as it once was. They are

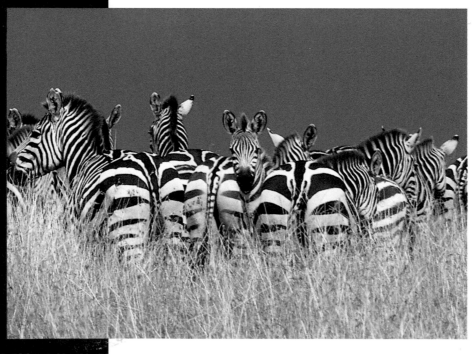

Zebras in the grasslands of the Serengeti in Africa (above).

The vast Empty Quarter of Saudi Arabia (right).

places where, because of remoteness, hostile climate, difficult terrain or, in a few cases, historical accident, there has been little human development. There is an overriding sense that nature still prevails, for all are truly wild places.

In their landforms and ecology, the places chosen here give full display to the forces and creations of nature. The colossal power of Earth's movements is evident in the tropical Highlands of Irian Jaya, where mountains have been thrust so high that ice forms on their tops. The island remains of Krakatau bear witness to the awesome forces unleashed when volcanoes erupt. Other places demonstrate how climate acts on topography to shape the landscape. Glaciers from a previous age, for example, have gouged their mark into the rugged relief of Fiordland. Insights into the wildlife communities of places such as Ellesmere Island show how plants and animals manage to adapt to the harshest of environments.

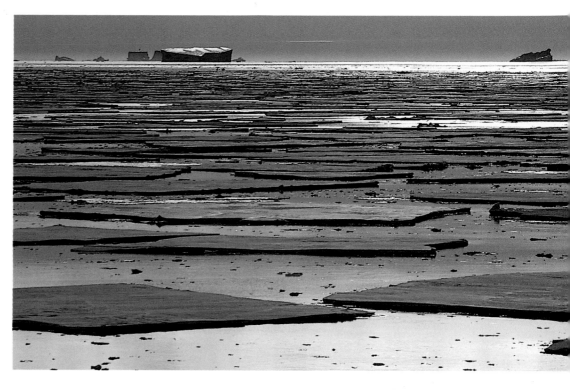

The desolate icy wastes of the remote Antarctic Peninsula (above).

Though nature rules in these wild places, humans are by no means absent. Small numbers of people live in many of the featured places. Some lead a settled existence; others, such as the Bedouin tribes of the Empty Quarter, are nomadic. In some wildernesses people enter temporarily to gather the resources – people such as the harvesters of honey and wood who travel into the Sundarbans. But whatever the human presence, it is of a form that does little to alter the wild character of the land. The people's story is one of adaptation to an often harsh environment rather than of attempts at domination.

Selected areas are featured in the main part of the book. As the gazetteer shows, many more exist. Nevertheless, wilderness regions today are rare and becoming rarer. In Europe, and in most densely settled parts of the globe, true wildernesses are few and those that exist survive only because they are strictly set aside for nature. Elsewhere, great sparsely populated tracts of the Earth remain, but even these are ever more likely to bear the imprint of humans as world population grows and the demand for land and resources continues to increase. Already some of the wild places in this book are under threat – Lake Baikal, for example, from the pollution of its waters, Tai National Park from logging around its periphery. Some will undoubtedly be despoiled or tamed in the future, but with concerted international action, we *can* continue to preserve most of these treasures of the wild.

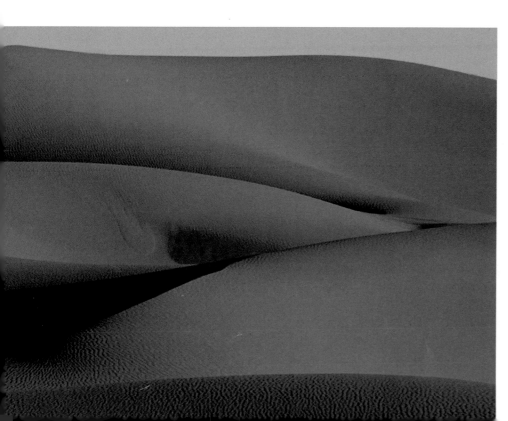

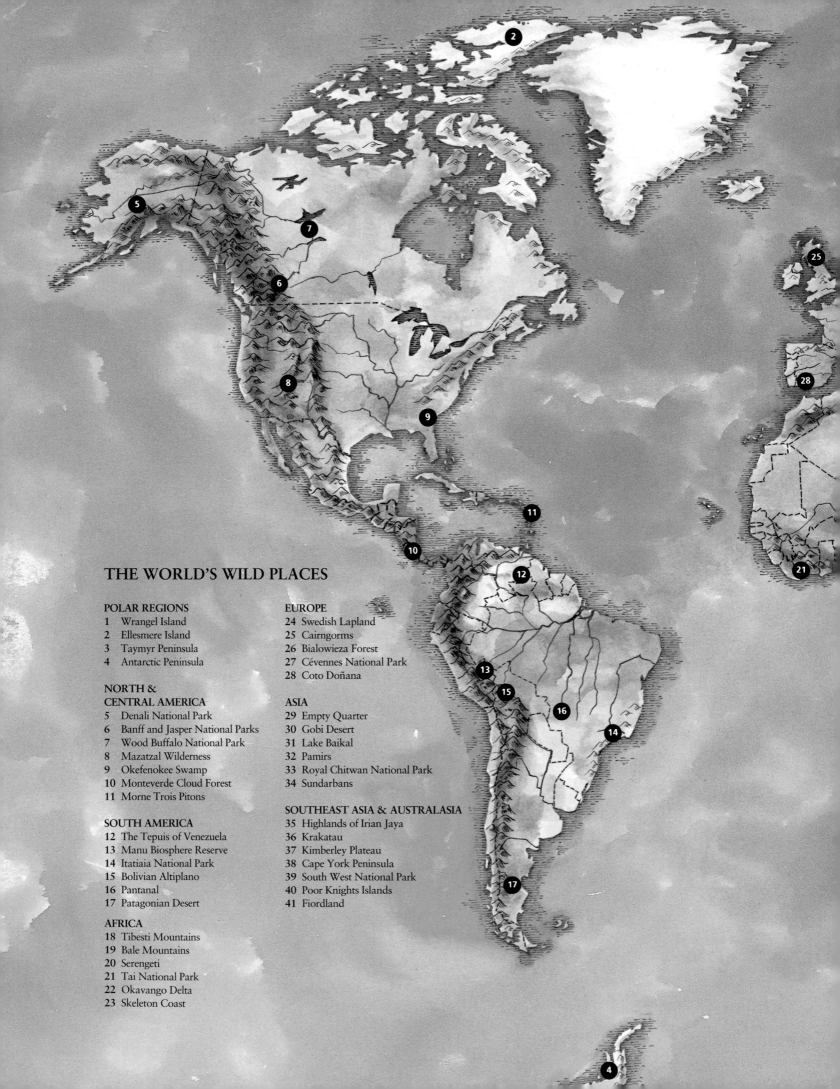

THE WORLD'S WILD PLACES

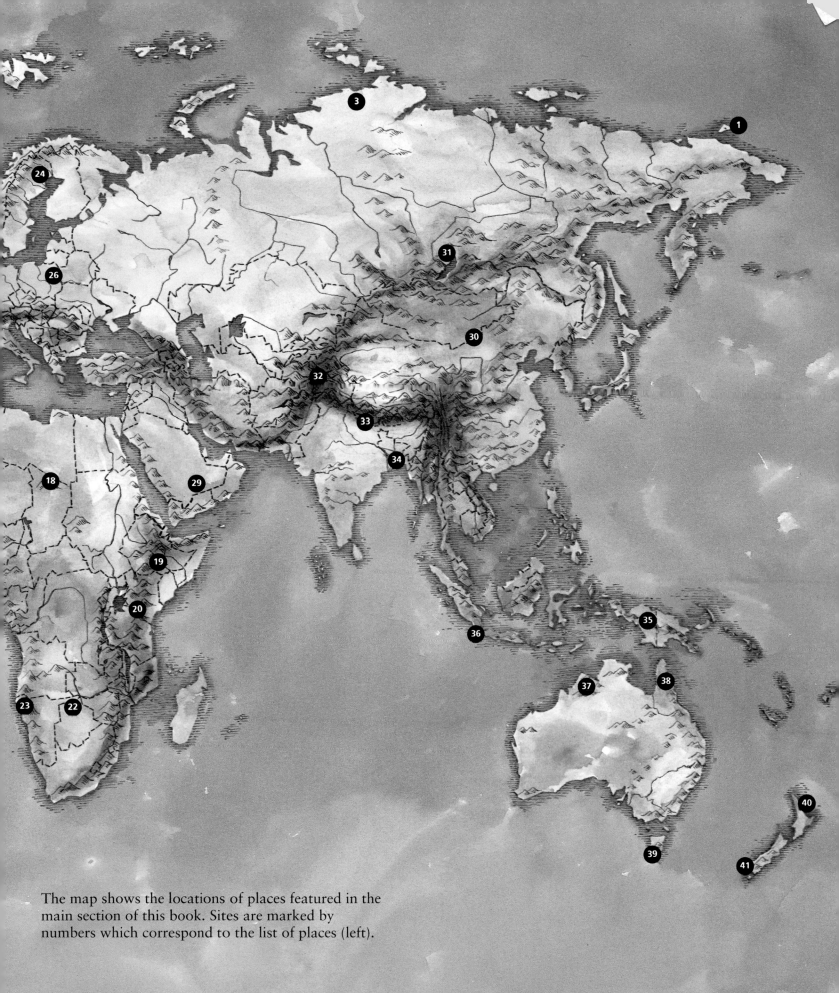

The map shows the locations of places featured in the
main section of this book. Sites are marked by
numbers which correspond to the list of places (left).

WRANGEL ISLAND

"An uninhabited polar wilderness, isolated from the rest of the world"

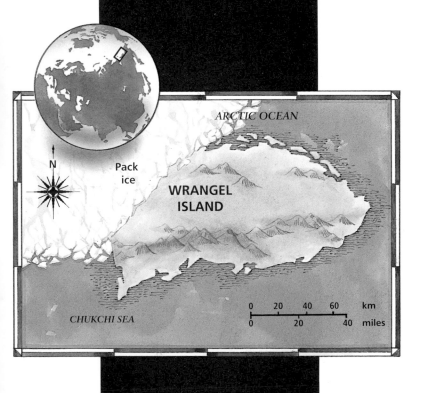

ARCTIC OCEAN

Pack ice

WRANGEL ISLAND

N

CHUKCHI SEA

| 0 | 20 | 40 | 60 | km |
| 0 | | 20 | | 40 | miles |

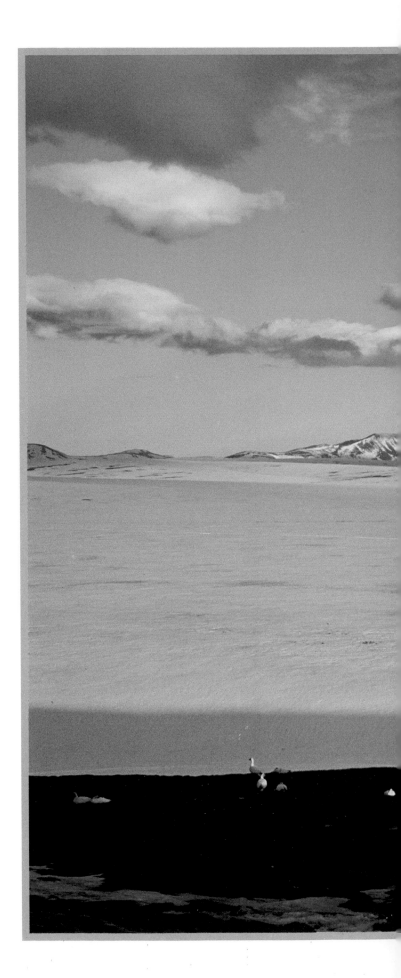

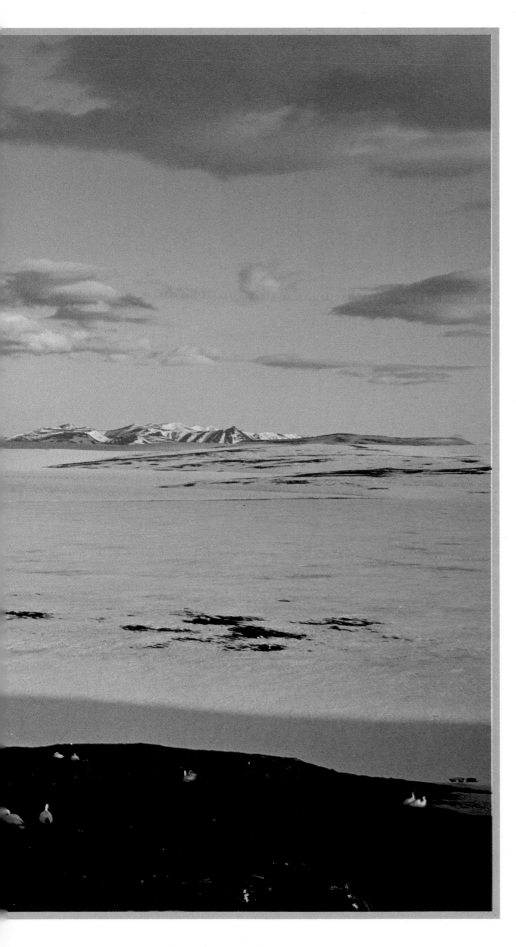

A remote outpost in the Arctic Ocean, Wrangel Island lies off the coast of Siberia. It is located near the limit of permanently frozen ocean surface, and approach by sea is made treacherous even in summer by shifting pack ice. In the cold dark winter, a platform of solid sea ice several miles wide seals the shores of this uninhabited polar wilderness, making it still more isolated from the rest of the world.

About 78 miles (125 km) in length, the island seems to guard the entrance to the Arctic above the narrow Bering Strait that divides Siberia from Alaska. Wrangel takes its name from a Russian explorer, who knew of its existence but never had the chance to glimpse its desolate shores. In the 1820s, while mapping the northeastern Siberian coast, Ferdinand Wrangel noted flocks of birds flying out and back across the icebound sea. Local Chukchi people confirmed the belief that there must be land somewhere to the north in the frozen wilderness.

But such was the isolation of the island that it was not definitely sighted by Russians until 1849. When explorers finally reached its shores, they found a pristine, remarkably ice-free land – a wild haven not just for huge numbers of migratory birds, but also for true Arctic wanderers such as walruses and polar bears.

Unlike many other islands of the High Arctic, Wrangel does not have any permanent ice cap nor any glaciers. Thin winter snow covers its undulating mountain chains and coastal lowlands, and deep, windblown drifts may accumulate

Remote Wrangel Island is a haven for *wildlife. Lesser snow geese migrate to the island in their thousands in summer, finding safe nesting sites and plentiful food on the ice-free tundra.*

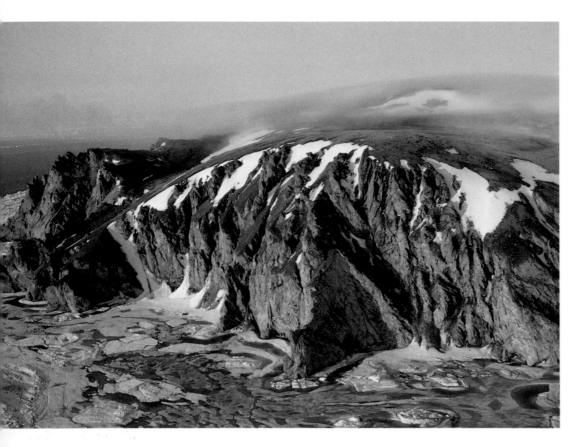

numbers. Especially numerous are brent geese, common eiders, knots, turnstones and gray plovers.

Wrangel is also the only place in this part of the Arctic where large colonies of lesser snow geese nest. By May these graceful white birds can be seen in the air all over the island, traveling to and from colonies shared by many thousands of pairs. Snowy owls often nest alongside the colonies in what seems to be a deliberate strategy for mutual protection against nest-robbers. The watchful geese provide early warning when marauding gulls, skuas and Arctic foxes approach, then the owls swoop in to drive the intruders away.

Along the rocky coasts of the island, birds gather in even greater concentrations. The best sites are crowded with nesting guillemots, cormorants, kittiwakes and other birds that constantly wheel in the sky around their cliff-ledge haunts. At least half a million seabirds throng Wrangel's coast at the height of the Arctic summer, finding abundant food in the surrounding waters as some ice thaws.

The break-up of the coastal ice also allows sea mammals to swim inshore, where the water is shallow and food easier to find. As soon as openings in the ice appear, so do bearded and ringed seals. By July walruses, too, are hauling themselves onto traditional beaches to court, spar, mate and raise their pups. Wrangel Island is one of the most important breeding areas for walruses in the world, in some years attracting as many as 80,000 of these hefty, tusked sea mammals.

Another spectacular animal, the polar bear, also breeds on Wrangel. Protected by its thick fur and layers of subcutaneous fat, the polar bear rides on ice floes and braves the freezing water for short swims as it searches for prey. Its principal victims are seals, which it catches on the ice or

in the valleys, but the relative warmth of summer is enough to melt away most of the snow each year.

During the brief Arctic summer, numerous rivulets and streams take meltwater down through ponds and marshes to the coast. The rugged tundra landscape through which these streams flow is painted mostly in shades of russet and brown with scant, patchy vegetation rarely growing more than about 4 inches (10 cm) in height. Among these diminutive plants are some flowering species – types of poppy, meadow grass and cinquefoil, for example – that are unique to the island.

The small size of the plants is both a result of the short growing season and an adaptation to the climate. Ground-hugging plants are less exposed to winter gales and are better protected from intense cold. The hardiest plants, such as mosses and lichens, can grow outside the valleys and lowlands, but even they cannot survive on the highest ground of the

Thin summer ice around Wrangel reflects mild conditions in comparison with the island's ice-age past. Its peaks, once part of a great mountain chain, were worn down and smoothed by thick ice sheets that covered the land.

island. There, not even the thinnest covering of soil exists, just shards of rock debris. These lie loose on the surface in summer, but are locked together by the permanent frost underneath.

Before the snows have fully melted on Wrangel Island, summer visitors are already winging into the sheltered grassy valleys and shoreline plains ready to begin nesting. These birds must arrive early if they are to complete their breeding cycle. By the end of August, worsening weather will have driven most of them away again. Though the trip across to Wrangel is too arduous for many species that nest in Siberia, those that do extend their journey north come in large

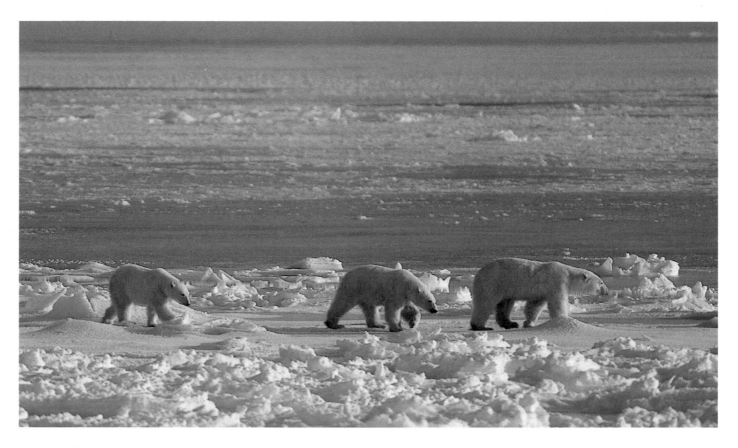

waits to club with its paw when they surface at breathing holes.

By November, when winter returns to Wrangel, a few hundred bears will have made their solitary way inland to occupy lairs on snowy hillsides. Many are pregnant females, and during the midwinter darkness, they give birth to their cubs under an insulating blanket of snow. Not until April can the cubs emerge into the gentle spring sunshine.

A few thousand years ago, very different creatures roamed Wrangel Island – the wooly mammoths. These prehistoric, elephantlike beasts were generally believed to have died out worldwide at the end of the ice age, more than 10,000 years ago. By that time, rising sea levels had cut the island off from the mainland.

But in 1991, paleontologists found some much more recent remains on the island. These indicate that mammoths could have lingered undisturbed in this lonely wilderness until as late as 2000 B.C.

Up to 300 polar bears return winter after winter to denning areas in the interior of Wrangel Island. For the rest of the year, bears like this mother and her well-grown cubs (above) are wanderers on the polar pack ice.

A knot of guillemots finds space on a Wrangel cliff alongside a noisy colony of black-legged kittiwakes. The continual din from nesting seabirds shatters the peaceful desolation of the island in the summer months.

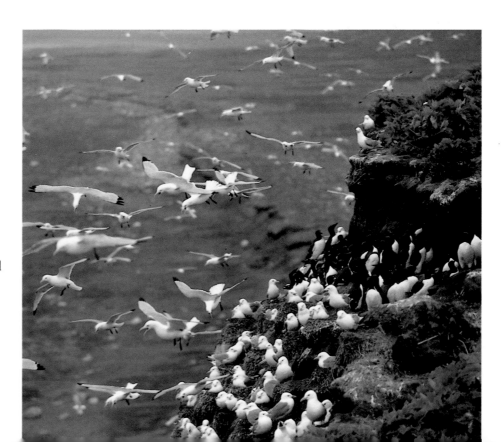

Ellesmere Island

"A truly forbidding place, one of the great wildernesses of polar lands"

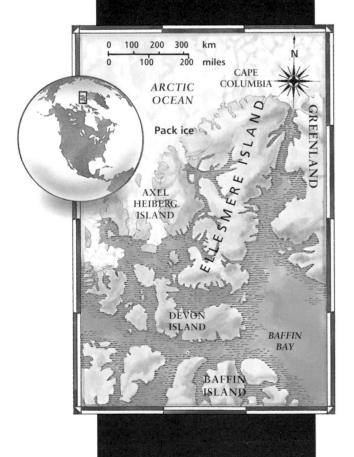

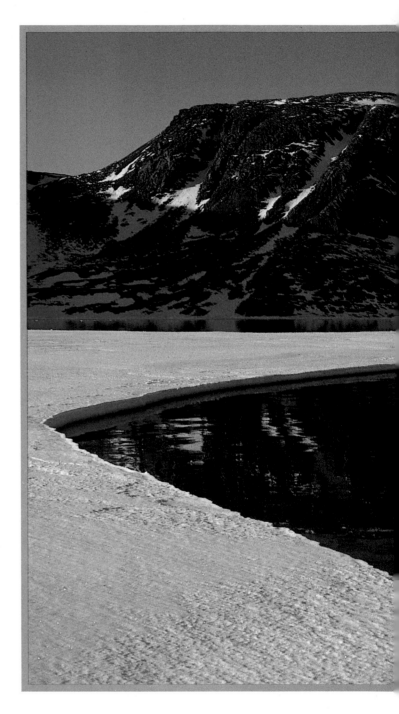

Ellesmere Island's bleak, rugged interior is no place for the lonely. The most northerly of Canada's Arctic lands, it lies 2,500 miles (4,000 km) from Canada's main cities. Though it is the size of Great Britain, this beautiful but empty land is home to just a few hundred people, clustered into a handful of tiny settlements and research stations along the coast. Intense cold, scant vegetation and

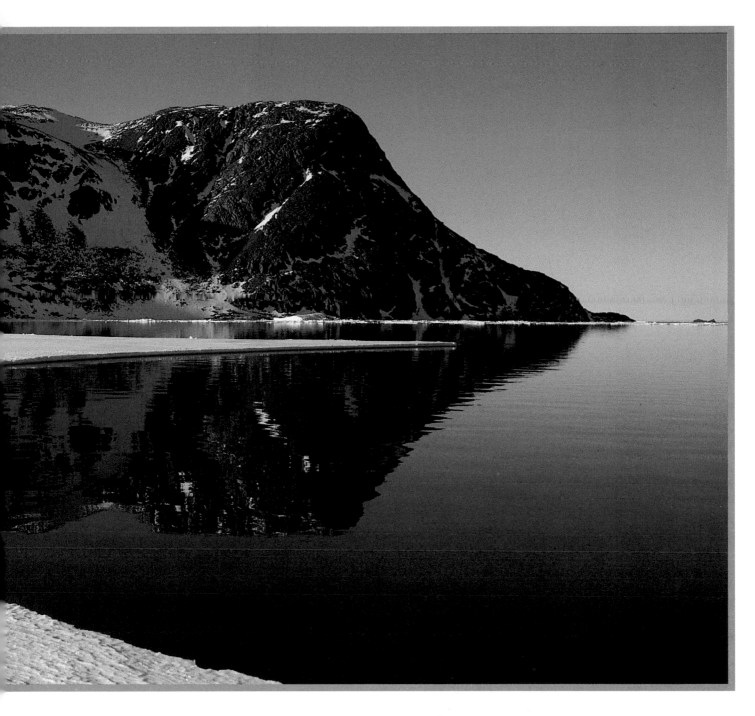

the prolonged darkness of the Arctic winter combine to make the island a truly forbidding place, one of the great wildernesses of the polar lands.

Conditions on Ellesmere are governed by latitude. Straddling the 80th parallel, the island lies almost at the top of the world. Its northernmost point, Cape Columbia, is less than 500 miles (800 km) from the North Pole. Only the extreme tip of Greenland is nearer. At this latitude,

the seasonal effect on climate caused by the tilt of the Earth as it orbits the sun is dramatic. For most of winter, the sun never rises above the horizon. The land is plunged into continual darkness that lasts up to five months in the north of the island. For a similar period in summer, the sun remains in the sky, dipping daily toward the horizon, but never below it.

Long months without sunshine make the Ellesmere winter exceptionally

Ellesmere is the most northerly and mountainous of the Canadian Arctic islands. Ice caps cover the higher ground, and for much of the year snow whitens the entire landscape.

cold – average midwinter temperatures are well below –22°F (–30°C). Even at midday in summer, the sun is so low in the sky that it does little more than take the chill off the air. Average

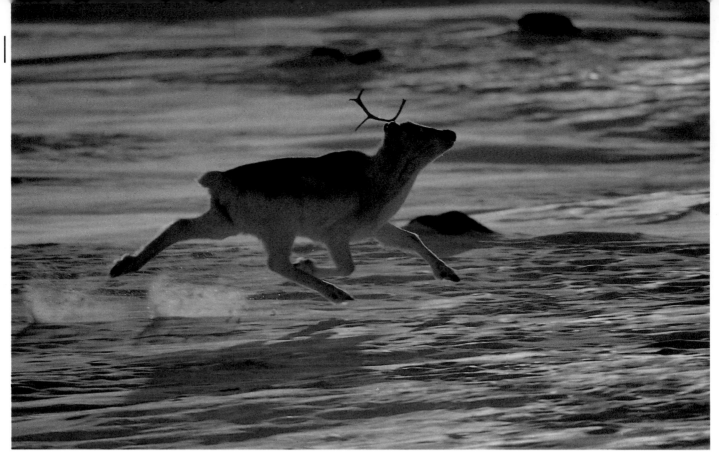

summer temperatures on the island are only just above freezing.

Year-round pack ice (frozen surface layers of the sea) fills the Arctic Ocean to the north and the straits and channels to the west. Only to the south and in the narrow strait separating Greenland to the east does the coastal water become clear for shipping in summer. Inland, huge sections of higher ground are covered in permanent ice caps. Snow whitens the ice-free land, the arctic tundra, for nine months each year. Ironically, however, Ellesmere's environment is classed as desert. Over most of the island, only about 2½ in (65 mm) of snow falls per year – enough to coat the ground, but less moisture than the Sahara Desert receives yearly as rain.

Survival on Ellesmere Island is difficult. Archaeologists have found traces of ancient Inuit (Eskimo) settlements on the island and even evidence that there may have been some trading with Viking adventurers in the 12th century. The island probably served as a migration route between islands to the southwest and Greenland. But until the tiny modern Inuit settlement of Grise Fjord was founded on the south coast in 1953, nobody had made a permanent home on the island for 250 years. The only visitors were Inuit hunters and a few scientists and explorers.

The fate of one expedition underlines the harshness of Ellesmere. In 1883, having failed to receive relief supplies by ship for two years running, an American expedition party which had been exploring the northern part of the island retreated south in desperation, amid gales, ice and blizzards. When they reached the emergency stores they were seeking, they found only meager supplies with yet another terrible winter to face abandoned. By the time they were rescued the following summer, only 7 of the original 25 had survived.

Harsh though the dark winter may be, Ellesmere in the light of summer presents a majestic face. As the light strengthens and the snow thaws, the landscape revealed is one of towering mountains up to 8,500 feet (2,600 m) high, vast ice caps, glaciers, rugged stony plateaus, and an emerging flush of green in the valleys. Magnificent fiords indent the coast, and icebergs drift menacingly offshore.

Peary's caribou is the smallest of all the races of caribou and one of the island's most enchanting inhabitants. But life on Ellesmere is tough for these deer, forcing them to wander far afield in search of meager vegetation, which they expose by scraping the snow aside with their hooves.

The landscape is one of vast, open tundra. No trees can exist here – only dwarf willow shrubs manage to survive the rigors of winter. Various lichens, mosses, grasses and small herbs such as saxifrages and Arctic poppies, however, relieve the bleakness of the tundra and provide a lifeline for wildlife. In sheltered valleys the plants cover the ground thickly, creating pockets of relative plenty.

On the richest parts of the tundra, animal life appears in summer – if not in the variety present in warmer climes, then in an abundance that may still seem hard to reconcile with the harshness of winter. But most creatures have done their best to avoid the Arctic winter. Some come out of hiding; others arrive from more clement winter quarters. Hardy

"Harsh though the dark winter may be, Ellesmere in the light of summer presents a majestic face"

VERDANT VALLEYS

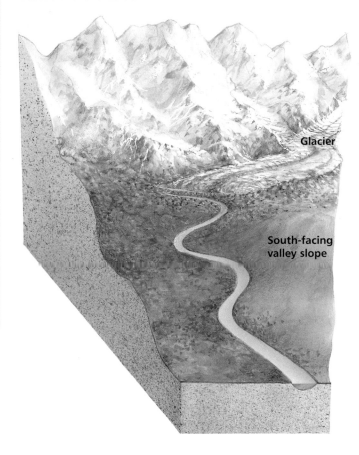

Glacier

South-facing valley slope

On clear summer days, sheltered valleys on Ellesmere can become oases of warmth in a chilled land, with temperatures rising from time to time as high as 68°F (20°C). The sun is continually low on the horizon, and south-facing slopes become effective suntraps. Snow melts away quickly on them, and pockets of surprisingly lush greenery can develop.

insects, among them butterflies, emerge from winter dormancy in the soil and mosses. Great numbers of birds, such as plovers, sandpipers, ducks, geese, waders, terns, auks and skuas, fly in from lands far beyond the Arctic to nest and feed in the tundra, along rivers and lakes, and on the coast. Shortly after breeding is complete, they retreat south again.

Only the few mammal species resident on the island remain active as winter sets in. Lemmings, Arctic hares and Arctic foxes do not hibernate – if they did they would probably freeze to death. As the blizzards start to swirl, caribou paw snow aside to find forage. When winter darkness falls, life is grim indeed.

Musk oxen, protected by shaggy coats, move up onto the upland plains, where at least the strong winds blow some of the snow cover away and allow them to find morsels of plant food. Arctic wolves may rely a good deal on scavenging. They trek far and wide in the gloom to find the bodies of musk oxen and other mammals that have succumbed to the severity of winter in this wild island of the High Arctic.

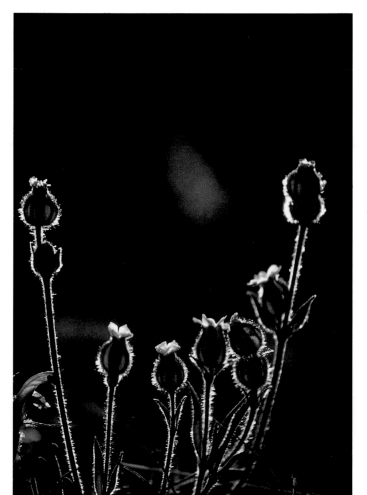

Arctic poppies prepare to unfurl their flowers in the precious warmth of summer, adding their delicate beauty to the harsh grandeur of Ellesmere's tundra. The petals attract hardy insects emerging from winter dormancy, though they may also suffer the nibblings of Arctic hares.

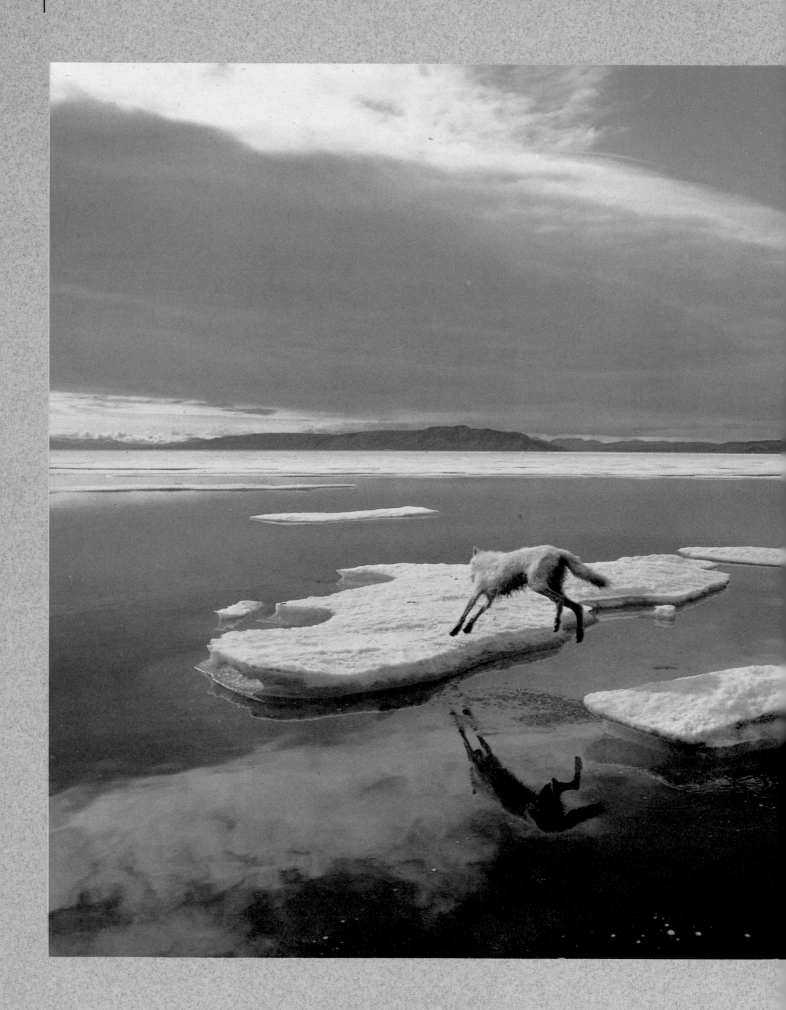

THE ARCTIC WOLVES OF ELLESMERE

In the wilderness of Ellesmere Island, far from the prejudice and persecution meted out to them in settled lands, Arctic wolves hunt and breed without menace from the gun.

But life is by no means easy. The thick white fur of the wolf is testament to a landscape gripped by intense cold, and though the diet is broad – wolves hunt or scavenge for musk oxen, caribou, lemmings and ground-nesting birds like the ptarmigan – prey is so thin on the ground that each pack needs a territory of perhaps 1,000 sq. miles (2,600 km²) if it is to find enough food.

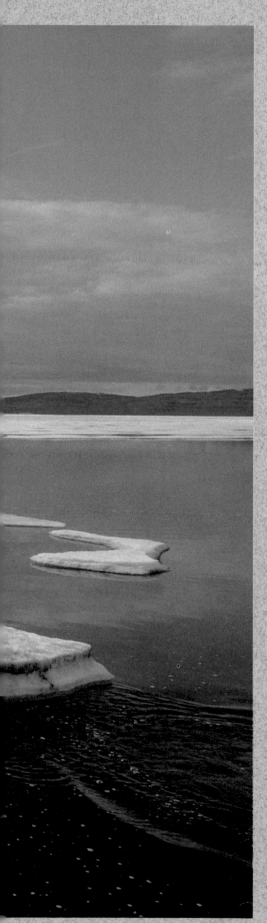

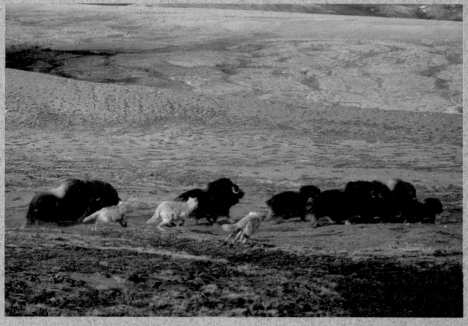

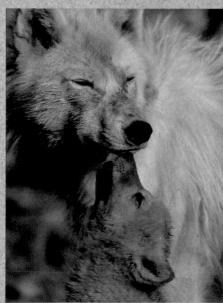

Leaping between drifiting ice floes, a male Arctic wolf patrols the edge of his territory (left). Coastal areas are valuable to a wolf pack, providing plenty of opportunities for scavenging and the chance to hunt for resting seals.

Musk oxen form a defensive ring when attacked, with the adults' horns facing menacingly outward (above).

Adults in the pack share the responsibility of looking after pups (right).

THE TAYMYR PENINSULA

"Views can be breathtaking, especially in winter when the northern lights illuminate the dark snow and frozen waterways"

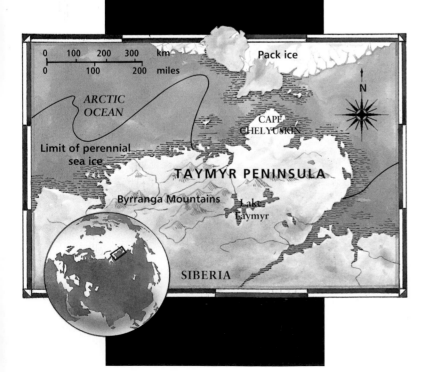

Bordered by ice-filled seas, raked by terrible blizzards and plunged each year into four months of perpetual darkness, the Taymyr Peninsula reaches farther into the Arctic than any other part of Siberia. Cape Chelyuskin, its northernmost point, is the closest any continent gets to the North Pole. It is a part of Russia that has long deterred even the hardiest of settlers, and its coastal region was one of the last in Siberia to be explored.

Still virtually devoid of people, Taymyr has enormous vistas of open

tundra, crossed and dotted by myriad rivers, pools and lakes. Its views can be breathtaking, especially in winter when the atmospheric extravaganza of the northern lights, or aurora borealis, delicately illuminates the dark snow and frozen waterways.

Tundra stretches across the entire northern rim of Russia, sandwiched between the great Siberian forests and the Arctic coast. At Taymyr, with its extension deep into the Arctic, this tundra belt assumes its greatest width, forming an enormous block of treeless, windswept land the size of

Germany. The peninsula is largely flat or undulating, although a ridge of low, worn mountains, the Byrranga, crosses its center and in places forms precipitous crags.

As throughout the Arctic, the ground underfoot is frozen solid by permafrost – subsoil that remains below freezing point throughout the year. In this region of Siberia, probably because of the severity of past glaciation, the deep freeze penetrates far underground, as much as 1,000 feet (300 m) into the subterranean rock strata. In winter,

when temperatures can plunge below -58°F (-50°C) at times and gales can drive snow across the land for days on end, the entire landscape of Taymyr lies frigid and white. But summer sunshine not only melts away most of the snow, but also warms the surface of the soil enough to thaw the top 4 inches (10 cm) or so of frost.

Without this annual melting, the short tundra vegetation would not be able to survive and grow. In fact, compared with the grip of winter, summer on Taymyr is surprisingly warm, averaging 46°F (8°C) in July and rising to an exceptional 86°F (30°C) in places on still, sunny days.

The great latitudinal span of the Taymyr Peninsula creates varying conditions from north to south. In the far north, where the climate is coldest, vegetation is scant and there are large patches of bare ground. Only the hardiest Arctic animals eke out an existence here. The most numerous are those typical Arctic rodents, the lemmings. Two kinds live on the peninsula, the collared lemming and the Siberian lemming, digging holes in the snow for shelter during the icy winter.

Farther south, across the Byrranga Mountains, the ground is more thickly covered with mosses, lichens, sedges, grasses and dwarf shrubs. Particularly abundant is "reindeer moss" – actually a type of branching lichen that grows in tight mats up to 6 inches (15 cm) high. As its name suggests, the moss is a staple food of reindeer or caribou, which spread north across the peninsula in summer

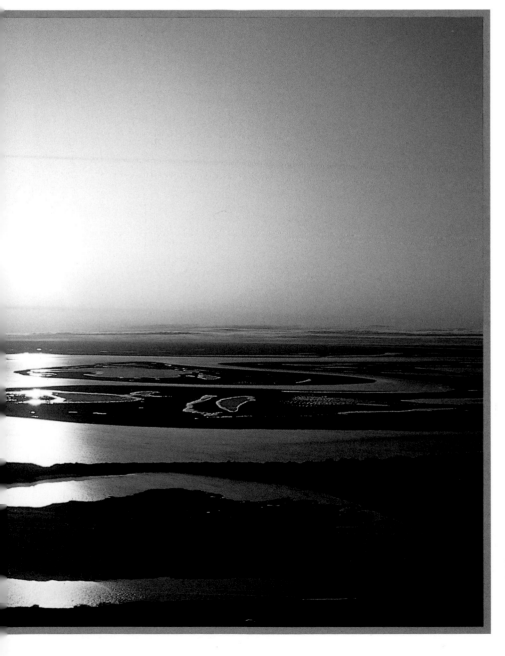

The lonely Taymyr Peninsula lies *farther north than any other part of mainland Russia. Tundra and shallow summer water stretch for immense distances across its open terrain. Apart from a line of low mountains crossing its center, there is little in this vast land to break the horizon.*

in herds thousands strong. Up to half a million of them may be present in all, making Taymyr one of their main strongholds in Siberia. By September, each herd begins to trek south again, often shadowed by a pack of wolves.

Along their route south, the surrounding vegetation becomes steadily thicker as the moss tundra blends into the zone of shrub tundra. The soil becomes a little deeper and more peaty, and dwarf forms of birch and alder – 3 feet (1 m) in height – form thickets over large areas. They provide good nesting sites for small tundra birds such as snow buntings which, when they appear in early May, are among the first of the summer migrants to the peninsula.

Everywhere, especially in this southern half of the peninsula, water seems to be abundant. Melting snow and soil frost swell the winding rivers and shallow lakes. At this time, Lake

Every spring, *once the winter snows have thawed, herds of caribou or reindeer trek deep into Taymyr to find fresh feeding pastures. Here they fatten themselves on the lush tundra vegetation, a diet complemented by birds' eggs and the occasional lemming. Females calve in the relative warmth of June, each rearing a single young that is up and running within hours of birth.*

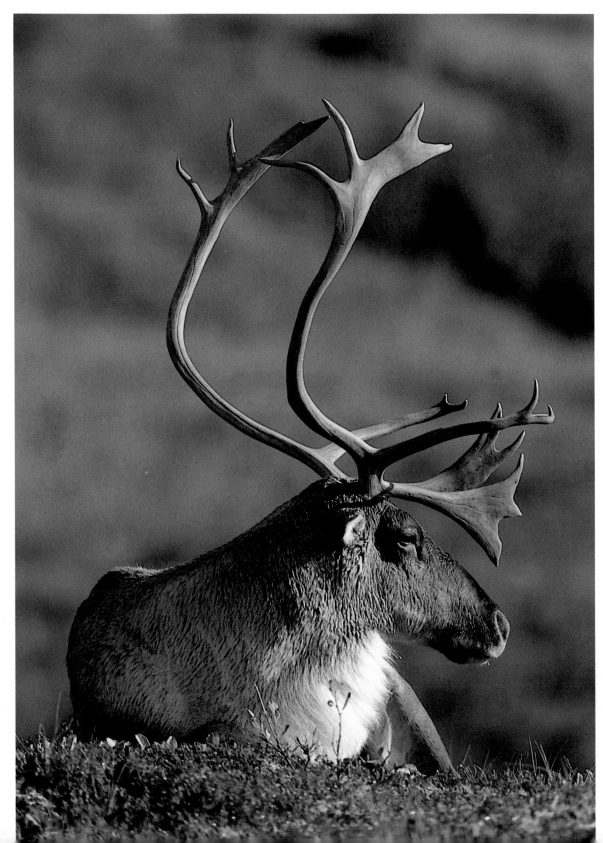

Taymyr in the center of the peninsula gradually doubles in surface area to 1,780 sq. miles (4,600 km²) though it is nowhere deeper than 85 feet (26 m). Over flat areas, the soil holds the meltwater like a sponge, since permafrost prevents the water from percolating downward, and the ground becomes sodden and marshy.

One of the characteristic effects of permafrost in tundra zones is to pattern the ground. Complex cycles of freezing and thawing heave up the soil, move and sort debris, and create angular fissures. On level terrain, they make the ground seem drawn into polygonal sections, sometimes disarmingly regular as if traced by giant human hands. The polygon rims tend to be higher than their centers, allowing ponds that accentuate the patterns to form in each.

All this fresh water and marshland, bordered by bright-flowered meadows, attracts untold numbers of nesting birds. During the warm days of continual sunshine, they can forage at any time. Gulls and terns glimmer white in the air, at times twisting and turning as piratical skuas harass them to relinquish their food. Many spectacular fowl nest close to the water, among them white-billed divers, Bewick's swans, king eiders and long-tailed ducks. The most beautiful is surely the red-breasted goose, a threatened species for which the peninsula is the single most important breeding area.

By the time the last migratory birds have left, the caribou, too, are well advanced on their terrestrial migration. Some linger through winter on the tundra, but most head away from the peninsula deep into

the forest margins, where food is easier to come by. At the southern limit of the peninsula, stunted larches about 10 feet (3 m) high appear. These pockets of trees, surrounded by open tundra, are the northernmost forests anywhere on the planet.

TUNDRA PERMAFROST
Deep permafrost benumbs the tundra soil, but in the brief summer the surface thaws enough for plants to grow in this "active layer." Because surface water cannot penetrate the permafrost and drain away, the ground becomes marshy in summer and pools develop.

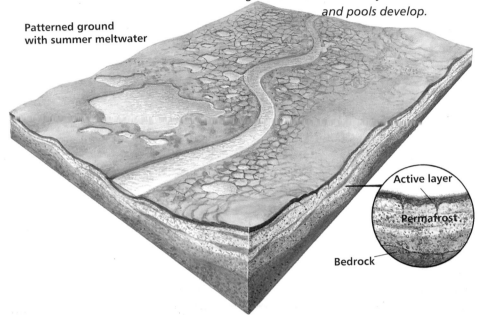

Patterned ground with summer meltwater

Active layer

Permafrost

Bedrock

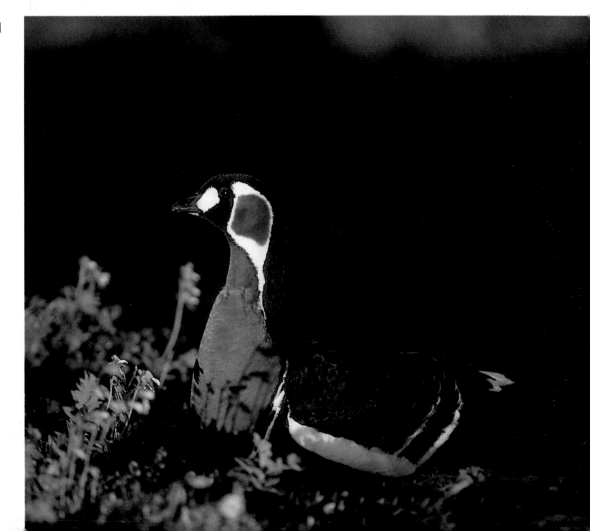

The red-breasted goose breeds on Taymyr. Small flocks of the geese appear at ice-free lakes and rivers in June, ready to make nests on mounds and clumps of vegetation.

THE ANTARCTIC PENINSULA

"Life has a firmer foothold here than elsewhere on Antarctica"

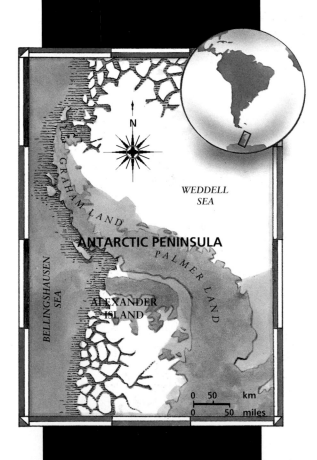

Antarctica has the harshest climate of all of the Earth's wildernesses – it is colder, drier and windier here than anywhere else in the world. But one part, the Antarctic Peninsula, which stretches out across the Antarctic Circle to within 600 miles (1,000 km) of South America, has a slightly less severe climate than the continental heartland. Surrounded by the

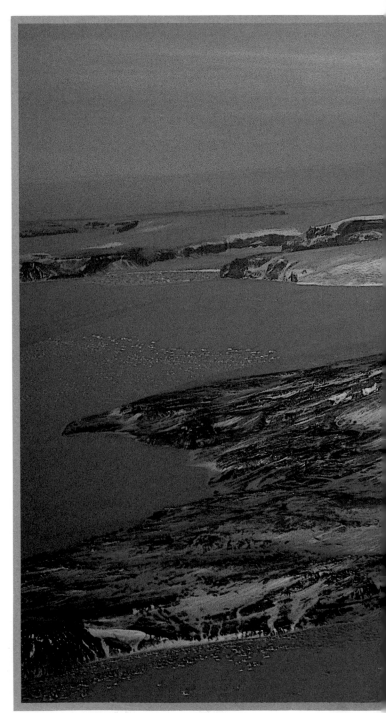

moderating influence of the ocean, the peninsula is a little warmer and more humid than the rest of the continent and, as a result, plant and animal life has a firmer foothold here.

The backbone of the Antarctic Peninsula is a chain of mountains that begin to rise in western Antarctica. They run the entire crooked length of the peninsula, raising it to heights of nearly 11,500 feet (3,500 m) in the loftiest sections. Geologists regard these mountains as an extension of the South American Andes, and it has been suggested that a land bridge once connected the two continents.

Palmer Land, the poleward section of the peninsula, is a curving finger of land up to 155 miles (250 km) wide between the Bellingshausen and Weddell seas. The ice sheets that cover most of its interior form a

On the wild and desolate Antarctic Peninsula, realms of mountain, ice and ocean converge. Here, where exposed rock interweaves with icebound terrain and snows melt briefly in summer, a few species of plant and animal struggle to survive.

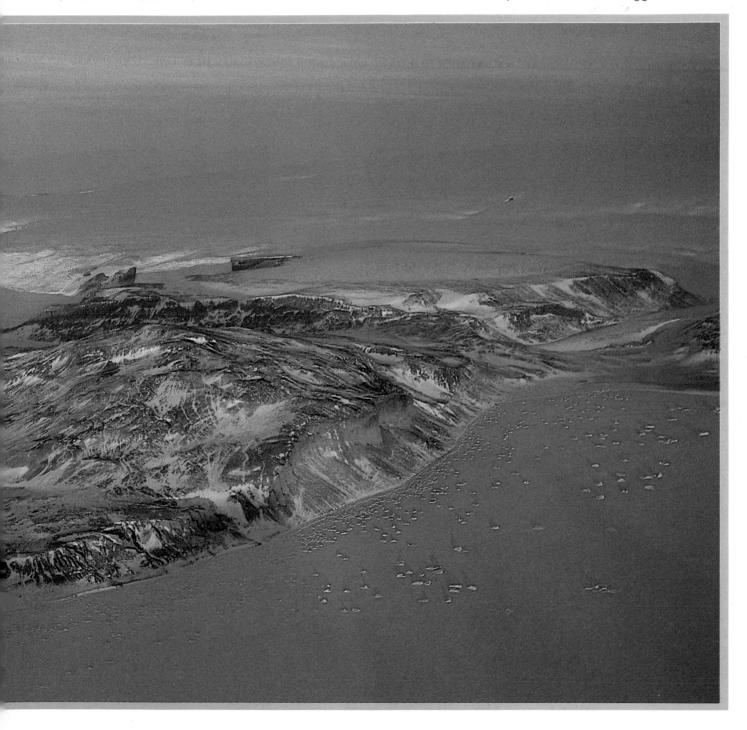

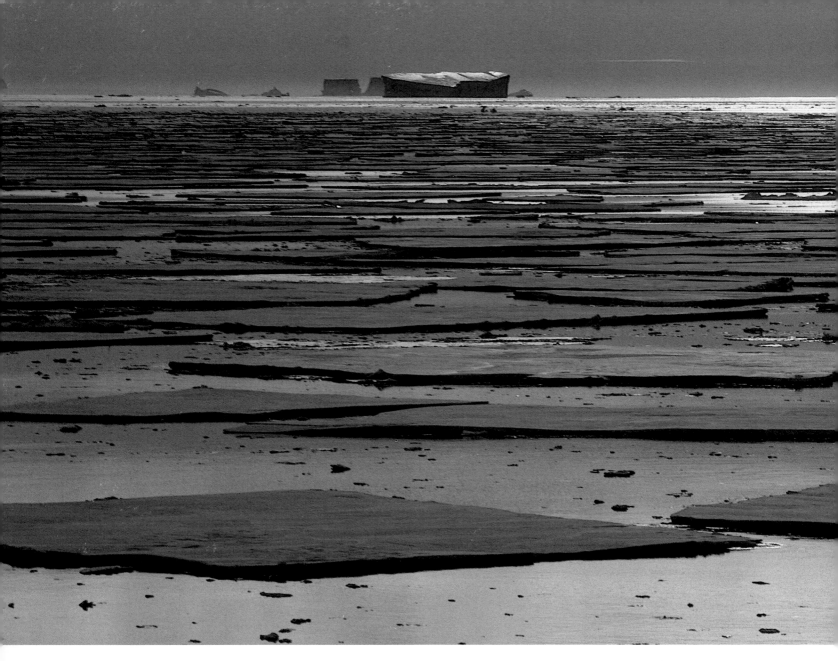

AN OCEANIC CLIMATE

Like a giant spur on the fringe of Antarctica, the peninsula thrusts out into the oceanic zone. Its climate is made slightly warmer and moister than that of the rest of the continent by the heat-retaining effect of the ocean and the greater humidity of the sea air.

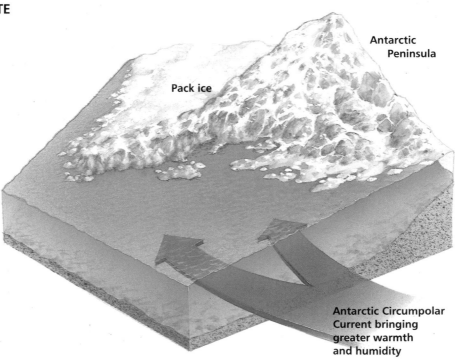

Pack ice

Antarctic Peninsula

Antarctic Circumpolar Current bringing greater warmth and humidity

***Treacherous sea** ice forms around the Antarctic Peninsula during the long and bitter polar winter (above). These frozen rafts of sea water form vast, unstable plains that are interrupted only by mountainous floating icebergs.*

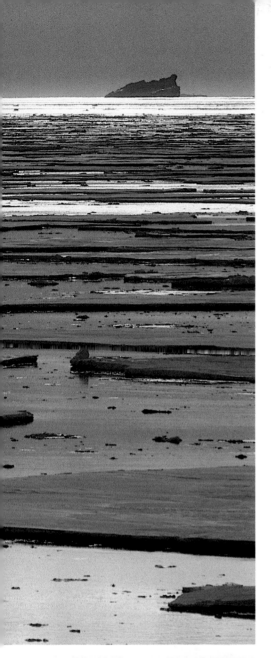

plateau more than 6,500 feet (2,000 m) high. Graham Land, the northern section juts from it like a recurved talon. Only 25 miles (40 km) wide in places, it rises from the sea in steep cliffs leading to snowbound peaks. Glaciers flowing from the mountains to the sea have sculpted deep valleys and indented the coastline with fiords.

Islands flank both coasts of the peninsula, separated from it by deep straits and channels. Many, like the giant Alexander Island west of Palmer Land, are locked for most of the year within huge ice shelves (floating platforms of glacier ice) or pack ice (frozen surface layers of the sea). Only the western shore of Graham Land is relatively free of sea ice through the Antarctic winter.

Nevertheless, the peninsula's icy climate is the mildest in Antarctica – though its nickname "the banana belt" stretches the point too far. In the north, temperatures may creep above freezing point even in winter, and it can be 59°F (15°C) in the peninsula on a midsummer's day. The average for the year is about 27°F (-3°C) compared with an average of -58°F (-50°C) at the South Pole. The peninsula also receives much more precipitation than the rest of Antarctica, which is classed as desert. Most of the continent receives only 2 inches (50 mm) of moisture in the form of snow in a year, but the peninsula has ten times this amount.

Such conditions make it possible for two species of flowering plant to survive here – the only ones known in Antarctica. But in general, the dominant plants are diminutive, hardy kinds. Cushions of moss and liverworts appear on ice-free rocks along the shore, and tiny fungi lace the pockets of soil. Smears of algae can even spread across snow and ice, staining it green or red with their pigmentation.

The most abundant and successful plants of all are the lichens. About 350 kinds occur in Antarctica, well adapted to the extremes of climate. Most ignore the rigors of winter by becoming dormant, closing down the processes of life to conserve their resources and prevent damage by freezing. But in summer they begin photosynthesizing, making the most of the slanted sunshine. They plaster exposed rocks all over the continent, even some isolated peaks that poke above the ice sheet close to the pole. Though many are black or gray, others are bright orange and green, bringing splashes of color into the peninsula landscape.

The dwarf "forest" of Antarctic plants is home to wildlife of a similar scale. The only truly terrestrial animals that can cope with Antarctica

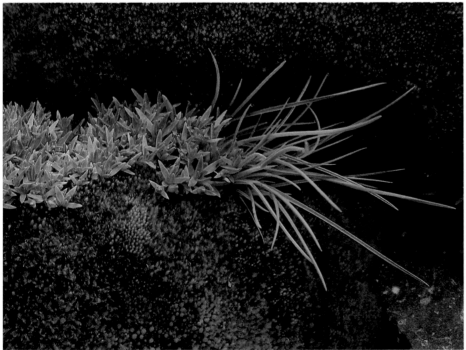

Only two types of flowering plant grow in the whole of Antarctica – the Antarctic hair grass and the pearlwort. Both grow near the coast on Graham Land, usually on rocky, north-facing slopes from which snow thaws more easily in summer. The grass tends to grow in clumps, but occasionally forms a closed turf over the surface.

are either microscopic or of small insect size. They include protozoa, rotifers, roundworms, lice, fleas and gnats. Mites and springtails barely a millimeter in length cluster on plants and under rocks and forage on fungi and algae or, in some cases, on each other. The predatory mite *Rhagidia gerlachei* eats adult springtails and the

Gentoo penguins bask in the muted light of the Antarctic sun. Like Adélie and chinstrap penguins, gentoos nest on rocky and tussock-covered slopes on the peninsula, but in winter they move out beyond the expanding margins of the sea ice.

eggs, and is one of many creatures that zoologists suspect have a form of antifreeze in their body fluids – a substance that stops them from freezing rigid at winter temperatures as low as -30°F (-34°C).

Bigger animals are not permanent residents in Antarctica. They may use it as a base for resting and nesting in summer months, but spend most of their time either in or over the ocean. Seals swim in the waters off the peninsula and haul up onto the beaches in summer to give birth and rear their pups. Millions of birds, including petrels, gulls, terns and blue-eyed cormorants, flock to nesting colonies on the rocky coasts

and islands. Rich waters full of krill and fish provide them with plenty of food for their young. Four kinds of penguins breed in the area, and brown skuas and snowy sheathbills lurk among the colonies ready to steal eggs and chicks.

Most birds move away – even from the peninsula – in winter, but the emperor penguin holds out against adversity. Colonies of these birds, which are 3 feet (1 m) tall, huddle together on the ice fields of Palmer Land through the long, dark winters. Males take the first three-month shift, each bird incubating a single egg between its feet and its abdomen, followed by the females,

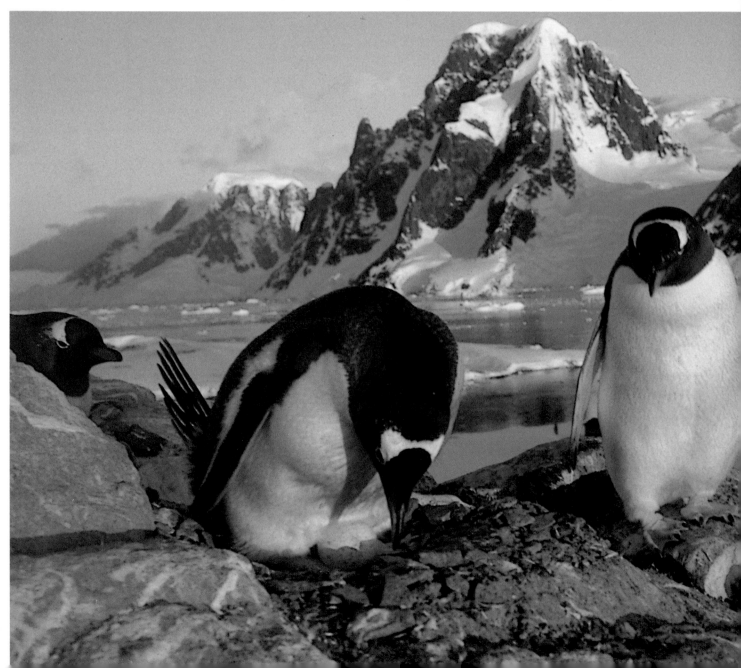

which return from the sea when the chicks are about to hatch. The male emperors then make the long journey across the ice to feed in open water.

There has long been a sparse human presence in Antarctica. Sealers operated in this region for most of the 19th century, but the greatest impact came with intensive whaling in the 20th century. Factory ships moved into the sheltered waters, processing stations were built on the shores, and harpoon gunners soon brought about a collapse in the great whale population. Though the industry has now been banished, the blue whale, which was hunted almost to extinction in the southern oceans, has

"The only true land animals that survive on Antarctica are of microscopic size"

scarcely begun to recover. The most likely cetaceans to be seen today around the peninsula are killer whales cruising offshore, waiting to snatch penguins and seals.

Now the sealers and whalers have gone, but the scientists have moved in. Research stations and bases are concentrated on the peninsula, the most hospitable and accessible part of

the continent, representing 10 nations in all. These bases reflect the desire of many countries to establish an official presence in – and therefore a stake in the future of – Antarctica. Some have already brought pollution to the fragile polar continent, but for now at least, this barren but beautiful land remains one of the greatest of all wildernesses on Earth.

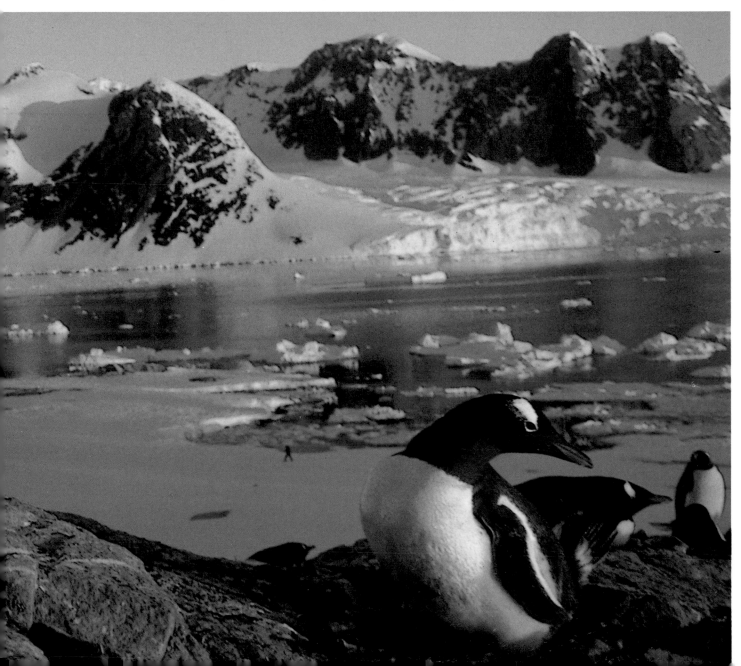

DENALI NATIONAL PARK

"Mount McKinley, North America's highest peak, crowns Denali's rocky majesty"

A magnificent expanse of subarctic wilderness, the Denali National Park and Preserve spreads its stark mantle of pristine snow and jutting rock over an area larger than the state of Massachusetts. Across this vast virgin landscape, which covers more than 6 million acres (2.5 million hectares) of the interior of Alaska,

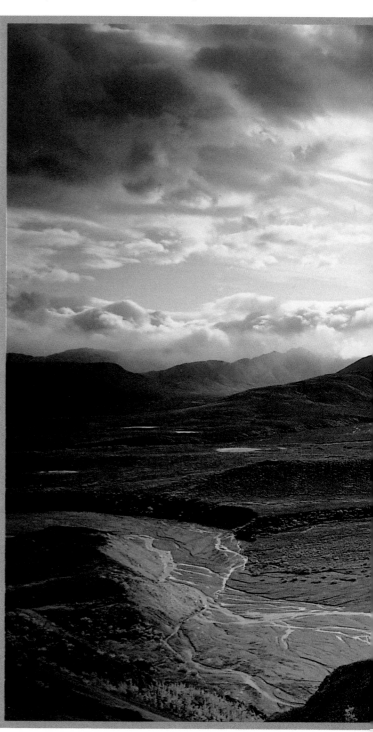

The foothills of Mount McKinley stand as a massive backdrop to the wandering rivers and vast expanses of heathlike tundra of Denali.

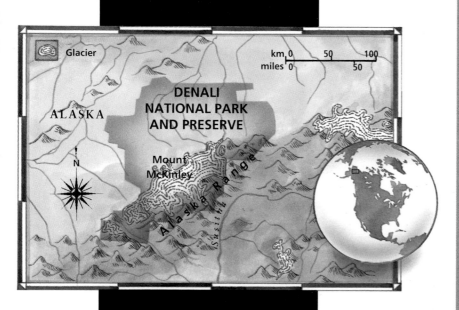

Glacier

km 0   50   100
miles 0   50

ALASKA

DENALI NATIONAL PARK AND PRESERVE

Mount McKinley

Alaska Range

Susitna

N

roam herds of migrating caribou and Dall sheep, pinpricks of life in the enormous emptiness. And Mount McKinley, North America's highest peak and perpetually shrouded in snow, crowns its rocky majesty.

Athabascan Indians knew the mountain as Denali, "the High One." It forms the apex of the awesome 600-mile (1,000-km) Alaska Range, a natural barrier that separates Alaska's rugged interior to the north from the coastal lowlands to the south. The bulky, looming range dwarfs the surrounding panorama of treeless tundra and sparsely wooded taiga, threaded with braided, meandering rivers that originate in its own glaciers. The south peak of Mount McKinley juts higher than any other point in North America, rising 20,340 feet (6,200 m) above sea level in an astounding vertical sweep. In addition, its north summit ranks as North America's second-highest peak at 19,455 feet (5,930 m).

Solid ice hundreds of yards thick blankets the granite and slate core of Mount McKinley, and the permanent ice fields that cover more than half

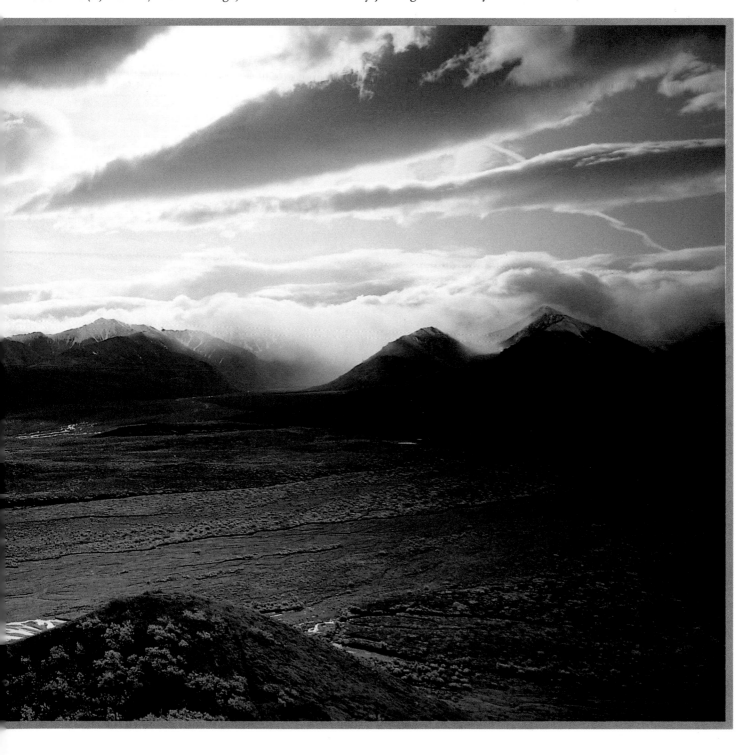

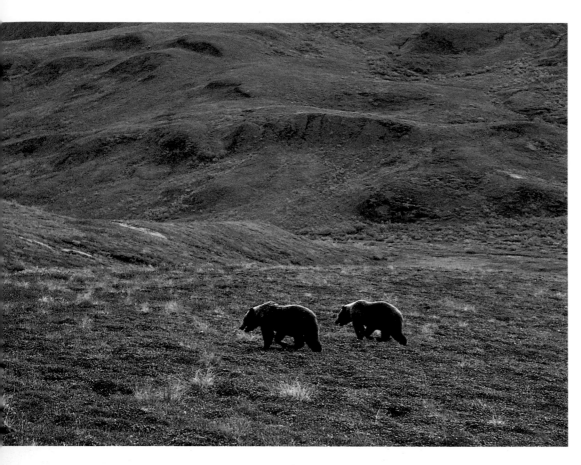

In the vast wilderness of Denali, *grizzly bears roam far and wide in search of plants and berries to eat as well as prey. A full-grown grizzly stands up to 7 feet (2 m) tall and weighs up to 850 pounds (390 kg).*

"*During the brief summer season, the rocks burst into glowing color as flowers bloom in amazing profusion*"

the mountain feed a myriad of glaciers, which surround its base. Even in summer, temperatures are severe; in winter, temperatures on the mountain plummet below –94°F (–70°C) and slicing winds gust in excess of 150 mph (240 km/h).

Both of Mount McKinley's peaks, located on the Denali Fault which is the largest break in the crustal plate in all of North America, are still rising. Geologists now think that Denali may encompass up to 7 blocks of unrelated land, while Alaska itself may be composed of as many as 32 of these crustal blocks called terranes. Denali's seven terranes formed independently, in different places around the globe, but over eons of time the Earth's tectonic plate movements drove them together.

The arrival here, 100 million years ago, of one such block, made of volcanic islands, may have given rise to the Alaska Range, whose geological faults and folded rock

formations provide the evidence of its ancient birth. The monumental collisions and grindings would have produced spectacularly violent earthquakes and volcanic eruptions. Geologists now know that the pressure to fold these rocks into such high and bulky mountains came from the Kula Plate pushing beneath Alaska for 100 million years.

As a result of these thunderous birth pangs, Denali's wildlands display a fabulous rainbow of rocks. The Polychrome Pass, from which grizzly bears are often sighted, takes its name from the bright palette of colors of its folded rock. Cathedral Mountain and other lesser peaks are reddish, and Igloo Mountain, which is ice-free in summer, has masses of loose rock fragments, or talus, that display a wide range of hues.

After the continental ice sheets retreated about 10,000 years ago, centuries passed as a fragile layer of topsoil gradually accumulated and the slow process of revegetation began. Above the permafrost – permanent subsurface ice that has remained frozen for thousands of years – this thin cover of soil thaws just enough in summer to support successful plant growth. Two major types of plant community now exist in Denali – tundra and taiga.

Tundra may be moist or dry. On moist tundra, tussocks of sedges and cottongrass or dwarfed shrubs, such as birches and willows, carpet the ground. Dry-tundra plants occur in patches, sometimes dotting rocks at higher elevations. During the brief summer season, the rocks burst into glowing color as an amazing profusion of blossom attracts the insects that will help the plants reproduce before winter returns.

Taiga means "land of little sticks" in Russian, and the name aptly characterizes the tree growth close to the Arctic Circle. Denali's taiga, which mainly clings to the river valleys, is composed largely of white and black spruce trees, interspersed with quaking aspen, alder, balsam poplar and the white, or paper, birch. Open areas of taiga fill with shrubs – blueberry, willow and dwarf birch. In these desolate wildlands, the limit of tree growth occurs just 2,700 feet (820 m) above sea level, nearly 18,000 feet (5,500 m) below Mount McKinley's summit.

Much of Mount McKinley's character remains a secret of the wilderness, since the mountain is often wreathed in cloud. On a few summer days, the clouds briefly lift or part to reveal its hulking, snow-clad shape, perhaps still trailing enshrouding streamers of mist.

By contrast, the open, rolling lowlands of Denali National Park and Preserve seem tame at first sight. Shallow-bedded and laden with glacial flour – the liquid suspension

of rock pulverized to powder by the grinding ice masses as they flow over the land – the rivers wander across the broad, flat valleys at will. They can dam themselves in a matter of hours with their own sedimentary load and sometimes set new channels overnight. All may appear calm, yet a grizzly bear may suddenly disrupt the tranquil scene, revealing the wild

The tundra in the fall glows with low-growing but brilliantly colorful foliage. Dwarf shrubs such as bunchberry, bearberry and Labrador tea (below) create swaths of red and gold across the land. In their brief growing season, these plants provide food for a multitude of tiny voles and rodents as well as the many birds that migrate north to nest in Denali.

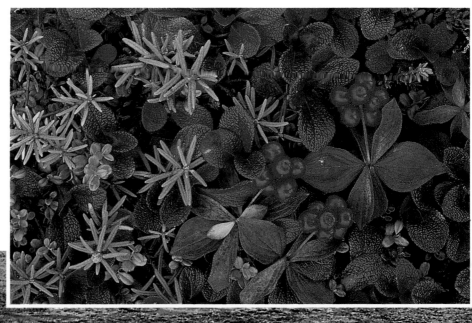

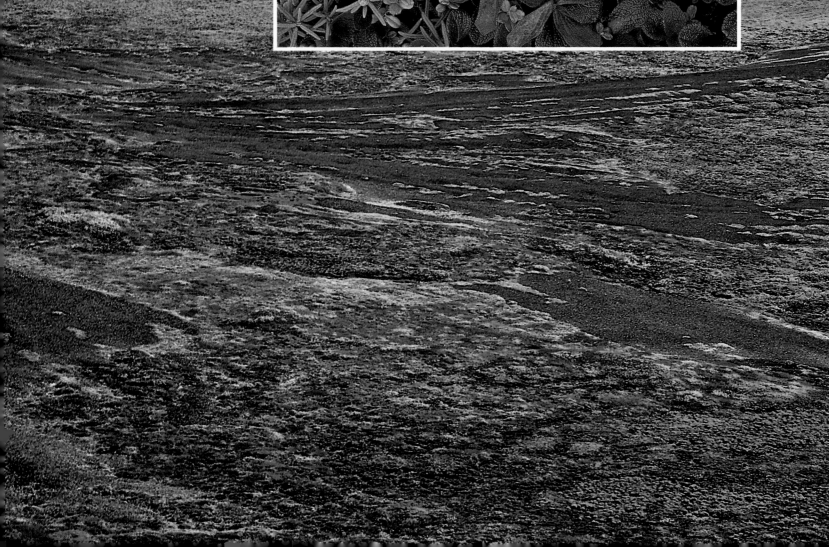

elements in the sprawling landscape as it nonchalantly turns over huge chunks of tundra to lift the roof off the Arctic ground squirrel's burrow.

The grizzly's prey is also known as the parka or "parky" squirrel because the Indians of the Alaskan interior used its pelts to make winter parkas and lined the hoods with the pelts of long-haired wolves. But in their private wilderness drama, squirrels and wolves meet on different terms. While a wolf would rather make a feast of a Dall sheep or caribou calf, it often chases down the plump ground squirrel for a quick meal. Wolves may hunt alone in summer; in winter, they generally hunt in packs and often prey on moose, whose escape is hampered by deep snow in the willow thickets where they graze.

When the tundra and taiga are snowclad, little life moves across the severe landscape. Exceptions are ptarmigans, well camouflaged by their white winter plumage, as well as snowshoe hares and the owls and lynxes that hunt them. Slow-moving porcupines remain active, too, protected from most predators by their coat of quills. Occasionally, a lithe weasel will burrow under the snow and kill a porcupine by attacking its vulnerable underbelly.

Every summer, large populations of migrating birds cover the vast distances from Siberia, Central America and South America to breed in Denali. Many of these summer visitors feed on the hordes of mosquitoes and other flying insects that spring from the temporary fecundity of the moist tundra. Like subarctic plants, these insects must mature and reproduce quickly before winter clamps its deadly cold on them once again.

But the grizzlies, so called because of the grizzled appearance of the gray flecked coat, are perhaps the most potent symbols of Denali's wild seclusion. Hundreds of these bears, among North America's most formidable animals, inhabit the park.

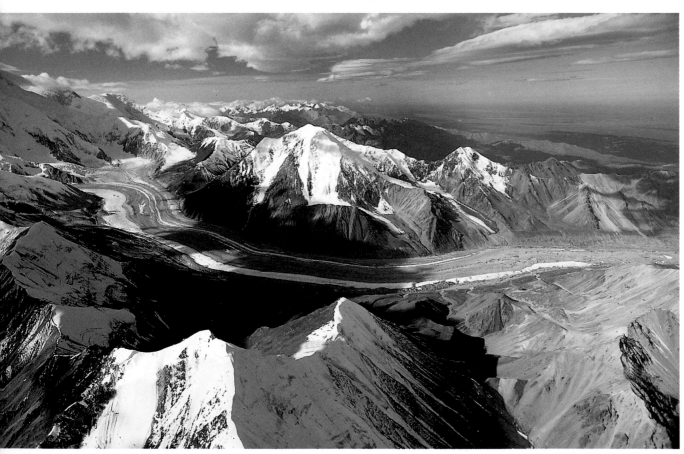

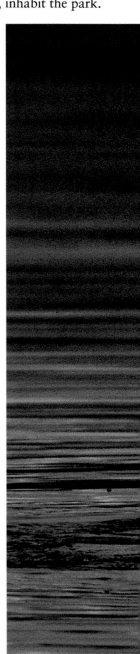

Like the frozen river that it is, the huge Peters Glacier gathers tributaries as it carves a path from its source deep in the Alaska Range. But a glacier's tributaries do not merge into one; they remain separate, as the lengthwise striations here reveal.

Spreading antlers drip water as this moose, which has been feeding on succulent underwater plants, surfaces to keep a watchful eye on its surroundings. Moose also browse on dwarf willows and other low-growing tundra shrubs.

They have no natural enemies – only humans unnaturally armed with high-powered rifles can destroy them. Although bears, like cats and dogs, belong to the carnivore group of mammals, they tend increasingly toward omnivorous eating habits. The grizzlies in Denali subsist on berries and small plants such as vetch, as well as on ground squirrels, the calves of moose or caribou, and occasional carrion – the decaying carcasses of animals that have been killed or that have died as a result of disease or old age.

Grizzlies usually hibernate through the harsh winter, and females give birth to their cubs in underground dens during this period. When they first emerge into the dazzling spring sunshine with their cubs, female grizzly bears are at their most dangerous, prepared to defend their young against all enemies.

Despite their great size, ferocity and agility, grizzly bears do not hold absolute power over Denali's landscape. A full-grown Alaskan moose will stand its ground against a hungry grizzly, and a female protecting her calf will chase the bear away. The largest members of the deer family, Alaska moose can weigh 1,800 pounds (820 kg) and stand more than 7½ feet (2.3 m) high at the shoulder; a bull moose's antlers alone may spread 6½ feet (2 m) and weigh an incredible 90 pounds (40 kg). So even a predator as feared as the grizzly bear must exercise extreme caution to avoid injury.

Stunning contrasts heighten the thrilling impact of Denali: grizzlies feed on the tiny vetch, Mount McKinley's cloud-splitting peak towers over a lowland of vulnerable plants. And if Mount McKinley symbolizes the permanence of Denali's wilderness world, the youthful rivers and leaping streams exemplify its renewable vitality. Little altered by human intervention, here is a self-determined wilderness that retains its natural integrity.

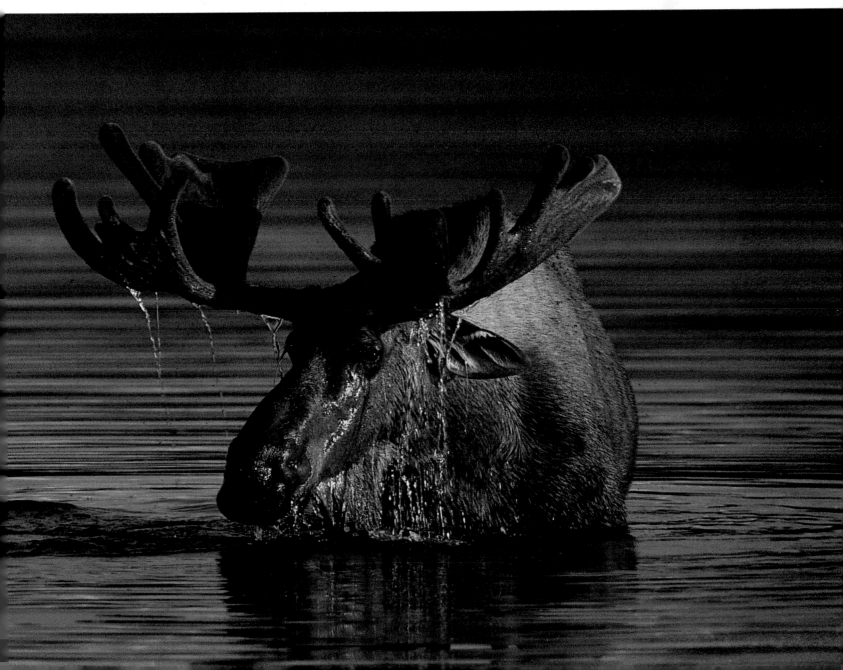

BANFF & JASPER NATIONAL PARKS

"Shining mountains rise above the valleys in matchless grandeur"

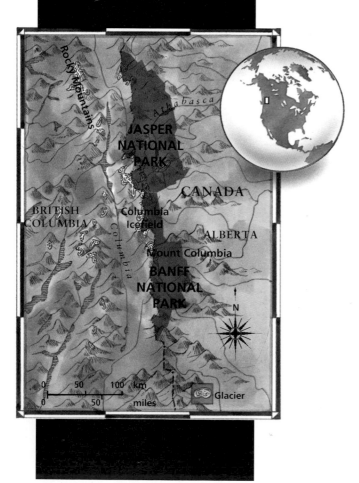

On the crest of the Canadian Rocky Mountains, the alpine peaks of Banff and Jasper National Parks pierce the sky at every point of the compass. Shining, skyscraping mountain walls rise above the valleys in matchless grandeur, like immovable bulwarks of nature damming the horizon. These

A breathtaking sunset over the snowcapped peak of Banff's Mount Rundle is dramatically mirrored in clear lake waters.

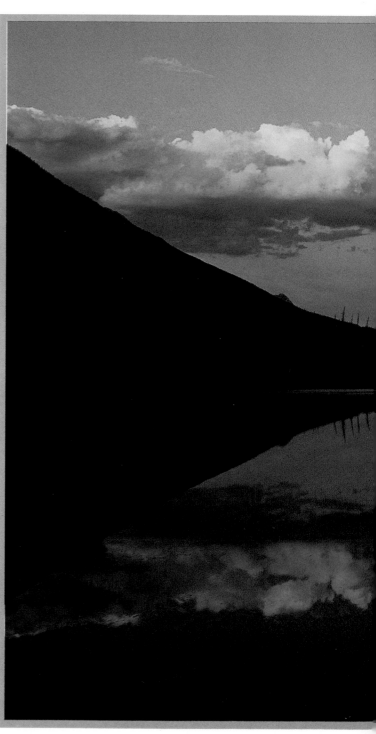

spectacular, adjoining parks straddle the border between Alberta and British Columbia in western Canada and between them cover a total area of some 6,760 sq. miles (17,500 km²).

Sediments of shale, dolomite, sandstone, limestone, quartzite and slate fuse here in the Canadian Rockies to form North America's upper spine, a skeleton so awesome that the Colorado Rocky Mountains seem puny by comparison. West of the Canadian Rockies' crest, great geological fault zones splinter the broad valleys. Most prominent is the Rocky Mountain Trench, a fissure from 2 to 10 miles (3 to 16 km) wide in the Earth's crust which separates the Rockies from the older western ranges in British Columbia. The massive proportions of this trench, 800 miles (1,300 km) long in Canada alone, and of the Purcell Trench, which joins it 200 miles (320 km) north of the Canadian border, seem to create a three-dimensional mirror of the mountains of Banff and Jasper, as deep as the cliffs are high.

At the crest, summit shales more than 12,000 feet (3,700 m) above sea

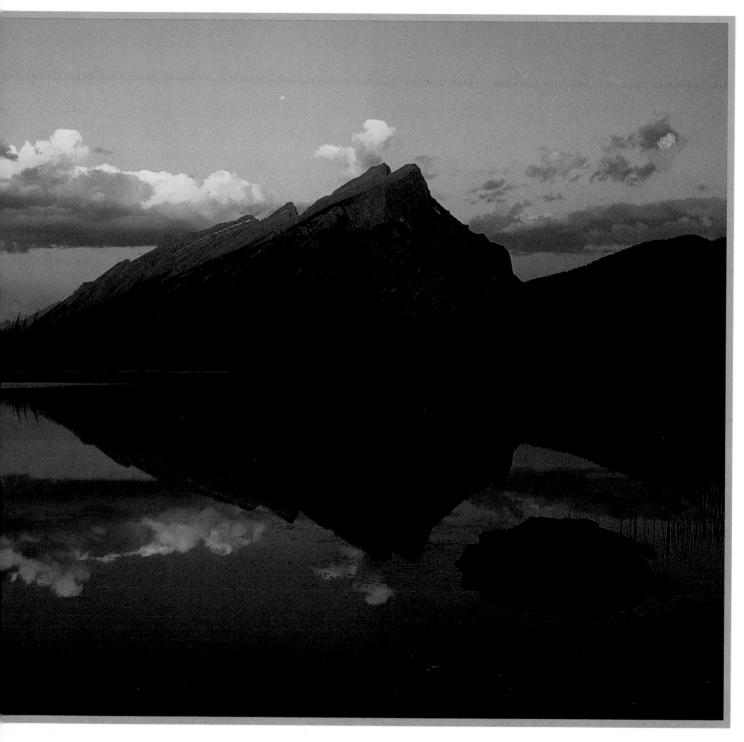

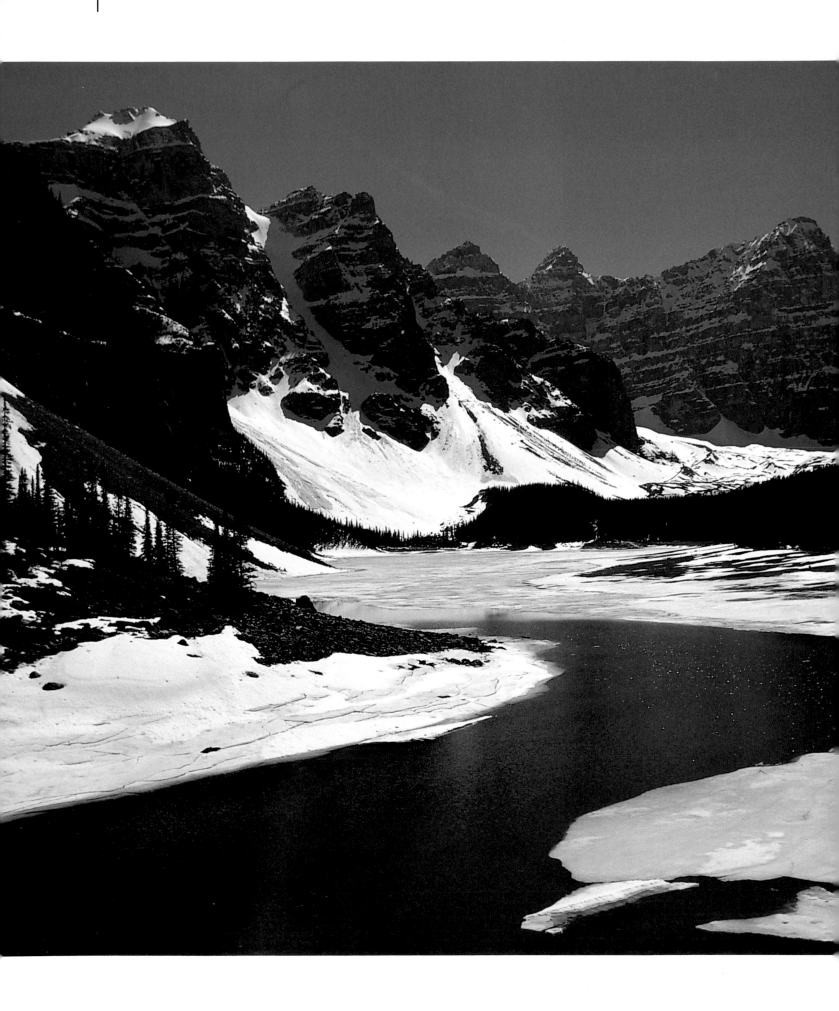

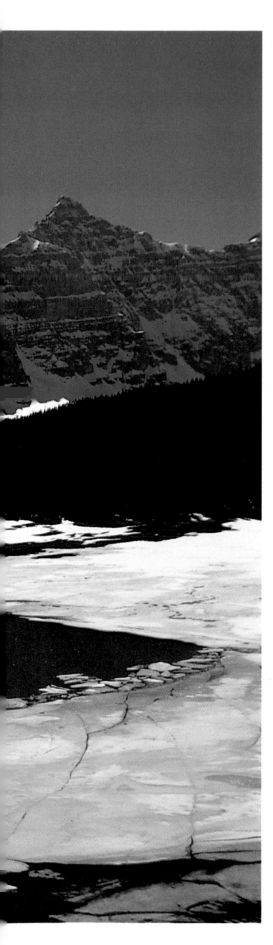

level are stacked like oversized sedimentary pancakes. Their striated massifs and undulating cliffs tilt hazardously from the vertical, while their horizontal surfaces run for miles, as if they could link the ancient past to the unknown future.

The Rocky Mountains stretch more than 3,000 miles (5,000 km), extending northward from central New Mexico through Canada and across Alaska. They reach their highest point – 12,972 feet (3,954 m) – on Canada's Mount Robson, 48 miles (77 km) northwest of Jasper. For most of their length, the Rockies define the Continental Divide, the great watershed separating the rivers that drain into the Pacific Ocean from those that drain into the Atlantic and Arctic oceans.

At the heart of the Canadian Rockies, in the middle of the Banff and Jasper parks, lies the immense Columbia Icefield, a remnant of the great ice shield that blanketed most of Canada 10,000 years ago. Not a single glacier but an astonishing assembly of them, Columbia's 100 sq. miles (250 km²) of icefield smother the mountains and dig deep into their

valleys with tentacles of alpine glaciers. Up to 2,500 feet (750 m) thick at some points, the icefield is buried under about 200 inches (500 cm) of snow every year. Its featureless white surface is gashed by gaping crevasses. Glacial meltwater at the foot of such crevasses is kept from freezing only by its own rushing motion.

Forged by a process that echoes the formation of sedimentary rock, glacier ice is composed of snow crystals that compress under their own cumulative weight and harden. The tremendous pressure of the glacier's weight against the steely bedrock of the mountains creates friction, which heats the lower surface of the glacier and melts it just enough to lubricate the entire glacier's forward motion.

From the Snow Dome of the Columbia Icefield, endless meltwater flows in all directions: via the Columbia River to the Pacific Ocean, via the North Saskatchewan River to Hudson Bay and the Atlantic Ocean, and via the Athabasca, Slave and MacKenzie rivers to the Arctic Ocean.

Jasper's Athabasca glacier is moving in two ways at once. It is

When warmer climates force a glacier into retreat, a natural dam results from the debris at the glacier's head. Copious meltwaters collect and can form lakes such as Moraine in Banff (left).

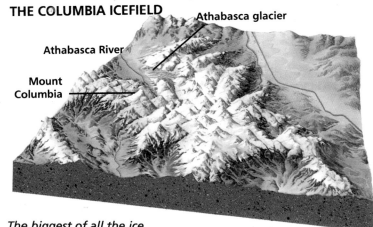

THE COLUMBIA ICEFIELD

Athabasca glacier

Athabasca River

Mount Columbia

The biggest of all the ice caps in the Rocky Mountains is the Columbia Icefield in the Banff and Jasper parks. Its ice mass reaches to a depth of 1,000 feet (300 m) in places and feeds so many rivers that it is known as the hydrological apex of North America.

receding gradually because it is melting faster than the accumulation of new snow at its head can replenish it. However, since the glacier is still 1,000 feet (300 m) thick in places and fed by substantial annual snowfall, its retreat is extremely slow.

Simultaneously, Athabasca glacier is sliding down the mountain, and, for the first few miles of its flow, the meltwater may not be water at all. Glaciers flow as frozen rivers, similar to fields of molten lava. As Athabasca's ice flows over cliffs, rocks as big as railroad cars split from its face and crash to its base – if these frozen lumps were to split off a glacier and tumble into tidal waters, they would be called icebergs.

Not everything moves at the lumbering pace of glacial ice – a yard or so a day. An avalanche of snow can streak downhill at 100 mph (160 km/h), pushing and compressing the air in front of it into tornado-force blasts that snap mature trees like matchsticks. Rocks also respond to the force of gravity. Blocks of soft sedimentary rock routinely weather and break loose, fanning out from the base of the mountain in vast fields of debris called scree or talus.

The mountainous wilds of Banff and Jasper are a haven for rare bighorn sheep. Once common from New Mexico to British Columbia, bighorn now dwell only in isolated pockets of wilderness, to which they have adapted by developing spongy footpads that give them a firm foothold on bare rock. While they summer in the highlands, harsh winter conditions force them down to the foothills, where domestic stock now graze. Safely hidden from predators among the rocky crags, bighorn sheep easily fall victim to the diseases of domestic livestock, and overcrowding also threatens them with disease.

During the mating season, male rams, weighing up to 250 pounds

"Rocks as big as railroad cars split from the face of the Athabasca glacier and crash at its base"

(110 kg), vie for breeding rights by butting heads. The horn-splitting crashes can be heard half a mile away, and the stately combatants often turn from their confrontations with bloody noses and rolling eyes. But nature has bestowed some protective safeguards on the bighorn sheep. To withstand the repeated head to head clashes, the sheep's skull is porous and double-layered, and thick facial hide absorbs and cushions the blows.

Banff and Jasper also harbor the mountain goat, whose smaller, spiky horns and whiter, long-haired coat distinguish it from the bighorn. Both animals live off the meager mat of alpine vegetation that is briefly exposed by summer's snowmelt – a mixture of dwarf plants, mosses and ground cover that have adapted to the thin soil, brief growing season and harsh surroundings. Certain high-mountain plants, such as alpine buckwheat, grow masses of tiny hairs on their leaves and stems; the hairs block or slow the passage of the wind over the plant and thereby restrict its loss of moisture.

Life throughout these harsh wildlands is arranged in layers that are determined by the growth of vegetation. On the highest meadows live mammals such as marmots and

pikas, or conies, grazing among the grassy pockets of scree and talus. Smaller pikas, sometimes nicknamed rock rabbits, gather grasses and sedges and make little caches beneath rocks, where in winter they eat their carefully stashed hay beneath an insulating blanket of snow.

The next mountain layer belongs to the sheep and goats, and not far below them are the elk, properly called wapiti. Most regal of the large mammals here, these members of the deer family are second in size only to the moose and are distinguished from other deer by their size, yellow rump and the dark mane around their neck. Elk weigh more than 800 pounds (350 kg), and a male's antlers can have a spread of more than 5 feet (1.5 m).

Bulls that grazed the alpine slopes together peacefully through the summer become fierce adversaries when they descend to the valleys in the fall and begin to assemble their harems. For weeks, they parry and shove, bugling majestically and eventually lowering their horns and charging rivals at full speed. Repeatedly victorious males are reduced to exhaustion by the mating season and rendered uncharacteristically vulnerable to bears. Sometimes the bulls' antlers lock inextricably during combat, and both beasts starve to death.

No more sustained stretch of stunning alpine scenery graces the North American continent than that of Banff and Jasper, where towering snowy peaks are reflected in forest-rimmed alpine waters. Lake Louise in Banff displays an almost magical serenity. Draped in glaciers, Mount Victoria rises solemnly behind it, forming a somber backdrop; from certain vantage points, the mountain and its icy cloak appear to rest delicately on the lake's surface.

But this is not gentle country. The rugged nature of these mountain-encrusted parks has helped them remain truly wild lands.

A sure-footed mountain goat (below) wanders the craggy slopes of Banff and Jasper in search of plants to graze on. The goat's straight spiky horns distinguish it from the curled horns of the bighorn and Dall's mountain sheep.

Ever watchful for predators such as eagles, hoary marmots have a warning cry that has earned them the name of "whistle pigs." In spring and summer, marmots feed voraciously on mountain plants to build up layers of fat to last them through the long winter hibernation.

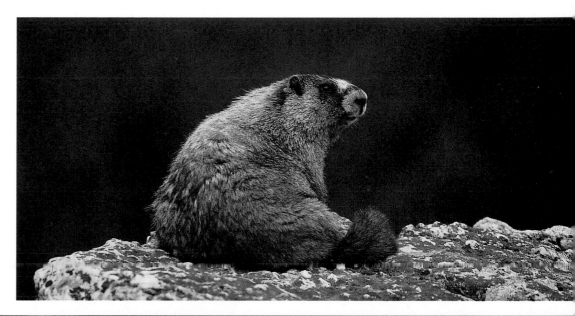

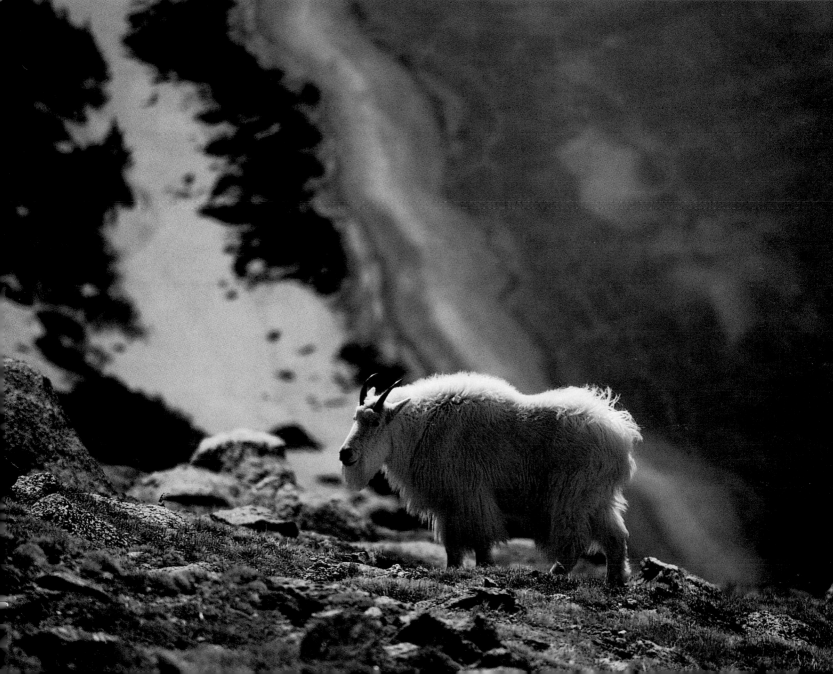

MOUNTAIN LIONS OF BANFF & JASPER

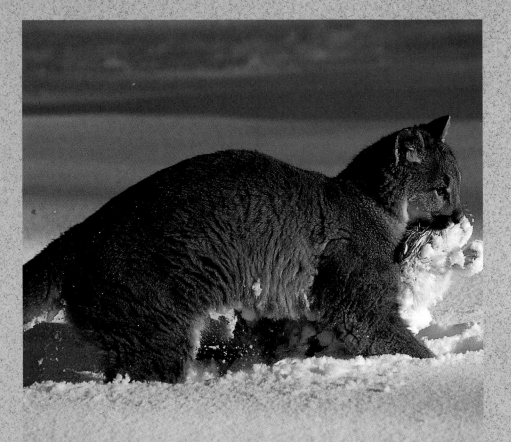

The biggest members of the cat family in North America, mountain lions survive in habitats as diverse as the snowy parks of Banff and Jasper, the parched deserts of the southwestern United States, and the humid subtropical conditions in Florida. Female mountain lions measure up to 8 feet (2.4 m) long, including tail, and males are up to 9 feet (2.7 m).

Mountain lions are stealthy solitary animals which hunt mostly at night and are seldom seen. Deer are their main prey, and one large kill can last a lion several days. In Banff and Jasper, the lions also hunt hares, beavers, mountain goats and sheep. Unlike other big cats, mountain lions do not roar. They utter long and unearthly howls which echo around the remote wildernesses in which they live.

Female mountain lions give birth to one to six young, usually two, in a sheltered den. They care for their cubs alone and teach them how to stalk prey and become powerful killers.

The mountain lion can run fast, but only over short distances. It generally stalks its prey, then makes a final dash to pounce on its victim, killing it with a bite to the neck. Mountain lions are also good climbers and may take cover in a tree to watch for prey.

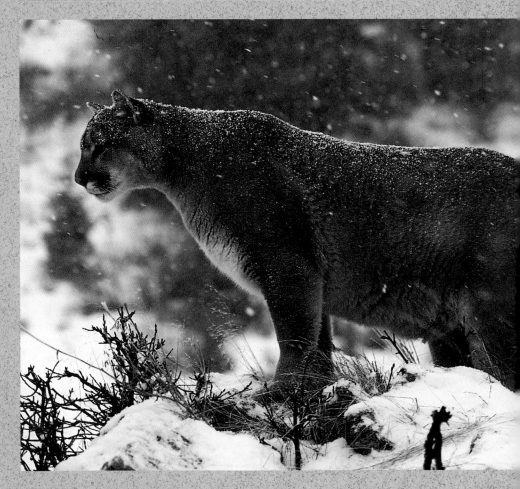

A snowshoe hare falls victim to a mountain lion (left). Like its smaller cousin the lynx, the mountain lion hunts year round through the rugged winters of Banff and Jasper.

Cougar, puma, panther and painter are just some of the names by which the mountain lion is known over its range – the widest of any mammal in the Americas.

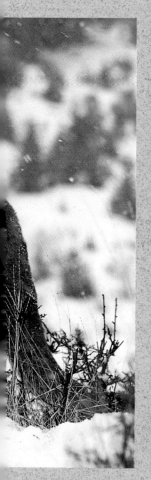

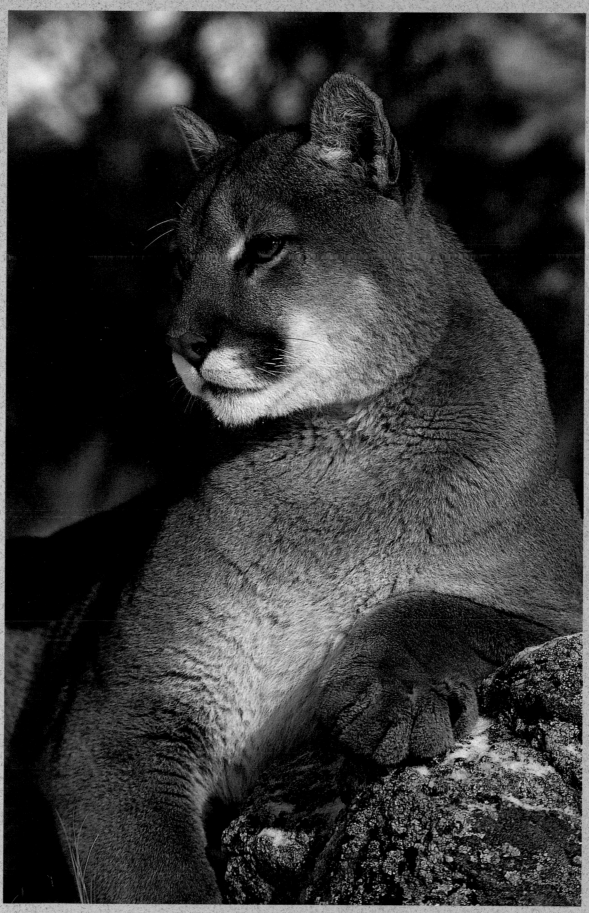

WOOD BUFFALO NATIONAL PARK

"A wetland wilderness of astonishing variety"

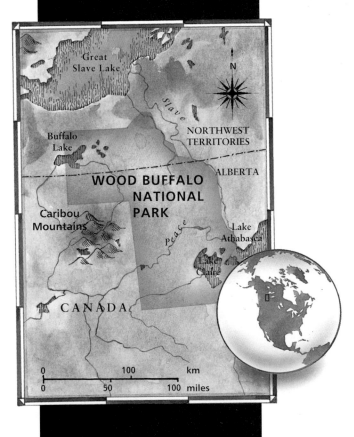

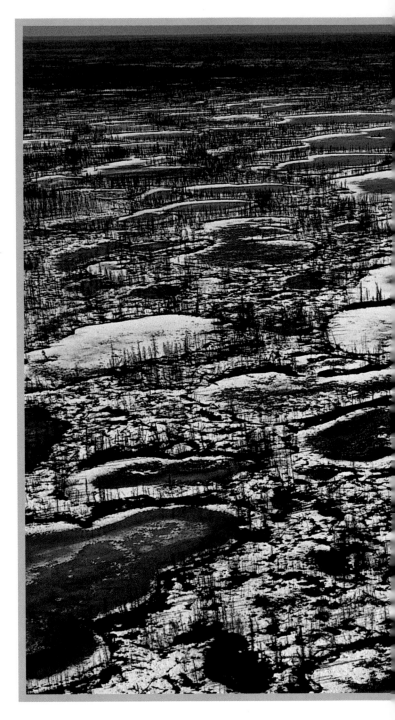

Wood Buffalo National Park is the living definition of big. Originally set aside as parkland to protect the wood buffalo from extinction, it is so spacious that its herd of five to six thousand bison, the largest free-roaming bison herd in the world, can virtually disappear in its vast plains. Larger than all of Switzerland, eight times bigger than

A vast expanse of land with abundant surface water makes the wildlands of Wood Buffalo a natural haven for wildlife.

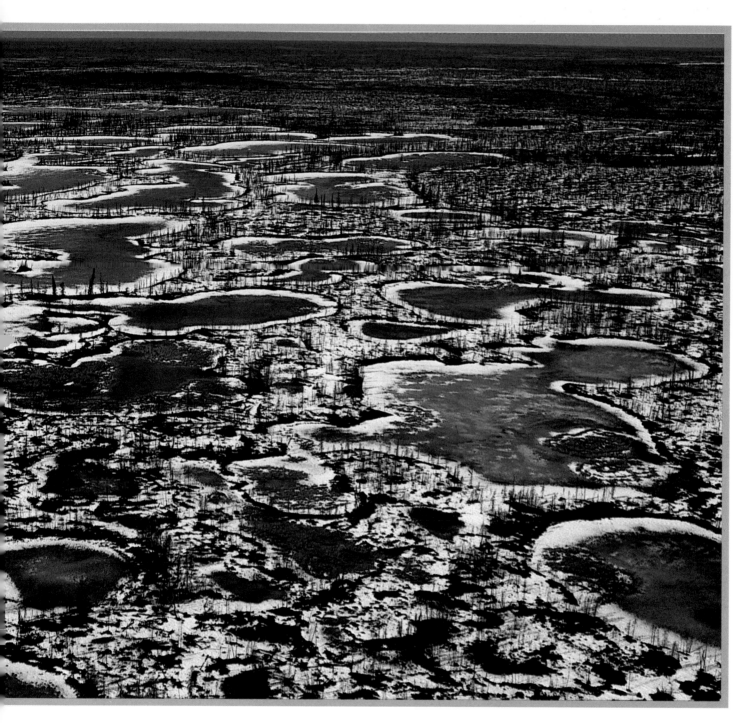

Yellowstone National Park in Wyoming, Wood Buffalo is Canada's largest park and the second largest in the world. It covers 17,400 sq. miles (45,000 km²), straddling the boundary between the provinces of Alberta and the Northwest Territories south of Great Slave Lake.

Three separate and magnificent wild environments could be created from Wood Buffalo's parklands.

Its rugged uplands feature sprawling, fire-scarred forests of spruce, pine and aspen, characteristic of extreme northern latitudes. A fertile plateau, pocked with bogs and embroidered with meandering streams, unrolls at the lower elevations. Finally, the Peace-Athabasca Delta, one of the world's largest freshwater deltas, encloses shallow lakes, marshes and the continent's largest grass-and-

sedge meadows in a wetland wilderness of astonishing variety. Situated in the park's southeastern corner, the immense delta abounds with waterfowl in spring and summer. Converging here from four North American flyways, the swans, ducks and geese seasonally number more than a million birds.

Much of Wood Buffalo rests on a bedrock of limestone and gypsum, water-soluble rock that dissolves in seeping rain and groundwater, leaving the underground terrain perforated with sinkholes, sunken valleys and complex networks of caverns and subterranean rivers.

In brilliant contrast to the underground caves' mysterious darkness are the dazzling salt-encrusted white mud flats and saline meadows in the southeastern section of the park – the only such landscape in Canada. As the salty water emerges from underground springs and flows across the plains, it evaporates, leaving behind salt and other dissolved minerals on the land. During dry years, salt mounds nearly 6 feet (2 m) high form around salt springs. Salt-tolerant plants grow in these saline meadows. While most plants die in salty environments, several species here excrete the excess salt they accumulate instead of succumbing to it.

Summer is brief in Wood Buffalo, and both plants and animals rush to complete their reproductive cycles before winter returns. The burst of plant life provides food for the clouds of insects which in turn feed migratory birds – and pester bison, moose and other mammals. Dark-furred moose, with branching

UNDERGROUND CAVES AND CAVERNS

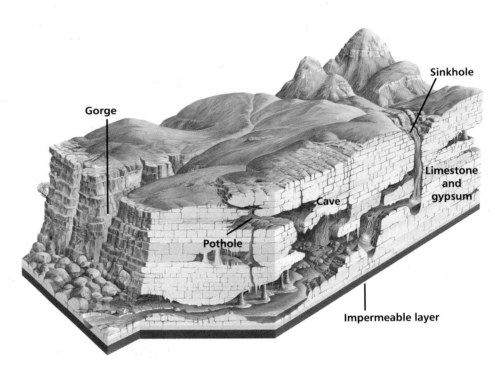

antlers that span almost 6 feet (2 m), thrive in Wood Buffalo's watery lands, browsing on waterside grasses as well as underwater plants in ponds and lakes. Moose represent a large proportion of the diet of timber wolves. These powerful predators hunt moose in packs, generally testing several animals before deciding which one to pursue.

In addition to the moose, the lush grasses of the Peace-Athabasca Delta support most of the park's bison, along with numerous muskrats and beavers. The industrious muskrats take the watery environment as they find it, but beavers alter nature by damming the waterways to create their own safe havens in which to store their food. These large rodents build lodges of mud, sticks and logs which are impenetrable to wolves.

If this varied magnificence were not enough to make this wild place

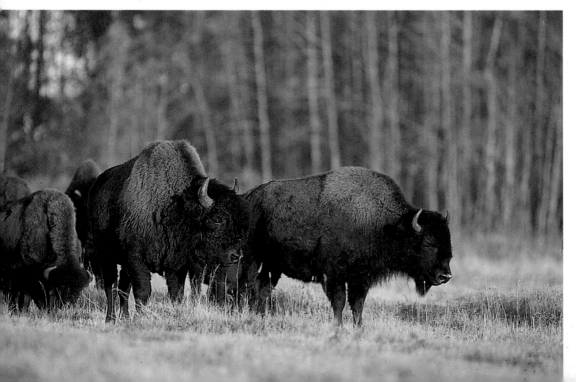

Wood buffalo are the larger woodland-living cousins of plains buffalo. Although they weigh up to 2,000 pounds (900 kg), these creatures can disappear like magic among the trees.

Black bears spend much of the winter in dens hidden beneath trees or in hollow logs. In spring they emerge to search for food such as berries and eggs as well as small mammals and insects.

The karst landscape in Wood Buffalo is considered the finest example of this kind of terrain in North America (left). The underground structures characteristic of karst are created as water seeps down from above, gradually sculpting the gypsum and limestone into caves, caverns and potholes, sometimes with waterfalls and rivers running through them. Some caves grow so large that they collapse, creating depressions known as sinkholes.

Rare whooping cranes nest and lay *their eggs far from civilization in the wild swamplands of Wood Buffalo (right). There are few such undisturbed wetlands left in North America – a fact that has contributed to the decline in numbers of this graceful bird.*

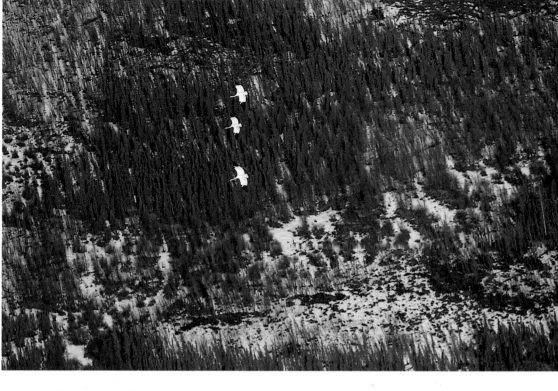

exceptional, Wood Buffalo also contains the only natural nesting ground of the endangered whooping crane. In the 1940s, the entire population of this species dwindled to a mere 17 birds; today, roughly 140 whooping cranes live in the wild, and another 50 or so birds are protected in captivity.

The cranes are white with black-tipped wings, stand 5 feet (1.5 m) tall and typically mate for life. Each year they migrate more than 2,500 miles (4,000 km) from the southwestern United States to breed here. And no smaller habitat would allow them to survive – the territory of each pair of cranes can be anything from 230 to 1,000 acres (93 to 400 ha). In the hospitable muskeg, or level swamp, of Wood Buffalo, they can scatter widely to breed and find ample space to construct large nests of cattails and bulrushes.

In spring the cranes lay two large eggs, which they incubate for 30 days while feeding on marsh plants, frogs and fish. The eggs hatch about two days apart, but the second, younger chick rarely survives. Like many other birds, the parent cranes, accompanied by a single fledgling, leave Wood Buffalo in mid-September to undertake the six- to eight-week flight back to Texas. As the northern winter sets in, bison, ptarmigans and timber wolves are left to reign over this vast domain once again.

Winter is harsh. Temperatures may fall to -40°F (-40°C), and the sun peeps only briefly over the horizon each day. When snow shrouds the landscape, the feathers of ptarmigans, which do not migrate south, turn completely white to lend the bird protective camouflage. Every season, the land and its inhabitants shift and change to accommodate each other, and every year the immense wilderness of Wood Buffalo renews its unique character.

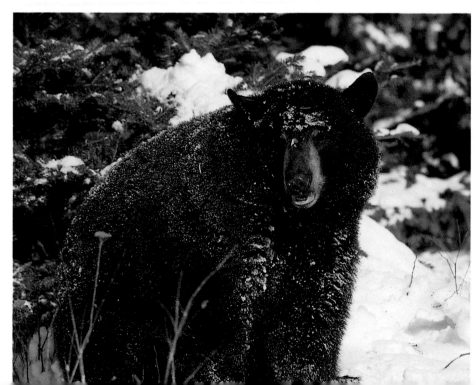

MAZATZAL WILDERNESS

"Inaccessible canyons and sheer-walled cliffs characterize this rugged wilderness"

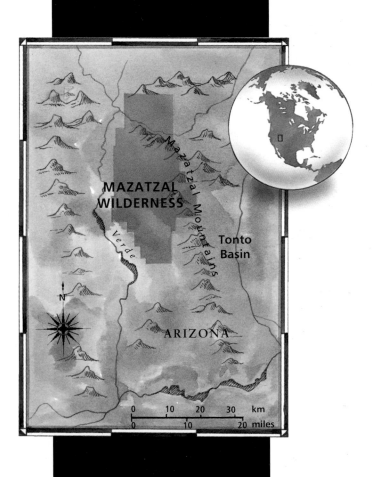

Hells Hole, Lousy Gulch, Suicide Ridge, Poison Canyon, Hardscrabble Mesa. Only a landscape of the cruelest elements and wildest unyielding nature would generate harsh names such as these, and it is little wonder that they belong to the canyons and gullies of the Mazatzal Wilderness. A vast, empty spread of

A mass of prickly pear cacti typifies the inhospitable nature of this harsh desert land. Yet in the cooler mountains beyond, Douglas firs thrive.

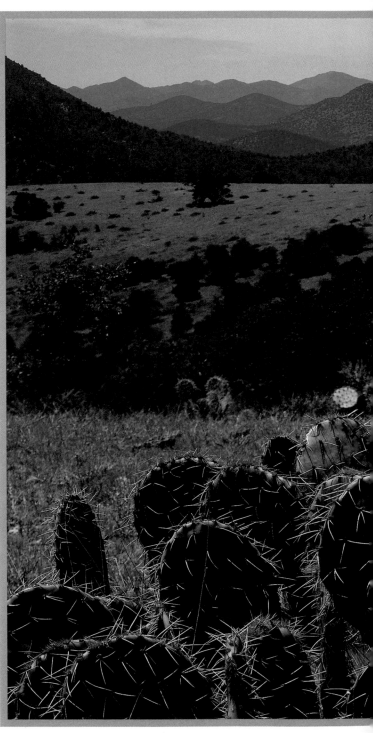

205,000 acres (83,000 ha) in the arid center of Arizona, Mazatzal sprawls eastward from the Verde River, climbs the rugged Mazatzal Mountains, and then plunges to the depths of the Tonto Basin.

The state's largest designated wilderness and one of the largest in the Southwest, Mazatzal's very name reflects its character. Pronounced "madda-zell," the name is either Apache or Paiute and means "the land between" or "the space between." When the original Apache or Paiute residents held up four fingers, representing the mountain peaks, the space between the fingers was termed "maz-at-zark."

The Mazatzal Mountains reach a height of nearly 8,000 feet (2,440 m).

Almost all of the southern part of the range is composed of old granitic rock, dating back at least 600 million years to Precambrian times. In the higher eastern portions of the range, outcrops of extremely hard rhyolite and porphyry jasper rocks form steep slopes that resist wear. By contrast, the western side slopes more gently, and at lower elevations the old rocks

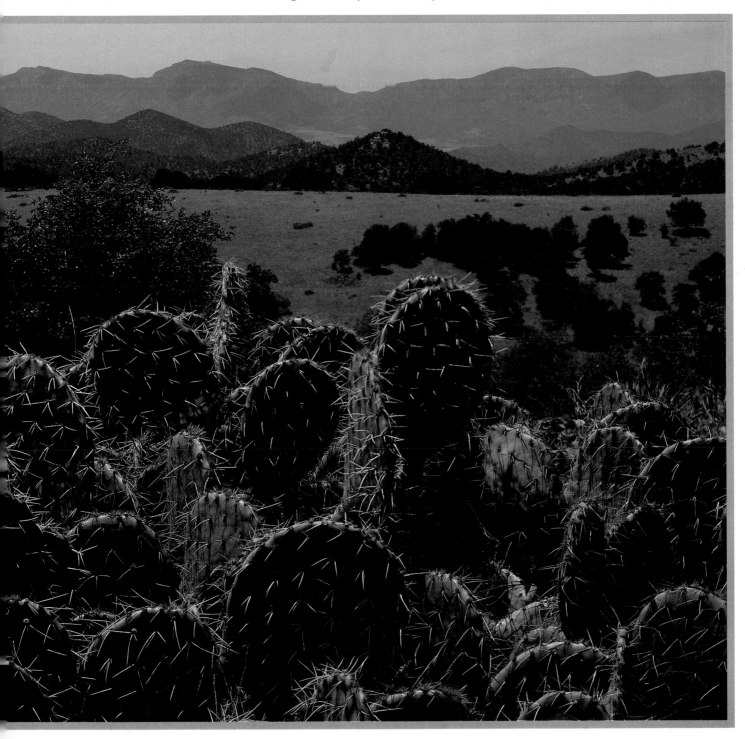

are covered by volcanic flows and other volcanic material.

Although Mazatzal is surrounded by semi-arid lowlands, the mountains create islands of more temperate life. On the uppermost vegetation zones are trees such as ponderosa pines and even Douglas fir – a species usually associated with more northerly climes. The presence of the fir here dates back to the ice ages when its range was forced south. But when the continental ice sheets retreated from this region at the end of the last ice age, only high elevations were cool and moist enough to support northern species such as the Douglas fir. These mountain forests of temperate plants are now, in a sense, stranded in this desert land.

The lowest point of Mazatzal, only 2,100 feet (640 m) above sea level, is at the edge of the Sonoran Desert, simmering in temperatures that can rise above 110°F (43°C) in the summer months. Some summers, the temperature exceeds 100°F (38°C) for as many as 80 days in a row. The Sonoran is one of five North American deserts and the only one that extends to an ocean, meeting the Pacific at Baja California.

Humans must struggle harder than plants to survive the searing heat of Mazatzal. It can take a full day to travel on horseback between one waterhole and the next, and the water may not be potable once it is found. Even the water standing in an animal track may come to look attractive.

With its curved limbs raised to the open sky, the saguaro cactus is the area's most characteristic species, perfectly adapted to its desert existence. The roots of the giant cactus are never farther than 3 inches (7.5 cm) from the desert surface and radiate from the cactus's base almost exactly as far as the main stem is high. Through specially adapted root hairs that grow in response to moisture, the roots can soak up as much as

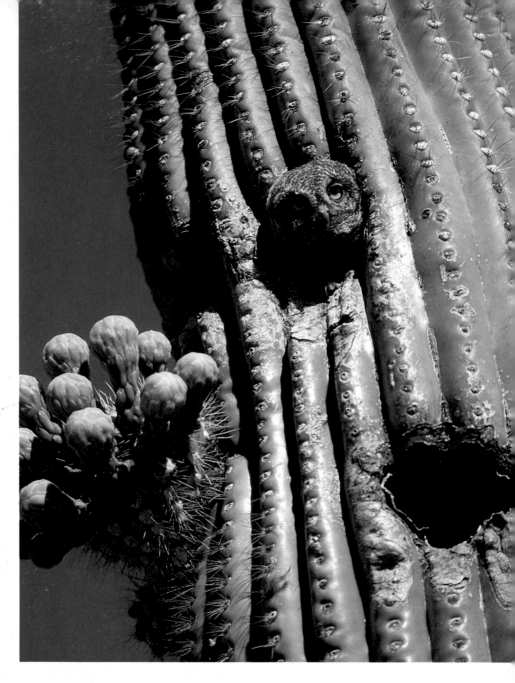

165 gallons (750 liters) of water during a single downpour, enough to sustain the saguaro for a full year. If it survives lightning, wind and occasional frost at the northernmost limit of its range, a saguaro may live to 175 or even 200 years of age, and a 150-year-old specimen may grow 50 feet (15 m) tall.

The saguaro offers shelter to myriad forms of life, day in and day out. Like an apartment building with many stories, it provides varied ecological niches and nesting habitats in close proximity. Gila woodpeckers and their cousins, the gilded flickers, dig holes for their nests in the saguaro's trunk and larger branches. Well insulated by the plant's thick

A saguaro cactus provides a variety of feeding, nesting and shelter sites to an array of desert wildlife. This nesting screech owl claims a hole that was probably drilled out by a gila woodpecker in search of food.

walls, these holes are much cooler in summer and warmer in winter than the air outside.

The woodpeckers excavate new nest holes each year, and their vacant apartments are quickly occupied by sparrow hawks, American kestrels, cactus wrens, screech owls, elf owls and even honeybees. Red-tailed and Harris hawks construct their bulky exterior nests on this cactus, too.

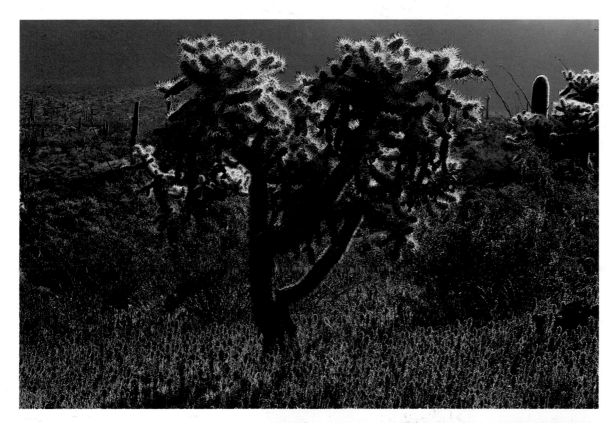

In bloom after recent rainfall, colorful owl clover carpets the ground around a spiny cholla cactus.

The roadrunner (below) runs rather than flies when chasing prey such as rattlesnakes and lizards. This fast-moving bird can reach speeds of up to 20 mph (30 km/h) and kills its victim with a blow from its sharp beak.

Mazatzal's larger animals include coyotes, black bears and mountain lions, or cougars. These big cats were once widespread in North America, but three centuries of relentless hunting has brought them to the brink of extinction. The species now benefits from the protection provided in wildernesses such as Mazatzal. Here mountain lions can roam, relatively undisturbed, preying mostly on wild deer.

The numerous coyotes and black bears are omnivorous, with a taste for carrion as well as for victims they have hunted themselves. Coyotes eat plants, insects, rodents, birds and reptiles. Agile black bears devour all of these, plus copious quantities of the berries of the manzanita bush.

Although its wild, forbidding lowlands usually vary from dry to bone-dry in climate, Mazatzal blooms vividly after the spring rains with yellow brittlebush, owl clover, blue lupines, golden poppies and a host of other wildflowers. But nature guarantees nothing in this desert

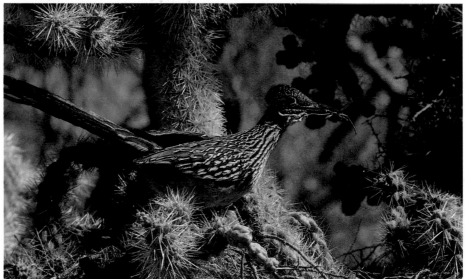

setting, so some flowering plants have prepared themselves for the unreliability of the rains by coating their seeds with germination inhibitors. Until enough rain falls to wash away this coating and assure moisture for the plant's complete reproduction cycle, the seeds will not germinate. Some lie dormant waiting for rainfall for 70 years or more without losing their fertility.

Ironically, Mazatzal can suffer from too much water. When flash floods occur, the steep mountain gorges collect more rainwater than the floors of dry stream beds, known as washes, can absorb. Tumbled boulders and broken cottonwood trees attest to the freakish power of water, whose unpredictable presence proves the wild, unbridled nature of this rough land.

OKEFENOKEE SWAMP

"A brooding stillness wraps the swamp in mysteries as dense and seductive as its vegetation"

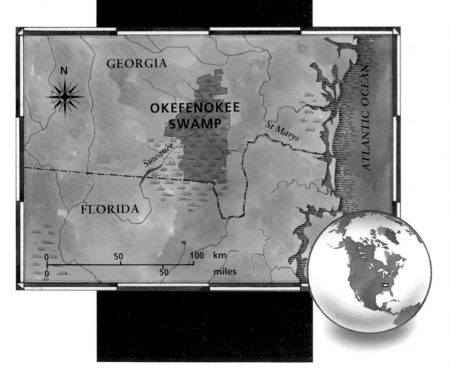

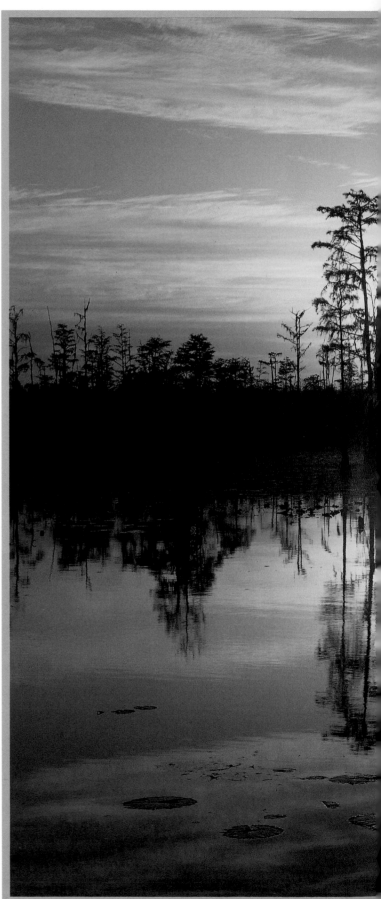

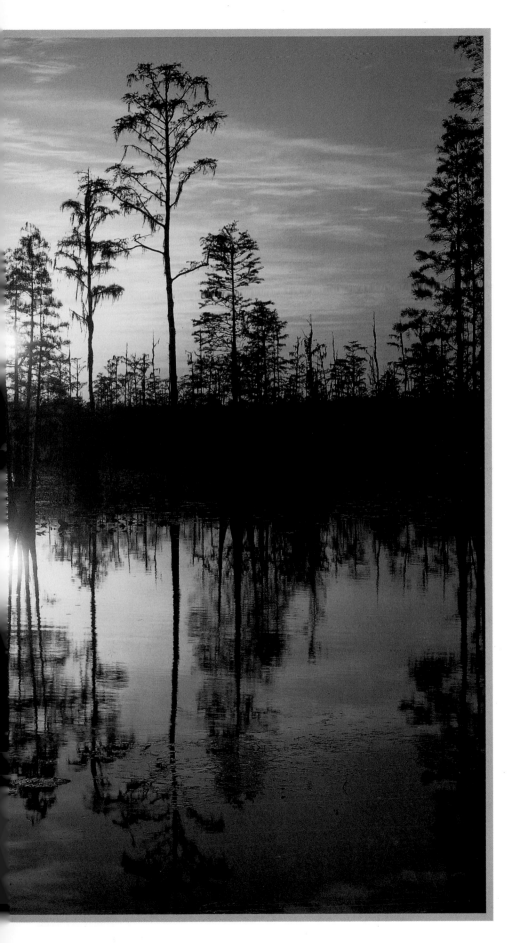

Dark and tangled, echoing eerily with the bellow of alligators and the cackle of cranes, Okefenokee Swamp is the largest freshwater wetland in the contiguous United States. The swamp itself and its nurturing watershed cover roughly 600 sq. miles (1,500 km²) of southern Georgia and northern Florida. The dark water shines like a polished mirror, reflecting the twisted cypresses and elegant water birds, and a brooding stillness wraps the swamp in mysteries as dense and seductive as its vegetation.

Perhaps because it seems so impenetrable, the swamp has become a wilderness of misnomers, with its title and two of its three major habitats mislabeled. More than a swamp, which by definition contains standing water, Okefenokee qualifies as a watershed, since it gives rise to two rivers, the St. Marys and the Suwannee. Its so-called prairies, characteristic watery expanses of vegetation, are actually marshes, and its cypress bays are not bays but dense forests, once logged for their bald cypress trees which usually grow in standing water. The third major habitat, however, is just what its name implies, pinelands of slash and loblolly pine that cannot tolerate standing water.

The present ecological character of Okefenokee was formed 250,000 years ago when the Atlantic Ocean shoreline was 75 miles (120 km) west of today's swamp. An extensive sandbar, eventually about 40 miles (65 km) long, emerged off the coast, and a shallow lagoon formed just

Reflections in Billy's Lake double the dazzling display as low-angled evening sunlight bathes the Okefenokee Swamp. This isolated wilderness is a haven for a variety of wildlife, including huge American alligators.

west of it. After the ocean receded, draining the lagoon, it left behind a shallow sand basin in which Okefenokee Swamp developed. Today's swamp lies about 45 miles (70 km) inland and is shaped like a large, shallow bowl or saucer with two small spots – the outlets of the St. Marys and Suwannee rivers – low on its rim. Its elevation ranges from 105–130 feet (32–40 m) above sea level; by comparison, the Everglades in southern Florida never rise more than 8 feet (2.5 m) above sea level.

Okefenokee is renowned for its peaty brown waters, known as blackwater, with their uncanny, mirroring surface. Over the span of the swamp's existence, blackwater has developed as dying plant life continually drops into the water of the swamp and decays, forming masses of peat. The slowly decomposing peat then releases acids collectively known as tannin, which hangs suspended in the water and gives it a brown cast like that of strong tea, rendering the surface highly reflective.

The submerged layers of peat average from 5 to 10 feet (1.5 to 3 m) in thickness, yet the gases that derive from organic decomposition and become trapped beneath the peat layers sometimes push them to the water's surface and set them afloat. A floating mat of peat may provide a home for airborne seeds that germinate, root and grow on it. Twisting around water-lily roots and those of other aquatic plants, the roots of the new plants anchor the floating peat securely to the bottom and transform the raft into a floating island of decayed vegetation on which even full-size trees may grow.

One meaning given to the name Okefenokee – a local Native American word – is "trembling earth," which refers directly to the floating islands in the swamp that have taken root and become

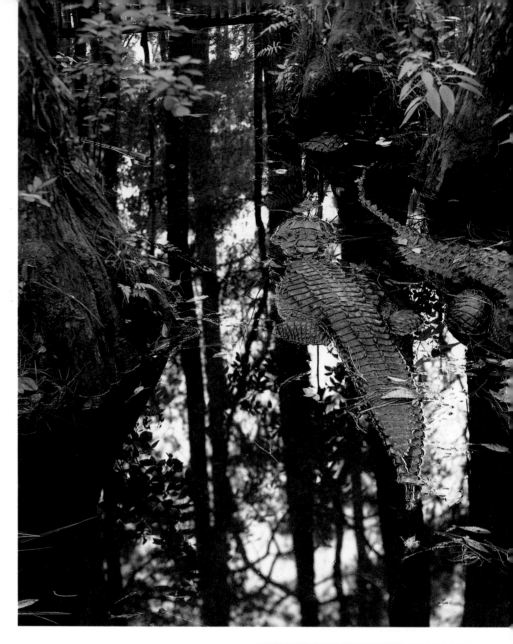

stationary. The sensation of walking on such a rooted peat island, locally called a "house," has been compared to walking on a water bed.

The other islands that grace Okefenokee are firmly rooted in the distant geological past rather than in botanical decay. Approximately 70 islands are known throughout the swamp, 60 of them large enough to have names. The larger, outlying islands at the edge of the swamp are draped in thick pine forests, while cypress trees cover the small islands deep in Okefenokee's interior.

Many of the larger islands are actually the fragmentary remains of ancient ocean sandbars that took shape during the ice ages before continental ice sheets ground the massive North American rock to

"No creature can be confident that almost imperceptible stirrings in leaves will not explode to reveal the death-dealing jaws of an alligator"

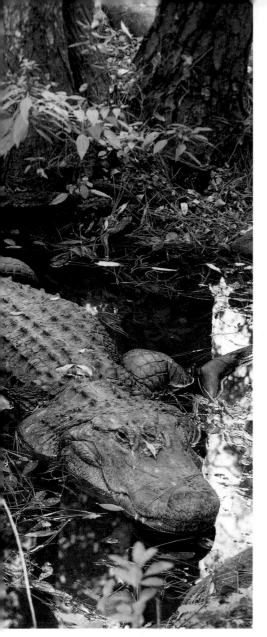

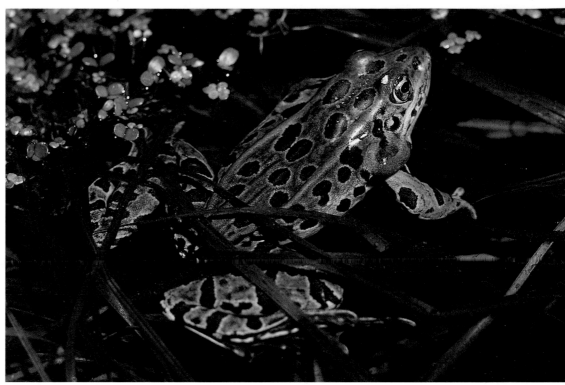

Alligators at rest can look like fallen versions of nearby swamp trees, but these great reptiles can charge with surprising bursts of speed to seize unwary deer at the water's edge. The bellowing roar that often accompanies a charge sounds eerily prehistoric.

Leopard frogs are among the multitudes of amphibians whose croaking calls fill the air in the Okefenokee springtime. They are preyed on by everything from alligators and snakes to stalking herons and ibises.

granular material. As pieces were washed seaward, the relentless tossing of the waves reduced them still further, breaking the grains into sand. Vast quantities of this sand were deposited on what was then the relatively shallow offshore continental shelf. Today, this shelf is the coastal plain in which nestles the gently curved saucer of Okefenokee.

Where sand rather than peat lines the floor of Okefenokee Swamp, clear water sparkles in the dappled light, but the absence of minnows proves that clear waters are not the rule here. In fact, no minnows at all are found in Okefenokee, despite the fact that 9 species live in the river drainages surrounding the swamp, and 69 species have been identified throughout Georgia. Moreover,

though they are regionally abundant, few species of the sunfish family inhabit the swamp. No natural physical barriers prevent the upstream migration of these missing species into Okefenokee, and all species of fish found in the Okefenokee waters are also found in the rivers and streams of the surrounding coastal plain. But the swamp's waters are, on average, significantly more acidic than the surrounding waters, and fish experts have discovered that some of the missing species avoid waters of such acidity.

The 40 or so fish species that do inhabit the swamp include the chain pickerel, largemouth bass, warmouth, gar, mudfish and mosquito fish, and while the range of species may be limited, the numbers of fish are

staggering. As its name suggests, the diminutive mosquito fish has evolved through a direct relationship with the insect whose breeding females bite warm-blooded creatures, including humans, to extract the blood they need for their reproduction process. Mosquito fish feed in turn off the insects' abundant larvae.

Historically, the Florida panther was the major predator of the white-tailed deer that thrive in the swamp. Now this big cat is extremely rare in all of its former range, but there are plans to introduce more animals into Okefenokee and create a protected self-sustaining population there.

Another awesome Okefenokee predator takes the occasional deer but feeds primarily on snakes, fish, turtles and other small swamp

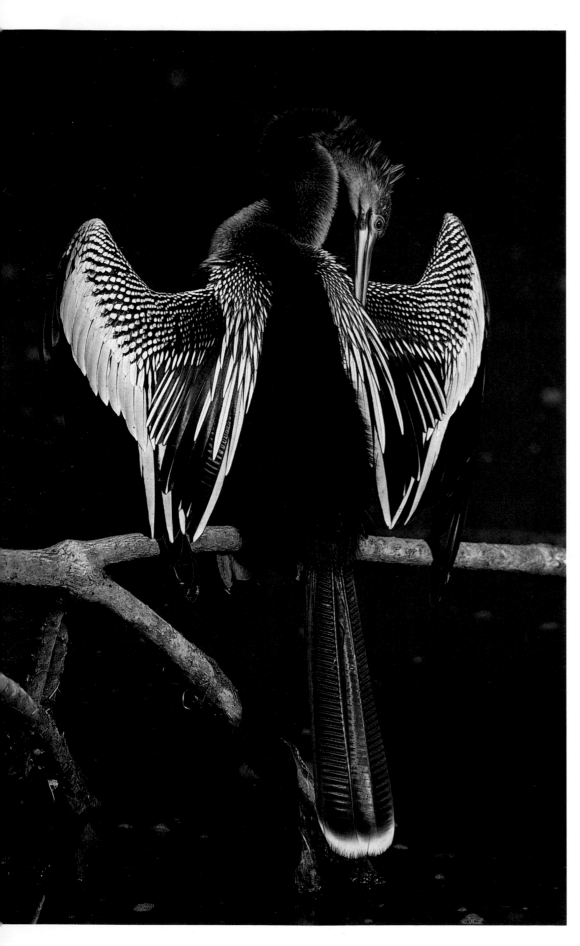

animals. The American alligator is one of Okefenokee's most ancient animals whose lineage goes back 200 million years to the days when scaly creatures, from lizards to dinosaurs, ruled the Earth.

Alligators dominate the swamp's aquatic life today. As opportunistic feeders, they will eat almost any of the swamp's inhabitants, including their own young, and forage onshore as well as in the dark waters. No stalking shorebirds – herons, egrets, ibises – or swimming muskrats can ever be confident that the almost imperceptible stirrings in nearby leaves will not suddenly explode to reveal the death-dealing jaws of a predatory alligator.

Although a mere 6 inches (15 cm) long when hatched, alligators can grow to be 12 feet (3.5 m) and weigh more than 650 pounds (300 kg). These seemingly slow and clumsy creatures are normally observed basking in the sunshine, but they can move with extreme speed and attack with great power. When subduing their prey and in the males' courtship battles, they roll rapidly in the water, turning their bodies into mighty levers to augment the vicelike grip of their elongated jaws.

Another group of predators reinforces the swamp's aura of mysterious wildness in a different manner entirely. Three carnivorous plants – pitcher plants, bladderworts and sundews – sustain themselves in part by eating insects, a predilection determined by their habitat. Meat eating enables them to grow in soil

Perched motionless with wings partly spread, this anhinga is drying out its feathers; they lack the water-repellent oils that keep the feathers of most water birds from getting soaked. Known locally as water turkeys, anhingas evolved from woodland-dwelling ancestors.

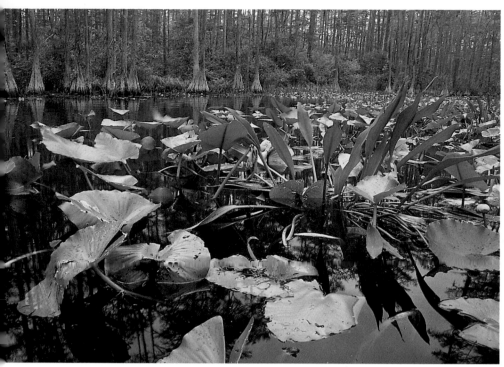

FLOATING ISLANDS

Large-leaved spatterdock lilies cover large areas of Okefenokee's water surface (left). They grow on the mats of peat that float on the water and give the Okefenokee Swamp its special character. The peat mats form from deposits of plant matter that settle on the swamp bottom. Gases emitted during the decaying process can force the peat upward and create floating islands where plants, and even trees, can take root (below). The average thickness of the peat islands is about 5 feet (1.5 m), but in places they are as much as 15 feet (4.5 m) deep.

that is too low in nitrogen to sustain plant life. In order to gather the nitrogen they need to survive, pitcher plants and sundews use attractant fluids, and the bladderwort employs entrapping air sacs to lure hapless insects into its grasp. Pitcher plants resemble straightened cornucopias, but function in reverse. Stiff hairs lining the cone allow insects to travel down it, but not up again; eventually they drown in the pitcher's pool of fluids, and their soft body parts are absorbed into the plant's tissues.

At present, only 15 percent of Okefenokee is composed of the open, watery prairies that define its swamp-like character. The geological saucer is slowly and inexorably filling with organic detritus, the remains of a vital botanical ecology. It is therefore possible that at some time in the future, Okefenokee Swamp could transform itself into a relatively dry landscape, sliced by creeks and rivers, where the earth no longer trembles. But for the present, its tea-colored waters remain, and provide a unique home for a remarkable collection of North American wetland wildlife.

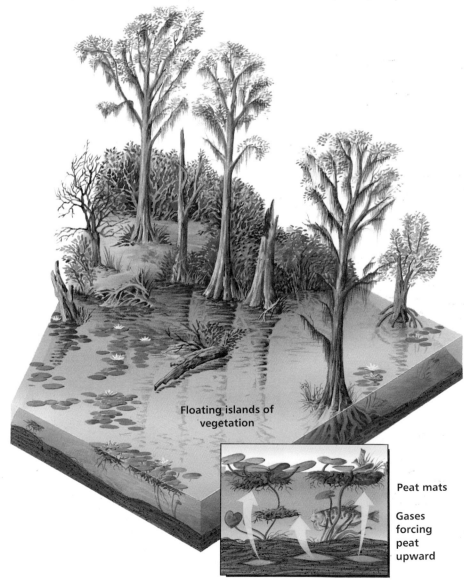

Floating islands of vegetation

Peat mats

Gases forcing peat upward

MONTEVERDE CLOUD FOREST

"An abundance of life unrivaled in the western hemisphere"

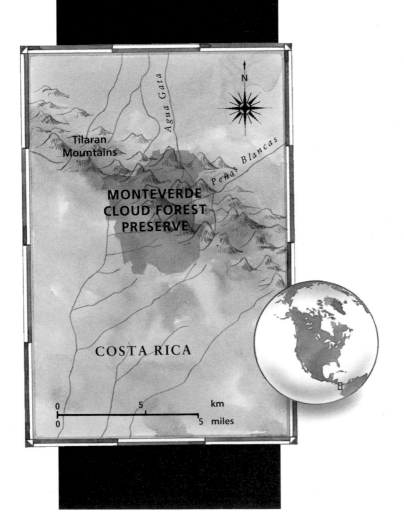

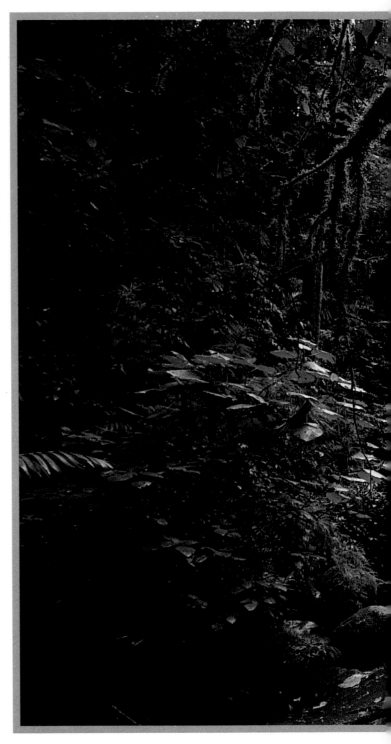

Perched high in the Tilaran Mountains in the north of Costa Rica, the Monteverde Cloud Forest Preserve is a luminous wilderness of exquisite orchids, sluggish sloths and exotic parrots. This tiny wilderness covers only about 20 sq. miles (50 km²), but contains an abundance of life

In this Costa Rican cloud forest, where streams and rivers abound, there is an incredible diversity of plant and animal life.

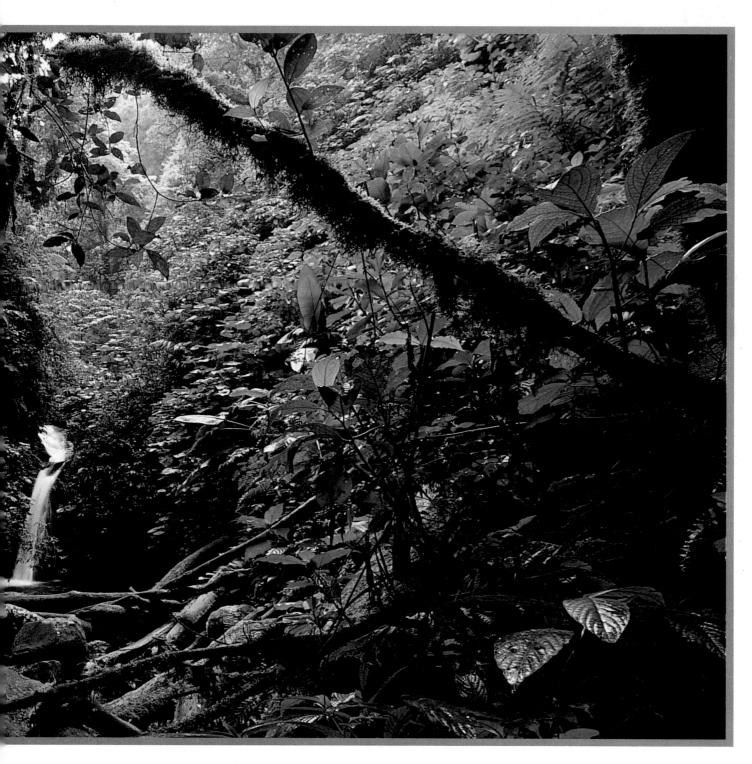

unrivaled in the western hemisphere. Nature itelf seems more fertile in this preserve, which boasts more than 2,500 species of plants including 200 different species of orchids alone.

Costa Rica occupies a narrow volcanic rise separating the Caribbean Sea and the Pacific Ocean at the midpoint between North and South America. It covers an area of about 19,600 sq. miles (50,700 km²) and includes two distinct coastal environments as well as watered mountain forests such as Monteverde.

As warm, wet air masses waft westward off the Caribbean Sea, the Tilaran Mountains force them to rise and cool. As a result, the air masses lose their capacity to hold and transport moisture, and they release it as precipitation which nourishes the forests below. Since the Caribbean air masses have lost most of their moisture by the time they reach the crest of the mountains, the western, Pacific, slopes of the Monteverde area, and of Costa Rica generally, are not as wet and verdant as their eastern counterparts. These western slopes become progressively drier as they near sea level, and their lower reaches support tropical dry forests; lower still, dry chaparral similar to that of southern California prevails.

Within the Monteverde preserve, the dense forest canopy all but blocks direct sunlight from the forest floor. So lush is the canopy vegetation that plants even grow on other plants.

Bromeliads, for example, thrive high in the canopy on the branches of trees. These members of the pineapple family create their own microhabitat in the forest, trapping and holding rainwater in their rigid, upthrust foliage. Like a hanging reservoir 200 feet (60 m) above the forest floor, a single bromeliad plant can become the focus of life for bats, salamanders, tree frogs, katydids, beetles, snails and spiders, as well as

the water-dependent larvae of insects such as gnats and mosquitoes.

More than 100 types of mammals and 400 bird species inhabit the tiny Monteverde preserve. The mammals form a varied menagerie of wild cats such as jaguars and ocelots, spider and black howler monkeys, three-toed sloths, banded anteaters and collared peccaries, which belong to the pig family. The birds include a flurry of brilliantly colored species of hummingbird, some of which are, without their tails, only the size of a human thumbnail.

Iridescent emerald and scarlet, the dazzling quetzal, Costa Rica's most spectacular bird, is endemic to the mountain forests of Central America and grows to about 12 inches (30 cm) in length. Overlying the main tail, long feathers called coverts provide an impressive train measuring some 35 inches (90 cm). At the end of the breeding season, male quetzals shed these long tail coverts the way some mammals shed their antlers, reducing their overall length considerably.

Tree-dwelling and solitary, the quetzal lives in the lower forest layers. Despite its striking color and spectacular train, it can easily hide itself in the forest, but its alert response to the loud calls of other quetzals, even to a tape recording of

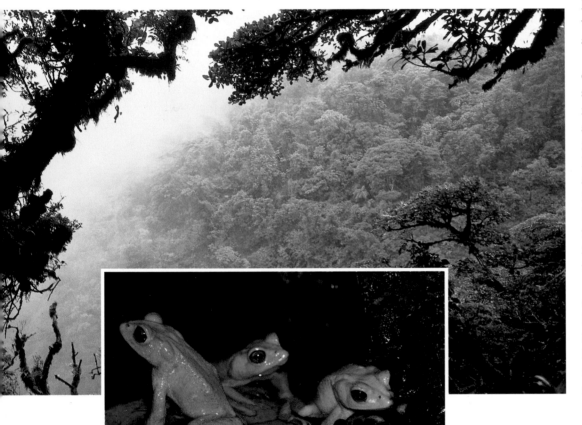

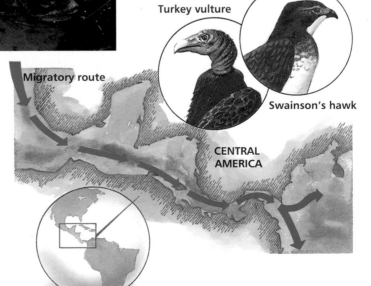

Cloud forest is a type of rainforest growing at high elevations. Because of the height and the constantly damp air, such forest is often swathed in clouds of mist and fog (top).

These jewel-like golden toads live in a small part of the Monteverde forest. Only the male toads are golden – their brilliant hue attracts the dark green or black females.

Migratory route

Turkey vulture

Swainson's hawk

CENTRAL AMERICA

BIRD FLYWAYS
Areas such as Monteverde are vital stopping-off points for birds migrating from North to South America. Many birds depend on strong thermal air currents over land and are forced to travel over the narrow strip of Central America.

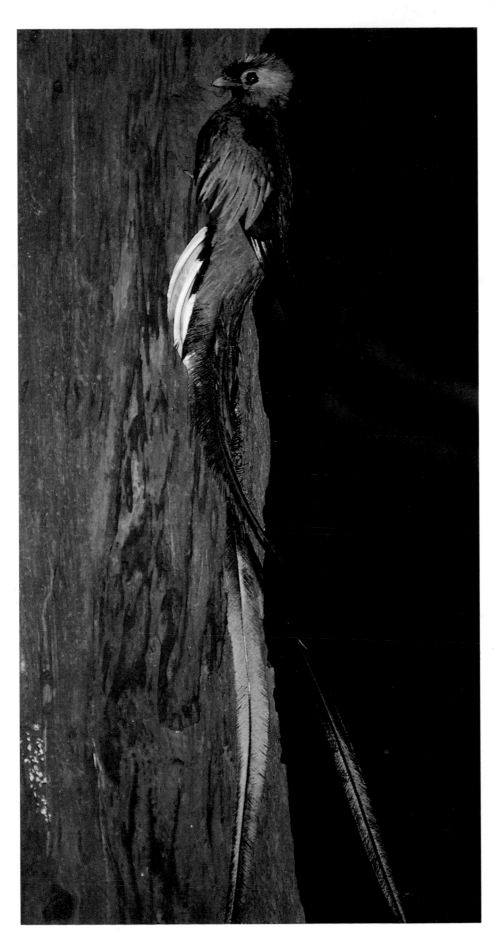

the clucking, reveals its presence to human and animal predators.

Among the largest South American parrots, scarlet macaws can be 33 inches (85 cm) long. These parrots are most often seen as pairs, but they do flock together in groups of 20 or so when moving from nighttime roosts to feeding sites. As the flock moves, pairs fly nearly wing to wing. Surprisingly little is known about the domestic habits of these macaws. They feed in the trees in near silence, eating nuts, fruits, berries and seeds and emitting their raucous, squeaking alarms only when they are disturbed and take to the air.

In complete contrast to the scarlet macaw, the three-toed sloth lives a life of near invisibility, conveniently clothed in a mottled gray fur coat that perfectly matches the bark of its favorite tree, the *Cecropia*. This sloth is so well adapted to life in the trees that its hair grows in the opposite direction from that of most mammals. The fur points downward for the efficient shedding of water when the sloth is hanging upside-down on its hooklike claws. The algae that live in the grooved hairs of the fur, tingeing it green, contribute to the sloth's effective camouflage.

In Monteverde's lush landscapes and constant climate, many animals and plants have evolved together, in a process called coevolution. The perfect match of the sloth's fur and the bark of the *Cecropia* tree is just one example, but nature's infinite sophistication can be seen everywhere in this ecological complex of cloud, forest, water and wildland.

With its showy plumage and long streamerlike tail coverts, the male resplendent quetzal richly deserves its name. Quetzals live in the cloud forest trees, where they search for fruit and insects to eat and make their nests in rotting trunks.

MORNE TROIS PITONS

"A mountainous and little-known land where dense vegetation seems to shut out the rest of the world"

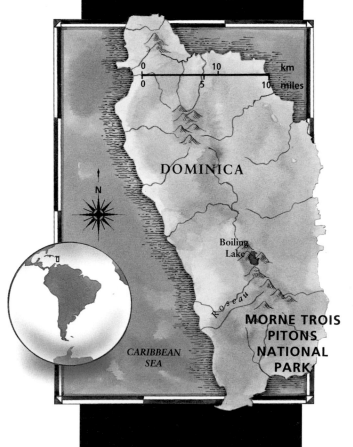

DOMINICA

N

Boiling Lake

Roseau

MORNE TROIS PITONS NATIONAL PARK

CARIBBEAN SEA

0   10   km
0   5   10   miles

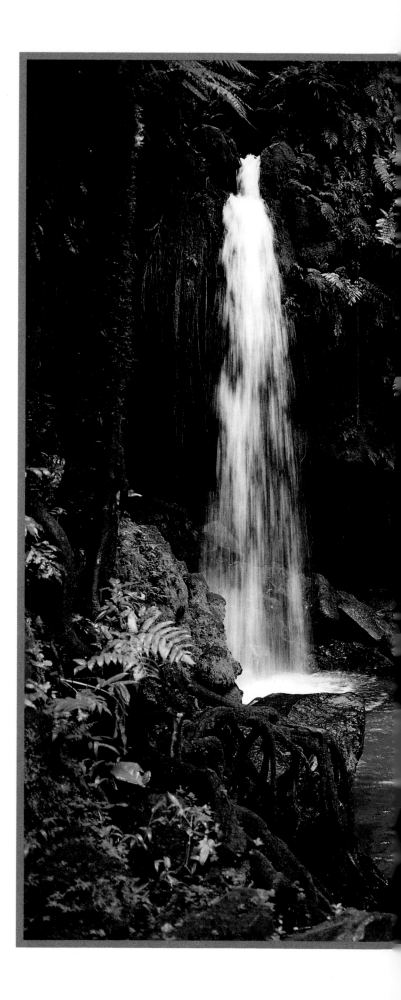

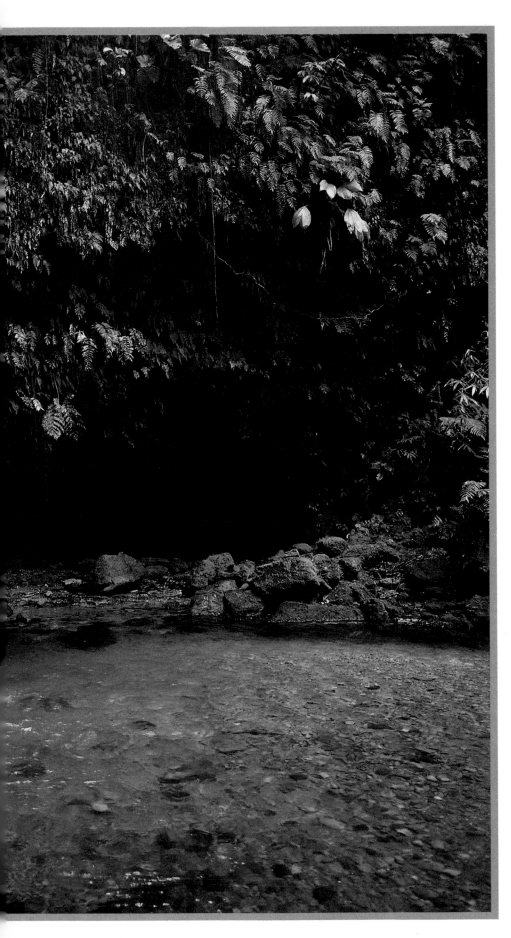

A paradise of verdant trees, brilliant birds and steaming lakes rising out of the Caribbean Sea, the island of Dominica houses the largest stand of island tropical rainforest in the Caribbean. More than 40 percent forested and the least developed of the five Windward Islands (the others are St. Lucia, St. Vincent, Grenada and Martinique), Dominica is a mountainous and little-known land.

Time seems to have stopped here. The island has no sandy beaches to lure the invasive tourist and no port to draw large ships, so much of Dominica remains unexplored except by the native Carib Indians. In its Morne Trois Pitons National Park, the dense vegetation seems to shut out the rest of the world.

Dominica's craggy cliffs are crowned by Morne Diablotin, which stands 4,774 feet (1,455 m) above sea level and marks the highest point in the Windward Islands. The rainforests of Morne Trois Pitons drift up to blue-green peaks that explain the island's nickname "Switzerland of the Caribbean"; at the highest elevations dwarfed forests, shaped by the wind, supplant the rainforest.

The mountainous interior of Morne Trois Pitons bursts with natural surprises. Giant ferns line the banks of the rushing rivers, and orchid plants grow on the trees, their bright colors glowing in the dim, nearly green light of the canopy. Among the most stately trees of the Morne Trois Pitons forests are the gommier or gumwood trees, named

Rainforests thrive in Dominica's Morne Trois Pitons National Park. Volcanic mountains force the trade winds to drop their moisture as rainfall, assuring a plentiful supply for the dense plant growth. Hidden in the forest are many waterfalls and deep clear pools – this one is known as the Emerald Pool.

for their aromatic gum, which grow to more than 100 feet (30 m) in height. Island people still fashion their traditional dugout canoes from this majestic species, and the national bird of Dominica, the endangered imperial parrot or sisserou, nests in holes high in the trunks.

Native to the island, the sisserou does not live naturally in the wild anywhere else in the world. It is one of the largest parrots, measuring up to 20 inches (50 cm) long with a fabulous 30-inch (75-cm) wingspan. The parrot's gorgeously colored wings are green and red, its tail and back a brilliant dark green; red eyes gleam in its iridescent head. A broad, deep violet band crosses the back of its neck, and its breast is bright purple. Sisserous feed while hanging head down – a posture well suited for plucking the fruit of the tall kaklin trees they seek out.

The wild population of sisserous now numbers only 50 or 60, and their continued survival is at risk. When Hurricane David ravaged Dominica and its forests in 1979, its 150 mph (240 km/h) winds threatened many native species with extinction. It levelled many of the gommier trees in which sisserous were nesting and blew the entire year's crop of nuts and fruit off many of the island's other trees. The parrots that escaped the lethal winds were driven down into the lowlands in search of food. Many were illegally captured and offered for sale on the black market as cage birds.

For the sisserous that currently haunt Dominica's higher mountain reaches, volcanic eruption looms as a permanent long-term threat. Dominica has never outgrown its volcanic origins, and the volcanic forces lurking below the island bubble to the surface perpetually in Morne Trois Pitons, particularly in the barren Valley of Desolation.

Noxious underground gases have turned its bare rocks every imaginable shade of red, yellow and brown, and minerals that have leached to the surface color the valley's waters both jet black and cloudy white. Volcanic ground vents give forth deafening roars, and a dramatic waterfall plunges over one end of the nearby Titou Gorge, a volcanic fissure that has filled with water.

Often hidden by its self-generating veil of water vapor, Boiling Lake in the Valley of Desolation is the world's

The aptly named Boiling Lake of Morne Trois Pitons is a flooded fumarole some 260 feet (80 m) wide in the bleak Valley of Desolation. Billowing clouds of steam rise from the seething waters of this eerie lake, which is kept bubbling by the volcanic heat beneath.

A BUBBLING LAKE

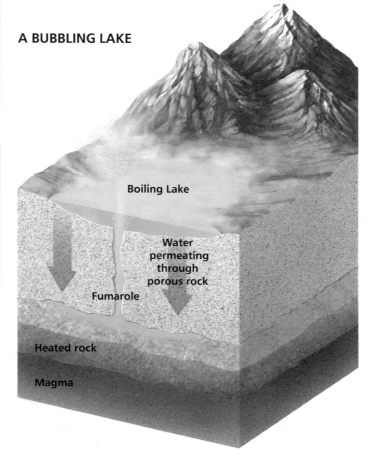

Boiling Lake

Water permeating through porous rock

Fumarole

Heated rock

Magma

In a fumarole such as Morne Trois Pitons' Boiling Lake, groundwater from the surrounding mountain region percolates through porous rock and is heated by the magma below. This super-heated water is then forced up through a vent to the surface as steam.

largest fumarole. Fumaroles occur where groundwater that has been excessively heated underground returns to the Earth's surface as steam, lacking enough moisture to flow as water. Where acid gases transform solid rock into clay, as at Boiling Lake, fumaroles bubble in wet mud; smaller, viscous fumaroles are known as mudpots.

Magma, a molten material which lies unusually close to the surface of Morne Trois Pitons, heats the subterranean groundwater deep in the Earth, where it is subjected to enormous pressure. As the steam pushes up toward the surface, however, the pressure on it slackens, and it expands with tremendous force, literally bringing Boiling Lake to a boil.

The abundant rainfall in Dominica is inextricably tied to its mountains, as the disparity between the rain on the coast and in the mountainous interior proves. On its windward coast, Dominica registers 70 inches (1,780 mm) of rainfall per year; the high mountains receive more than 236 inches (6,000 mm). This phenomenon is called orographic rainfall. The mountains force the moisture-laden air to rise and cool; as it does so, it releases its moisture as rain.

The liberal orographic rain that pours onto Morne Trois Pitons and other mountainous areas nourishes the complex ecology of this luxuriant island. Its natural riches are protected by the very wildness of the rugged, densely forested terrain that, so far, has kept the world at bay.

"Dominica has never outgrown its volcanic origins, and the volcanic forces lurking below the island bubble to the surface in Morne Trois Pitons"

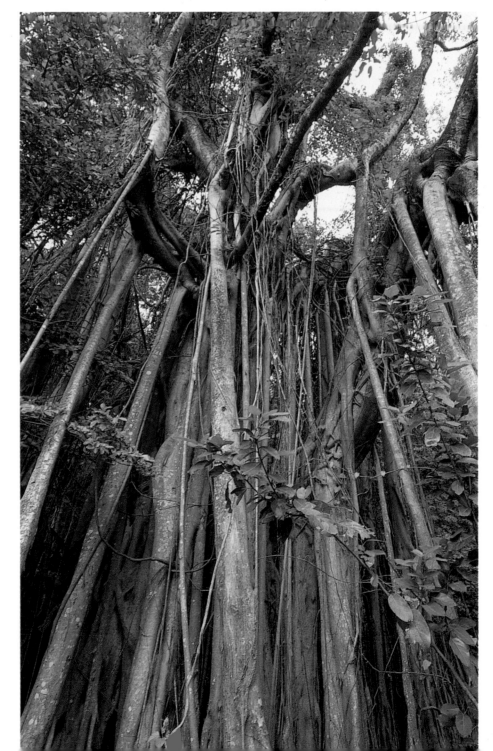

Roots of a giant fig stream earthward *like a forest of mini tree trunks. In fact, this fig cannot support itself structurally, but depends on the tree it parasitizes. It may eventually strangle the host tree, compressing its trunk until its cells can no longer transport water and nutrients.*

THE TEPUIS OF VENEZUELA

"Mysterious flat-topped mountains rise from this ancient wilderness"

The only way to penetrate the remote tropical forests of southern Venezuela is by river. About 400 miles (650 km) due south of Caracas on a tributary of the upper Orinoco, little can be seen from the water beyond the continuous green wall of the trees. But at a bend in the river, a huge rock suddenly looms into view. Blue in the

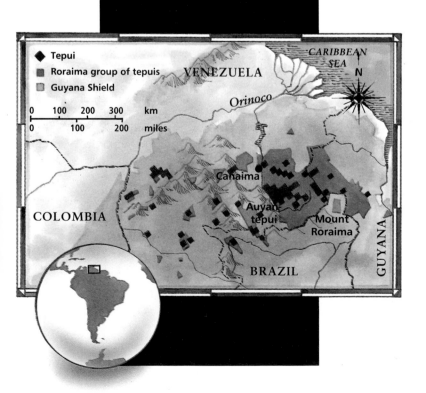

CARIBBEAN SEA

VENEZUELA

■ Tepui
■ Roraima group of tepuis
■ Guyana Shield

Orinoco

0 100 200 300 km
0 100 200 miles

N

Canaima

Auyan tepui

Mount Roraima

COLOMBIA

BRAZIL

GUYANA

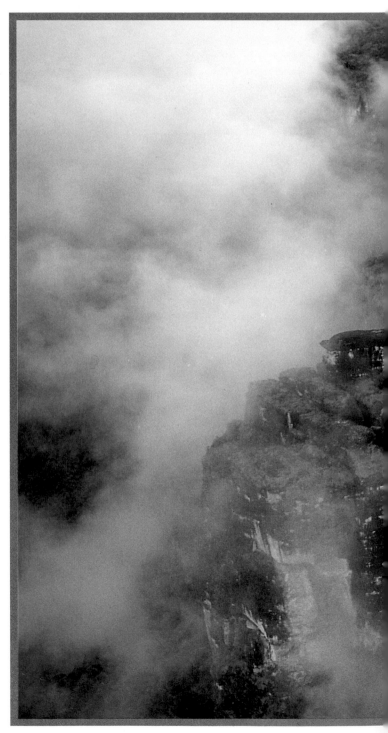

distance – it is some 30 miles (50 km) away – its sides climb sheer from the surrounding forest in one enormous step to a broad, level summit that is suspended hundreds of yards in the air. The extraordinary rock is Autana, and it is one of more than a hundred mysterious, flat-topped mountains that rise in this ancient wilderness region of South America.

Often described as rock towers, mesas or table mountains, they are best known by their local Penom Indian name "tepuis." The greatest concentration of them lies in and around the Canaima National Park of southeastern Venezuela, but others are scattered across the rest of southern Venezuela, the northern frontier of Brazil, Guyana and Surinam. All have

Enveloped in cloud, the rim of Auyan-tepui falls sheer to the forest far below. Auyan-tepui is the largest in area of scores of similar table mountains that rise like dislocated slabs of earth in the region south of the Orinoco River. The isolation and mystery of their broad summits have long inspired legend and adventure.

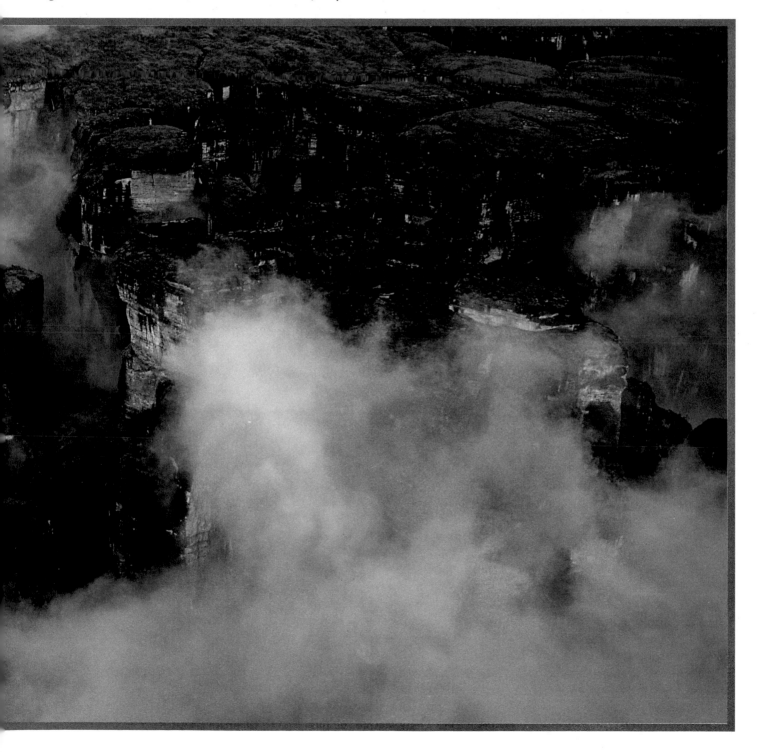

steep, perpendicular sides, rising as much as 5,000 feet (1,500 m) above the land beneath, sometimes in a single slope, sometimes in two or three giant steps. Their flat summits form elevated portions of land almost as isolated from one another and from the ground far below as islands in an ocean. Remote, awesome, often shrouded from view by swirling mist and cloud, many of these lonely summits have yet to be explored.

Autana is an outlying tepui, a long way from the nearest flat-topped peak. But from high viewpoints in Canaima, the shapes of tepuis of various sizes stud the horizon. The giant slab of Mount Roraima, at 9,220 feet (2,810 m) the highest of them all, commands the view to the east. Other much smaller tepuis, separated by miles of intervening land, stand like blunted pinnacles. It is as though an enormous scythe has been swept over the land, slicing away the tops from a range of scattered mountains.

The explanation for this dramatic landscape lies in its geological history. The rock of the tepuis is mainly sandstone with intrusions of crystalline material such as quartzite. Geologists believe the sandstone formed at least 1.8 billion years ago, making it one of the oldest sandstones in the world. (It directly overlies the so-called Guyana Shield, the oldest rock in all South America.) The layers of sandstone laid down by water and wind accumulated to a depth of up to 8,200 feet (2,500 m). Much later, these layers came to form a vast plateau surrounded by lower land.

When the plates of the Earth's crust carrying South America and Africa started drifting apart about 135 million years ago, the plateau was probably wrenched and fractured by these forces. Some blocks may have been lifted upward, while rivers crossing the plateau and tumbling down its sides cut deep valleys

between them, especially along the weakened fissures. As the climate became wetter, so erosion intensified. In time, the plateau became ever more dissected until all that remained were the isolated blocks of today.

Millions of years from now they, too, will have been eroded out of existence. Rainfall, already high in this region of South America, is often torrential on the tepuis. Air rising over the summits cools and sheds up

> "Remote, awesome, often shrouded from view by swirling mist and cloud, many of these summits have yet to be explored"

to 157 inches (4,000 mm) of rain every year, in cloudy drizzle as well as violent electrical storms. Streams etch deeply into the terrain and at the summit edge plummet over the rock wall on all sides. These numerous waterfalls carve backward into the tepuis as they cascade down to the lowland, and the sides of the rock are eventually eaten away.

From the surrounding lowlands, people have long viewed the flat

heights of the tepuis as worlds set apart from their own. Native legends have grown up concerning many of these cloud-shrouded peaks, and some, like Autana, are considered sacred. A remarkable cave runs straight through Autana, opening high in the rock wall on each side – a natural wonder said to be the home of a monster.

Nobody has yet found any monsters, but the isolation of the tepuis is strikingly reflected in their known flora and fauna. Around half of all the plant species that occur on them are endemic – they do not exist anywhere else in the world. They include hundreds of species of orchids, bromeliads and sundews, as well as shrubs and low trees. Many are confined to a single tepui.

Animals unique to the tepuis have also been discovered, including endemic insects, amphibians such as the minute toad *Oreophrynella quelchii*, and birds like the greater flower-piercer and the tepui spinetail. Because they are adapted to survive in the summit conditions, including a climate of cold nights and warm days, it is difficult for many tepui plants and animals to spread farther afield even if they could escape their highland fortress. For beyond the cliffs lie tropical lowlands with a dramatically different climate.

Even birds of the tepui summits would be unlikely to fly far from their home region. Yet there are birds living high on the tepuis with close relatives at least 435 miles (700 km) away in the Andes Mountains. The

Drenching rain on Auyan-tepui feeds Angel Falls, the highest waterfall in the world. In two leaps, the water plummets 3,212 feet (979 m) over the edge of the tepui, from the coolness of high altitude to tropical heat at the foot. The total drop is nine times that of Africa's Victoria Falls.

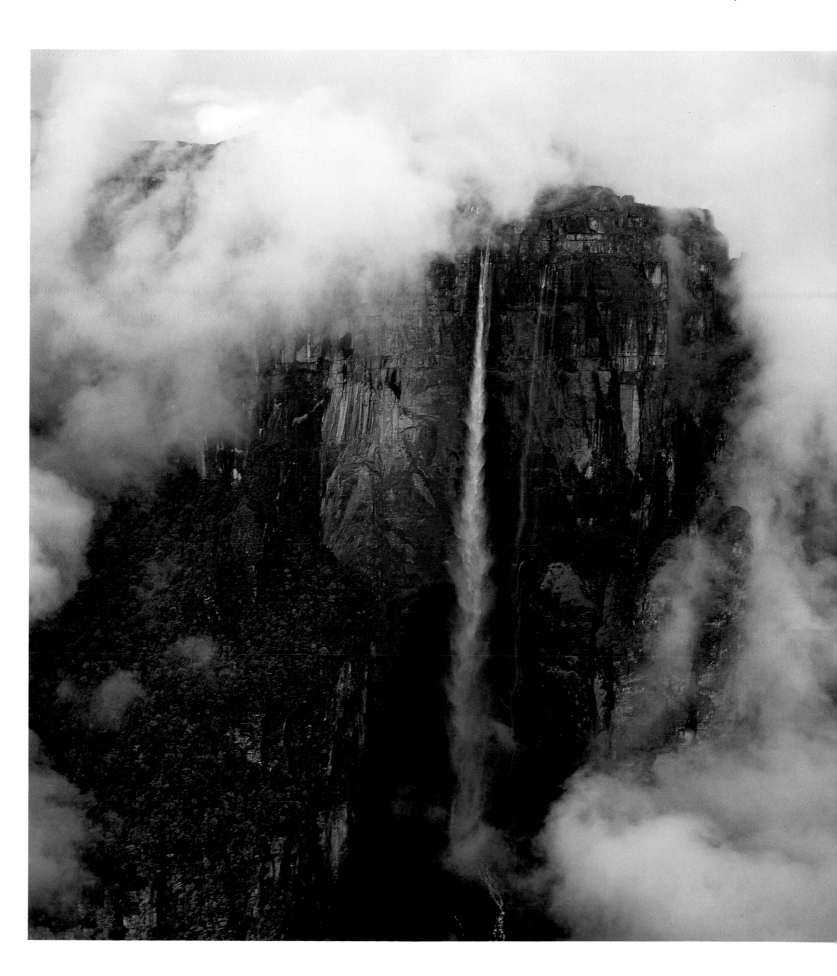

Paramo seedeater and the white-throated tyrannulet, for example, are widespread in the Andes, and both have distinct races out on the tepuis. But, as far as is known, no highland ever linked the tepui region with the Andes, so how could these normally sedentary birds have made their way across such a vast environmental barrier as the tropical plains?

The answer may be that, some time in the past, the barrier was not there. Changes in climate brought temperate conditions to the lowlands, and the birds naturally advanced across them. When the climate warmed again, the lowlands became unsuitable once more. Those populations living near tepuis retreated upslope to find the right conditions. Some reached the mountain tops and managed to survive, but in isolation.

Many tepuis rise abruptly from jungle-cloaked land. The forests continue onto the lower slopes, coating the wedges of weathered debris that skirt the cliffs. Even the cliffs themselves may be laced with vegetation clinging to crevices and ledges. The walls of Autana are thick with plant life in places and noted for the abundant tarantulas that patrol the vertical rock face in search of prey. As the cliffs rise ever higher, so the plants that cling to them need to be able to tolerate the cooler temperatures of altitude as well as a combination of murky daylight for much of the time and intense sunshine when the mists clear.

On most tepuis, the vegetation of the elevated summits looks quite different from that toward the bottom. Mount Duida which rises from the rainforests southeast of Autana is topped with low bushes, swamp patches and hardy cushion plants – a distinct contrast to the towering trees at its foot.

Dense, low vegetation also clothes much of Auyan-tepui, which lies within Canaima National Park. With

FORCES OF EROSION

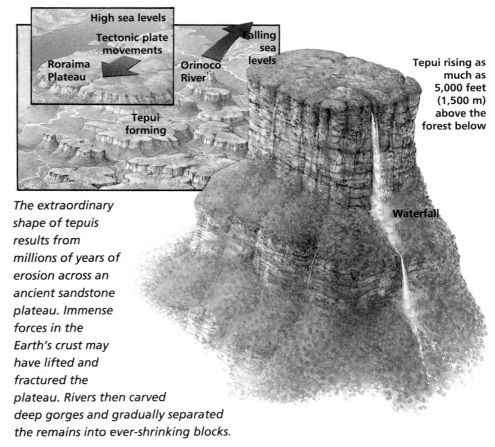

The extraordinary shape of tepuis results from millions of years of erosion across an ancient sandstone plateau. Immense forces in the Earth's crust may have lifted and fractured the plateau. Rivers then carved deep gorges and gradually separated the remains into ever-shrinking blocks.

a surface area of about 270 sq. miles (700 km²), Auyan-tepui is the most extensive of all tepuis. Streams racing across its broad summit have cut deep gorges into its heart, and one of them tumbles over its rim to form Angel Falls, the highest waterfall anywhere in the world. By the time the plummeting water has descended from the lofty heights to the tepui's forested base, most of it is a misty veil of spray.

Roraima and its neighbor Cuquenan, though higher, are not nearly so large in area as Auyan-tepui. Nor are they so well vegetated. Little soil exists on their blackened summits, and intense rainfall has leached most of the mineral nutrients from the weathering sandstone. Their surfaces are gnarled and weirdly sculpted, sometimes into almost impenetrable rock labyrinths, with

pockets of plant life lurking mainly in crevices and hollows.

In places, however, clumps of moss and lichen growing on bare rock create miniature platforms on which other small plants can secure an anchorage. Some have even evolved carnivorous habits. Given the paucity of nutrients available to roots, some plants use devices such as sticky traps and slippery pitchers to catch and digest insects instead.

Botanists are gradually learning more about the unique plant life of the isolated summits, but the animals of the tepuis remain little studied. Though a steady trickle of hikers now reaches the top of Roraima every year, great sections of the summit are yet to be penetrated. Meanwhile, some tepuis have still to receive their first human visitors. Who knows what mysteries await them?

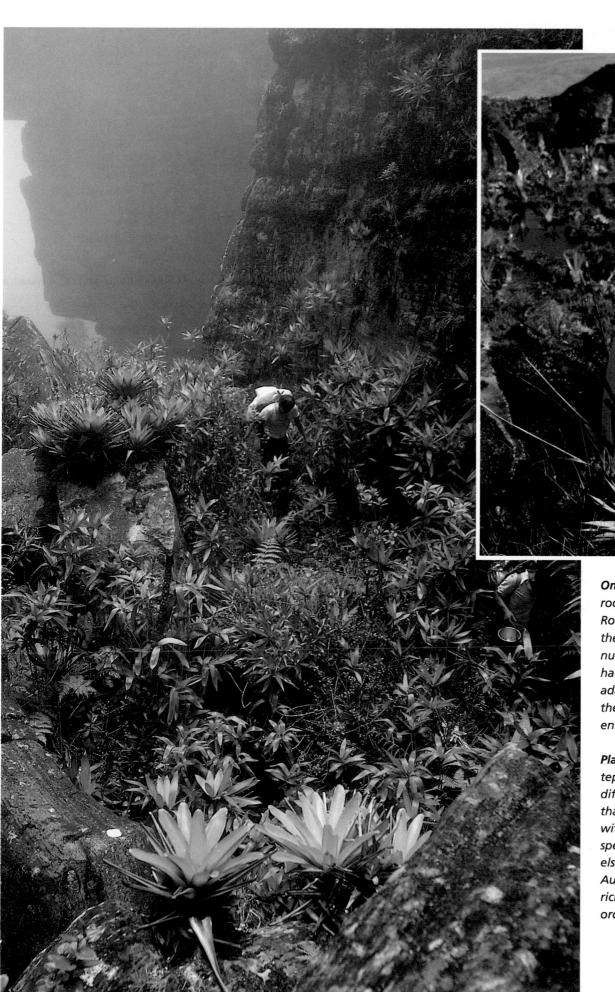

On the bleak, rocky surface of Roraima (above), there are few nutrients. Plants have special adaptations to their strange environment.

Plant life on tepuis is radically different from that down below, with many species unknown elsewhere (left). Auyan-tepui is rich in endemic orchids.

Manu Biosphere Reserve

"Dense virgin forest, with one of the greatest concentrations of wildlife on the planet"

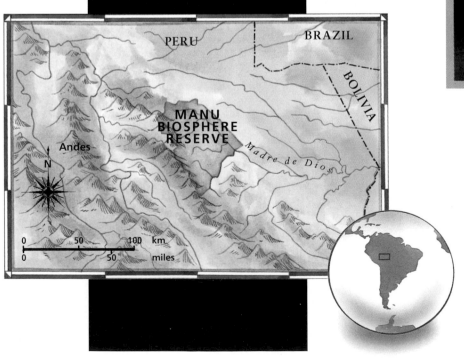

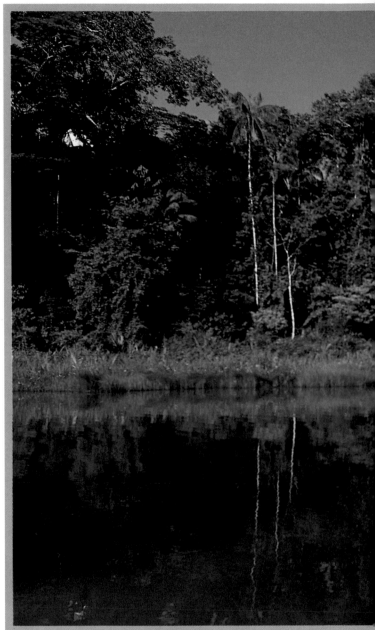

On the eastern slopes of the Peruvian Andes lies a region so remote and so little explored that archaeologists still dream of finding within it long-lost hoards of Inca treasure. But its true riches are of a biological kind. Mantled in dense, virgin forest, it has one of the greatest concentrations of wildlife diversity on the planet. This region of South America is of such global importance that the world body UNESCO declared it should become the Manu

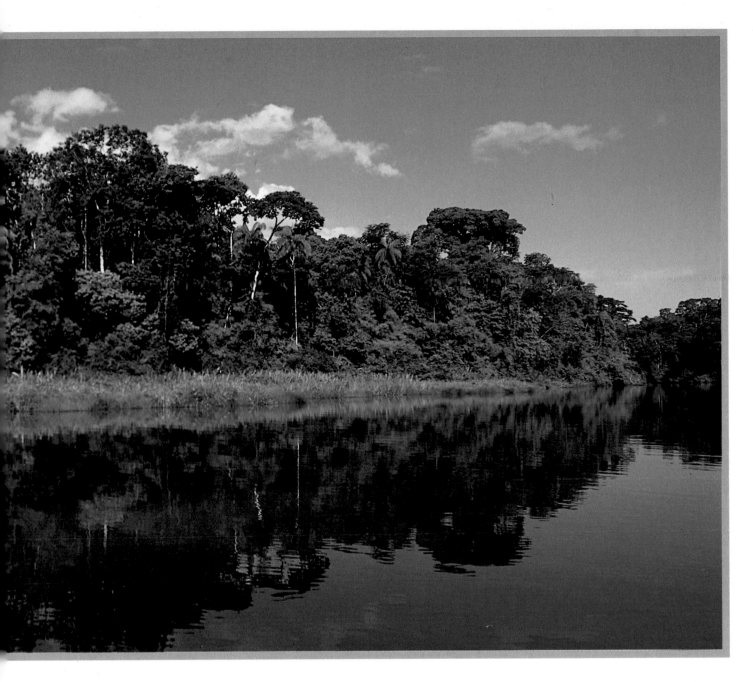

Biosphere Reserve, in recognition of its outstanding ecological wealth.

With an area of over 7,260 sq. miles (18,800 km²), Manu Biosphere Reserve covers part of the Upper Madre de Dios River basin, including all the lands drained by its major tributary, the winding Manu River. The headwaters of the rivers lie in the easternmost wall of the Andes, the Paucartambo Mountains. From the open and windswept slopes around these 13,000-foot (4,000-m) peaks, the streams fall rapidly into rugged valleys carved into the mountains' flank, filled with ever thicker vegetation and enveloped for much of the time in swirling cloud. These daunting slopes, it is conjectured, could still harbor somewhere the "Paititi" or "lost city" of the Incas. This legendary place is the secret refuge to which Inca people are supposed to have fled, taking with them treasures they saved when the Spanish pillaged their highland realm.

Eventually, the streams cease their turbulent plunge as they reach the

From its winding lowland rivers to its open mountain tops, the Manu reserve on the fringes of the Peruvian Andes is immensely rich in wildlife. It remains one of the most isolated and least explored parts of Amazonia.

foot of the Andes. The rivers become broad and deep and start to meander over flatter ground in the eastern half of the reserve. Their waters are destined to reach the Amazon River, and by now their banks are clothed in

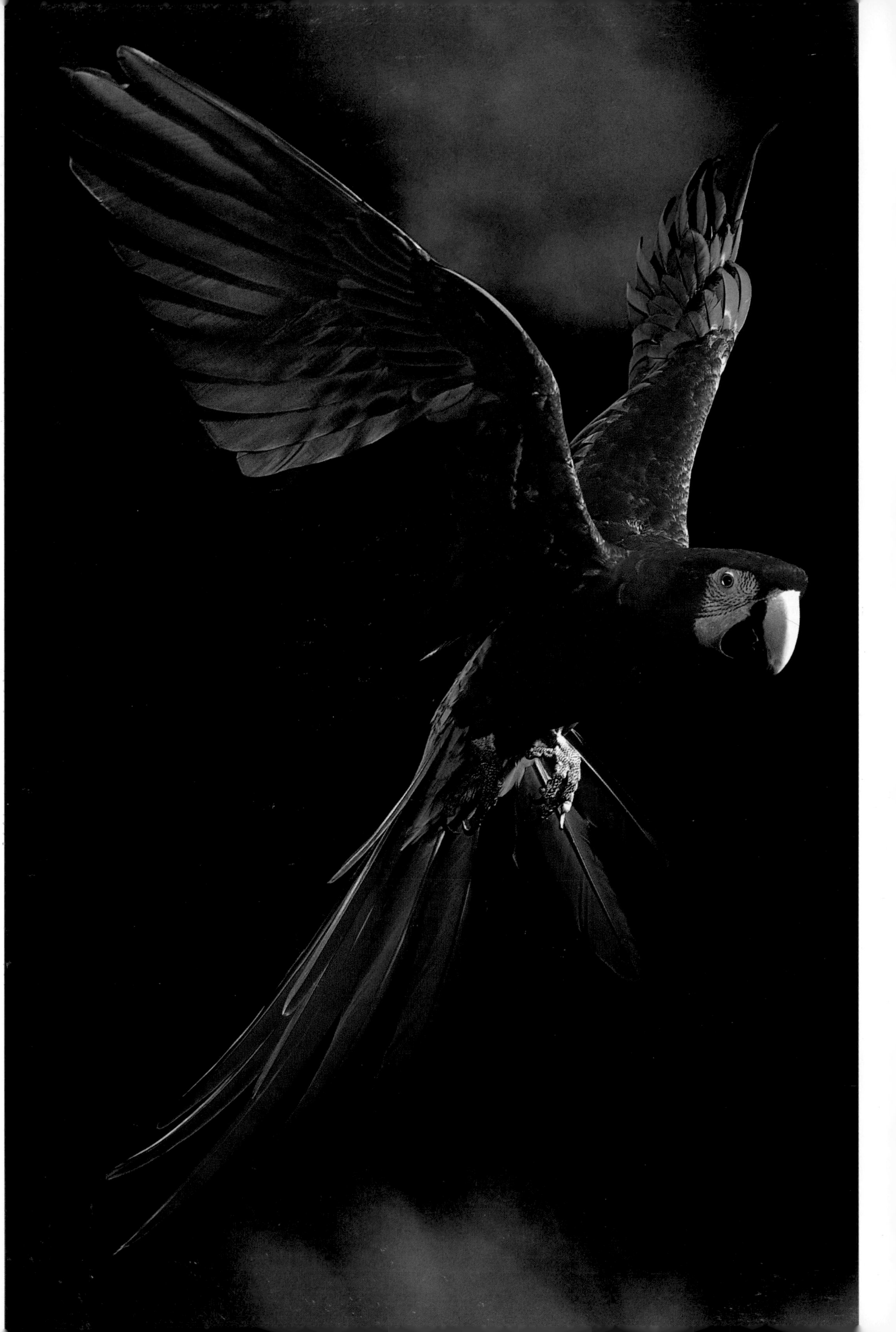

full lowland rainforest, one of the most pristine stretches of continuous forest in all the Amazon region. Few outside people have settled in the area of the reserve, and those scattered tribes for whom the forest has long been home, such as the Machiguenga, Kugapakori and Nahua, still lead for the most part traditional lives, with minimal adverse impact on their natural surroundings.

If one were possible, a roll call of the wildlife species that inhabit Manu would take in a huge proportion of the animals that exist in South America. Inventories of the reserve's fauna, even for larger animals, however, are far from complete. Estimates suggest that there could be 200 mammal species and as many as 90 different kinds of frogs. Bird species found throughout the reserve could number more than 1,000 – an extraordinary 550 birds have been recorded in one area alone. Fishes in the streams, rivers and lakes are highly diverse, and the number of different insects and other invertebrates could easily run to one million or more.

Yet it is not simply diversity that makes Manu so special. Because the forests and mountain slopes have suffered so little human disturbance and exploitation, animals becoming rare in other parts of the Amazon occur in much more healthy numbers in Manu. These include endangered species such as the giant otter, which hunts for fish in the lowland rivers,

and the harpy eagle, which is the reserve's symbol. This raptor is a giant among birds of prey, capable of snatching animals as large as monkeys and sloths from the treetops.

Some of the wildlife ranges widely over the park, from the lowlands up through the lower mountain slopes. This includes foraging and browsing mammals like the agouti and the red brocket deer, as well as hunters like the jaguar and the ocelot. The king vulture, a spectacular scavenging bird that relies largely on smell to detect its food, cruises conspicuously over both the lowland and upland forests. A few highly adaptable animals, among them the puma, occur from the plains right up to the high elevations well above the forest.

But most animals are not so flexible in their habitat preferences. Varying conditions in the reserve associated with different altitudes therefore bring changes in the mix of wildlife.

The flatter, lowland sections below about 2,000 feet (600 m) altitude are hot and humid throughout the year. Rainfall becomes heavier from October to April, but is always high, with frequent downpours from dark thunder clouds that gather over the landscape. Temperatures are around 75°F (24°C), rising to a stifling 97°F (36°C) on the warmest days.

Constant heat and moisture are ideal conditions for luxuriant plant growth, creating the richest of all land

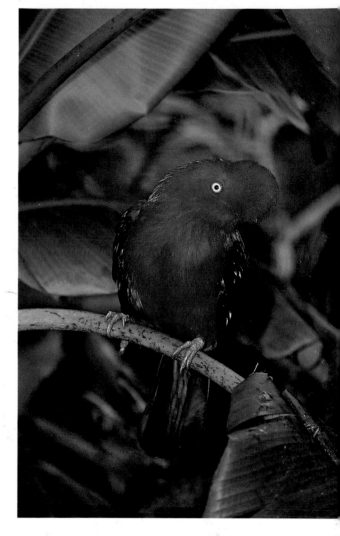

The Andean cock-of-the-rock, with its vivid plumage and curious semicircular crest, dwells in misty, jungle-clad ravines. While females watch, male birds perform dramatic mating displays. They leap into the air, whirring their feathers, flicking their tails and making loud calls.

The spectacular scarlet macaw (left) is one of several members of the parrot family that live in the Manu rainforest. Noisy flocks of macaws gather to feed at fruiting trees.

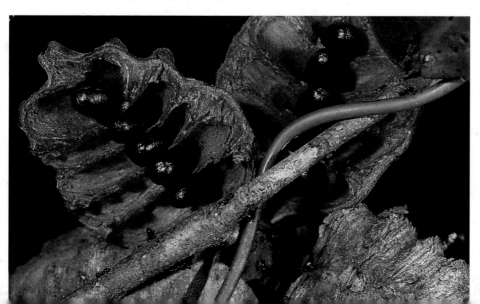

Colorful fruits attract numerous forest birds, which eat the flesh and later disperse the seeds in their droppings. These fruits have been split open to reveal their seeds (left).

habitats – classic tropical rainforest. Deep in the forest, away from the crowded, sun-soaked "jungle" that typically lines a clearing or river, the air is still and the light is muted. Tall trees rise with columnar trunks before spreading their branches and leaves at the crown to form a continuous green canopy up above. Varieties of cedar, mahogany and kapok mingle with hundreds of other tree species so that it is hard to find two of the same kind standing side by side. The largest have massive buttressed bases up to 10 feet (3 m) across and rise more than 200 feet (60 m) into the air.

Beneath the canopy, twisted lianas dangle from on high, creepers cling to the trunks and branches, and palms spread their fans. Down near the ground, cast in continual shade, thin saplings strive upward, and an untold variety of low-growing plants thrives scattered over the fallen leaves, twigs and other debris.

Though all levels of the forest abound in wildlife, it is the canopy, the forest roof, that harbors the greatest concentration. Here are the bulk of the leaves, fruit, nuts and

> *"Among the hundreds of tree species it is hard to find two of the same kind standing side by side"*

flowers – food for myriad insects and spectacular birds such as cotingas and toucans. Howler monkeys, whose loud calls echo through the forest, roam the canopy feeding largely on foliage. Hordes of plant-eating creatures attract legions of hunters that eat them or prey on one another, including spiders, tree frogs, lizards, boas, woodpeckers, hawks and bats.

Below them deer and tapirs browse on the undergrowth, and large ground birds such as tinamous and currasows scour the forest floor for fallen food.

Moving westward across Manu on to the lower mountain slopes, subtle changes appear in the rainforest habitat. A combination of steepening slopes, thinner soil and slightly lower temperatures makes it increasingly difficult for trees to grow to the heights they reach on the lowland. The canopy becomes less even, more light reaches the forest floor, allowing thicker undergrowth, and different types of flora have a chance to grow.

Eventually, the slopes reach a height where they are enveloped for much of the time in low cloud, bringing even more rain than in the lowlands. Temperatures, still hot by day, become cool at night, when the air is dank. Many of the trees seem twisted and stunted compared with those lower down, and their branches are typically laden with other plants such as lichens, mosses, ferns and beautiful orchids.

This is the cloud forest, home to an especially high diversity of small, colorful birds, including mixed flocks of tanagers that forage through the treetops for berries and insects, and various hummingbirds that sip nectar from the abundant flowers. It is also the stronghold of the vivid red and black Andean cock-of-the-rock, which nests in rocky ravines, and of the spectacled bear, which piles sticks on a tree fork to make its lair.

By an altitude of about 10,000 feet (3,000 m), the forests give way to an open landscape of tussock grasses and shrubs, with reedy pools on the flatter portions. This highland habitat, restricted to the southwestern limits of Manu, is known as "puna." Temperatures are low at this elevation – becoming frigid at night – winds are strong, and there is a marked dry season from May to September. To cope with the high

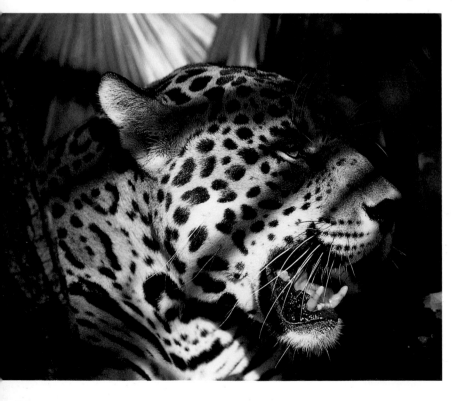

Solitary, stealthy and formidably strong, the jaguar is the top predator of the South American forests. It hunts mostly at night. Having stalked its prey, which may range in size from a ground bird to a tapir, the jaguar attacks with a mighty leap, aiming to clamp its powerful jaws around the neck of the victim.

mountain conditions, both plants and animals have to be hardy. Thick fur is an asset for small mammals like the mountain viscacha as well as for its enemy, the Andean fox. They share the grassy slopes with a deer that is becoming increasingly rare in the Andes, the Peruvian huemul.

Although the Manu Biosphere Reserve is remote, conservationists are fighting to keep it free from the pressures of logging, gold-mining and oil exploration that are already affecting regions along its borders. The challenge to keep Manu in its natural state means not only maintaining a refuge for endangered species like the huemul and the harpy eagle, but also preserving the entire ecological base of one of the richest forest lands on Earth.

Rivers snaking their way through lowland Manu shift course over the cenuries as they cut new paths and dump sediments transported from the mountains. Abandoned meanders form tranquil oxbow lakes, which make secluded havens for wildlife (below).

THE ZONES OF THE FOREST

Marked changes in vegetation appear with increasing altitude on the mountain slopes in western Manu. The constant heat that bathes the lowland rainforest gives way to cooler temperatures on the middle slopes. Fog and cloud commonly drape the forest here, the canopy of which is lower and less even. Higher still, conditions become too cold for forest trees to develop at all.

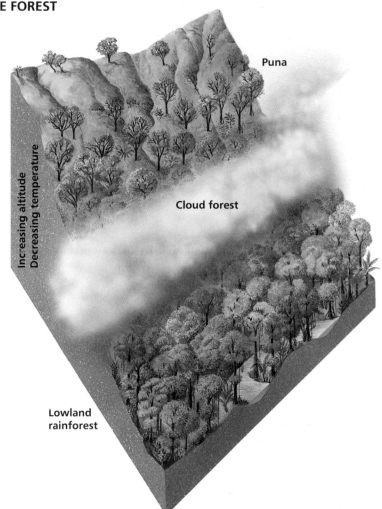

Puna

Increasing altitude
Decreasing temperature

Cloud forest

Lowland rainforest

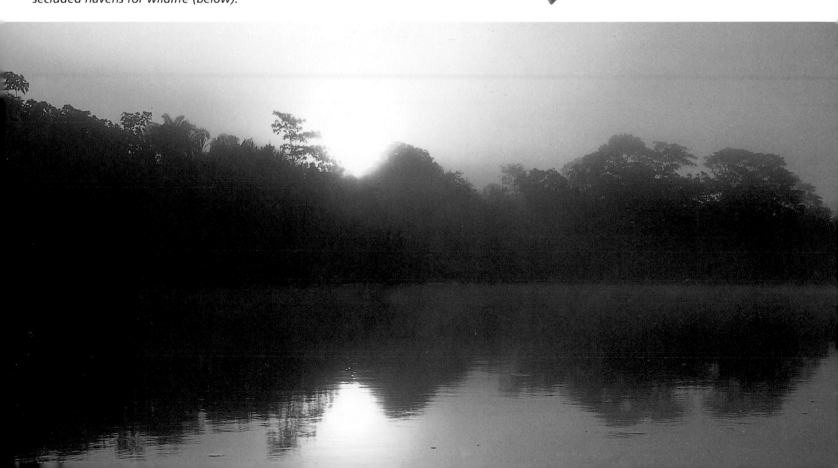

NATIVES OF THE AMAZON BASIN

Since time immemorial, the Amazon Basin has provided food and shelter for people scattered across its rainforests, riverside flood plains and fringing savannas. The many indigenous native tribes include groups such as the Kayapo of the south, the Jivaro of the west and the Yanomami who live in the north of Amazonia. Today, though most of the native cultures have been swamped by often disastrous contact with outsiders, some tribes still lead traditional lives, in close contact with the natural world around them.

Though lifestyles differ from tribe to tribe, most Amazonian people live by a combination of farming, hunting and gathering. Tribal villages are usually surrounded by garden plots cleared by slash-and-burn. When the soil is exhausted, the villagers move to new sites. Various weapons are employed in hunting and fishing, among them harpoons, bows and arrows, traps and snares. Poison-tipped darts are blown with lethal accuracy from long bamboo guns to fell groups of birds and monkeys high in the trees. Other food is simply harvested from forest plants.

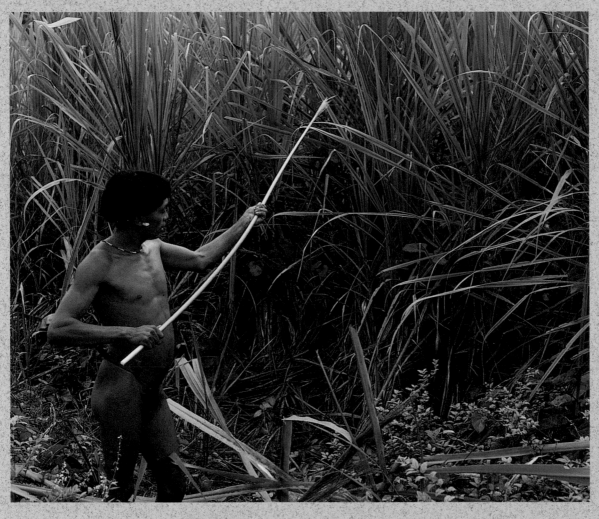

A Yanomami Indian prepares a riverside reed for use as a hunting arrow. The forest provides myriad food sources for the Yanomami people. Some, such as birds, monkeys, deer, tapirs and armadillos, have to be hunted. Others, including fruit, nuts, honey, caterpillars and beetle grubs, are simply harvested from the wild and stored in baskets and fiber pouches fashioned from forest plants.

Many Amazon peoples cultivate staple crops suited to the rainy tropical climate such as manioc, plantain and maize. Here, Yanomami women grate manioc to prepare bread for a funerary feast (right).

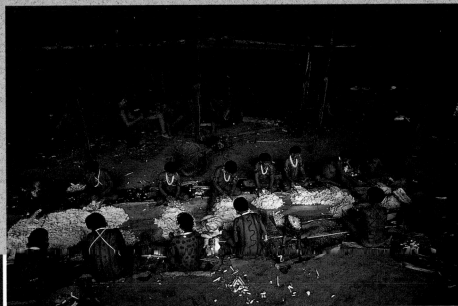

A Kayapo Indian fishes with a bow and arrow in the calm waters of the great Amazon River (below). Such a method of fishing requires patience, stealth and skill.

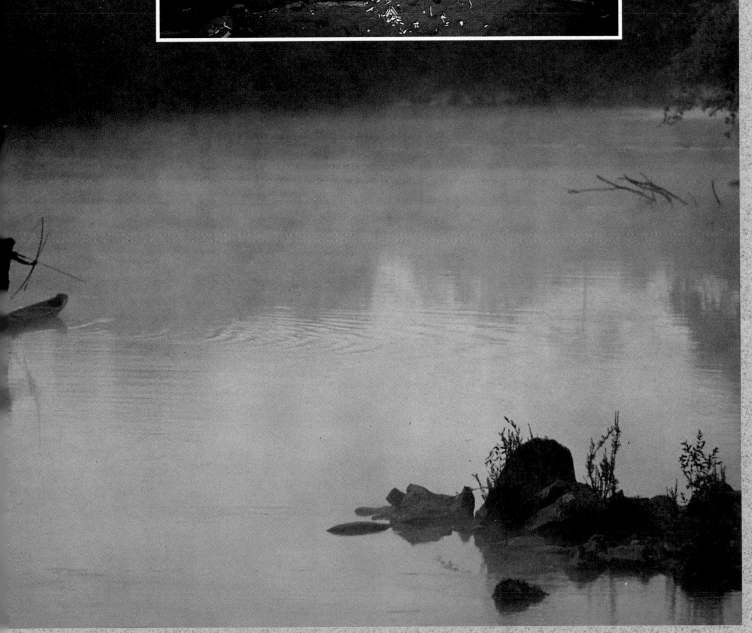

ITATIAIA NATIONAL PARK

"The call of the wild is ever present here, where parrots race across the treetops with raucous cries"

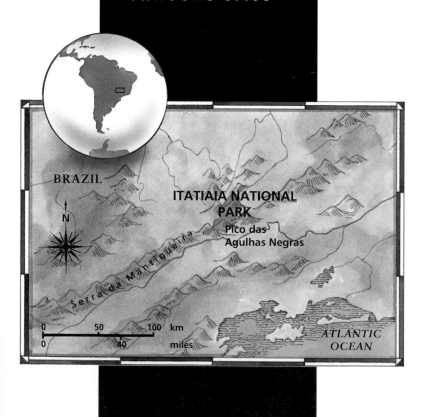

BRAZIL

ITATIAIA NATIONAL PARK

Pico das Agulhas Negras

Serra da Mantiqueira

N

| 0 | 50 | 100 | km |

| 0 | 40 | | miles |

ATLANTIC OCEAN

Set among rugged mountains, some 40 miles (65 km) inland from the coast of southeast Brazil, is the Itatiaia National Park. The park is renowned for its luxuriant tropical forest that sweeps up the hillsides, clings to steep valley walls, and crowds around every cascading stream.

Inside the forest, the call of the wild is ever present. In the early morning, when mist still hangs in the air, bands of howler monkeys challenge one

Lush and tropical, Itatiaia National Park encloses a precious fragment of Brazil's once extensive Atlantic Forest. Many of the forest's plants and animals are unknown outside the region.

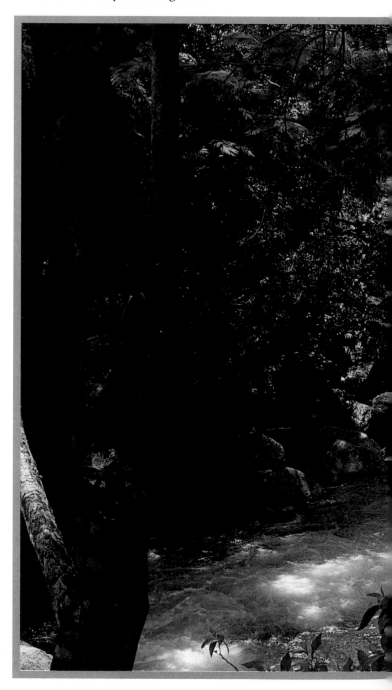

another across the valleys. Their haunting calls are not so much howls as deep roars like the sound of distant wind. As the sun rises, flocks of parrots and parakeets leave their roosts and race across the treetops with raucous cries. Later, the muted sounds of still noon are broken by the drilling of a woodpecker's beak, and at night the damp air echoes with the peeping calls of tree frogs.

A few centuries ago, sounds like these were commonplace far beyond the boundaries of Itatiaia. Where the bulk of Brazil's population lives today, a huge belt of dense forest used to carpet the plains and mountains abutting the country's eastern coast. Known as the Atlantic Forest, it was a type of ecosystem quite separate from, but no less exuberant than, the Amazon rainforest well to the north.

Charles Darwin was thrilled by the Atlantic Forest in 1832 during his epic voyage on HMS *Beagle*. He wrote: "Here I first saw a Tropical forest in all its sublime grandeur," and remarked upon "not being able to walk one hundred yards without being fairly tied to the spot by some new and wondrous creature."

But already, by Darwin's day, the forest was disappearing. Today all that is left are scattered remnants: precious wildernesses – like Itatiaia – mostly on mountainous land that is too steep for easy cultivation.

The 115 sq. miles (300 km²) of wild country that make up Itatiaia

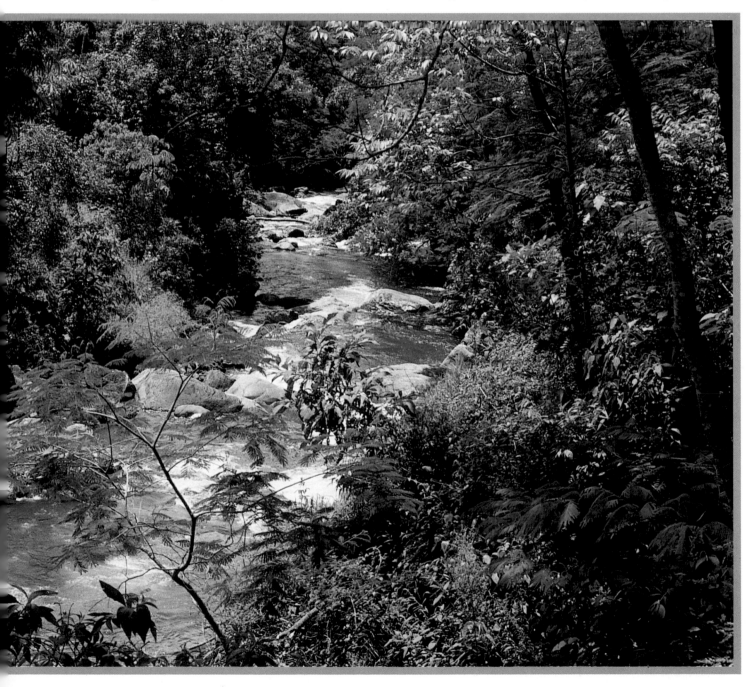

National Park lie within a large mountain chain, the Serra da Mantiqueira. An offshoot of the range, the Serra do Itatiaia, forms the central highest ground of the park, a cold, open plateau of grassland and bare granite rocks. Rainfall is plentiful for most of the year on the plateau, although it becomes drier in winter, when nighttime temperatures often drop below freezing. Clumps of grasses, thin-leaved bamboo, small shrubs and herbs grow here, providing cover from predators like the savanna fox for small birds, including the rufous-tailed antbird and the Itatiaia spinetail.

Far richer in terms of wildlife are the forests that spread across the bulk of the park to the north and south. At a height of about 6,000 feet (1,800 m), the upper limits of the forest are shrouded for much of the time in cloud. All the forested land of Itatiaia is montane forest, its appearance strongly reflecting the influence of steep slopes and high humidity.

Because of the mountainous nature of the land, the tree canopy is stepped rather than even, and there are more open patches than in a lowland rainforest, allowing pockets of ground vegetation to thrive. Some of the biggest trees, like the massive 130-foot (40-m) jequitiba-rosa, have space to grow horizontal branches and broad spreading crowns. Others

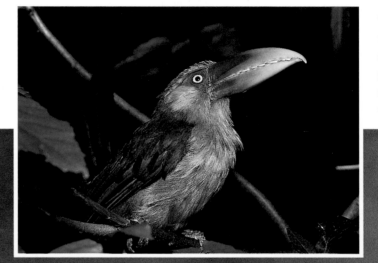

The saffron toucanet perches high in the forest, plucking berries and fruits with its colorful beak.

are prominent not for their size but for golden or violet blooms that, at a distance, coat the trees with vivid color against the green backdrop.

Palms and tree ferns are common in the forest, especially in the damper areas near the mountain streams. Patches of bamboo, however, are more common in drier, sunlit places and form extensive groves up toward the tree line. But the forests are most impressive for the incredible abundance of plants that establish themselves high above the soil, supported on trunks and branches. Plants with such a habit are called epiphytes. Many of these plants,

"An incredible abundance of plants grows high above the soil on tree trunks and branches"

including ferns, mosses and orchids, draw their moisture either from rainwater running down the tree bark or directly from the humid air through delicate dangling roots.

Bromeliads, however, store their own water supplies. The smooth radiating leaves of these large plants pack tightly together at the base to form a container for falling rain. Itatiaia is renowned for its bromeliads, three-quarters of which occur nowhere else but in the remaining fragments of the Atlantic Forest. They crowd at such density on the biggest tree branches that the stout limbs look in danger of collapsing under the weight.

Like many of the plants, a large proportion of the animal inhabitants

In early morning, and often later in the day, mists and cloud hang over the verdant landscape of Itatiaia. Much of the forest is on rugged slopes above 3,600 feet (1,100 m).

of Itatiaia are unique to the Atlantic Forest ecosystem. They include rarely seen animals of the treetops, such as the wooly spider monkey – the largest monkey of the New World – and the leaf-eating maned sloth, as well as bold, conspicuous creatures like the red-breasted toucan, which feeds largely on fruit and nuts.

Other inhabitants are much more widely distributed across the forests of South America, including ground foragers like the paca and the tapir, hunters such as the jaguar and ocelot and powerful raptors like the harpy eagle. As more and more rainforest is destroyed, protected parks like Itatiaia are an increasingly important refuge for such wildlife.

SAVING THE GOLDEN LION TAMARIN

With its vivid coloration and opulent mane, the golden lion tamarin is among the most celebrated, yet most endangered, of the Atlantic Forest's unique animals. It used to thrive in the lowlands near Rio de Janeiro, but today its wild population has dwindled to only 500 individuals.

Strenuous efforts are being made to protect the remnants of the monkeys' habitat. And, with the help of zoos around the world, Brazilian biologists have set up a special reintroduction program. Captive-bred tamarins have already been released into a protected area of the forest in the hope that they can survive and form a stable breeding group in the wild.

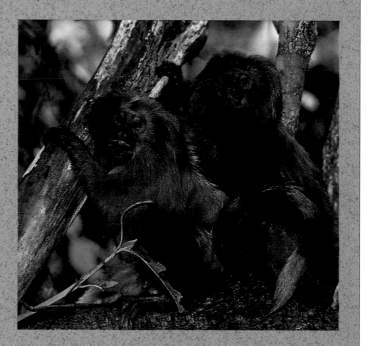

THE BOLIVIAN ALTIPLANO

"An immense level plain – a frigid desert of grass, bare earth and salt flats"

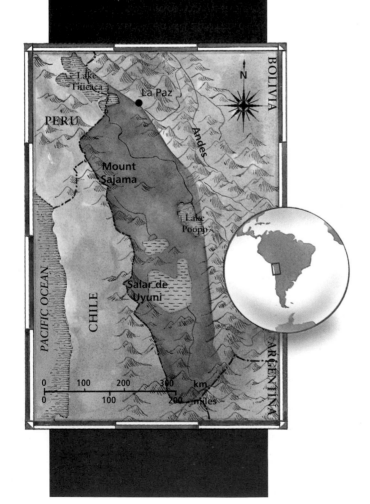

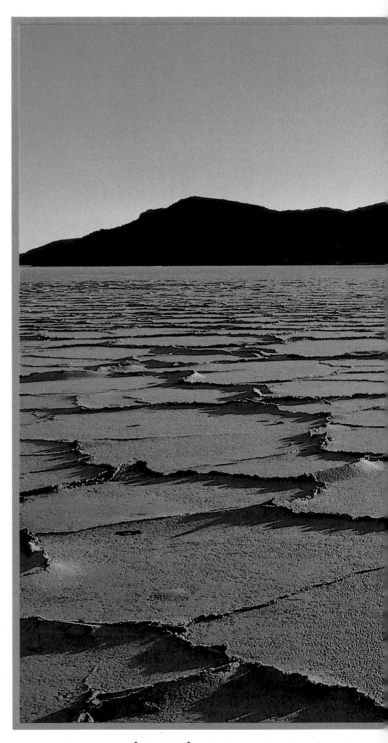

The Bolivian Altiplano lies in the central part of the Andes, where the great mountain range of South America is at its widest. Here, the parallel lines of peaks – the western and eastern cordilleras – stretch far apart, leaving a vast intermontane basin 500 miles (800 km) long and up to 80 miles (130 km) wide. The land

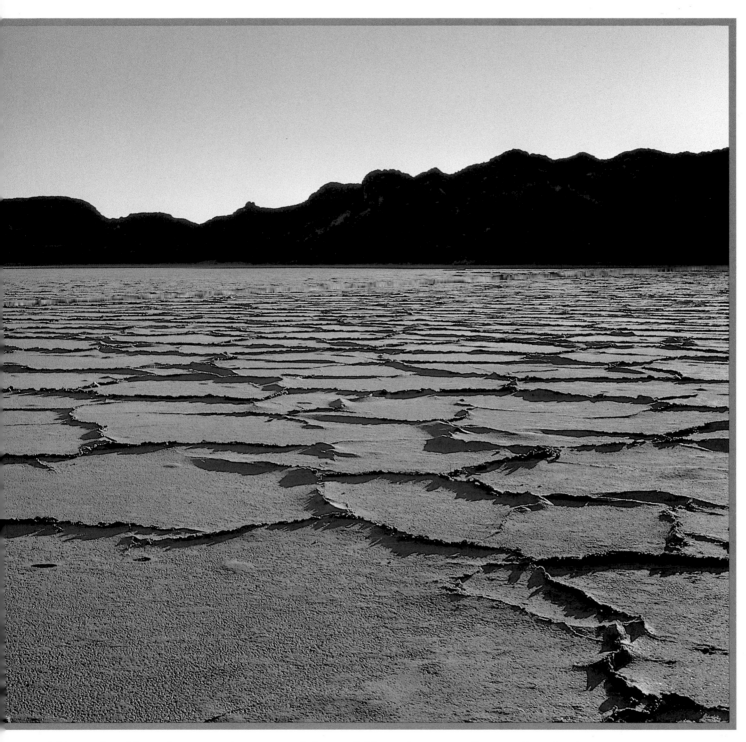

within, enclosed by volcanoes and peaks, is a world of the unexpected. Instead of rugged slopes and valleys, it is filled almost to the brim with an immense level plain – a frigid desert of grass, bare earth and salt flats.

The Altiplano's smooth surface is the product of millions of years of erosion and deposition. After the basin was formed, huge quantities of eroded material from the surrounding mountains were carried into it by wind and water, accumulating as layer upon layer of sediment. As more and more layers were added, those strata beneath were gradually squeezed to solid rock. In time, the infilling reached high enough to swamp the basin's underlying topography. The top of the deposits currently stands at

The Salar de Uyuni is a huge salt flat on the Bolivian Altiplano. Early morning light falling near its rim softens the glare from the salt plain and picks out its only surface features – geometric ridges just a few inches high. Intense evaporation across the bed of a dried lake produced the salt deposits, which are more than 23 feet (7 m) thick in places.

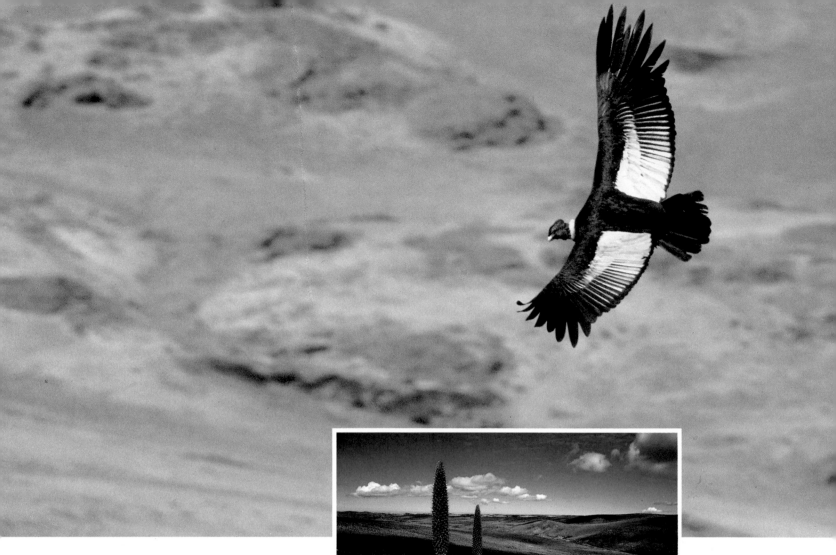

Giant puya plants are welcome shelter for creatures in this treeless landscape.

12,000–12,500 feet (3,650–3,800 m), forming a strikingly flat surface, broken only by a few ridges, hills and volcanic cones.

Conditions on the Altiplano are inhospitable indeed. During most of the year, rain seldom falls, and in the thin mountain air, strong sunshine quickly evaporates away much of the moisture from the occasional summer storm in December and January. After sunset, the air cools fast, to below freezing, and sweeping gales can chill the land at any time. The windy, cold, desert climate is reflected in the thin, dry soil across most of the region and the sparse vegetation.

In the north around Lake Titicaca, the weather and the soils are slightly better, and people have long been able to make some sort of living from the land. Yet compared with the fecundity of the forests just to the east across the mountains, life has a difficult hold even here. Apart from clumps of bunch grasses, which retain old leaves around the edge as some insulation against the cold, there is little plant life save hardy cushion plants and cacti. On a few scattered hillsides live colonies of the giant puya – a distant, slow-growing relative of the pineapple, with enormous bayonet-sharp leaves. It blooms only once before dying, growing a flowering spike that towers 30 feet (9 m) above the ground.

The Desaguadero, one of the few permanent rivers of the Altiplano, flows south through this region. The sole outlet of Lake Titicaca, it is a sluggish waterway continually depleted by evaporation in the strong sunshine and dry winds. It crosses decreasingly fertile land, flanked on each far side by the walls of the Altiplano. To the east, the snow caps of the cordillera gleam in the sunshine, their rugged heights home to condors. The mountainous horizon to the west marks the Chilean border and is studded with volcanoes, including the mighty Sajama which rises to 21,463 feet (6,542 m).

Eventually, the Desaguadero reaches shallow Lake Poopo. Large flocks of flamingoes, egrets, herons, ducks and geese feed here, their abundance in sharp contrast with the empty lands beyond.

Most of the water that reaches the intensely arid section of the Altiplano south of Lake Poopo soon soaks into the dry soil or evaporates away. Only

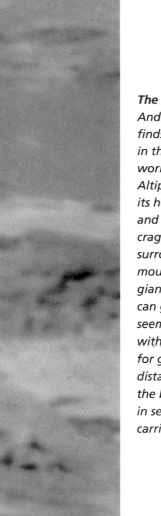

The majestic Andean condor finds sustenance in the harsh world of the Altiplano. From its home in lonely and inaccessible crags on the surrounding mountains, this giant scavenger can glide, seemingly without effort. for great distances across the bleak terrain in search of carrion.

SALT LAKES

The water of Altiplano lakes can be too mineral-rich for many aquatic organisms. But salt-tolerant algae do thrive in some places, staining the water vivid green, brown or red, and nourishing other creatures. Here, the calm waters of Laguna Colorada are colored reddish-brown by algae. Water loss from evaporation, with little replenishment in the desert climate, has left a concentrated broth of mineral salts. The glistening bergs of crystalline salt were probably formed during past phases of rapid evaporation.

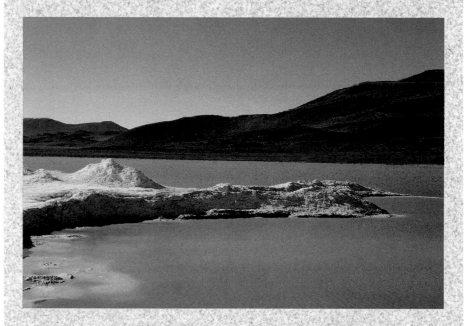

"Strange lakes laden with salt exist in the volcanic landscape"

when rainfall has been heavy do streams flow for any distance. But evidence of wetter times is obvious in the landscape, literally blindingly obvious in a series of salt flats, or "salars." In brilliant sunshine, the glare from these perfectly level plains of crystalline salt is dangerous to unprotected eyes.

The largest by far is the immense Salar de Uyuni, a sheet of salt of a whiteness more pure than driven snow. Several yards in depth, it is more than 80 miles (130 km) from rim to rim. It owes its formation to a humid time when the Altiplano was almost covered in water.

Around 15,000 years ago, the meltwater from ice-age glaciers and snowfields in the mountains created two enormous lakes, one in the north, one to the south. After the ice age, the lakes gradually dried out, leaving today's remnants – Titicaca in the north and Poopo in the south. The Salar de Uyuni was also part of

the southern lake's bed. Thousands of years of intense evaporation removed the overlying water but left its dissolved salts behind and continued to suck the ground beneath dry, bringing yet more salts to the surface. The same process continues today after occasional heavy rain storms spread a short-lived coat of water over the salar.

Strange lakes laden with salt but not yet dried out exist in the rugged, volcanic landscape that forms the southern fringe of the Altiplano. This scarcely inhabited arid zone of sand, gravel, banded rocks and bubbling geysers, lies at about 14,000 feet (4,250 m) above sea level. The chill is even more intense at this level, and few creatures are visible across the barren terrain. Only silent herds of vicuña, graceful wild relatives of the llama, wander the desert in search of scattered pockets of vegetation in this, South America's most singular and mysterious wilderness.

PEOPLE OF THE ALTIPLANO

The slightly more fertile north of the Altiplano is the homeland of the Aymara tribe, whose god Viracocha is said to have risen from Lake Titicaca to establish their ancient culture. Old traditions still remain in the lives of many modern Aymaras. These are reflected in the thatched adobe huts in which they live, in their herds of llamas and alpacas grazing the tough bunch grasses, and in the old, staple crops such as potato and oca tubers and quinoa grain that they harvest from terraced plots.

In a land of thin air, frosty nights, sun-baked days and fragile soils, life is unquestionably harsh, but the natives of the Altiplano seem to have evolved a physical hardiness to match their surroundings. Studies suggest that special features of their anatomy and physiology enhance the intake and passage of oxygen through the blood, an invaluable adaptation for toil at high altitude.

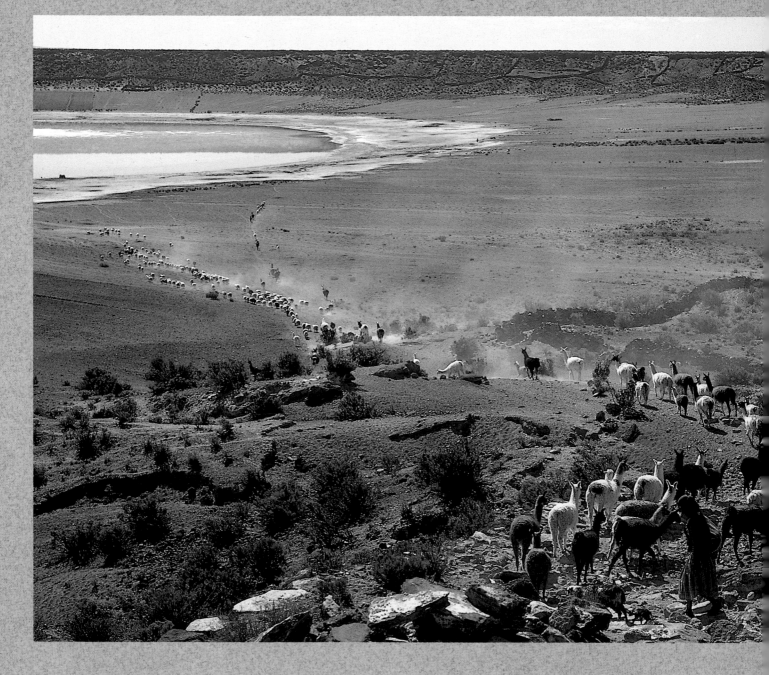

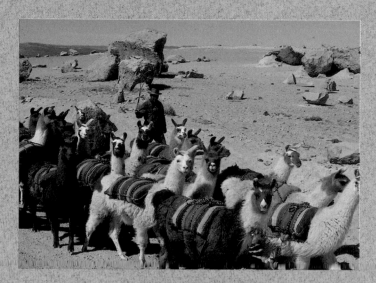

Llamas play a crucial role in the traditional life of the natives of the Altiplano. Hardy and dependable, llamas are beasts of burden as well as sources of wool, leather and meat. Even their dung is not wasted – it is dried in the intense sunshine and used as fuel for cooking and heating.

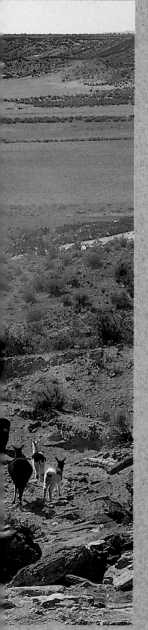

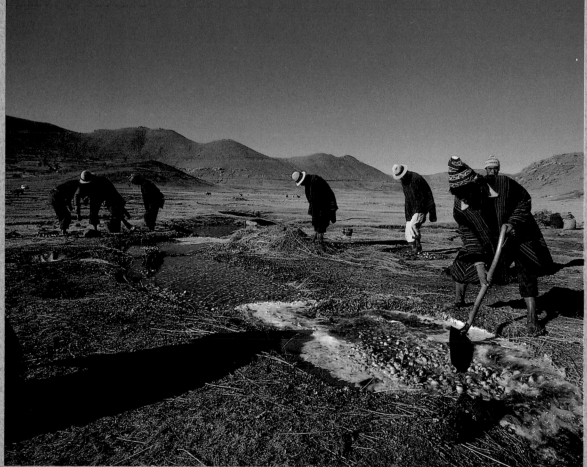

In spite of the harsh climate and thin soils of the Altiplano, tribal peoples have long made their home as farmers and herders in this uncompromising environment. The livestock they tend – llamas and alpacas – can find food even in volcanic deserts like this, where pasture is at best scant and coarse.

The potato probably had its origins as a crop plant on the Altiplano. Certainly it had been cultivated here for many centuries before it was discovered and introduced far afield by Europeans. Tolerant of dry soils and the bitter cold of night, it remains a staple crop of Altiplano people.

THE PANTANAL

"A maze of mingling habitats creates an extraordinarily diverse assemblage of life"

The lowlands known as the Pantanal form an enormous wilderness in the heart of South America. This flat, rain-fed region, laced with waterways and submerged beneath silvery sheets of floodwater for half the year, is one of the most evocative places in all the continent. The sweeping views and breathtaking sunsets are a backdrop for scenes matched only on the plains of Africa. Nowhere else in North or South America are so many animals

A mosaic of habitats including rivers, swamps, grassland and forests makes the Pantanal one of the richest wildlife havens in all South America.

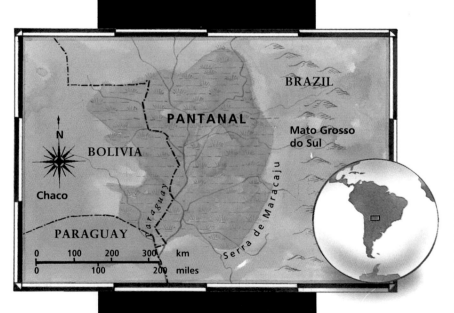

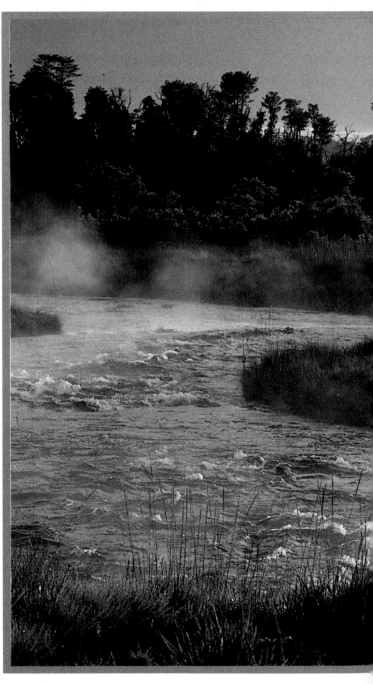

of such variety so spectacularly visible as in the Pantanal.

One reason for the exuberance of animal life is the sparse human settlement of the region. Because of the damp land and annual flooding, large-scale cultivation of the land is impractical, and access remains difficult. Giant cattle ranches lay claim to the land, but they are stocked at low density, and ranching has done little to change the essential character of the landscape.

But it is the natural shaping of the terrain that makes the Pantanal special. It straddles the border between Brazil and Bolivia and covers more than 75,000 sq. miles (200,000 km²) of lowland tropics. It is, in effect, a vast basin almost encircled by higher ground. Some of these surrounding lands reach heights of over 3,000 feet (900 m), yet the Pantanal is only 500 feet (150 m) above sea level.

Long ago the depression would have been much deeper and perhaps filled with lakes, but for thousands of years rivers from the surrounding highlands have deposited sediment in the basin. Today that sediment is 260 feet (80 m) thick in places and has created a flat surface across which rivers flow in channels in the dry season. But in the wet season the rivers' excess water spills across the basin. All the rivers flow into the River Paraguay, which divides the Bolivian third of the Pantanal from the larger section in Brazil.

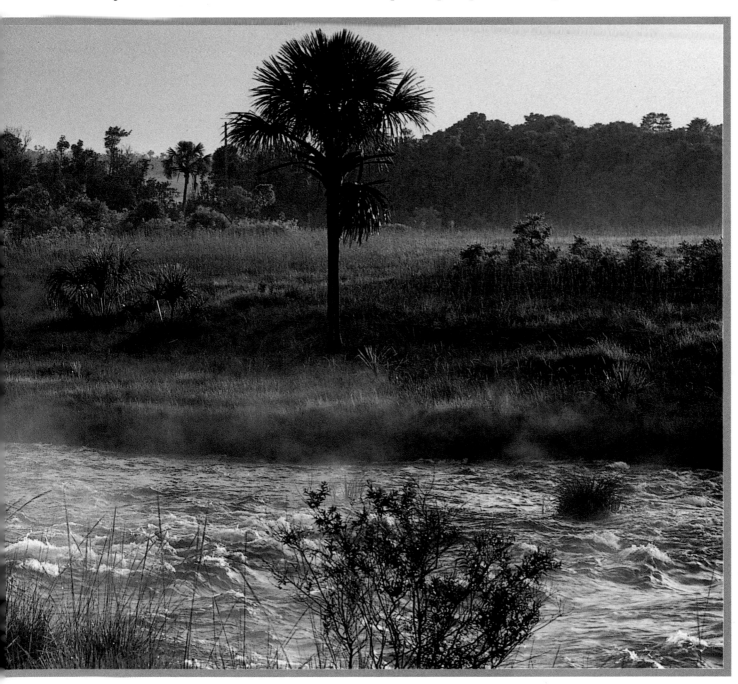

LAND OF
SEASONAL FLOODS

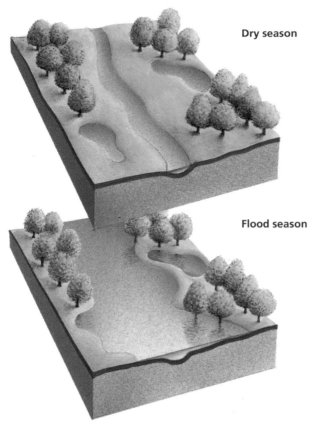

Dry season

Flood season

The landscape of the Pantanal changes with the seasonal floods. In the dry season, much of it is grassland broken by rivers and isolated pools. In the wet season, river levels rise and floodwaters spill across the land, leaving only islands of higher ground where trees and shrubs can survive.

Weed-choked *pools in the Pantanal are favorite haunts of caimans. The largest are 8 feet (2.5 m) from snout to tail.*

In geological terms the Pantanal plain is young, yet its newly formed landscape has been colonized by flora and fauna from all directions. Plants and animals from outlying regions such as the forests and swamps of the Amazon, the savannas of central Brazil and the thorn forests of the Chaco have all spread into the Pantanal, creating an extraordinarily diverse assemblage of life.

The Pantanal can support such variety because its landscape, though broadly level, is just uneven enough to create a maze of mingling habitats. The name Pantanal means "swamp." In truth, however, the region is a vast wetland mosaic of permanent rivers, pools, flood plains, patches of higher ground inundated only for short periods, and still higher ridges that are seldom, if ever, flooded.

The dry season in the Pantanal, when rains are few, runs from May to October. The floods gradually recede, and aquatic life becomes concentrated in rivers and around the diminishing pools. The permanent waters of the Pantanal are extremely rich in fish, ranging from small, colorful tetras to 30-inch (70-cm) heavyweights like the pacu. There are several species of piranha, most of which are plant-eaters, and large bottom-dwelling catfish, such as the surubim, which scour the mud for invertebrate prey.

Fish, especially piranha, are the mainstay of Pantanal caimans – the large crocodilians that spend much of their time around the swampy margins of the pools. Often seen wallowing and feeding alongside caimans are families of capybara. Resembling a giant guinea pig, this conspicuous rodent is the biggest in the world, with a maximum weight exceeding 130 pounds (60 kg).

The greatest spectacle of all is provided by the mingling flocks of water birds that crowd onto the dry season ponds to probe, sift and stab for prey. They include huge numbers

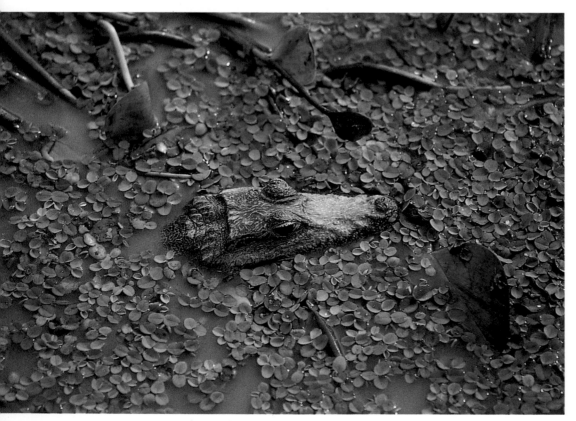

of egrets, herons, ibises and wood storks, as well as limpkins, which feed largely on snails, and lofty jabiru storks, symbol of the Pantanal.

On the flat ground surrounding the permanent waters, the soil becomes dry enough to support great fields of grass. These seasonal grasslands are the open savannas of the Pantanal, providing forage for fleet-footed pampas deer, marsh deer, peccaries (the New World equivalent of wild boars) and greater rheas (the "ostriches" of South America). Ants and termites make their nests on the grasslands, attracting giant anteaters and armadillos, and the numerous rodents and ground birds provide prey for maned wolves.

When danger threatens, many of the grassland creatures seek cover on the higher ground and ridges of the Pantanal. Generally free from annual flooding, these areas support thicker vegetation, with tall thickets in some places, groves of palms and even strips of dense forest, depending on the soil conditions. The trees and

palms form nesting and roosting sites for great numbers of Pantanal birds, among them egrets, cormorants, jabirus and hawks.

The rains come again in the wet season between November and April. The rivers draining into the Pantanal break their banks, and the grasslands soon become inundated, in places to a depth of more than 10 feet (3 m). Just

as the landscape of the Pantanal changes character during the flood season, so does its wildlife spectacle. Aquatic animals have the chance to spread. Now the dry land fauna must become more concentrated. Savanna and forest animals mingle on the scattered islands of high ground beyond the reach of the rising floodwaters in this watery wilderness.

A capybara with a large family to guard takes a wary look ahead for any dangers (right).

The biggest and most distinctive of the Pantanal's many water birds is the jabiru stork (below).

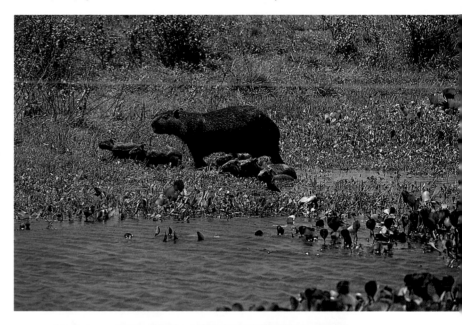

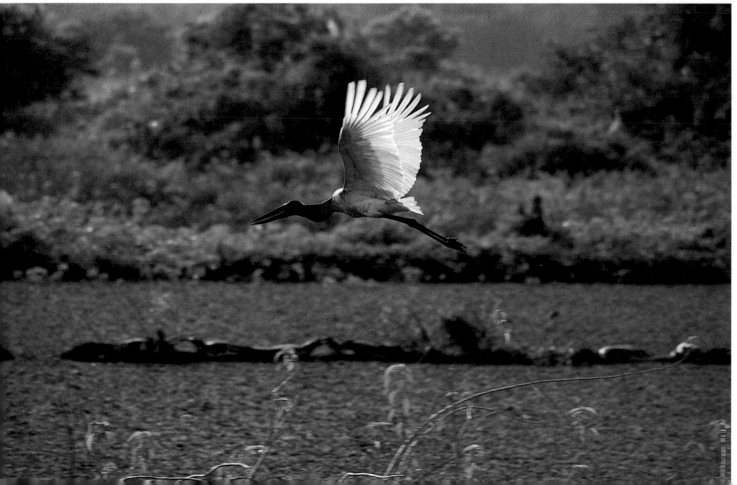

THE PATAGONIAN DESERT

"The last tapering segment of South America"

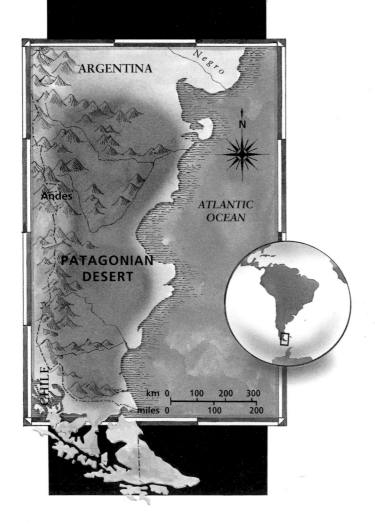

Across the level plains that fill Patagonia, rain seldom falls. The soil is dry and the landscape flat and treeless, often without feature until it blurs into the distance. Winds sweep across the arid ground, fanning choking clouds of dust and obscuring the horizon. Nights are cold and winter is harsh here, for Patagonia, the last tapering segment of South America, stretches farther toward Antarctica than any other continental land mass.

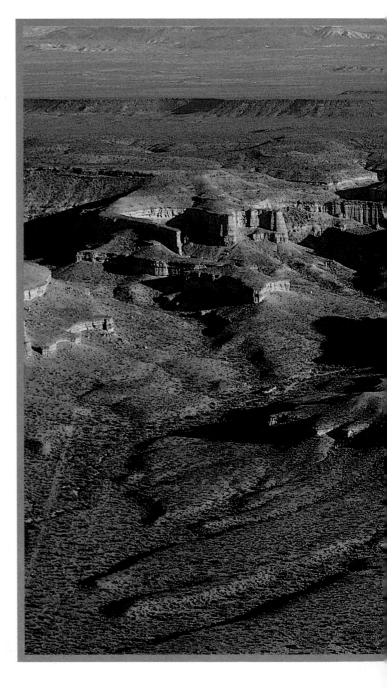

Such a bleak land offers so little comfort for people, that across its vast 260,000 sq. miles (675,000 km²), the Patagonian Desert has no major cities, just a few towns and roads, widely scattered settlements and thinly stocked sheep ranches. The rest is desolation.

Patagonia consists, in essence, of mountain and plain. The spine of the southern Andes runs along its western edge, dividing the narrow, mountainous strip of Chile from the much broader Argentinan Patagonia to the east. With the towering peaks as backdrop, the land rapidly levels out to the east into a complex of plains and valleys. The terrain descends until it reaches a continuous line of cliffs fronting the Atlantic. In the north, the land drops in a series of broad steps. Farther south, the pattern is less regular, with evidence of volcanic eruptions in dark sheets of basalt and hills of crystalline rock.

The past also reveals itself in the series of broad, deep valleys – many with steeply walled sides – that cut east through the Patagonian plains. The rivers that flow through them now are too small to have made such a dramatic mark on the landscape. The valleys were probably carved by

Vast empty landscapes of browns and grays, their harshness accentuated by stark hills, characterize the Patagonian plains. Though increasing numbers of people have settled in Patagonia over the last 150 years, immense stretches remain lonely and untamed.

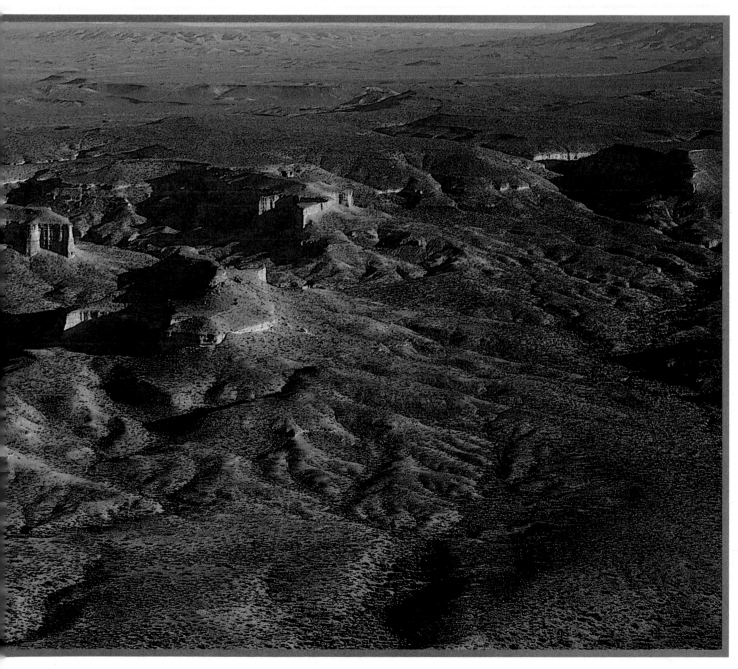

meltwaters pouring from the Andes during times when ice blanketed the heights much more extensively than it does today.

Giant glaciers ground down the flanks of the mountains then and gouged out basins at their feet. Today several of these basins are filled with large lakes. These lakes and the evergreen forests of southern beech that line the foot of the Andes are a haven for wildlife. Elegant waterfowl nest on the water's edge, and deer run in the woods in a scene of natural splendor very different from that of the desert close by. The rocky Atlantic coastline, with its rich waters

Ancient trees transformed into stone form these logs of petrified wood. Trees cannot grow on the arid plains today, but these dramatic fossils show that, long ago, the climate must have been much more humid.

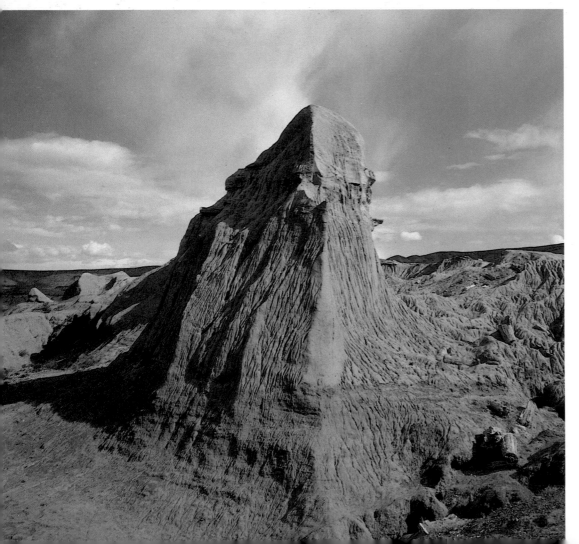

and swirling flocks of seabirds, that rims the desert over to the east, provides a similar contrast with the arid somberness of the plains.

The Patagonian Desert exists because the Andes rob it of water. The westerly winds that prevail over Patagonia bring thick cloud to the slopes of the mountains. As the air mass rises toward the cold summits, most of the moisture condenses out and falls in a concentrated belt of heavy rain or snow. The last reserves are spent on the eastern slopes, watering the beech forests at their base, but leaving the air that crosses the plains dry and virtually cloudless.

Most of the Patagonian Desert receives less than 8 inches (200 mm) of rain per year. The combination of dry air and warm sunshine over the plains also means that evaporation is high, intensifying the drought. The rivers fed by rain and melting ice in the Andes steadily diminish in volume as

they cross eastern Patagonia through their oversized valleys. Many of them flow intermittently, leaving their watercourses empty for long periods with just a few saline pools to show that water runs from time to time.

Not surprisingly, the vegetation cover of the plains is poor, becoming worse with increasing aridity from north to south. In the region close to the Rio Negro (the river generally regarded as the northern limit of Patagonia), the landscape is one of open bushland. Thorny thickets up to 7 feet (2 m) tall stand widely spaced over bare soil. In sandy areas, grasses predominate. Farther south, where the plants have to survive with a minimal water supply, the bushes become ever lower and more scattered. In many places, the ground is covered only with rounded gravel.

Toward the Andes, the desert proper changes to a zone of semi-arid steppe, where bunch grasses take over. But whether scrub or grass predominates, the scene across plain and plateau is one of evenly spaced, knee-high uniformity.

In such a desert, it is all the more startling to find rebellious signs of animal life – the tracks of a snake, the dismembered remains of a scorpion, the prints of egrets around a drying pool. Like all deserts, the arid plains of Patagonia have their fauna, hardy creatures that have adapted to tolerate the dramatic swings between warm and cold, and can get by with low moisture intake.

One of the greatest problems for a desert animal, especially on the open plains of Patagonia, is the lack of cover in which to take refuge and hide. Successful adaptation to desert conditions reflects this problem. The guanaco and the lesser rhea, a large flightless bird, have evolved the escape strategy of speed. Both can run fast when danger threatens; indeed, the guanaco can outrun a horse. Similarly, the mara, a rodent

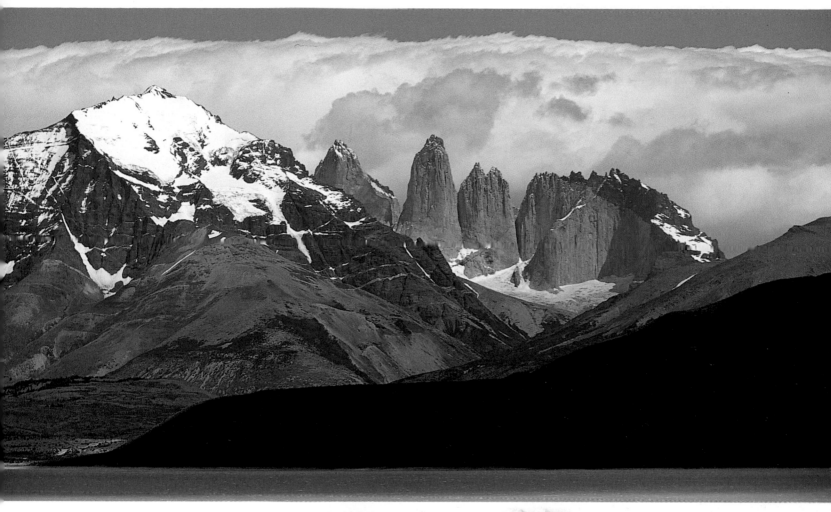

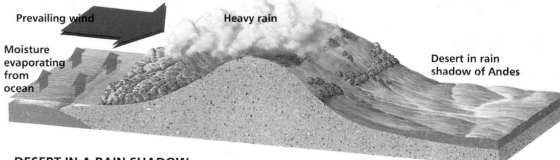

The towering pinnacles of the Paine Towers, part of the Patagonian Andes, are visible from far across the plains.

of the plains, has the long legs and body shape of a hare to help it race away from predators. The mara takes refuge at night in burrows dug in the earth. Several other animals depend more or less exclusively on the burrowing strategy to escape from danger, and have strong limbs and claws for digging. They include the pygmy armadillo, a type of rock rat and several species of tuco-tuco – compact, short-legged rodents that dare to make only brief foraging excursions above ground.

Predators of the desert, in turn, do their best to counter the defense strategies of their prey. The slender

DESERT IN A RAIN SHADOW

The Patagonian Desert lies in the rain shadow of the Andes. Air currents coming from the west are forced to shed almost all their moisture as they cross the mountains, leaving precious little for the plains to the east.

Patagonian weasel can pursue rodents into burrows, while foxes and the puma use a combination of stealth, ambush and speed to catch their quarry. The puma is fast and strong enough to hunt guanaco, as long as it can steal within range first, crouching as best it can behind low vegetation.

The most conspicuous hunters of the plains are the birds of prey, scourge of the tuco-tucos. Hawks and eagles employ the advantage of flight and acute eyesight to the fullest. Soaring high in the sunshine, they can scrutinize broad areas with little effort, the desert with its living secrets spread wide open beneath them.

THE TIBESTI MOUNTAINS

"Surrounded by blistering desert on all sides, this rugged terrain remains remote and wild"

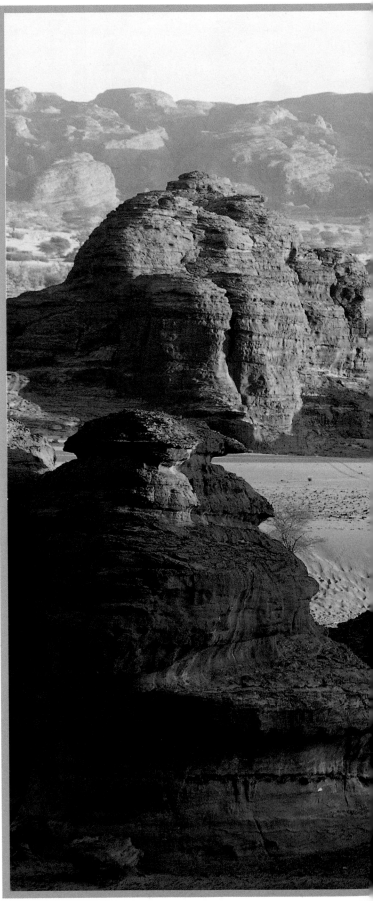

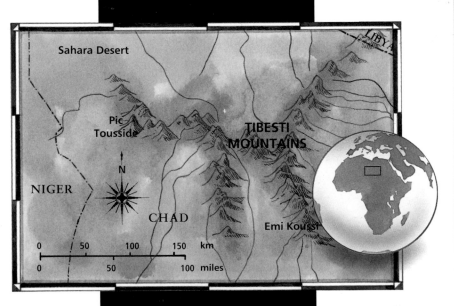

Sahara Desert

LIBYA

Pic Tousside

TIBESTI MOUNTAINS

NIGER

N

CHAD

Emi Koussi

| 0 | 50 | 100 | 150 | km |
| 0 | | 50 | | 100 miles |

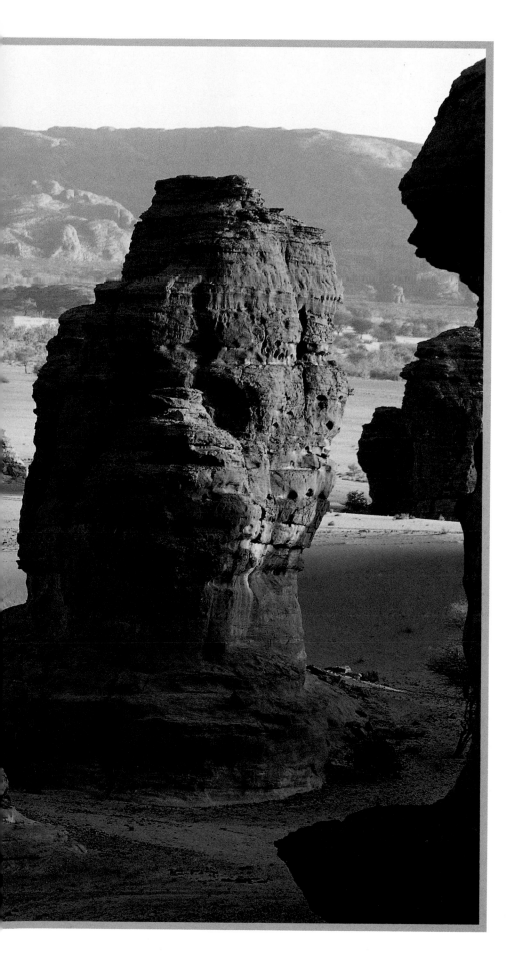

At the heart of the Sahara Desert lie the spectacular mountains of Tibesti. Visible from far away across the desert wastes, this isolated highland massif soars from rocky and sandy plains to heights of more than 10,000 feet (3,000 m) in a series of volcanic peaks topped with craters.

The Tibesti range covers an area greater than Switzerland, and its mountainous landscapes, though dominated by bare rock and desert dryness, are no less dramatic. From the summit of Emi Koussi, the tallest of the volcanoes, jagged crests and steep cliffs tinted with pink and violet stretch away to the north and west. Between them are broad platforms of land, some studded with curious rock towers and deep, dark ravines.

Surrounded by several hundred miles of blistering desert on all sides, this rugged terrain remains remote and wild. Once a hideout for raiders of camel trains, it has also long been a refuge and fortress for desert tribes fiercely resistant to outside control.

Though the Tibesti Massif lies within the hot desert, the mountains create their own modified climate. Temperatures are cooler at altitude compared with the desert plains, rarely rising to more than 68°F (20°C) by day, and dropping below freezing at night. Rainfall, though still sparse, is slightly higher than in the surrounding desert. Pockets of water collect in depressions, in the floors of craters and in the bottom of mountain valleys. Occasionally, heavy clouds build up over the peaks, sending stormwater through otherwise dry

A forbidding wilderness, the Tibesti Massif is a vast sandstone plateau, studded with the towering remains of giant volcanoes. The summits of the peaks are high enough for frost to form in hollows in the rocks at night.

> *"Tibesti was born of earth movements that uplifted ancient sandstone strata to form a plateau"*

valleys or "wadis." At these times, rock and mud debris is flushed into the valleys, and rainwater streaming from the massif can penetrate as far as 100 miles (160 km) into the surrounding plains of sand and stone.

The mountains, with their slightly more ample supply of water, are able to harbor more vegetation than the desert beyond. In addition to more than 300 species of small, drought-resistant herbs, grasses and bushes, the Tibesti has pockets of acacias and palms growing in its dampest sites. Surprisingly dense groves develop along some permanent streams.

Moisture and plant life support a simple community of animals. Seeds

BIRDS OF THE DESERT

Few birds are so at home in deserts as the family of plump, dovelike fowl known as sandgrouse. All the 16 species live in arid and semi-arid environments in Africa, Arabia and Asia. Two of these haunt Tibesti – the crowned sandgrouse and Lichtenstein's sandgrouse. Capable of fast, direct flight, they can travel large distances across the desert to visit waterholes and areas where seeds – their principal food – are plentiful.

The male sandgrouse has a remarkable adaptation to desert life. He has specialized belly feathers that can soak up water from pools rather like a sponge. This means he can bring water from distant waterholes back to the nest so that thirsty chicks can sip the precious moisture.

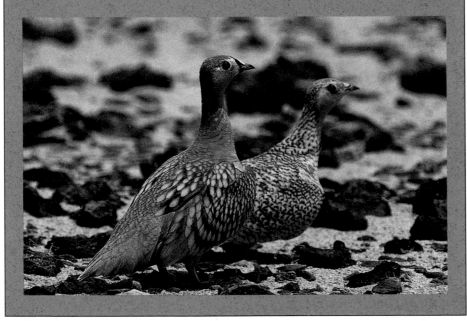

and other plant matter nourish desert rodents, including gerbils, spiny mice and gundis. Snakes and lizards are quite numerous, among them an insect-eating gecko that lives high in the mountains. Rock pools are visited for drinking and bathing by larks, sandgrouse and trumpeter finches. Doves, bulbuls and sunbirds live in the better vegetated areas, while white-crowned black wheatears snatch insects on the rocky slopes.

Among the most common larger predators are Rüppell's foxes, fan-tailed ravens, lanner falcons and tawny eagles. Barbary sheep, the hardy wild denizens of north Africa's mountains, are still fairly abundant in Tibesti, where they browse avidly on acacia leaves, flowers and even bark.

Nevertheless, Tibesti today is a predominantly dry, barren massif. Most of its surface is bare rock or rock fragments. But the area has not always been so arid. Global climatic cycles once brought more humid conditions to Tibesti. Higher rainfall in the past meant that Mediterranean oaks and pines grew on the mountains; the moisture nourished powerful rivers that carved much of the present terrain and dumped the eroded material across the surrounding lowlands.

Some of the rivers were big enough to reach the Nile and the Niger; others flowed into distant interior basins of the Sahara, where the water dispersed and evaporated. Numerous prehistoric rock paintings in the area show that antelopes and other animals more typical of the African savannas used to dwell around Tibesti, and the remains of crocodiles have been discovered in sediments at the foot of the mountains.

Evidence of a violent era much farther back in time exists in spectacular fashion in the relics of volcanoes high in the Tibesti Massif. Tibesti was born of earth movements that uplifted ancient sandstone strata

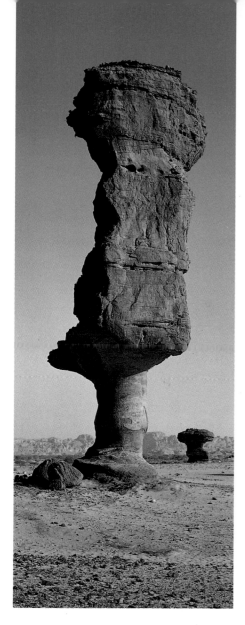

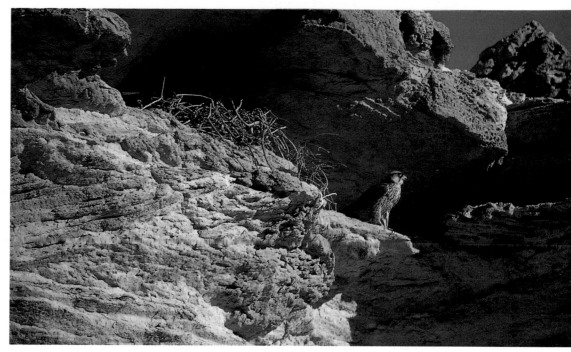

Grains of sand driven by strong winds abrade and undercut exposed rocks in parts of Tibesti, creating some spectacular and bizarre landforms. Water from occasional rainfall also plays its part in the shaping of the landscape, though less so now than in humid eras of the past.

The lanner falcon finds secure, sheltered nest sites on the rock faces of Tibesti. This powerful predator is the scourge of smaller birds, which it generally snatches on the wing. It also preys on small mammals, such as gerbils and spiny mice, and catches large insects including locusts.

to form a plateau. Probably at the same time, molten rock, or magma, from below the Earth's crust pushed its way upward through weaknesses in the plateau. Over millions of years, these volcanic outpourings built sheets and cones of basalt, tuff and lava on top of the sandstone. Today, most of the higher parts of Tibesti are built of volcanic rock.

At 11,204 feet (3,415 m), Emi Koussi is the highest peak – and one of the most dramatic. Its sides slope up evenly all around, then drop away suddenly into a vast, cliff-ringed crater roughly 12 miles (20 km) across and 3,000 feet (900 m) deep. The crater evokes a lunar landscape, but it was created not by a falling meteorite, but by eruptions from within.

About five million years ago, an enormous volcano began to develop.

Lava from a great subterranean chamber of magma poured from its vent and cooled on its flanks, building up a massive cone far higher than it is at present. Eventually, however, the emptying magma chamber could not support the weight of the cone above. The top of the cone began to collapse, probably in gradual stages, leaving the unmistakable imprint of volcanic self-destruction – a giant circular depression known as a "caldera."

Trou au Natron is a similarly spectacular caldera, just as deep and about 5 miles (8 km) in diameter. But its genesis appears to have been rather different. The volcano from which it originated did not build a tall cone, and its eruptions appear to have been more explosive. Indeed, it is believed that the caldera was

blasted into existence by a series of titanic explosions that blew rock away and caused the remainder to collapse. Chunks of debris weighing many tons have been found 6 miles (10 km) from the caldera.

Volcanic activity on such a scale has long ceased, but Tibesti is by no means completely quiet today. Gases and hot water still stream and bubble out of vents in Trou au Natron, evidence that magma remains not too far below. The mineral-rich springs have left blinding white deposits of carbonate salts across the crater floor. Elsewhere in the Tibesti heights, there are several other places where hot springs emerge, along with fumaroles, geysers and sputtering mud pools. All contribute to the savage beauty of this extraordinary mountainous island in the midst of the desert.

THE BALE MOUNTAINS

"The single largest area of high ground in all of Africa"

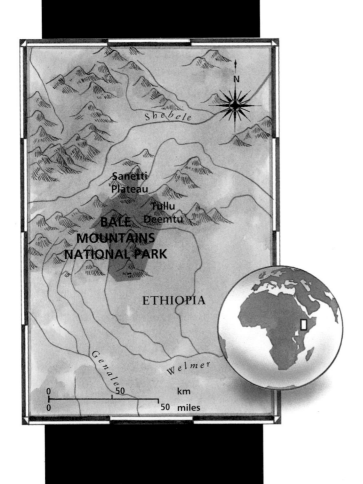

Ethiopia is a mountainous land. In a continent that is dominated by hills, valleys and plains, Ethiopia's rugged core stands in striking contrast. One of its loftiest and least explored sections lies toward the southeast: the frosty heights of the Bale Mountains.

These mountains form part of an upland mass cut off from the rest of

Red-hot poker plants make the most of the strong sunshine at high altitude on a grassy stretch of the Bale Mountains.

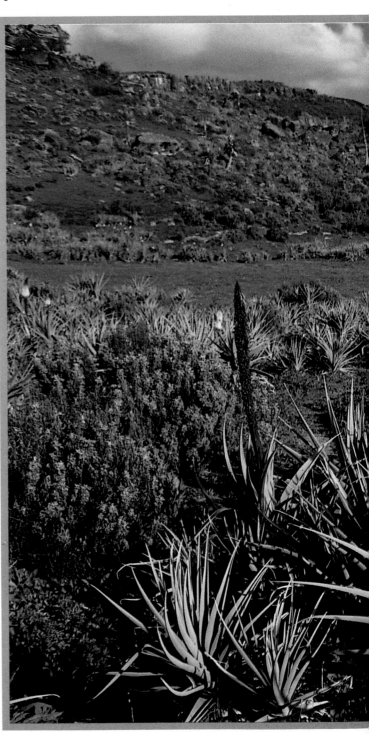

the Ethiopian Highlands by the
northern trench of east Africa's Great
Rift Valley. The mass is further cut
in two by a river valley, the upper
course of the Wabe Shebele. The
Bale massif lies south of this divide,
forming the single largest area of high
ground in all of Africa, with at least
400 sq. miles (1,000 km²) topping an
altitude of 11,000 feet (3,300 m).

From the open mountaintop, the
land falls away on all sides in steep
escarpments and narrow valleys,
cloaked in greenery. The vegetation is
fed by heavy rains deposited on high
by winds direct from the Indian
Ocean – from March to October, it
rains or hails on the summits almost
every day. The great Harenna Forest
spanning the southern flank is one of

the biggest stretches of mountain
forest left in Africa. It continues
downslope until it blends with acacia
woodland and savanna on the lower,
drier contours.

Tectonic wrenching of the Earth's
crust and upwelling magma from far
below combined to push Bale and the
rest of the Ethiopian Highlands up
out of the African plains long ago.

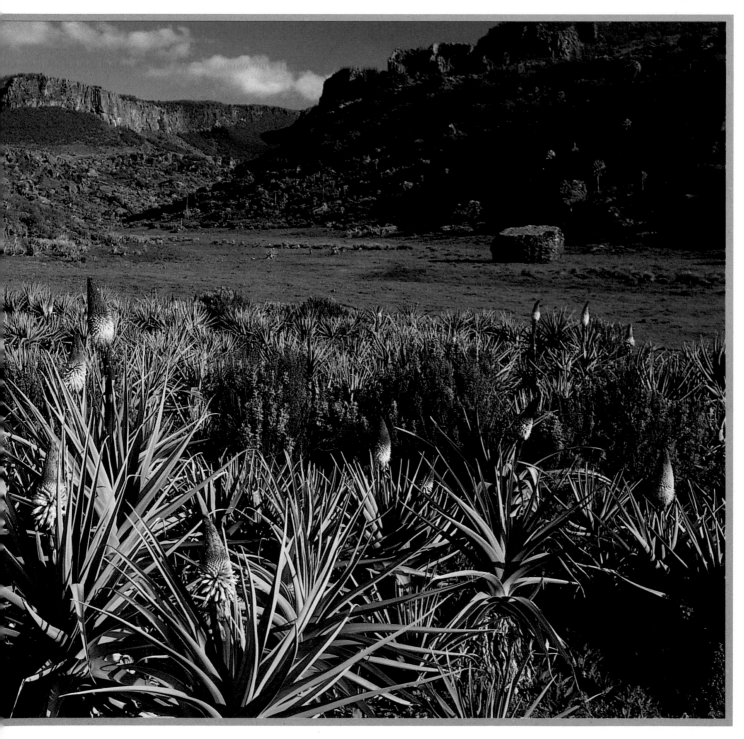

The huge bulge of rock so created was deeply cracked and fissured by the stresses. Other forces widened these fault lines, breaking up the dome and encouraging deep valleys to form between the mountain blocks. Immense splitting on a continental scale then rent the Great Rift Valley into existence, severing the highland dome completely.

As world climate repeatedly cooled during ice ages, ice caps formed on the Bale Mountains and brought tundra conditions to the slopes. Today, though the ice-age chill has long receded, nightly frosts on the tops split shards from exposed rock and create upheavals in the soil. Forests can grow on the slopes, but the heights remain too cold.

Partly because of its broad expanse of cold land, offering few sheltered valleys, the Bale massif has remained relatively free from human influence. While the rest of the Ethiopian Highlands has been severely degraded by the pressures of farming and settlement, the natural landscape of the Bale Mountains

remains more or less intact. In an effort to keep it so, a large section of the massif has recently been set aside as a national park.

From south to north, the park traverses the full range of habitats on the mountain slopes. Thick tropical forest of yellowwood, stinkwood, African olive and other trees on the lower slopes blends through clouds and mist to a belt dominated by reddish-flowered hagenia trees. Higher still, the landscape takes on a strangeness unique to high east African mountains. St. John's wort and heather predominate, but they are not the modest plants familiar in northern Europe. The varieties here grow to the size of trees and are draped in moss and lichens in the foggy, damp conditions.

A pattern of shrubby trees and glades gradually turns to open terrain across the highest ground. In places, especially toward the north of the park, fairly dense grass grows, dotted with colorful red-hot poker plants. But the high core of the massif, the Sanetti Plateau, is a bleak, windswept

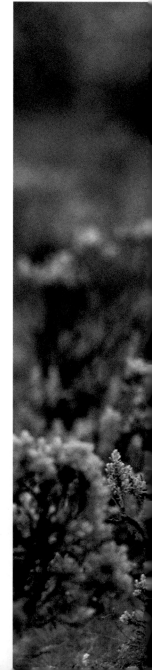

Simien jackals live in close-knit packs on the Sanetti Plateau. The pack works together to provide pups with food and protect them from danger, such as marauding birds of prey. Here a young jackal howls an alarm call to alert fellow pack members (right).

Giant lobelias thrive on the bleak Sanetti Plateau – the coldest, highest section of the Bale Mountains (left). At night, each cluster of spiked leaves closes up to protect the developing shoot of emerging flower heads from freezing conditions.

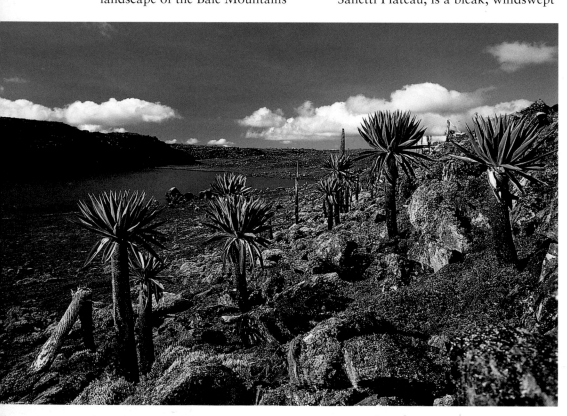

zone, reminiscent of moorland. More than 11,500 feet (3,500 m) high, the plateau is a gray-brown mixture of tussock grass and aromatic herbs such as lady's mantle and sage.

Most plants are ground-hugging to cope with the cold and the wind, but the mountains have another curiously oversized plant. Here and there, giant lobelias erupt from the diminutive ground vegetation of the plateau, with their thick stalks, spiked clusters of leaves and towering flower stems reaching up 16 feet (5 m).

On the flatter portions of the plateau, bogs develop, with small pools and lakes that are attractive to wildfowl. Some of them are birds familiar in other parts of Africa, like Egyptian geese, yellow-billed ducks and wattled cranes. Others, including white and black storks, drop into the high-altitude lakes for a rest during migration. But there are also birds that occur only in the heights of Ethiopia. The blue-winged goose spends all year on the pools and moors, its loose, thick plumage providing insulation from the cold.

The plateau and the grasslands are home to other animals unique to Ethiopia. Stately mountain nyalas, a type of antelope, have their stronghold in the north of the park, where herds a hundred strong sometimes congregate. They feed on the grasses and herbs by day, but retreat among the St. John's wort groves at night, where temperatures are milder. Simien jackals stalk the Sanetti Plateau, where they feed largely on rodents.

Bale also has its own species of hare, Stark's hare, and harbors a unique bird, the Rouget's rail. Indeed in the Ethiopian Highlands, and Bale in particular, a high proportion of animal species are endemic – they occur only here – a measure of the extreme isolation and unusual nature of these rugged mountains.

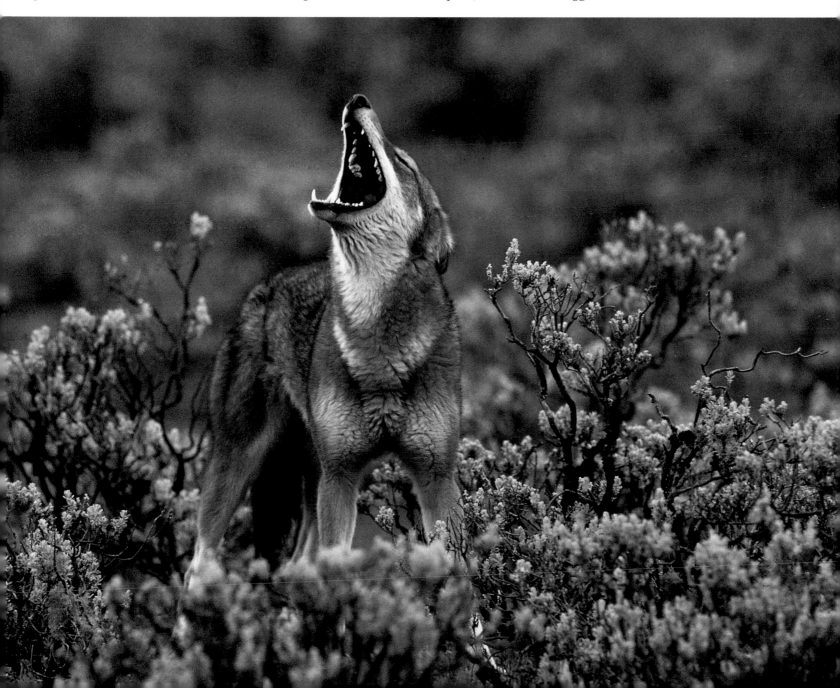

THE SERENGETI

"Immense flat plains of grass where large grazing animals exist in unparalleled numbers"

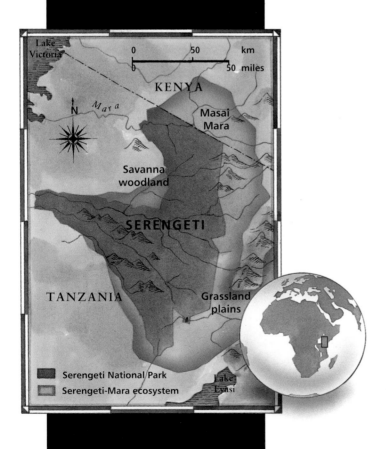

Serengeti National Park
Serengeti-Mara ecosystem

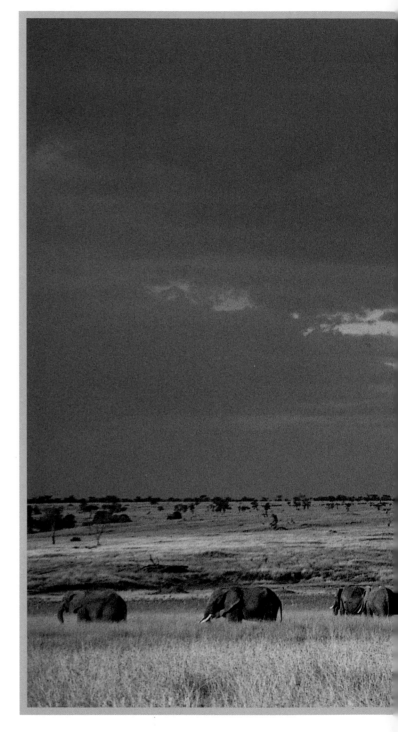

There is nowhere on Earth quite like the Serengeti. On this, the most famous of the east African plains, the herds of wild mammals easily outnumber those of any other place. The grazing animals can amass in such concentrations that they hide the ocean of grass beneath them. Yet, at other times, the same expanse of grass

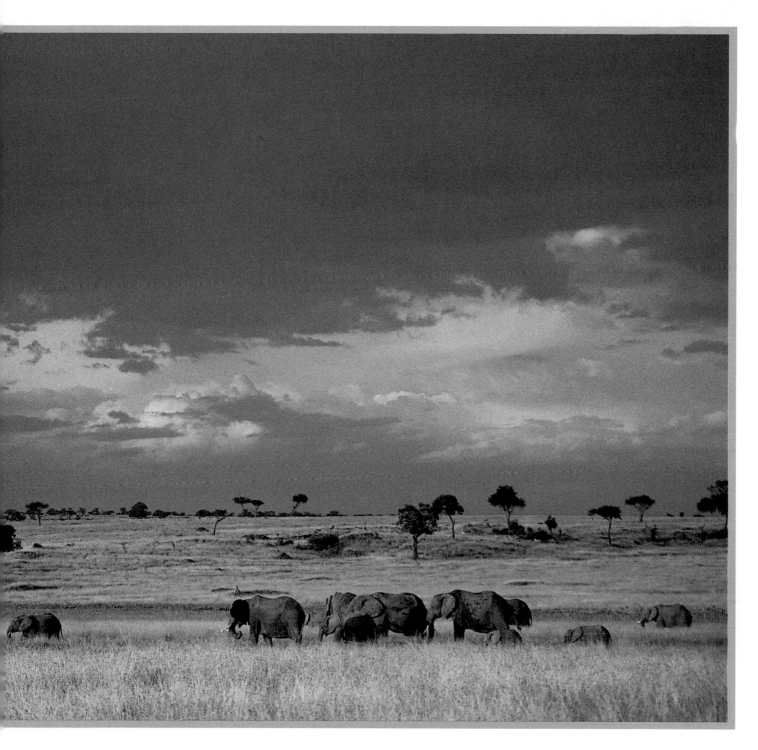

stretches seemingly empty as far as the horizon, abandoned by the herds whose instincts command them to wander with the seasons.

The Serengeti is a complex of savanna habitats, spread over a broad surface of volcanic soil, 5,000 feet (1,500 m) above sea level. The Serengeti National Park protects 5,700 sq. miles (14,750 km²) at its heart, but the full extent of the Serengeti takes in nearly twice this area. From Lake Eyasi in the south, flanked by highlands to the east and stretching toward Lake Victoria in the west, it reaches north to incorporate the Masai Mara Game Reserve across the Kenyan border. Immense flat plains of short grass in the southeast blend into areas of longer grass and

The Serengeti is one of the greatest remaining treasures of wilderness in Africa. Here, large grazing animals, such as the elephant for which the African plains are so well known, exist in unparalleled numbers. Unhindered by fences and farms, they can wander across the vast open grasslands and woodland savanna.

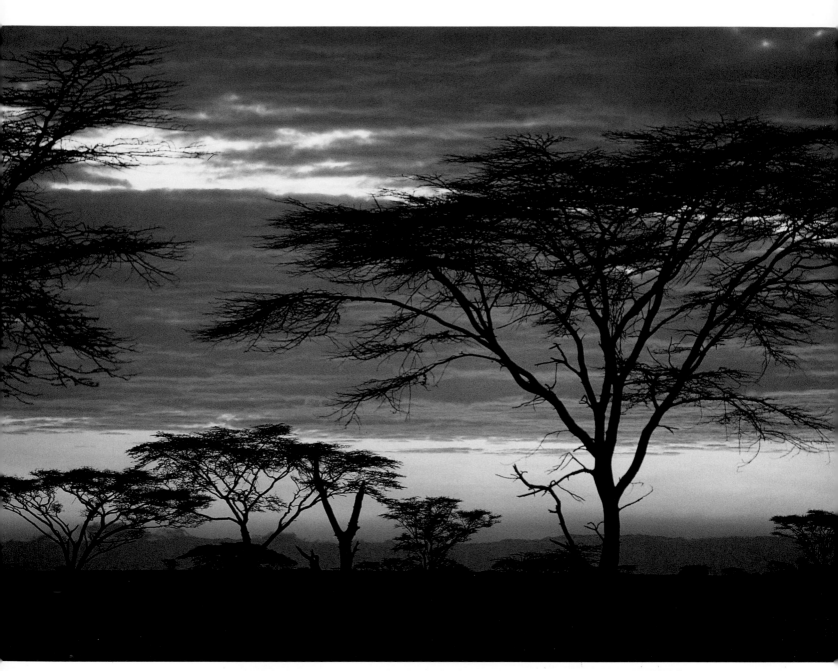

Rest takes up much of a lion's day, especially at times when prey is abundant and life is easy. Females do most of the hunting. Crouched low in the grass, they stealthily approach prey before springing to attack.

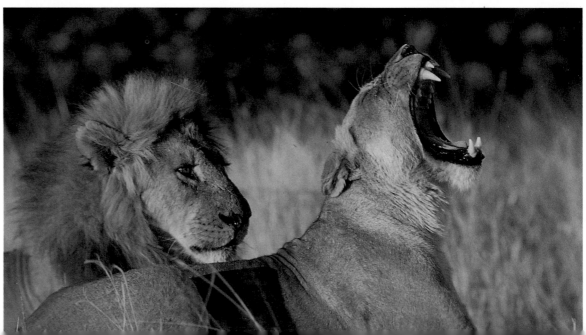

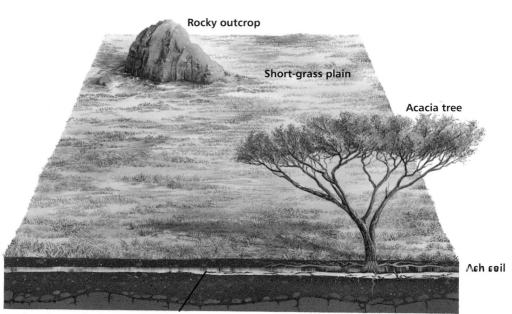

Rocky outcrop

Short-grass plain

Acacia tree

Ash soil

Hardpan layer of calcium carbonate

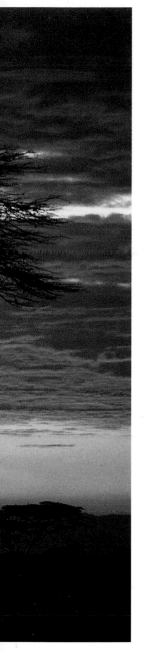

A LAND OF GRASS

Volcanic soils full of compacted ash underlie the vast expanses of grassland in the southeastern Serengeti. Grasses, with their fine, shallow roots, take hold readily in this soil, but bigger tree roots find it difficult to penetrate. They are further impeded by a rock-hard layer of carbonate deposits.

***The acacia is** one of the few trees whose roots do manage to break through the hard layers and establish themselves. Such trees stand out like sentinels on the grassy plain (left).*

then to the north and west turn into a broad swath of woodland savanna, where thorny acacias compete for space with the surrounding grass stems. Sometimes grasses take over, leaving acacias scattered in their midst; elsewhere the thorn trees crowd into tall thickets, with the shorter plants clumped patchily underneath.

Though the acacia woodlands bring variety to the landscape, greatly increasing its wildlife diversity, grassland remains the key to the Serengeti. Grass, and the small herbs

that grow among it, is the mainstay of the vast herds. It is food for some 1.5 million wildebeest and another million zebras, gazelles and buffaloes, and myriad other creatures, from termites to ostriches. The abundance of grass in the Serengeti, particularly in the almost pure-grass plains of the southeast, seems to be a product of the soil rather than the climate.

The plains themselves were built largely of wind-blown ash carried by prevailing winds from volcanic highlands to the east. Some of that ash formed hard concretions, with the grains bound so tightly together that tree roots now have difficulty finding a route through the soil.

The surface of the ash soil is highly porous to water. Rain passing quickly through the surface layer has tended to leach the calcium-rich deposits, dissolving out the mineral content and then depositing it again as a hard barrier of calcium carbonate 3 feet (1 m) or so below ground. Trees also have difficulty establishing themselves in these conditions because their roots are impeded, so space is left free for the short, flexible roots of grasses. The parts of the Serengeti closest to the parent volcanoes are those where the barriers to tree growth are at their most accentuated, and

grasses face the least competition for space.

Grass is wonderfully resilient, tolerant of fire damage, trampling and grazing. So long as grazing pressure is not too heavy, it can grow afresh time and again after its leaves and stems have been clipped away. This is because the plant's growing points are at the base and its oldest parts at the top, pushed ever upward by new growth below.

But even grass has its limits. Overtaxed pasture soon loses its productivity, especially if dry seasons rob the soil of precious moisture. Changing weather conditions in the Serengeti force the largest of the grazing herds to undertake epic migrations in search of fresh pasture. Their dramatic movements affect many of the other animals that share the Serengeti with them.

Wildebeest are the greatest of the mass migrants. In April, legions of them fill the southern short-grass plains. Many of the females have given birth only two or three months before and are busy nursing their calves. Yet within a month all will feel the stirrings of ancient wanderlust. The rains start to dwindle in the south, and the grassland begins to lose its verdant tint. Soon it will be dry and exhausted. Gradually, the animals become restless and start to move. Small herds walking in line join with others heading northwest, and as paths converge, the bigger herds coalesce.

Before long the wildebeest have amassed to form giant dark columns, streaming with singular purpose across the open plain into the longer grass zones and beyond. From the vantage point of a smooth rock outcrop – these large boulders rising like islands from the grass are a feature of the plains – half a million animals may be in view stretching for several miles to the horizon. As the wildebeest stream around the outcrop, noise fills the air and veils of dust settle around the small animals – perhaps agama lizards and hyraxes – that dwell on the rock.

Among the wildebeest and their calves, others join the procession toward better pasture. The stripes of zebras and the tawny coats of gazelles are readily visible. Though they are all grazers, there is little competition for food between the different animals. When the migrating herds pause to rest and feed, different feeding preferences are revealed. The zebras can cope with the fairly coarse tops of long grass; their chewing exposes more tender parts below. Wildebeest clip the sward further, leaving the lowest, newest growth for Thompson's and Grant's gazelles.

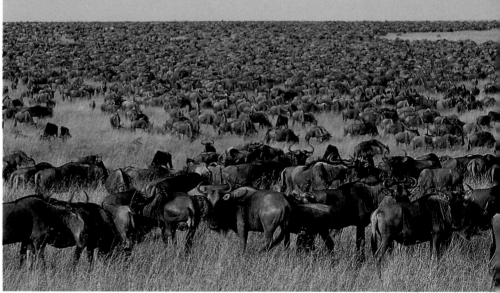

Plains zebras stoop to graze on long grass in the Serengeti (below). Their stomachs are adapted for digesting the tops of long grass – the oldest, toughest parts of the plant.

Wildebeest face many dangers on their annual migration. Perils such as predators, drowning and injury during stampedes claim an estimated 40,000 victims each year.

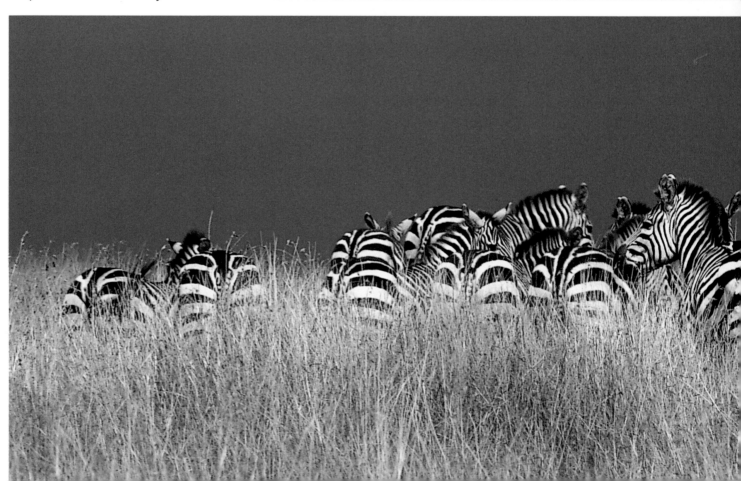

The plains through which the migrants pass are the permanent homes of other animals. Some are also grazers, but do not take part in the great migrations. Buffalo, hartebeest and topi tend to stay put and nibble what they can during the dry season. For some other animals, finding sustenance is hard work for most of the year, but the weeks when the herds are in the locality are a time of bonanza. Packs of hyenas living in the center of the Serengeti may be drawn 30 miles (50 km) or more from their denning area to take advantage of the glut of fresh meat.

The young herbivores, struggling to keep up with the herd and easily separated when the adults are frightened into stampeding, are among the most vulnerable prey. But adult animals are also picked off: sprightly gazelles often fall prey to cheetahs, wildebeest to hunting dogs and zebras to lions. If the supplies of food for such predators were constantly abundant, there might be many more of them. But lean times during the rest of the year, when they

"Dark columns of half a million migrating wildebeest stream with singular purpose across the open plain"

are left to hunt scattered prey – often consisting of smaller mammals and birds – serve to limit their numbers.

The wildebeest continue marching until they are well into the woodland savanna, some moving west almost to the flood plain of Lake Victoria. Here they may linger for several weeks in the company of impalas, elands and giraffes before continuing into the northern Serengeti where the dry season is relatively mild and good

pasture remains abundant. Their journeys force them to cross rivers, where the healthy size of the resident crocodiles shows the benefit gained from several weeks of easy hunting.

For many thousands of wildebeest, the long journey north does not finish till they reach the Masai Mara reserve. To do so, they have to swim across the Mara River. There are only a few suitable crossing points on the river, and great herds mass at these bottlenecks, nervously waiting for the first bold individuals to plunge into the water. The rest follow in a chaotic scramble. Having swum the breadth of the river, they clamber frantically up the opposite bank which is usually steep and muddy. On every crossing, the water becomes strewn with animals that have drowned or been trampled in the panic.

Wildebeest linger on the rich Masai Mara grasslands until October when the wet season returns. Then the wanderlust revives. As migratory birds escaping from the approaching winter in Europe and northern Asia arrive in the Serengeti, so the vast herds start to trek south again. By December those that have survived the hazards of the march are back in the southern plains, feeding on the fresh grass revived by the rains.

Conservation of the natural riches of the Serengeti has not been without problems. Some damage to the park and reserves has resulted from settlement nearby, and poaching has put severe pressure on some wildlife, such as the critically endangered black rhinoceros. But, at least for the time being, the Serengeti has few problems of competition for pasture between wild animals and livestock. No fences have been erected across the region to halt the mass seasonal movement of the animals. Once much more widespread in Africa, such wildlife spectacles have all but faded into distant memory. In the Serengeti, they live on.

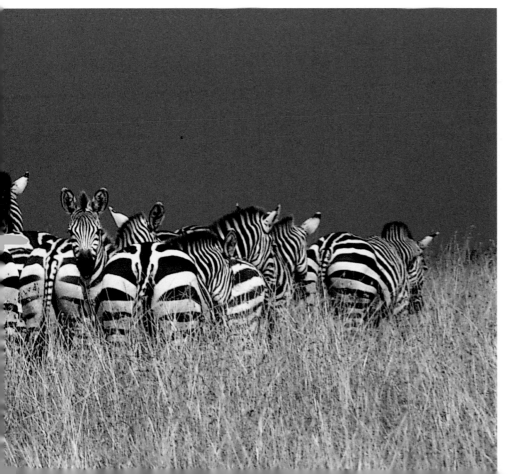

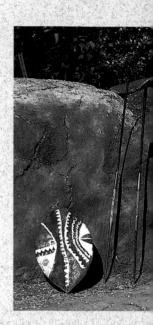

A Masai warrior displays his weapons outside a typical dwelling (right). All men become warriors after initiation into manhood. Once feared for their combat skills and cattle-raiding forays, the warriors' chief role now is to manage herds and ward off predators.

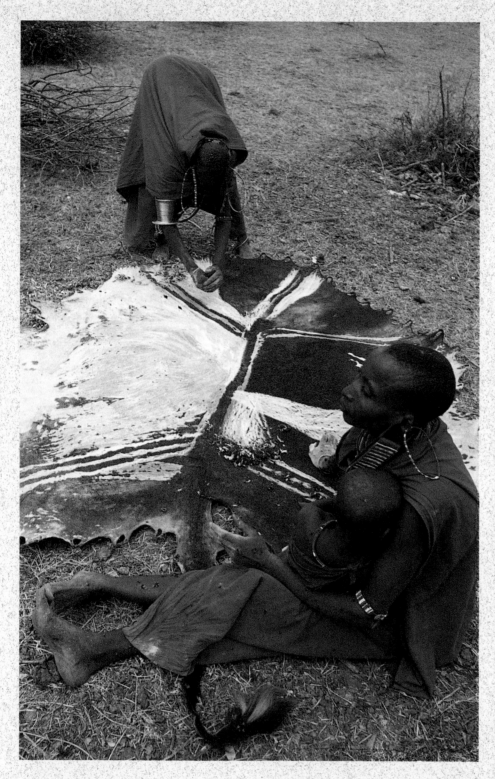

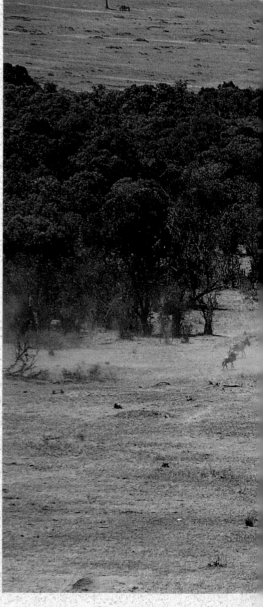

A Masai woman decorates an ox hide. Cattle are central to the subsistence, material life and customs of the Masai. Their blood, milk and meat provide food; their skins, horns and bones are used in many objects – decorative and practical; and their hides are also used to protect the mud huts in heavy rain.

The livestock herds of the Masai share the grassland plains with wildlife (right). Though overgrazing does occur more often today, the traditional way of life of the Masai is well suited to the fragile savanna. When a pasture becomes thin, each village takes its cattle and belongings to a new site.

THE MASAI

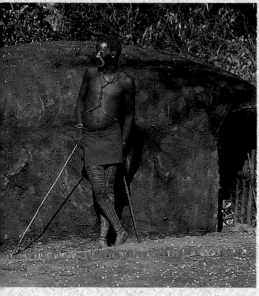

Grassy plains in Kenya and Tanzania are the homeland of the Masai. These people are renowned throughout Africa for their dignity and valor, for their adherence to tradition in lifestyle and values, and for their ornate crafts.

The Masai live by raising cattle, goats and sheep on the immense pastures that surround their settlements. Life revolves around the livestock and their need for food, water and protection from wild predators. The Masai move their villages with the seasons to make sure the herds have enough fresh grass.

The simple dwellings of the Masai are neatly in tune with the environment. Built from a framework of sticks packed with leaves and plastered with mud and dung, they are quick to make and proof against strong winds in the open terrain. The dung in the plaster is also an effective deterrent against termite attack.

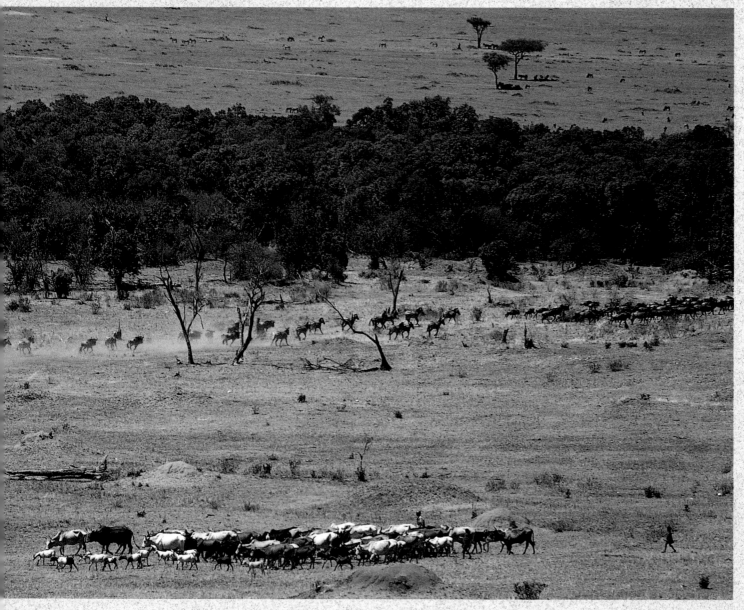

TAI NATIONAL PARK

"The remote forest interior offers a lifeline to the threatened wildlife of west Africa"

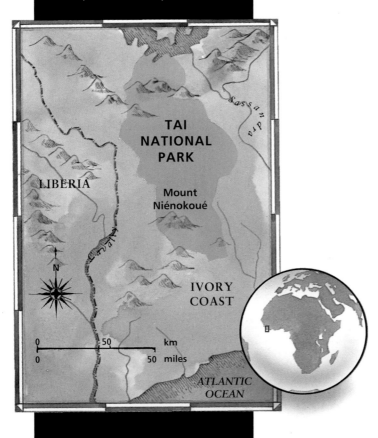

LIBERIA

TAI NATIONAL PARK

Mount Niénokoué

Sassandra

Cavally

N

IVORY COAST

ATLANTIC OCEAN

0   50   km
0   50   miles

West Africa's largest remaining stretch of virgin rainforest is contained in the Tai National Park. Beneath its sunlit canopy, in the eternal shade of the open floor, the forest feels hauntingly tranquil and all-enveloping. In every direction, trunks rise from the gloom far into the mass of greenery above. Vines and creepers hang from them

A curtain of greenery encloses the rivers and pools of the Tai rainforest. It droops right down to the water where creatures such as pygmy hippos wallow (right).

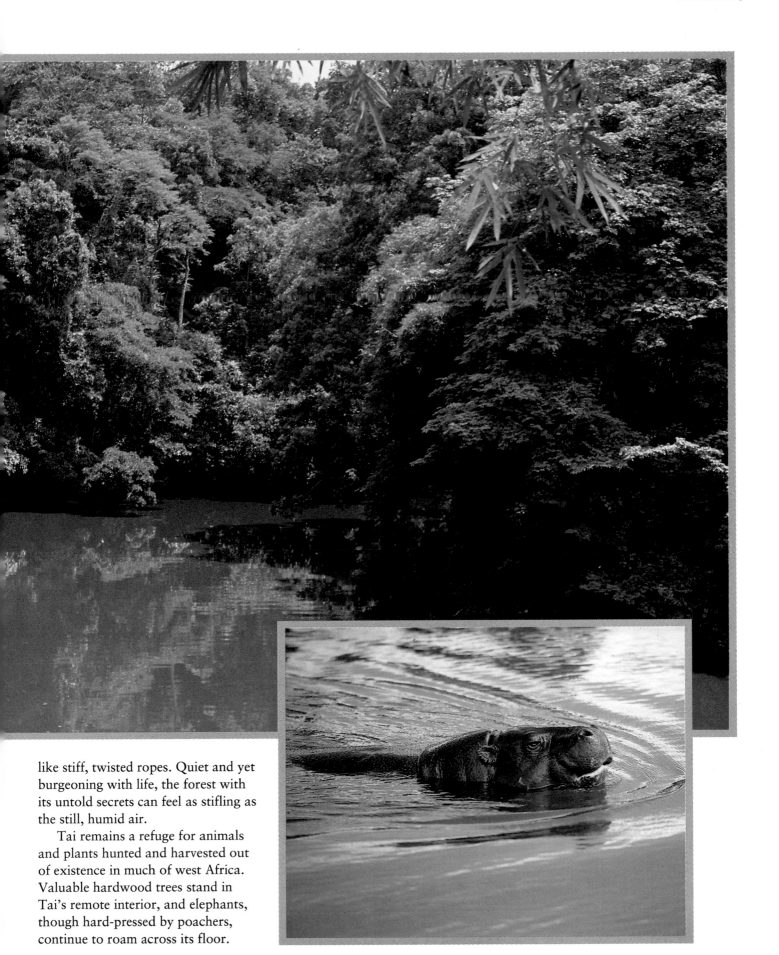

like stiff, twisted ropes. Quiet and yet burgeoning with life, the forest with its untold secrets can feel as stifling as the still, humid air.

Tai remains a refuge for animals and plants hunted and harvested out of existence in much of west Africa. Valuable hardwood trees stand in Tai's remote interior, and elephants, though hard-pressed by poachers, continue to roam across its floor.

Extending over some 1,350 sq. miles (3,500 km²), Tai National Park lies in the southwest of Ivory Coast, between the Sassandra River and the Liberian border. Its forest covers a lowland area of gently sloping plains and scattered hills. Mount Niénokoué, the highest point, is an isolated granite dome rising to 2,044 feet (623 m).

The luxuriance of Tai's vegetation is encouraged by conditions common to all true rainforests – constant heat and humidity. Temperatures average 80°F (26°C), with only minor variations through the year. Rainfall, though not as high as in central Africa, is still copious when compared with the rest of the continent. The period from December to February tends to be drier than the rest of the year, but no month is without rain.

Uninhibited by seasonal change, the plant life of the forest is in a constant state of growth. Flowers and fruits are ever present. The great bulk of tree foliage lies in the canopy, where the crowns of medium-sized species mingle. Scattered bigger trees, with massive columnar trunks often buttressed at the base, push unbranching through the canopy to emerge like sentinels in the sunlight above. The diversity of plant life is wondrous – there may be 600 different species of trees alone.

It is in the canopy and emergent trees that animal diversity is also at its most staggering. Here teem innumerable beetles, bees and spiders, lizards, snakes and tree frogs. The calls of birds flocking around a fruiting tree echo from on high, breaking the tranquillity of the forest.

The Diana monkey lives high in the forest trees. Here, in the cooler hours of dusk and dawn, it forages for buds, leaves, insects and even bird's eggs, as well as fruit. Very active and noisy troops of up to 30 of these monkeys sometimes race through the trees.

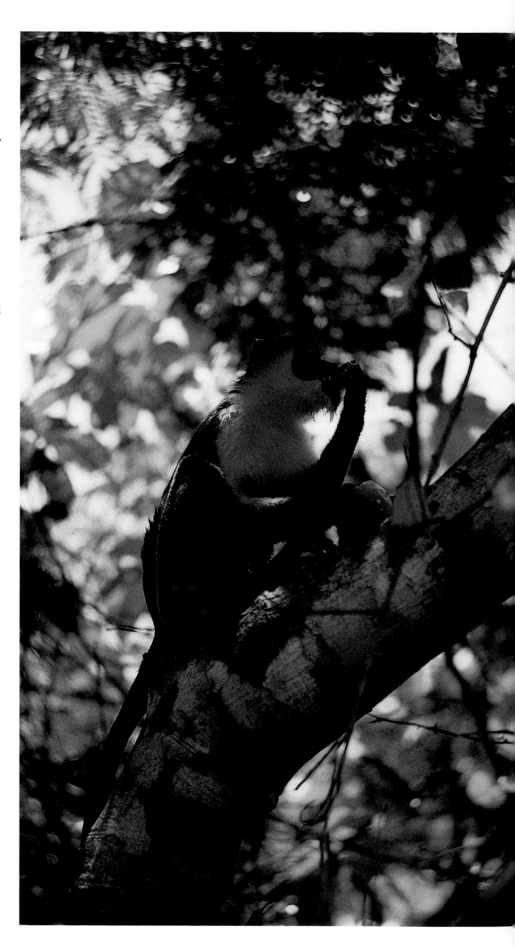

> *"The diversity of life is wondrous – there may be 600 different species of trees"*

FOREST SOIL SYSTEMS

Rainforest soil is generally poorer than that of a temperate forest. Heavy rainfall leaches soil nutrients beyond the reach of roots. But fallen leaves decompose rapidly, and trees spread their roots just under the litter to reabsorb as many nutrients as possible. Buttresses give these shallow-rooted trees extra support.

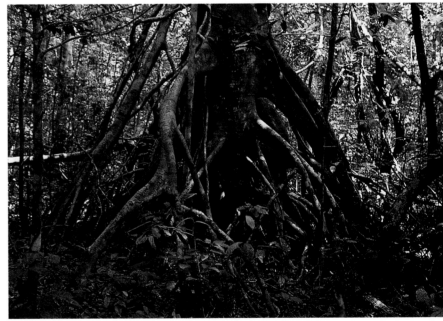

Tropical rainforest

Temperate forest

Buttress

Rapid recycling of nutrients from fallen debris

Slowly decomposing leaf litter

Nutrient -poor soil

Nutrient -rich soil

Ripe fruit can attract visitors from some distance across the forest – it is not unusual to find parrots, fruit pigeons, hornbills and barbets feeding alongside one another. Several different species of monkeys may also converge, chattering and feeding, at the same site, among them red, green and pied colobus monkeys, sooty mangabeys, and vividly patterned Diana monkeys.

The ground layer of the Tai forest, with its thin mantle of shade-adapted vegetation, its fallen trees surmounted by moss, ferns and fungi, and its dark recesses at the bases of tree trunks, seems a distant world from that of the canopy suspended 100 feet (30 m) above. Most canopy animals fear to venture from their lofty home, while many of the creatures found at ground level cannot climb high. At night, many of the latter emerge from hiding to browse on low-growing plants and sort through the leaf litter on the forest floor. Among the rare animals for which the park provides refuge are the giant forest hog – the biggest of all wild pigs – and the pygmy

A tangle of stilt, or prop, roots extends down to the ground from the lower part of the trunk of this rainforest tree. These probably help support the tree and incidentally create excellent hiding places for the creatures of the forest floor.

hippopotamus – the comparatively diminutive cousin of the hippo.

A few predators such as leopards and golden cats hunt for prey both on the ground and in the trees. These cats are good climbers and can make surprise ambushes by leaping down onto prey. The rare but conspicuous chimpanzees also roam from forest floor to canopy. Troops of chimps tend to feed by day, sifting through

ground debris for edible items, chewing leaves in the understory, or climbing high to pluck fruit – their favorite food – from the canopy.

For the chimpanzee and other threatened wildlife of west Africa, the remote interior of the Tai forest offers a lifeline, a precious chance of survival. So long, that is, as the logging and poaching that threaten its fringes can be kept at bay.

THE OKAVANGO DELTA

"The biggest inland delta in the world and a glittering jewel in the heart of southern Africa"

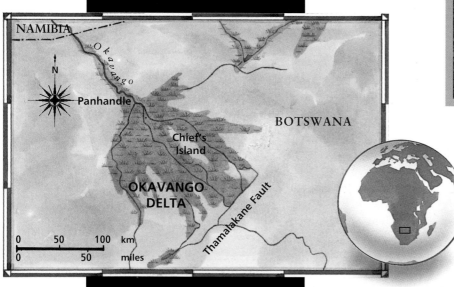

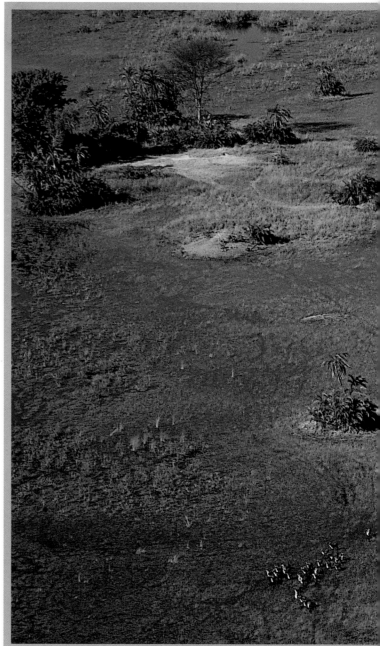

The Okavango River is doomed to perish. As it heads south through an ever-drier landscape of sand, thornbush and pallid grasses, little replenishment arrives to counter the toll of evaporation. Unlike most desert streams, however, the Okavango refuses to die a quiet, shriveling death. It ends, instead, in a blaze of glory. While it still has vigor, the river spills its waters into a giant, spreading fan. The radiating

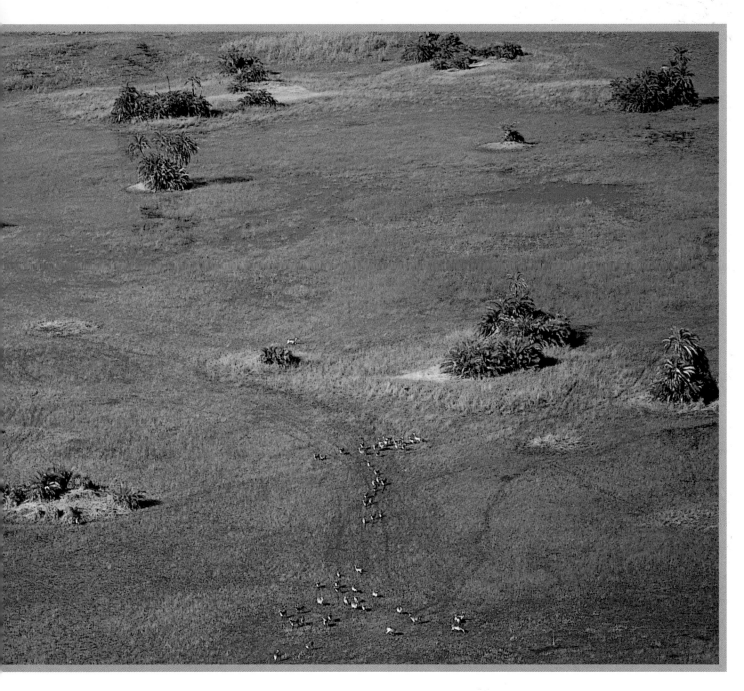

waterways feed a maze of shallow backwaters, lagoons and swamps, bringing sparkling vitality to the desert plain. The river's death-throes have created the biggest inland delta in the world and a glittering jewel in the heart of southern Africa.

From the west, in the ocherous expanse of the Kalahari Desert, the delta lines the horizon with distant, beckoning turquoise. The blue of the water blends with the green hue of thick vegetation – crowded stems of reeds, sedges and grasses and luxuriant swaths of trees and palms. With good reason, the Okavango is likened to an oasis. Not only does it support a wealth of permanent wildlife, but it also draws thirsty and hungry wanderers from far and wide, especially when receding floodwaters leave green pastures in their wake.

The Okavango Delta lies on an immense sandy plain within an ancient inland basin. The waters that feed the Delta flow into the basin from the highlands of central Angola and head steadily southwest for 700 miles (1,100 km) into northern Botswana. There, earth movements have created a system of geological

Red lechwe feast on new shoots springing from the flood plain grasslands of the Okavango Delta. A fertile, well-watered haven in the midst of the desert, the Delta is one of Africa's richest wildlife areas.

faults that seem to have remodeled and interrupted the water's path. First, the Okavango River is channelled between two parallel faults, where it forms the so-called Panhandle of the Delta. As it emerges from these, it meets further fault lines that help to break up its flow into divergent channels. A few of these continue through the Delta and beyond until they meet the Thamalakane Fault, which has created a sand-covered rock barrier some 125 miles (200 km) long. The remnant streams change direction and combine as they follow the foot of the natural dam, before passing through a breach in the fault as a single, ever-dwindling waterway.

As the Okavango River spills out of the Panhandle to form myriad smaller, shallower streams, so it drops most of its sediment load. An estimated two million tons of sand and silt is dumped into the Delta every year. Much more could have been deposited at times in the past when the river was larger and probably ponded back by the Thamalakane barrier. In time, as the stream channels have repeatedly

> *"The yearly flood tide has a dramatic impact on the landscape and ecology of the Delta"*

become blocked by sediment and been forced to find new courses, this has caused the Delta to build outward as well as upward, ramifying into the complex fan-shaped pattern of wetland that covers more than 6,000 sq. miles (15,500 km²) today.

This wetland is an intricate mosaic of reedbeds, swamps and areas of open water, dotted with patches of higher ground where trees and other dry land vegetation can grow. Moreover, it is a changing mosaic.

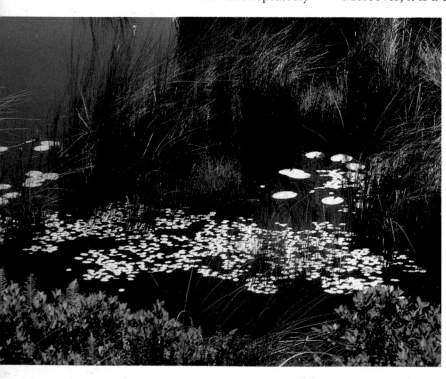

Aquatic plants thrive in the tranquil backwaters of the Delta. Only a few of the 80 or so species of fish in the Okavango chew at the leaves of water plants, but the red-breasted bream is one that can make short work of young lily leaves such as these.

Oxbow lakes – old meander loops cut off from the stream flow – testify to the transitory paths of water passage as erosion and deposition continually rework the surface. In recent times, one entire channel has largely dried up because its input has been diverted elsewhere in the Delta.

Islands and their vegetation change character as shifts in water levels expose or submerge more than before. Reeds trap sediment, so building up ground beneath them, and even Delta animals can bring about change. The mound-building habit of termites helps to establish islets, while the movements of hippopotamuses and elephants can break up banks and wear new water channels through reedbeds.

Toward the south of the Delta, the islands are larger, the land drier and the permanent swampland less extensive. This marginal zone of the Okavango is even more changeable. It has broad areas that are clothed with grass for much of the year but inundated when the Okavango waters make their small but influential annual rise. At this time the total wetland area can increase by some 2,300 sq. miles (6,000 km²).

The yearly flood tide in Okavango may be a sluggish event – the advancing high waters take about five months to pass from the Panhandle to the southern flood plain – but its impact on the landscape and ecology of the Delta is dramatic. As the flood-tide passes slowly through the different zones of the Delta, it replenishes oxygen in stale waters and redistributes nutrients. It also defines cycles of vegetation growth and provides the triggers and checks that govern the lives of the Delta's wild inhabitants.

The Okavango Delta has its rainy season from November to March, but the angry skies and scattered showers add little to the water levels. Real change begins to come toward the end

AN ANNUAL FLOOD TIDE

Every year the Okavango River, fed by heavy rainfall in its northern reaches, brings an enriching flood tide to the Delta. Rising waters spread out across flat grasslands to the south, greatly increasing the Delta's size. They also stir up and spread out nutrients from mud and soil and re-oxygenate stagnant pools.

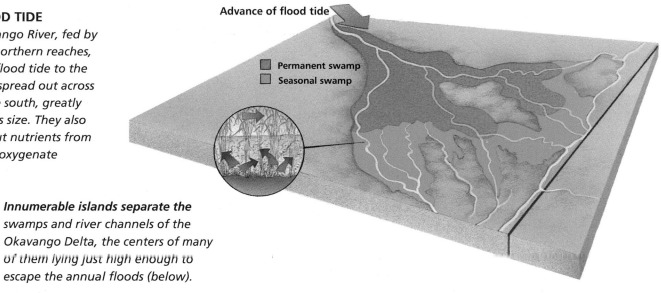

Advance of flood tide

Permanent swamp
Seasonal swamp

Innumerable islands separate the swamps and river channels of the Okavango Delta, the centers of many of them lying just high enough to escape the annual floods (below).

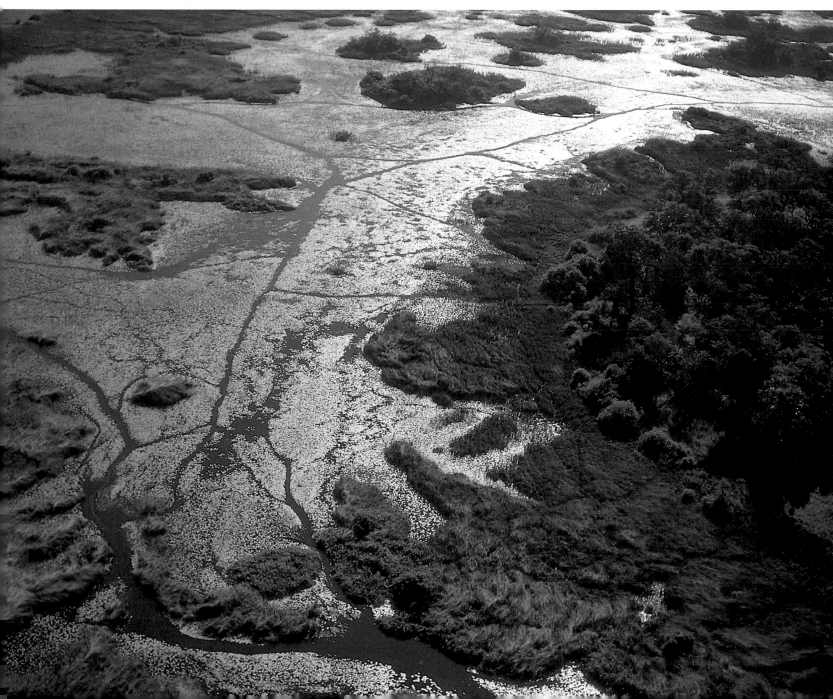

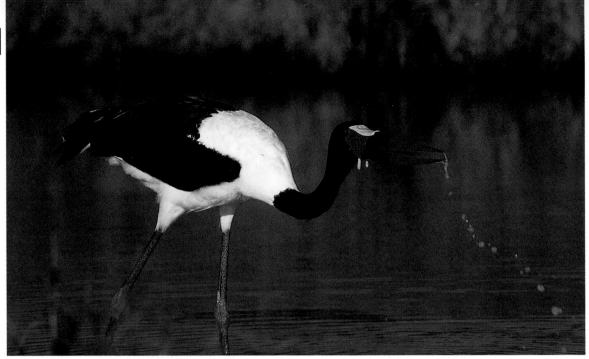

The saddlebill stork is a frequent visitor to the southern Delta during the flood season. As it wades through the shallows, it keeps its eyes firmly fixed on the water, ready to lunge with its bill at any sign of movement.

of the season, when more sustained rainfall across central Angola feeds the river downstream. The swollen river races first into the Panhandle, where it cuts its path through more or less continuous swamp dominated by tall papyrus stems and willowy palms.

As the river rises and washes over its banks, the swamps become replete with well-oxygenated water, in which aquatic plants and invertebrate animals thrive. Newly flooded land at the swamp margins becomes calving ground for sitatungas, the specialist antelope of the swamps, and huge numbers of migratory catfish wriggle into the shallows to spawn.

Large animals have difficulty moving through the swamp – the dense papyrus impedes them and the loose, spongy rootmats give little support underfoot. The sitatunga has large hooves that splay out as it treads over the mats, spreading its weight. Few predators can pursue it into its watery haven, although it does fall victim to the big crocodiles that lurk by the river.

As the flood tide crosses out of the Panhandle, it spreads over the much wider area of the Upper Delta. Yet there is still enough water in the swollen channels to flush through the swamps here, rehydrate drying reedbeds and lap up the sides of islands. Papyrus no longer dominates

the vegetation. Instead there is a mixture of reeds and sedges in water of varying depth, with high grass on flood plains and belts of lofty trees fronting the islands. Lazy waterways branch from the main channels, meandering sometimes into tranquil lagoons, where hippopotamuses spend their days and fish eagles, reed cormorants and otters hunt for fish.

Across such a habitat, flight is a tremendous asset, and it is little surprise that airborne creatures are among the most prominent of the Delta. Bats scour the waterways and dart over the reeds at dusk, snatching night-flying insects such as moths and mosquitoes. By day, the swamps are alive with bees and dragonflies, kingfishers and herons.

Thickets of water fig covering islands in some of the larger lagoons provide food for doves and parrots and harbor boisterous mixed colonies of storks, ibises, herons and egrets. Breeding in the colonies is timed so that the chicks hatch after the high waters have subsided. Fish and other prey are easier to catch when they are concentrated in shallower water.

For the fish, on the other hand, the flushing flood stirs up nutrients and opens up new foraging sites as the level rises. Many of the colorful cichlid fish of the Delta spawn during

high water so that their young can take advantage of the good feeding.

The flood tide still has not reached the southern margins of the Delta, where the flood plains remain covered with grass. It is dry season in the nearby Kalahari, and these precious Delta pastures have attracted grazing animals not just from the fringing acacia woodland but also from a large surrounding area of northern Botswana. The Delta now has peak numbers of zebras, buffaloes

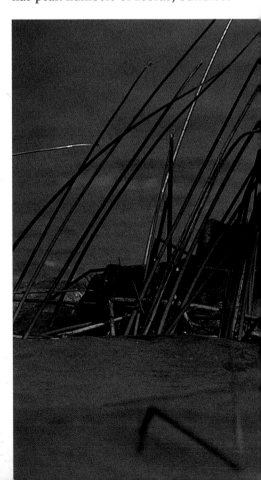

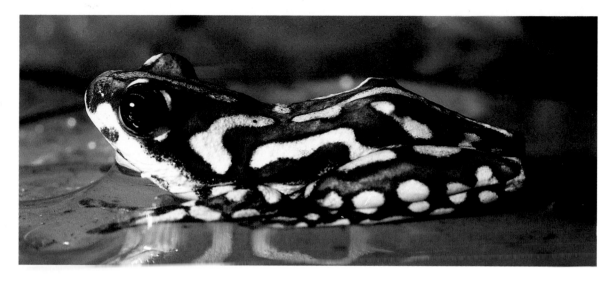

The tinkling calls of painted reed frogs add to the chorus of nocturnal life in the swamps. Male frogs are at their most voluble in the mating season from September to April when vying for the attention of females.

and elephants. They are accompanied by herds of wildebeest, giraffes, sable antelopes and impalas. Warthogs and chacma baboons are common, and the glut of game provides easy pickings for lions, hyenas and hunting dogs.

But the advancing tide front is creeping through the last stage of its journey. Soon it reaches the grassy plains and slowly spreads a sheet of shallow water across the flat terrain. Spawning fish wriggle among the drowned blades and, as the flood water becomes enriched with nutrients – from dead insects, dung, seeds and rotting grasses – many more will arrive, pursued by hunters such as the African pike. Dormant lily bulbs sprout from the submerged soil as they and other aquatic plants take their turn from the grasses. The new shoots provide food for geese and for the red lechwe – another of the Delta's characteristic antelopes.

Though most of the mammals are pushed from the flooded grasslands of the southern Delta, many retreat only into the bands of woodland, from where they can still emerge to slake their thirst from the fresh supply of water. The big nomadic herds of grazing animals tend to linger around the edges of the flood, concentrating on the grassy remnants before heading out into the wider Kalahari. In a few weeks, the floodwaters start to drop once again, and the tidal cycle of the great Okavango Delta turns inexorably on.

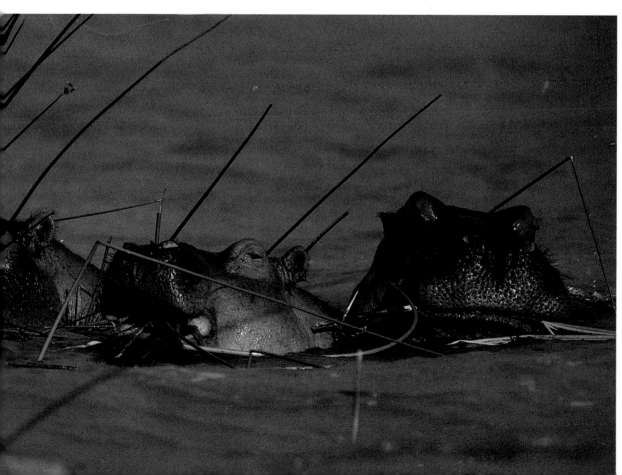

Hippopotamuses loll in lagoons in the deeper waters of the Delta by day. At night they emerge onto islands to crop the grasses. Their well-worn paths from water through swamp to dry land provide easy passage through otherwise impenetrable reedbeds for various creatures, including crocodiles.

PEOPLES OF THE OKAVANGO DELTA

Tribal villages lie scattered throughout the Okavango Delta, beside river banks or on sandy islands. People have lived in the area for thousands of years, drawing on the abundant food resources of this extensive swampy wilderness.

For all, life revolves around the waters. The rivers are places to drink, bathe and fish. They are the principal travel routes, and their annual floods renew the fertility of the soil for cultivation and for grazing animals.

The different tribal groups present in the Okavango – the River Bushmen or Banoka, the Bayei, and the Hambukushu –

share many of the same techniques for subsistence in the Delta. In addition to farming, people gather edible plants and hunt for meat in the swamps and woodland. Long ago, River Bushmen perfected the use of concealed pits dug along trails to trap game. They fish, using nets, hook and line, traps and spears. In shallow water, Okavango fishermen sometimes poison fish by throwing in dried and ground toxic bark from a local tree.

Travel is generally by shallow dugout canoe, carved from a single tree trunk and propelled either by pole in the shallows or by paddle in deeper water.

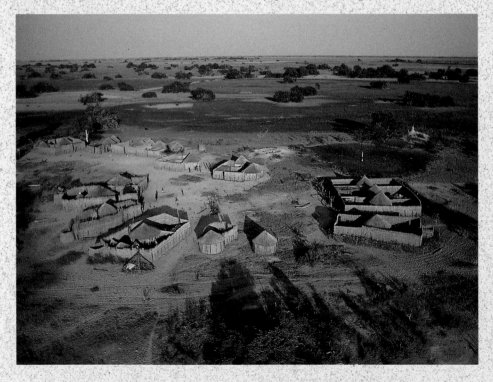

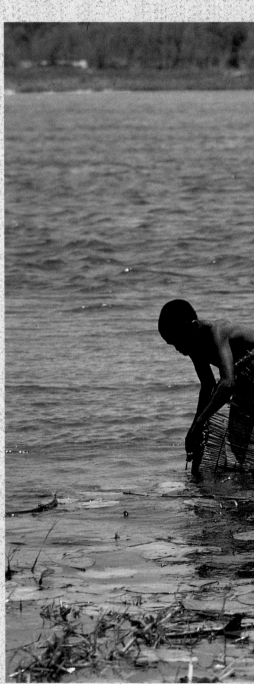

A small tribal village in the heart of the Okavango shows the neat construction of Delta dwellings, built from swamp vegetation. The grass-thatched huts are surrounded by fences of long, sturdy reeds carefully bound and trimmed. Most villages have cultivated plots and cattle pastures nearby.

Bayei women use *elegant, funnel-shaped baskets for catching fish (below). After placing the baskets side by side in the water, the women wade toward them from upstream, flushing fish into the traps.*

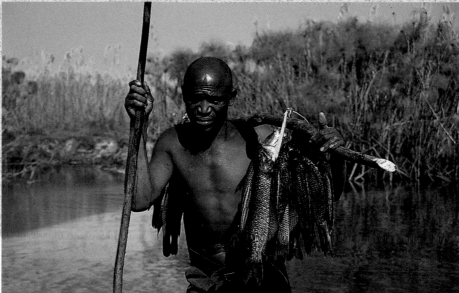

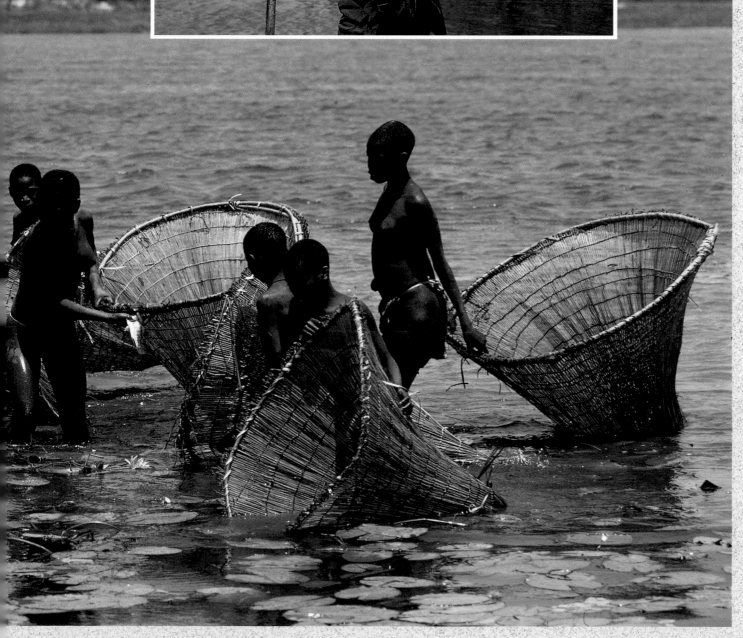

All the peoples of *the Okavango are skilled at obtaining the Delta's most abundant protein source, fish. Here, a River Bushman displays his catch, all snatched from the water by spear (left).*

THE
SKELETON
COAST

"A desert land of parched rock and shifting sands fronting a fogbound sea"

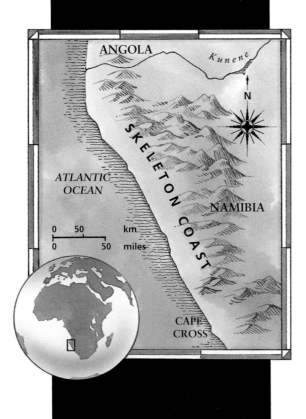

ANGOLA

Kunene

N

ATLANTIC OCEAN

NAMIBIA

S K E L E T O N   C O A S T

0   50   km
0   50   miles

CAPE CROSS

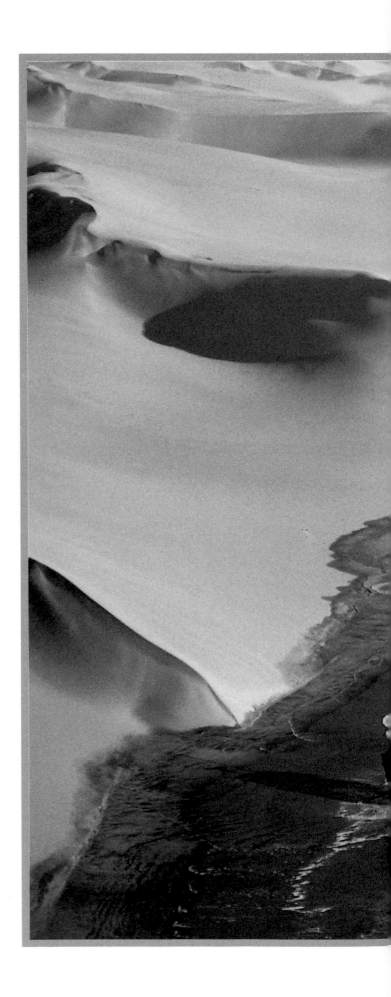

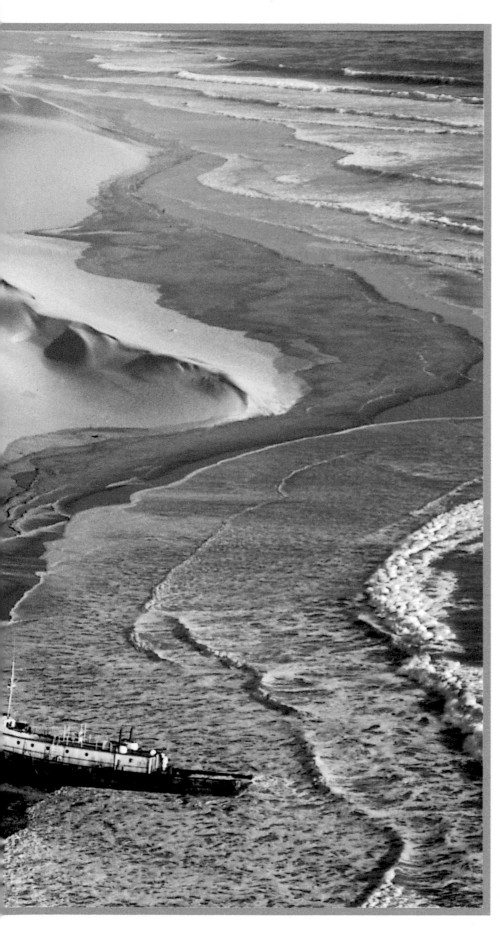

Few places in Africa evoke such an image of desolation as Namibia's infamous Skeleton Coast. The coast remains, to this day, lonely and forbidding – a desert land of parched rock, gravel and shifting sands fronting a treacherous fogbound sea. Its skeletons are the broken bones of foundered ships as well as the remains of long-dead castaways found half-buried in the sand. Yet there is life in this barren landscape, life that is surprising and ingenious in its adaptations to the environment.

The Skeleton Coast lies in the north of Namibia, running from Cape Cross up to the frontier with Angola. Most of it lies within the Skeleton Coast Park, now a designated wilderness zone. Part of the 1,250-mile (2,000-km) long Namib Desert that fringes the coast of Namibia, the landscape is harsh but beautiful. Rugged brown hills of exposed rock sandblasted by the wind are backed by a distant chain of mountains.

Around the hills stretch broad, gravel-strewn plains with low-lying salt pans and undulating fields of sand. A number of valleys and deep gorges crossing the park mark the courses of rivers from the highland interior. Only one of these, the Kunene, is perennial. Others reach the sea regularly during rainy periods inland, but many disappear before they traverse the desert strip. Though these river courses are dry on the surface for most of the time, water usually lies underground within reach of plant roots, and in places rises to the surface as permanent waterholes.

Sand dunes run inland from the coast. Molded by the wind, they form

On even the brightest day, the Skeleton Coast can be swathed in mist. This treacherous coast claims many victims. Here, a deserted ship lies abandoned to waves of advancing sand dunes.

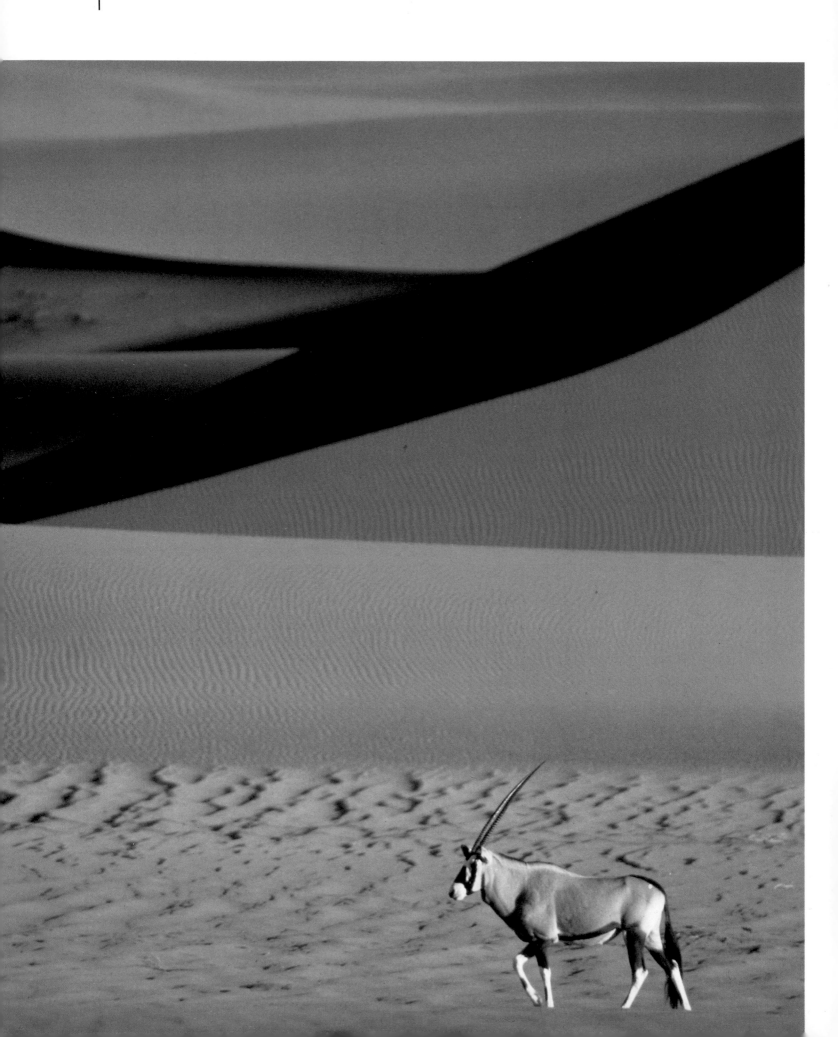

long ridges, ripples and elegant crescent-shaped dunes known as barchans. Some dunes are anchored around rocks and bushes, while others creep forward as grains of sand are blown over their crests by the wind. Barchans move the most rapidly; some advance up to 50 feet (15 m) across the desert every year.

Given the Skeleton Coast's tropical latitude, the water offshore is surprisingly cool, generally below 59°F (15°C). The chill is meted out by the cold Benguela Current, which flows up from Antarctica and sweeps along the west coast of Africa. The current gives the coastline its most characteristic feature – persistent fog. As warm, moisture-laden air from more westerly parts of the ocean meets the cold air above the Benguela Current, it cools and condenses much of its water vapor. Dense banks of fog usually hang offshore like a giant curtain, hiding the ocean beyond.

For mariners skirting the shore, this sea fog has always been a terrible curse, capable of cutting all visibility in seconds. Temporarily blinded, and on a sea with strong currents and heavy swells harboring hidden reefs, many have run their ships aground.

Even today, with the aid of navigational equipment, ships are still lost now and again along the Skeleton Coast. In times past, castaways from the shipwrecks faced little chance of rescue before thirst and hunger took their toll. It can still take several days for people lost in the desert to be rescued.

Lack of water is the worst problem. Although the sea fog makes the coastal air humid, the layer is too

A lone gemsbok roams the Namib Desert in search of food. It rarely drinks but gets all its moisture from the plants it eats. One of the driest of all deserts, the Namib receives no more than 1 inch (25 mm) of rain a year.

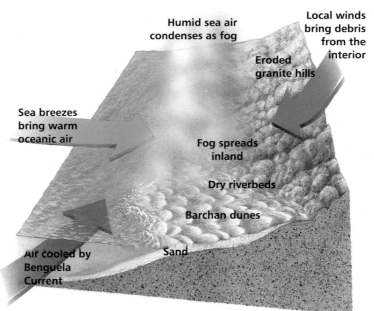

Humid sea air condenses as fog

Local winds bring debris from the interior

Eroded granite hills

Sea breezes bring warm oceanic air

Fog spreads inland

Dry riverbeds

Barchan dunes

Sand

Air cooled by Benguela Current

thin to create rain, and wider climatic patterns mean that the area seldom receives rain clouds. Just a few light showers fall from year to year and these evaporate swiftly in the burning heat of the day.

For castaways, the fruitless humidity of the coastal zone must have seemed all the more frustrating

> *"Dense banks of fog usually hang offshore like a giant curtain, hiding the ocean beyond"*

FOG OVER THE DESERT
Billowing curtains of fog form as warm, damp Atlantic air condenses over the icy Benguela Current, which travels up from the Antarctic Ocean. In early morning, the fog spreads inland, bringing precious drops of moisture to the barren desert.

at night and in the early morning. After sunset, the desert air quickly cools as the heat of the day escapes into the atmosphere. In some places temperatures drop close to freezing. The humid air near the coast becomes damp with condensation like the air offshore and soon fog develops onshore. The desert fog thickens and gradually spreads. By dawn, thick mists cover the desert for about 30 miles (50 km) inland, swirling into

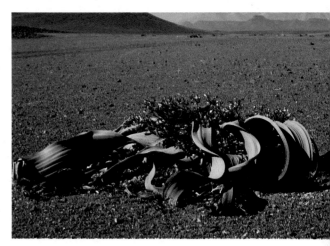

The welwitschia plant has long ribbon-shaped leaves which curl over the ground. The millions of tiny pores on each leaf, normally kept shut to conserve moisture, open up when nighttime fog condenses on the plant.

valleys and drifting over hills. Once the sun starts to rise again, the air warms once more, and the land fog gradually disappears.

The extreme aridity of the Skeleton Coast makes the sight of an elephant or even a lion strolling across the desolate landscape all the more incongruous. Yet this seemingly inhospitable desert harbors a remarkable range of wildlife. Animals more at home on the African grasslands manage to survive along the river valleys, relying on the waterholes to slake their thirst when the riverbeds are dry. Elephants, giraffes, zebras and antelopes travel these vegetated corridors, browsing

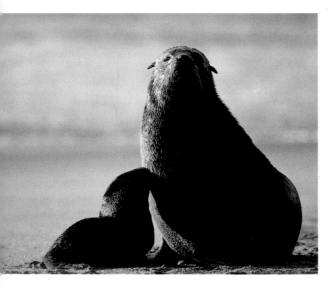

Cape fur seals come ashore in their thousands at Cape Cross on the Skeleton Coast to give birth to their young and remain there for up to two months until the young are strong enough to brave the sea.

on trees and bushes such as acacia and mopane whose roots draw on underground water reserves.

Lions sometimes lie in wait for prey around watering sites. Troops of chacma baboons have even colonized dry, rocky gorges with tiny erratic water supplies. Normally, these monkeys need to drink daily, but

observations of one group have shown that they have learned to survive without drinking for more than three weeks, if necessary, by reducing activity to a minimum.

Away from the valleys, on the rocky plains and dunes, true desert conditions demand special adaptations in plants and animals. Some plants such as grasses and herbs sprout only when chance rains dampen the desert soil, engaging in a race against time to grow and flower before the water disappears.

But the desert is best known for the plants that exploit its nighttime fogs. The ganna is a common straggly bush which usually traps around it a hummock of windblown sand; its roots then readily soak up fog and dew deposited over the dune. Desert lichens, which are abundant on rocks and gravel, remain dry, brittle and dull until the fogs sweep over them. Then they quickly soften, and their colors become vivid.

Some of the most remarkable of all desert animals live on the dunes. These seemingly barren seas of moving sand have their own hidden ecology, based on mere trickles of incoming nutrients and moisture. Ants, termites and beetles scour the sand for organic material blown from inland and from river valleys. They, in turn, sustain a web of burrowing predators such as scorpions, lizards and snakes.

Some of the dune animals "drink" the morning fog that rolls in from the sea by lying exposed near the dune crest and letting the moisture condense on their bodies. Snakes and lizards lick the precious drops from their skin; the sidewinder viper simply flicks its tongue over its coils. Other animals manage to obtain all the moisture they need from the plants or prey that they eat.

Through ingenious adaptations, wildlife manages to thrive in this most unusual of deserts, but the Skeleton

"These seemingly barren seas of moving sand have their own hidden ecology, based on mere trickles of incoming nutrients and moisture"

Coast has always been a harsh place for people. Few native tribes have ever penetrated the desert proper. European explorers came to the region from the 15th century, but did not linger long.

The 20th century has seen the arrival of prospectors and mining companies looking for diamonds and other minerals. Most of these operations proved uneconomic, and their facilities are now abandoned to the desert. The disfiguring imprint of human intruders who have come and gone – deserted huts, shipwrecks, bones – serve as testament to the wild seclusion of the Skeleton Coast.

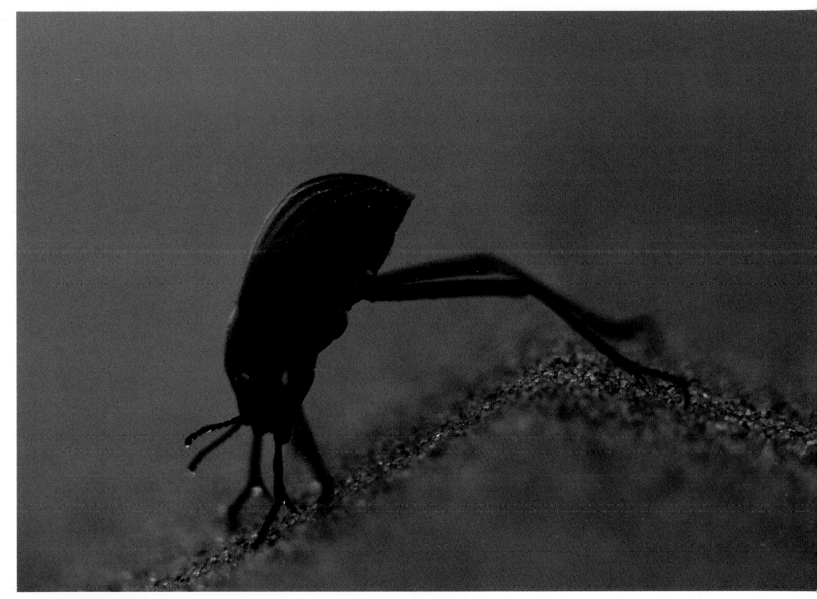

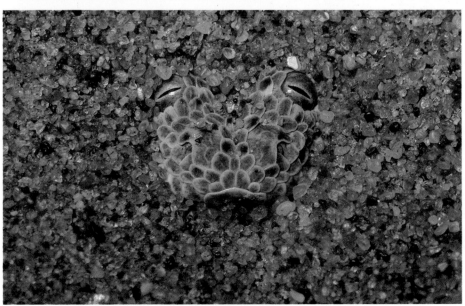

Half-hidden in the sand, a sidewinder viper lies in wait to ambush a passing cricket or web-footed gecko. The snake's mottled coloration helps it stay perfectly camouflaged.

A darkling beetle balances precariously on its head, so that the early morning fog condensing on its body trickles down into its mouth. These precious drops are the only direct source of moisture that the beetle can obtain in the parched desert.

SWEDISH LAPLAND

*"An immense
wilderness
with a harsh
and remote
beauty,
unchanged
for thousands
of years"*

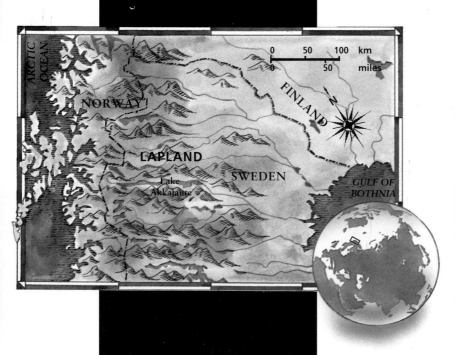

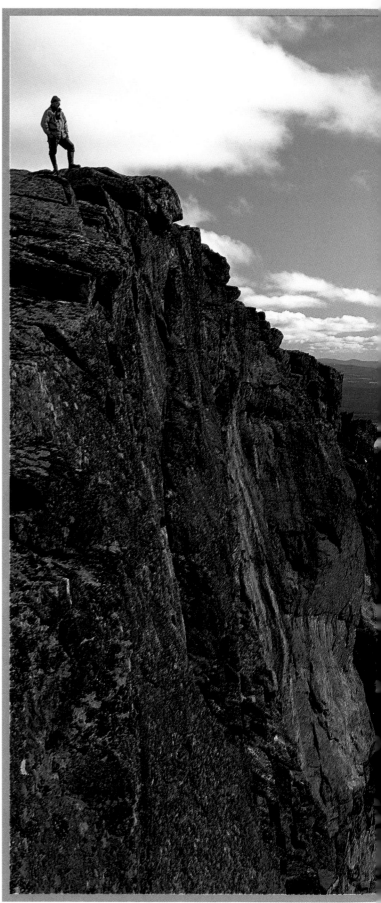

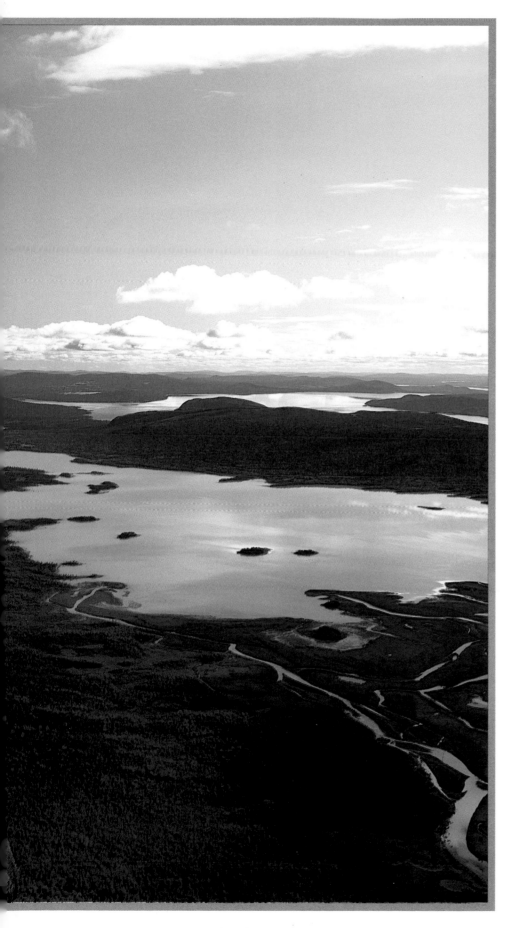

Sweden's vast northernmost county, occupying almost a quarter of the country's entire area, contains some of Europe's wildest scenery. The land sweeps down from the snowfields and craggy peaks of the western mountains in a long, wide slope toward the Gulf of Bothnia to the east. Glaciers, lakes and torrential rivers cut deep parallel grooves across this slope, running from northwest to southeast. As the terrain changes levels, it encompasses snow-covered summits, alpine tundra and deep-carved valleys, descending finally to virgin pine forests, lakes, peat bogs and marshlands.

Much of Lapland is north of the Arctic Circle, and its inhabitants, animal and human alike, have become adapted to a life of long, cold winters and short, cool summers. The few encroachments of the modern world – the mining towns and the tourist centers – are dwarfed by the immensity of the wilderness, and huge areas of Swedish Lapland retain a harsh and remote beauty that has remained unchanged for thousands of years.

The present shapes and forms of the land were sculpted as the great ice sheets of the last ice age retreated northward 10,000 years ago. Relieved of the huge weight of the ice, the crust beneath rose upward. Subterranean forces heaved and tilted the ancient plateau, thrusting the Scandinavian peninsula above the waters. Melting glaciers left behind a rocky detritus which dammed rivers and streams to form the elongated lakes typical of northern Sweden.

Rocky mountain crags look down on vast river systems snaking across the flat plains. In this wild and desolate landscape of Swedish Lapland it is possible to travel for weeks without seeing another human being.

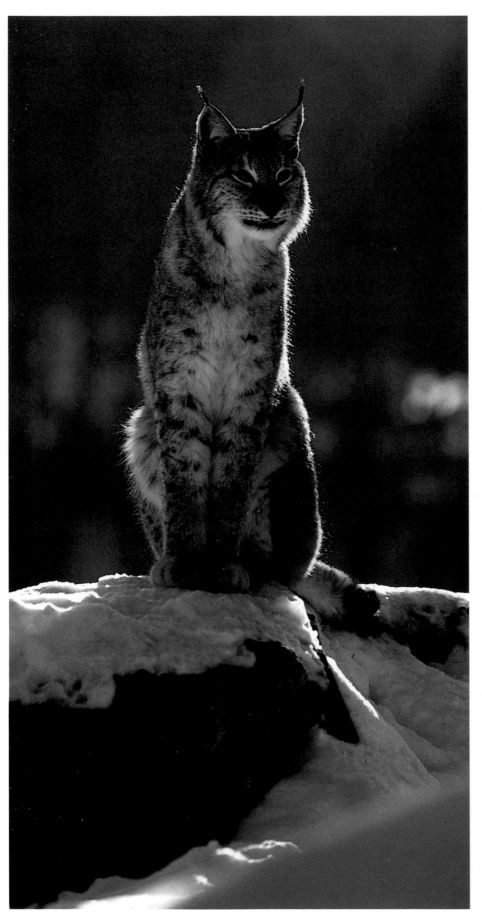

Much of Swedish Lapland is occupied by national parks, which are really wildernesses within a wilderness. They cover a vast area and contain a variety of landscapes rich in plants and animals. Three parks – Stora Sjofallet, Sarek and Padjelanta – are grouped together in the northwest, next to the Norwegian border. Together the parks comprise Europe's largest protected wilderness, with a total area of some 1,292,850 acres (523,200 hectares).

In Stora Sjofallet, steep mountain ranges flank Lake Akkajaure, and primeval forests of Norway spruce and Scots pine in the east of the territory give shelter to large mammals such as bears and elks. Sarek has 90 peaks of more than 5,900 feet (1,800 m) and close to 100 glaciers. Remote and difficult to access, the Sarek land ranges from steep river valleys forested with birch to alpine tundra and rocky peaks. The largest of the parks, Padjelanta, has a wide, rolling mountain character, with lakes bordered by alpine meadows and grassy heathland.

Central Lapland, which includes Muddus National Park, is a region of forests and peat marshes. Its bird sanctuaries shelter more than 100 species, from water birds to golden eagles, and its extensive wetlands are home to otters as well as water shrews and voles. Farther south is the Peljekaise National Park, established to protect the mountain birchwoods that glow with heathers and flowers in spring and summer.

Plant life varies with altitude on the rugged Lapland slopes. Lichens are the only plants that flourish in

The lynx once lived all over Europe, but Swedish Lapland is now one of its few remaining refuges. In these remote mountainous and forested lands, this stealthy hunter preys on hares, birds and even young reindeer.

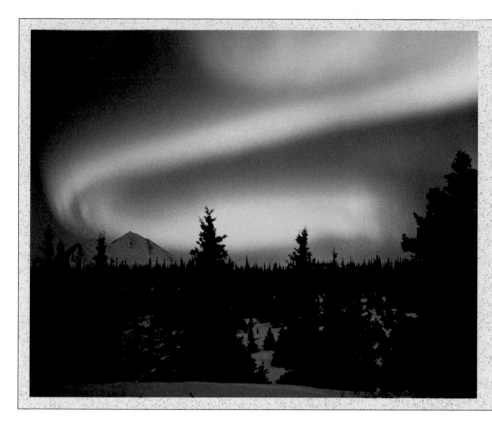

NORTHERN LIGHTS

The aurora borealis, or northern lights, is a dazzling display of shifting colored light that illuminates the polar night sky.

The phenomenon is caused by solar winds, carrying charged particles, streaming toward Earth from the Sun. The magnetic field of the Earth is shaped like a doughnut, with the holes over the poles. Charged solar particles pour down through these holes and react with the atmosphere's nitrogen and oxygen molecules to produce the colorful lights.

Solar flares periodically boost the density of the particles, leading to particularly spectacular displays. A similar phenomenon occurs in the southern hemisphere.

the upper alpine zone above 4,000 feet (1,200 m). Their success attests to the lack of airborne pollutants in the cold, clear air. The lower alpine zone beneath this level supports a scrub growth of dwarf willow, and the next zone down, the subalpine, is typified by birch forests. Lower down still is the coniferous zone, with its forests of pine, spruce and fir. Hardy plants such as blue mountain heath, mountain aven and three-leaved rush carpet the ground in the subalpine and lower alpine zones.

The mountain uplands of Lapland are the territories of many birds of prey. Golden eagles, rough-legged buzzards, gyrfalcons and snowy owls all hunt there. Water birds found in the marshes and lakes include lesser

white-fronted geese, red-necked phalaropes and whooper swans. The larger wild mammals are becoming increasingly rare in Europe, but the Lapland wildernesses provide refuges for bears, elks, and almost extinct wolves. Wolverines and lynxes still stalk the forests and woods.

Swedish Lapland has until now managed to survive the predations of industry and tourism, and its parks are among the most successful in Europe. The long, dark winters and the harshness of the Arctic terrain have undoubtedly contributed to the preservation of this icy land.

In the highlands of northwest Lapland, well above the Arctic Circle, land over 3,300 feet (1,000 m) is treeless, covered with vast stretches of wind-scoured permanent snow. The few plants that can survive grow close to the ground.

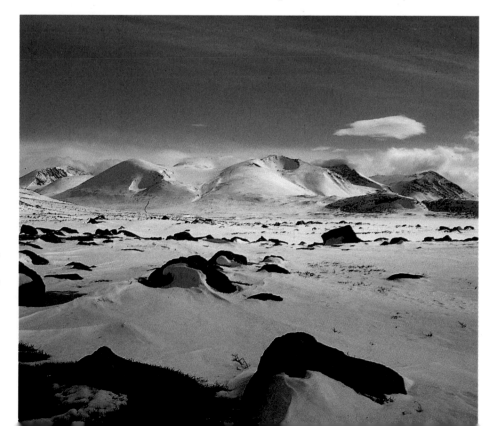

THE SAMI OF LAPLAND

Northern Scandinavia has been home to the Sami, as the Laplanders prefer to be known, since prehistoric times. Their ancestors may have been Stone Age hunters from central Europe who followed the retreating glaciers northward. There are currently about 60,000 Sami in Scandinavia, 17,000 of them in Swedish Lapland.

Some Sami became fishermen, others settled into forest communities, and still others adopted a seasonally nomadic life managing great herds of reindeer. The herders work to an eight-season year.

In April, known as springwinter, the Sami watch over the reindeer as they wander far over the snow-covered plains, digging through the snow for lichens. Spring sees the herds heading for the mountains where the cows give birth to their calves, and in springsummer and summer proper, the herds feed on abundant mountain vegetation. In autumnsummer, the herds are driven down to folds at the foot of the mountains for slaughter,

and through autumn the meat is preserved or sold. The reindeer stay close to the woods during autumnwinter, gradually moving farther afield in search of food as winter closes in.

The 3,000 or so Sami who still depend on reindeer speak their own language and organize their own village communities. They survive in their harsh environment as robustly as the reindeer by which they measure their wealth.

In August and February, the Sami hold ceremonial fairs, dressing up in their bright tunics, hats and boots, and buying and selling traditional wares as well as reindeer calves (below). Reindeer are the wealth of a Sami family.

The Sami once had a completely nomadic life-style, moving with their reindeer between winter and summer pastures. Nowadays, most people live in permanent homes while some of the young men do the herding (right).

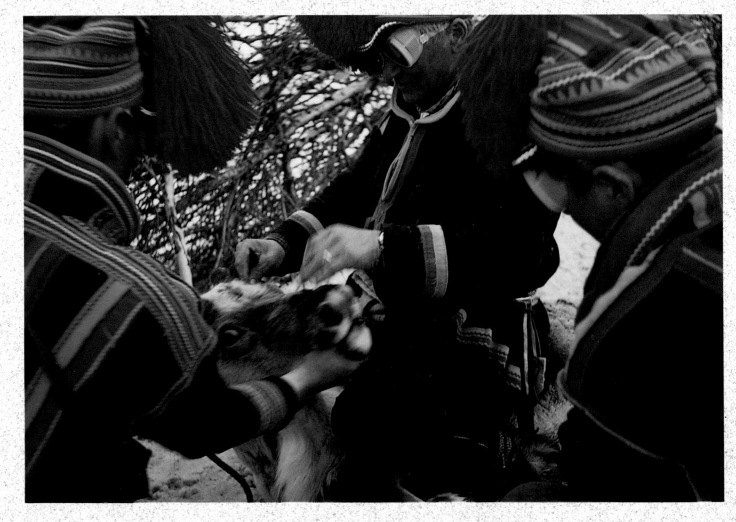

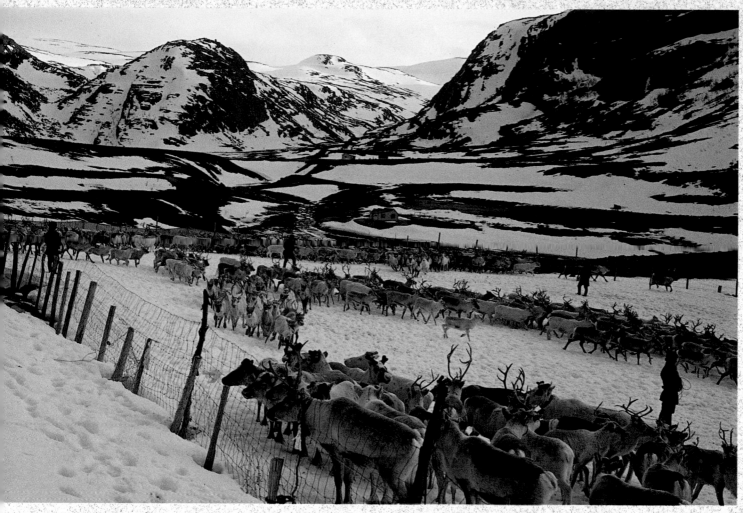

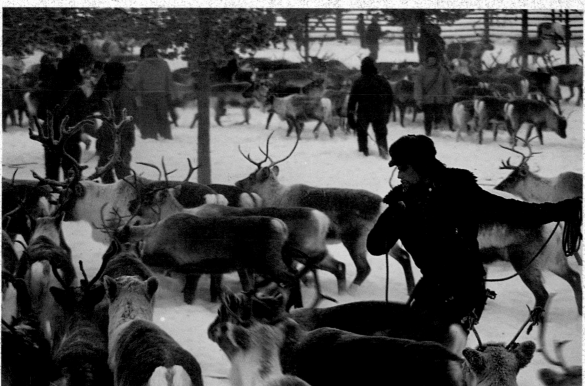

Reindeer are rounded up annually so that herders can mark their calves with earcuts or identifying brand marks. This is necessary since herds spread out during winter movements and can easily become mixed with another family's animals.

THE
CAIRNGORMS

"Below the plateaus, cliffs and sweeping moors of the high mountains are primeval pine forests"

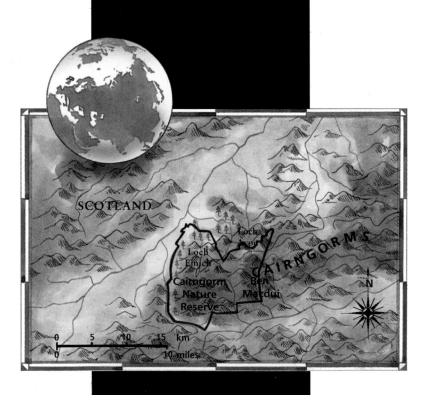

Bounded by great river systems, riven by steep-sided glens, and skirted by the remains of ancient forests, the Cairngorms are Britain's largest mountain region. This mighty granite mass in the Scottish Highlands is landscape on a grand scale, dwarfing all human activity.

In this uncompromising terrain, climate and landform conspire to create regions of daunting remoteness. For much of the year, the upper peaks and glacier-scoured slopes are brilliant with snow and ice. People make seasonal incursions to ski, climb, hunt or fish, and then hurry away again, leaving the lochs and rivers to ospreys and otters, the forests and mountains to eagles and deer, the snows to hares and winter-plumaged ptarmigan.

On the broad humps of the high mountain summits, no fewer than six of them more than 4,000 feet (1,200 m) high, bright sunshine can turn into gales and blizzards with frightening swiftness. More snow falls on the Cairngorm plateau than on any other mountain region in Britain; and, in high, shadowed fissures on the summits, snow can persist through to August or even September.

Below the plateaus, cliffs and sweeping moors of the mountains, the Cairngorms contain remnants of the great primeval pine forests that once covered well over 2½ million acres (1 million hectares) of Scotland. For 5,000 years and more, the pine forests formed a tree line up to an altitude of 2,000–2,100 feet (600–640 m) on the Cairngorm plateau.

Scots pines have grown in the Cairngorms since the end of the last ice age. These resinous trees, armored with great slabs of rough bark, flourish in mineral-deficient soils and provide food and shelter for a wide range of mammals, birds and insects.

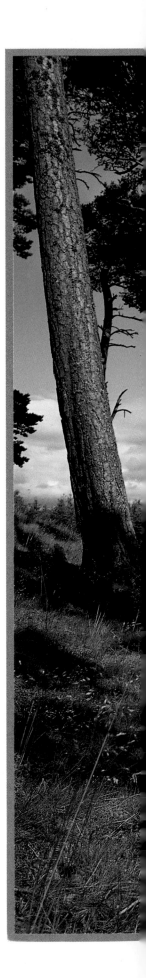

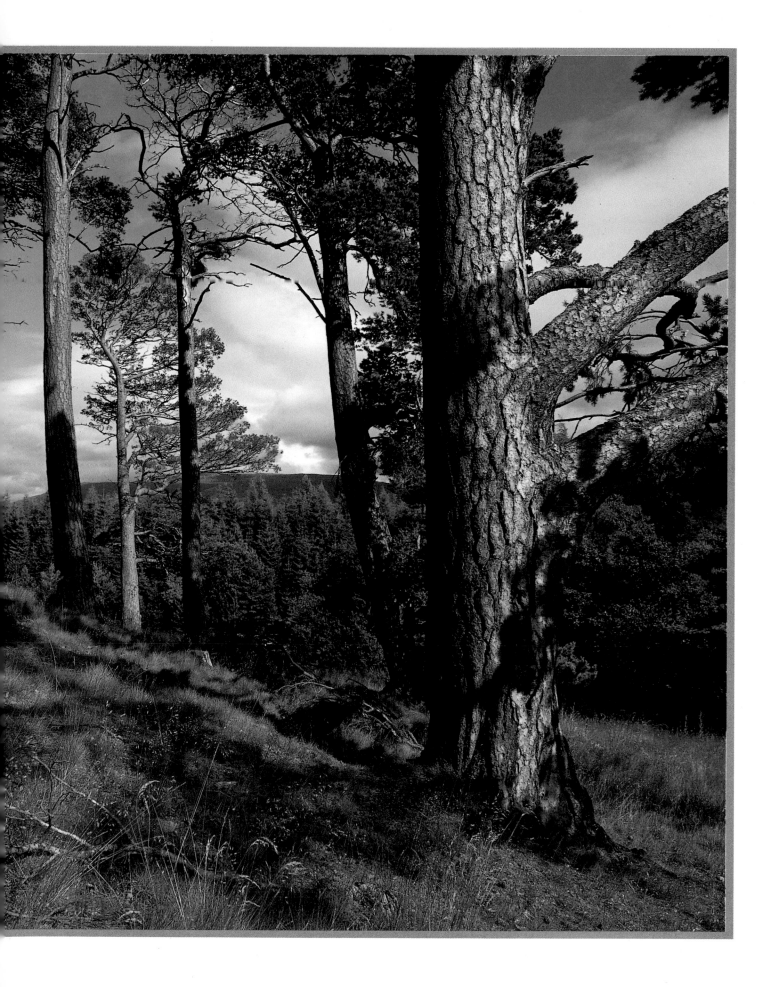

But from the 16th century onward, the majestic trees were burned to clear land and, later, felled for industrial furnaces. Now only 20,000 acres (8,000 hectares) of natural forest survive, scattered throughout the highlands, particularly on the slopes of the Cairngorms. The Scots pine, which thrives in poor soils and harsh climates, still dominates. The remaining stretches of trees vary from groves of straight-trunked giants almost 100 feet (30 m) high to twisted, wind-stunted trees of no more than 10 feet (3 m) on exposed slopes near the tree-line limit.

These old pine forests of the Cairngorms are found mainly in a curving swath that takes in Glen Feshie in the west, Rothiemurchus in the northwest and the Abernethy Forest in the north. There are forest pockets here that have never been controlled or managed in any way.

Unlike modern pine groves with their rows of uniform, geometrically planted trees, the ancient forest tracts contain open glades where the sun can penetrate the dense top cover. Here, birch, juniper, rowan and aspen grow among the craggy pines, and small plants such as heather and crowberry thrive on the forest floor. Once again, contrasts with commercial plantations are apparent – the ancient forest patches are noisy with birds such as the crossbill, which feeds on the seeds of the Scots pine.

Above the tree line, moorlands and peat bogs sweep up toward the rounded mountaintops. The retreating ice masses and glaciers of the ice age have left their mark on the Cairngorms, where the ice cap was once 2,850 feet (868 m) thick. The ice deepened the river glens, filled lochs with meltwater and terraced the sides of valleys with deposits of gravel. The moving ice also left behind thick layers of clay, sand and gravel which became fertile beds for the great forests.

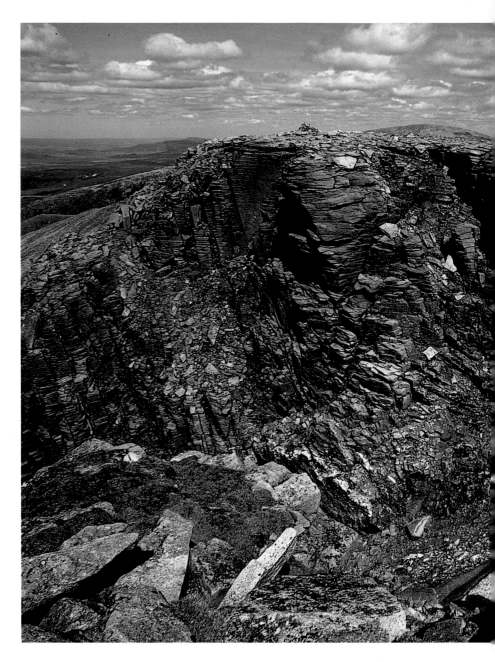

Ice also carved the amphitheater-like bowls called corries high in the northern and eastern faces of the mountains. Prevailing winds blew snow from the plateau which accumulated in hollows on the mountains. As the climate worsened and temperatures dropped, the compacted snow turned into ice and formed small local glaciers. These gouged the corries out of the mountainside, pulverizing rock and then carrying it away.

The great highland plateau of the Cairngorms consists of several

Thousands of icy winters have shattered these granite summits, already scraped bare by glaciers. Here, on the summit of Cairn Gorm, 4,000 feet (1,200 m) above sea level, few plants or animals can survive.

clusters of high, domelike granite summits, divided by deep glens. Most impressive of these deep divisions is the valley called Lairig Ghru. This great rift lies between the summits of Braeriach, Cairn Einich, Angel Peak and Cairn Toul, to the west, and

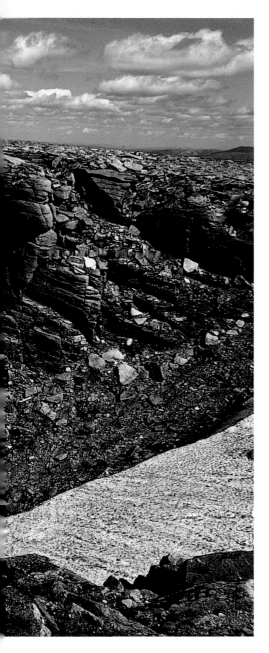

VALLEYS SHAPED BY GLACIERS

The Cairngorms owe their rounded forms to the action of glaciers during successive ice ages. The weight of slowly moving ice, aided by the hard debris of fractured rock borne with it,

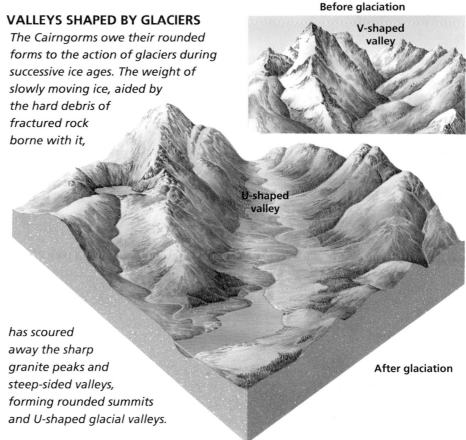

Before glaciation

V-shaped valley

U-shaped valley

After glaciation

has scoured away the sharp granite peaks and steep-sided valleys, forming rounded summits and U-shaped glacial valleys.

Cairn Gorm and Ben Macdui, highest of the peaks at 4,692 feet (1,430 m), to the east. Beyond Glen Derry, on the easternmost edge of the plateau, lie the high masses of Beinn a' Bhuird and Ben Avon.

South of the entire massif, the glens of Dee, Lui and Quoich run down into the east-flowing Dee which forms the Cairngorms' southern boundary. Rivers surround the whole region. The Feshie in its great forested glen is the western boundary, while the mighty Spey delineates the northwest margin as far north as the Abernethy Forest. The Avon flows along the east of the plateau, running north from its source on Ben Avon.

Above the forests and woods around the lower slopes of the mountains, the land becomes bare and unprotected, and the plants that survive there have to be able to cope with freezing gales and months of snow cover. Most of these Arctic alpine species grow close to the ground and literally keep a low profile. Some, like alpine mouse ear, have wooly leaves to keep out the cold. Others, such as the stonecrop, have waxy leaves to conserve moisture and withstand severe weather. Ling, or heather, is the most common moorland plant-cover, turning great expanses of the hills up to about 4,000 feet (1,200 m) purple in August. Above the heather is a zone of mosses, deer grass and stiff sedge, and on the highest levels, where the ground surface is a mixture of patchy earth and shattered rock, tough plants

"Retreating ice deepened the river glens, filled lochs with meltwater and terraced the sides of valleys"

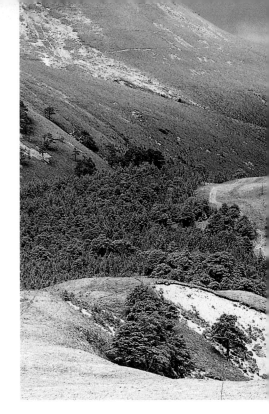

such as mat grass and three-leaved rush predominate.

Wildlife thrives in the ancient forest remnants on the lower slopes of the Cairngorms. Herds of red deer feast through the good weather on grass and heather, lichens, mosses and blaeberries. But the swift onset of the long winter drives them down from the open ground to the resin-scented shelter of the trees, where they wreak havoc on pine seedlings.

The appetites of the increasing herds of red deer are causing problems for the Scots pine. Mature trees grow ever larger, but there is no regeneration in the form of seedlings to replace the old trees as they fall. Many of the current Scots pine woods consist of mature trees that were seedlings some 200 years ago, when there were more humans and fewer red deer, and the herds that existed had a greater range of woodland to use in winter. New afforestation lands are usually fenced, which forces the deer increasingly into the unfenced ancient forest areas. Forest management could redress the balance and maintain the survival of both species.

Roe deer do not move around in large herds like the red deer. They stay instead in family groups or travel singly as they roam the slopes browsing on small shrubs such as bilberries. Reindeer became extinct in the 12th century, but had previously lived in the region. In 1952 a domesticated herd of reindeer was brought from Sweden to an area near Aviemore in the Cairngorms. The introduced herd is now living successfully in the wild, feeding mainly on mosses and lichens.

The old forests provide one of the last protective environments for the red squirrel, which has been usurped across most of Britain by the gray squirrel, introduced from North America. Red squirrels are natural inhabitants of coniferous forests,

and pine nuts are a favorite item in their diet. Other increasingly rare mammals still holding out in the Cairngorm pine forests include the wildcat and the pine marten. The otter, too, is found along forest rivers.

The wide and windy summits of the Cairngorms are home to several species of mountain birds. The dotterel, a member of the plover family, winters in north Africa, but migrates to the far north to breed and nest. The birds start to arrive in the Cairngorms in May, though many continue northward to nest well within the Arctic Circle, where they favor sea-level sites. In the Cairngorms, dotterels nest on the high mountain tops, the smaller males sitting on the eggs while the females congregate in groups away from the nests. The snow bunting, like the dotterel, is a rare bird and nests high in rocks and cliffs of the summits. There are maybe 30 pairs nesting in the whole of Scotland.

Another mountain dweller is the ptarmigan, which can survive in the severest of conditions, often roosting in holes in the snow. One nest found in the Cairngorms was at an altitude of 4,400 feet (1,340 m). The ptarmigan has a brownish plumage in the summer, with black barring and white wings. In winter it is all white. It feeds on flowers, shoots, berries and seeds of mountain plants.

But perhaps the most interesting bird found in these mountains is the capercaillie, with its spectacular courtship ritual. This large relative of the grouse became extinct in the 18th century, but was successfully reintroduced into the Cairngorms in the 1830s with Swedish stock.

In the spring, usually before dawn, male capercaillies begin their courting display by emitting a long series of clicks and rattling noises, mixed with hisses and gurgles. Moving into an open glade on the forest floor, a dominant male, resplendent in

colorful blue-green plumage, with red skin patches over his eyes and bristly feathers on his throat, spreads his great fan of a tail, holds his head high, and leaps into the air. Hen capercaillies assemble to watch the display from their roosts, and other males also enter the arena to perform their own, similar displays.

Around 33 pairs of strictly protected ospreys nest in the Scottish Highlands. In the Cairngorms, they nest at Loch Garten and Loch Morlich and, despite the predations of human nest robbers, they continue to thrive. The ospreys overwinter in Africa, migrating north in early spring to reach Scotland in March. One of the great sights of the Cairngorms is that of an osprey beating over a loch on its 5-foot (1.5-m) wingspan, before plunging into the water, wings held high, to seize a fish.

Despite some increase in tourism and winter sports, the Cairngorms, most of which have now been made a National Nature Reserve, are still one of the wildest mountain regions in Europe. Good management could mean that this area, with its awe-inspiring snow-covered summits, ancient forest lands and abundant wildlife, remains the unique and wild place it is at present.

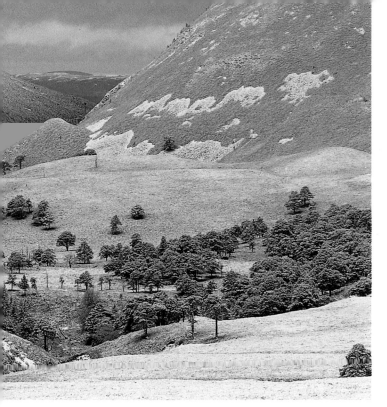

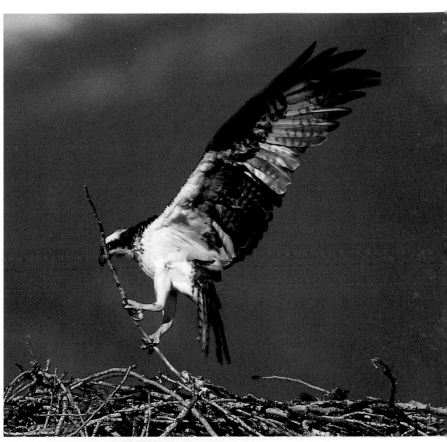

The moorland slopes of this broad pass through the mountains look down on a fertile wooded valley.

The capercaillie nests among the heathers on the forest floor and feeds on berries, leaves and insects (below).

Ospreys build their nests at the top of Scots pines, returning to the same nest year after year (right).

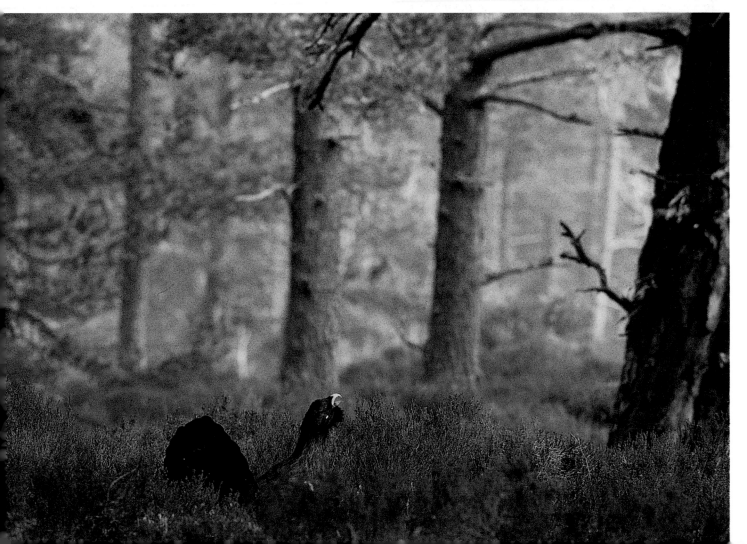

BIALOWIEZA FOREST

"A remnant of the huge primeval forest that once covered much of lowland Europe"

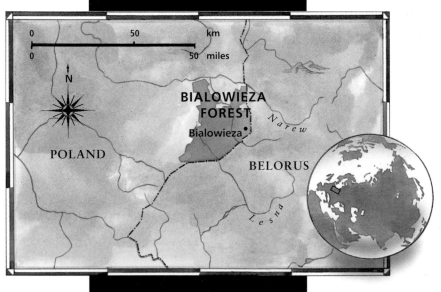

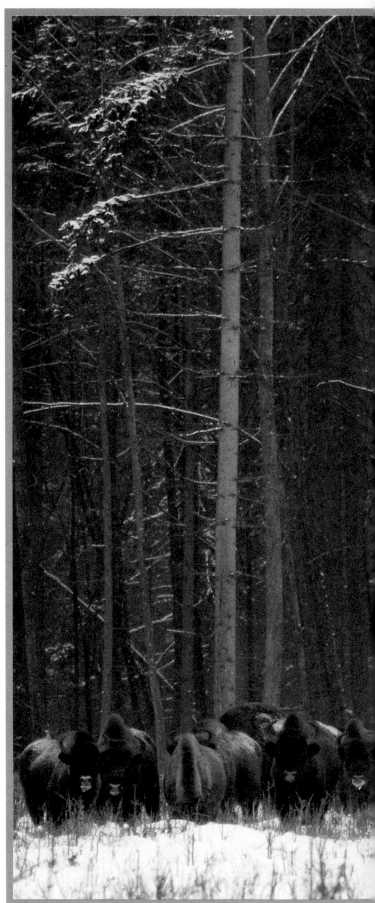

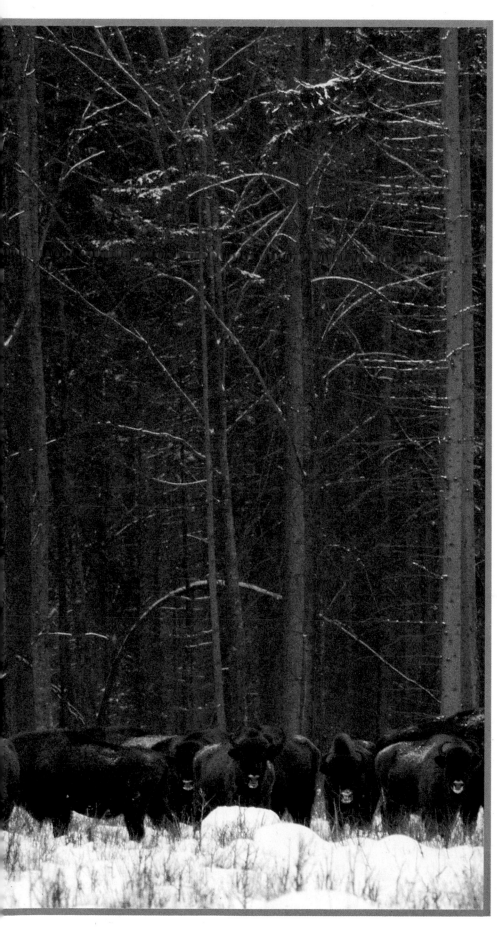

A living link with prehistory, the great Bialowieza Forest is the largest surviving region of primeval mixed-tree forest in Europe. It preserves the conditions which must have existed throughout many European forests two thousand and more years ago. Great oaks, hornbeams and pines create a dense, high ceiling that excludes the sunlight. This dark, shadowed gloom is occasionally relieved by glades where a thinner leaf cover lets through a green light.

Although it covers a total area of 460 sq. miles (1,200 km²) straddling the border between northeastern Poland and the Republic of Belorus, Bialowieza is but a tiny remnant of the huge forested tracts that once covered much of lowland Europe. The strictly protected Bialowieza National Park on the Polish side of the border constitutes some 13,000 acres (5,300 hectares) of the entire forested region. Internationally, the park is thought important enough to be a United Nations Biosphere Reserve and has been designated a World Heritage Site by UNESCO.

The forest is deliberately left untouched to preserve its virgin state. Ancient trees lie where they fall, to be overgrown by climbing plants, mosses and fungi. There is a rich, pungent dampness in the air, and the forest floor is frequently waterlogged. Peat bogs and marshes form open areas among the trees and along the banks of streams and rivers. This park is one of Europe's best inland wetlands.

The survival of the Bialowieza Forest is due to a long tradition of

A remaining fragment of ancient European forest, Bialowieza is a haven for small herds of bison. The animals graze on trees and bushes as well as ground plants. A full-grown bull is a powerful animal and can weigh more than 2,200 pounds (1,000 kg).

> *"King of the forest, the European bison looms out of the shadows like a dark ghost from an earlier age"*

protection going back to at least the 15th century. Generations of rulers – first the dukes of Ruthenia and Lithuania, then the kings of Poland, and finally the tsars of Russia – claimed the forest as their personal hunting grounds. Local inhabitants were forbidden to enter the forest lands to hunt or gather firewood.

By the beginning of the 19th century, the Bialowieza Forest was

Bialowieza contains broad-leaved and coniferous trees at all stages of growth. Flourishing in the rich earth, saplings shoot up tall and thin as they reach for the sky beyond the forest canopy.

already the last refuge of the European bison, which had once flourished from the Atlantic coasts of Europe to the China seas. Displaced by forest clearances across the continent, the last few hundred bison survived in the dark and impenetrable glades of Bialowieza – culled only by royal hunting parties – until the revolutions and wars of the early 20th century brought the first real threat for half a millennium to the forest and its inhabitants.

World War I saw the cutting of millions of cubic yards of ancient timber and the decimation of game, including the bison, for meat. The national park was created in 1921,

too late to save the last forest bison, which was shot in the same year. That would have been the end of the story for this primeval beast had there not existed around 60 bison which had been donated to various zoos and private game reserves.

A breeding program, using animals originating from the Bialowieza herd, was begun in 1929, and the first small herd was released back into the wild in 1956. There are now more than 250 wild bison living in the park in the Polish sector of the forest, and a somewhat larger herd in the Belorus sector. The European bison has a humped back, broad head and a tangled mane that includes a beard. Its horns are shorter and broader than those of its American cousin.

The forest is the green lung of a country which has had a bad record of industrial pollution. It is bracketed by the headwaters of the Narew and Lesna rivers, tributaries of the Bug, and the deep, rich soil nourishes immense trees, some of them 500 years old. Oaks and limes soar to 130 feet (40 m) in height, topped only by giant spruces 160 feet (50 m) tall. In total, some 26 species of tree contribute to the forest's great mass. There is also an abundance of flowering plants, with more than 550 species representing over 25 percent of the country's flora.

The birdlife of the forest reflects its physical makeup and the great range of available foods. Five different varieties of woodpecker noisily work the trees for grubs and insects, while the glades, swamps and river meadows are the domain of predators which include eagle and pygmy owls, black kites, goshawks, honey buzzards and several species of eagle. Warblers live among the water plants, and flycatchers and finches feast on the teeming insect life.

Deep in the protected heart of the park, creatures that have disappeared from most of Europe still live and

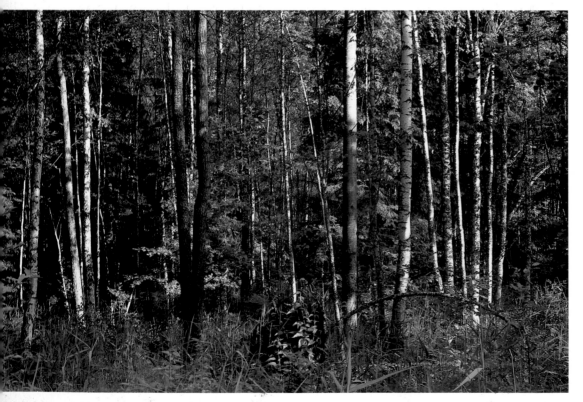

breed and graze and hunt, as they have done for thousands of years, safe from human intervention. Lanky elk wade through the marshes to feed on lush tangles of water foliage. Families of wild boar, guarded by huge old patriarchs, rip up the black soil for roots. Wolves and lynxes slip through the trees like wraiths, seldom seen by visitors. In the rivers, otters prey on the two dozen varieties of fish, while rare European beavers fell saplings and build their dams and lodges. Beavers have succeeded in crossing the border back into the Polish part of the forest after disappearing from there in the early part of this century.

Another great rarity is the stocky tarpan horse, a wild ancestor of the domestic horse, which became completely extinct early this century. Selective breeding of cross-bred zoo specimens has produced an animal which closely resembles the original tarpan, and a small herd is being raised within the park.

But the bison remains the great success story of the Bialowieza Forest. These great beasts are quietly thriving in the depths of this remote reserve. The undisputed kings of the forest, they loom out of the shadows like dark ghosts from an earlier age. The historical record of the European bison goes back to cave drawings of the last ice age. The great triumph of Bialowieza is that it is possible to step into the dark glades of this primeval forest and come face to face with a majestic creature that roamed identical forests in the time of our own Stone Age ancestors.

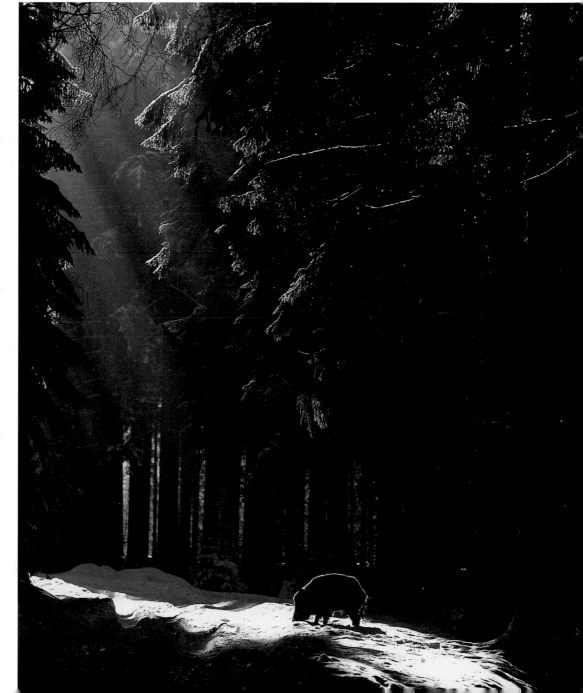

Ancient stumps and fallen trunks crowd alongside seedlings, saplings and mature trees. There is no artificial forest management.

Once the prey of royal huntsmen, who preserved the forest for their sport, the wild boar now lives peacefully in glades deep in the forest (right).

CÉVENNES NATIONAL PARK

"Granite mountains and limestone plateaus share a wildness and grandeur"

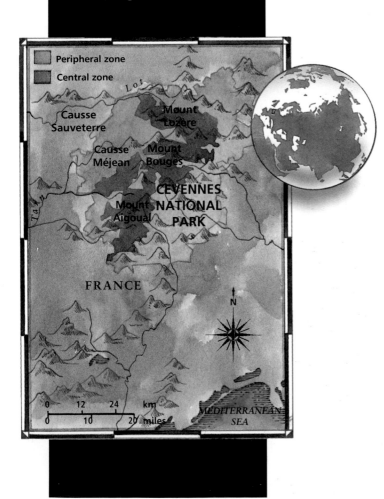

- Peripheral zone
- Central zone

Lot

Causse Sauveterre

Mount Lozère

Causse Méjean

Mount Bougès

Tarn

CÉVENNES NATIONAL PARK

Mount Aigoual

FRANCE

N

0 12 24 km
0 10 20 miles

MEDITERRANEAN SEA

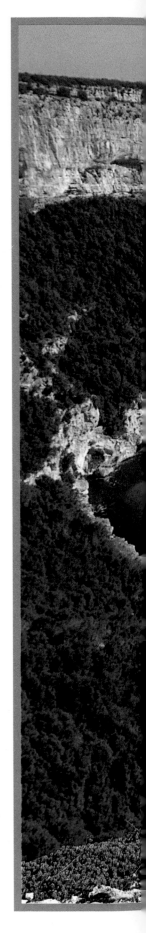

The Massif Central is a huge highland territory, covering one-sixth of France's total area, which stretches from the Loire in the north down almost to the Mediterranean in the south. Situated in the extreme southeast of the Massif Central is the Cévennes region, a thinly populated area of granite mountains and limestone plateaus. These two landscapes are completely different in character, but share a wildness and grandeur that make this a natural site for the country's largest national park.

The park, established in 1970, has a central protected zone of 225,894 acres (91,416 ha) surrounded by a peripheral zone. Some 600 villagers still live in the protected zone.

A great fault-line scarp running roughly southwest to northeast divides the Cévennes into two major watersheds and climatic zones. North and west of this line, the rivers flow toward the Atlantic and the climate is oceanic and alpine, with strong winds in the high country and icy winters. South and east of the scarp, the streams feed rivers flowing into the Mediterranean. The eastern slopes enjoy a Mediterranean climate, with hot summers and extremely wet winters and springs.

The mountains of the scarp are forested with pine, chestnut, fir, oak and beech below their rocky summits. Their lower slopes of meadow and heath blaze with wildflowers in spring, but in winter the granite and schist tops are hostile wildernesses of wind, rain and snow. Remote and

Swollen in spring with melted snow and rain, several of the great rivers in the Cévennes have carved deep gorges in the limestone cap. Unpolluted and difficult of access, these river gorges are an ideal refuge for wildlife such as beavers and otters, as well as for rare birds of prey.

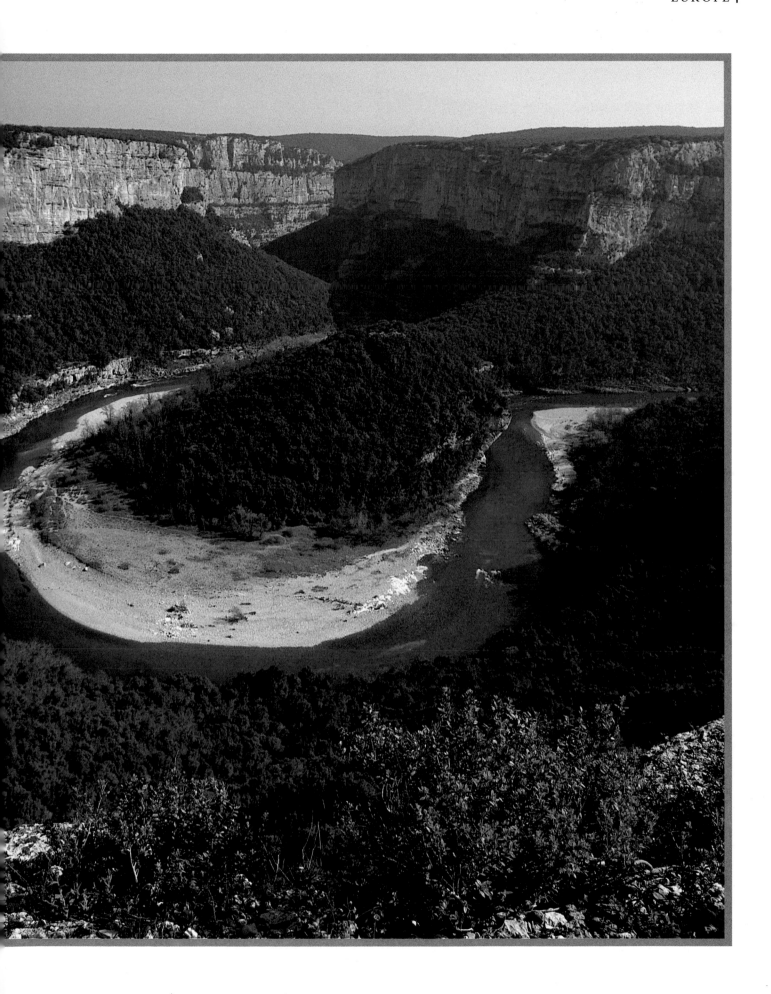

wild, these uplands have historically been a refuge for fugitives and guerrilla fighters and are now an ideal sanctuary for wild creatures.

West of the scarp, in the Atlantic watershed, the landscape changes dramatically. Instead of the ancient granite and schist bedrocks of the mountains, a much more recent limestone surface caps the strange plateaus of the Causses region. In fact, this is one great plateau, divided into a series of "causses" by the deeply carved gorges of the rivers flowing west toward the Atlantic Ocean.

The Causses are windswept table-lands with sparse vegetation and no surface water. Winters here are bleak and bitterly cold. The dry summers can be bakingly hot. In the fall torrential rain soaks straight down through the permeable limestone until it reaches a water-resistant layer over which it can run. Over millennia, the mildly acidic rain has eaten out subterranean networks of rivers and caves in the soluble limestone. Within these caves, dripping water has deposited minerals leached from the rock to build fantastic structures of stalactites and stalagmites.

"Historically a refuge for fugitives and guerrilla fighters, these uplands are now an ideal sanctuary for wild creatures"

The peaks lying along the central scarp of the Cévennes each has its own character. Mount Lozère is in the north of the park, a huge granite mass with a wide mound of a summit where the bare upland grass slopes are interrupted by piles of gigantic granite boulders. The decline of grazing has encouraged heathers and shrubs to begin the long task of recolonizing the dense grass mat of

the upper slopes. Lozère is the region's highest peak at 5,574 feet (1,699 m), with stunning views over the entire Cévennes hill country to the south.

Mount Bouges lies just southwest of Lozère. The north-facing slopes of Bouges are granite, and well forested between 1,640 and 4,600 feet (500 and 1,400 m). Evergreens are the predominant trees, interspersed with beech forests. The southern slopes of the mountain are of schist, and the terrain is typical of the Midi, with steep, sun-bleached ravines, and groves of chestnut and scrub oak.

Mount Aigoual means "the watery mountain" and lives up to its name. Its annual rainfall of 89 inches (2,250 mm) makes it the wettest place in France. Occupying the southwestern end of the scarp, Aigoual bears the brunt of the rains released as the Atlantic and Mediterranean air currents converge. The climate here is Mediterranean on the southern side, with steep valleys and chestnut groves. The long, dry summers are in marked contrast to the deluges of winter.

To the north, the mountain is rich in conifers such as Scots and Austrian pine, Norway spruce and larch. The slopes on Aigoual's northern side are far less steep than those on the south and extend to meet the limestone plateaus of the Causses.

The limestone cap of the Causses was laid down when the region was covered by sea in the Jurassic age. Nowadays, the only water to be found is deep in underground caves and channels, or in the rivers that swirl through the deep gorges to divide the limestone like the slices of a cake. In the park, the Causse Sauveterre lies

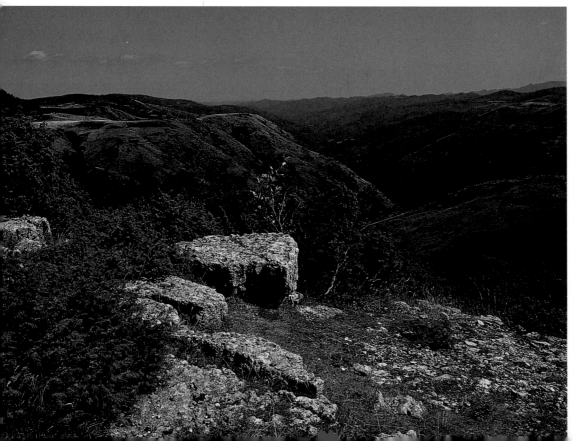

The exposed plateaus and moorlands of the Cévennes region suffer severely cold winters. The plants which do manage to survive among these gale-blasted mountainous outcrops are hardy and stunted.

between the rivers Lot and Tarn, and the Causse Méjean lies between the Tarn and the Jonte. The River Tarn runs through a spectacular series of steep-sided gorges towering above the rushing river for more than 30 miles (50 km) on its way west. Despite harsh extremes of winter and summer weather, the Causses put on tremendous displays of wildflowers in the spring, including wild tulips, pasque flowers and dwarf daffodils.

The centuries-long erosion of wild habitat in the Cévennes gradually led to the extinction of some wildlife species, but there has been an effort over the second half of the 20th century to reestablish some of them. The mountains and gorges are ideal environments for some of the larger soaring birds, and both griffon vultures and bearded vultures (also known as lammergeiers) have been reintroduced into the park.

Other reintroductions include red deer, roe deer and European beaver. By the beginning of the 20th century, the beaver had become almost extinct in France, but from a small population surviving on stretches of the Rhône, it was brought back to several regions, including streams in the Mediterranean watershed of the Cévennes. In 1977 the beaver was introduced to waters on the other side of the scarp.

The steep, rocky terrains of the Cévennes in all their diversity have preserved it from the excesses of commercial exploitation and tourism, It remains an impressive wilderness as well as a superb wildlife reserve, with a wide spectrum of upland habitats and landscapes.

Snow and rain soaking through the porous surface of the Causses have created cathedral-like caverns. Water seeping into these caves dissolves calcium and mineral salts, redepositing them as stalagmites and stalactites.

THE LAMMERGEIER

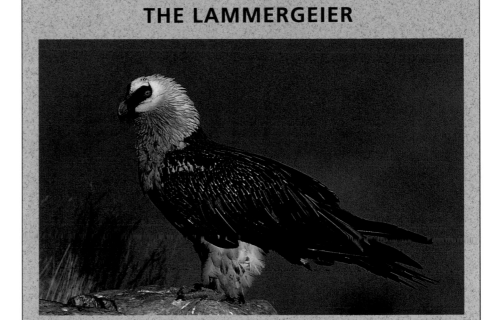

The magnificent lammergeier lives in remote mountainous areas of Europe, Africa and Asia. Now rare in Europe, lammergeiers had disappeared from the Cévennes, but have been successfully reintroduced into the park, where they are strictly protected.

Lammergeiers, also known as bearded vultures because of the bristles on each side of the beak, soar on their long, narrow wings over the precipitous river gorges of the region. Like most vultures, they do not usually kill prey, but feed on carrion – the remains of dead animals. They often shatter the bones of carcasses to get at the marrow they contain by dropping them from a great height onto rocks below. Lammergeiers also kill small rodents and birds.

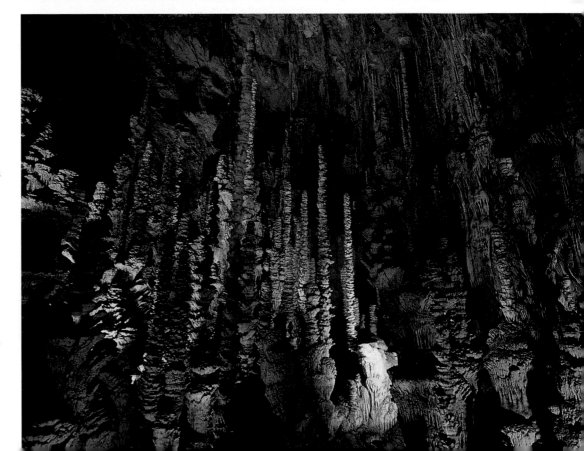

COTO DOÑANA

"Winter rains flood the great plain to create marshes stretching as far as the eye can see"

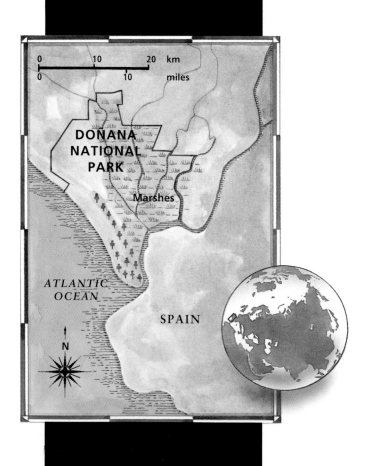

A magnificent wilderness of coastal dunes, marshes, scrubland and sandy heath, the Doñana National Park, in the province of Huelva, is Spain's largest protected park. The region, covering more than 292 sq. miles (757 km²), was once the delta of the Guadalquivir River, which forms the park's southeastern border. A constantly growing sandbar, sculpted into moving dunes by the prevailing

The tranquil and undisturbed wetlands of Coto Doñana provide seashore, dune, flood plain and forest habitats for a wide range of birds and reptiles.

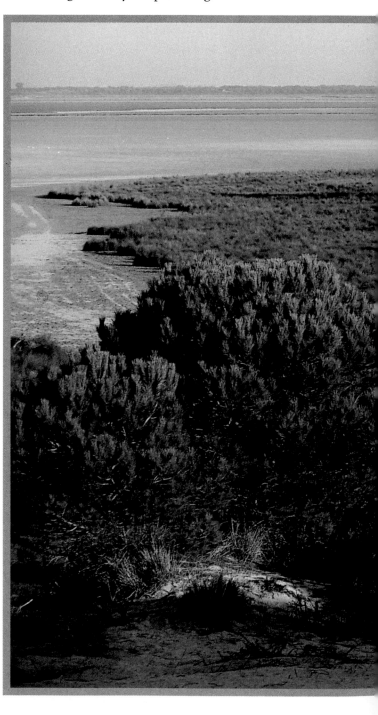

winds, has sealed off most of the delta from the sea, creating a unique barrier. This sandbar contains the vast marshes which make the Coto Doñana park perhaps the most important wetland site in Europe.

When the autumn and winter rains flood the great flat plain to a uniform depth of some 12–24 inches (30–60 cm), the marshes, or *marismas,* of the Coto Doñana stretch as far as the eye can see. Small islands known as *vetas* stay dry throughout the year, providing nest sites for many birds.

But at the height of summer, the marshes dry out in the blistering sun, reminding visitors that this corner of Spain is Europe's closest point to the African continent. What in the wet season was an area of hundreds of square miles of shallows is reduced to three long, canal-like, permanent bodies of water – once delta arms of the Guadalquivir – a few permanent lagoons, some stagnant pools and vast expanses of rapidly baking mud. The reduced waters in the pools can become so contaminated by concentrations of bacteria that they are lethal to water birds.

The great dunes of the Doñana sandbar vary in width between 330 feet (100 m) and 3,300 feet (1,000 m) across the base. Little by little, these dunes are migrating inland as their peaks and ridges are broken down by

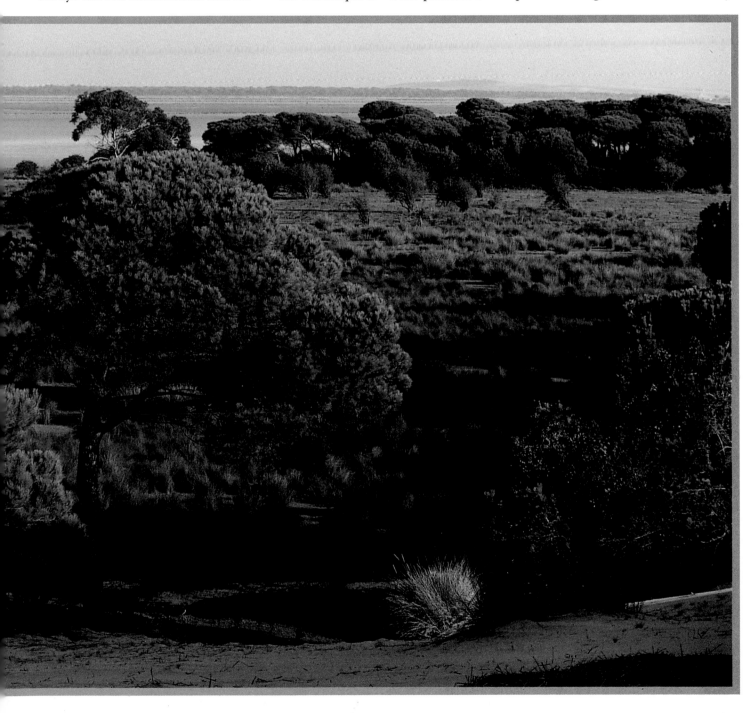

winds from the sea. Each year they can move as much as 20 feet (6 m), and anything in their path is buried. Even the sturdy stone pines in the woodlands that border the dunes sometimes fall victim to the sand. The dunes form a barrier all around the tree, eventually burying it completely.

Doñana's proximity to the narrow Strait of Gibraltar makes it a vital gathering, resting and feeding ground for birds which need to take the shortest possible migratory route between Africa and the European mainland. Large-winged birds such as kites and eagles are not able to make the long ocean crossings undertaken by some migrants – they need to rest during journeys by gliding. To do this, they require the thermal currents that are created only over land to carry them high enough to glide without losing too much altitude.

The Doñana National Park is, therefore, particularly rich in large birds of prey, some of them extremely rare. The most celebrated – and the most rare – is the imperial eagle. These majestic birds, with wingspans of up to 82 inches (210 cm), pair for life, and return to the same nest each year. There are at least 15 pairs of imperial eagles in the park – one-third of the entire Spanish population. Other birds of prey include booted eagles, short-toed eagles, red, black and black-winged kites, Egyptian vultures and griffon vultures.

Practically all known species of European waterfowl appear in Doñana during the winter and the main migration periods. The rich wetlands have become even more important to these visitors as other marshy regions of the Spanish coast have been drained for agricultural purposes. Rare crested coots breed in the park, and flocks of flamingos come in winter to feast on the shrimps of the brackish lagoons.

Doñana is also renowned for its populations of herons, egrets and

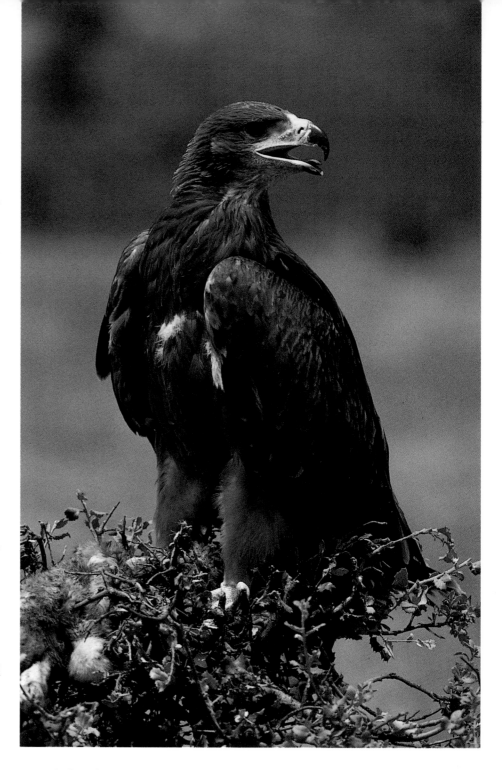

spoonbills. The cork oaks, which thrive on the acid soils of Andalusia, are favorite nesting trees of these social birds, which gather in noisy colonies in the tree tops.

The successive wet and dry environments of Doñana suit reptiles as well as birds, and the park is home to the spur-thighed tortoise and two species of terrapin, as well as many snakes and lizards. Short-toed eagles, armed with tough head feathers to ward off venomous bites, feed on the snakes.

The rare Iberian imperial eagle has one of its few remaining refuges in the Coto Doñana, where it nests on cliff ledges and at the tops of tall trees. It soars high on its broad wings in search of rabbits, which are its main food.

An abundance of predators is always a good sign in any wild environment, since it indicates flourishing populations of prey creatures. Doñana is one of the final refuges of the Iberian lynx. More

LAND OF SHIFTING DUNES

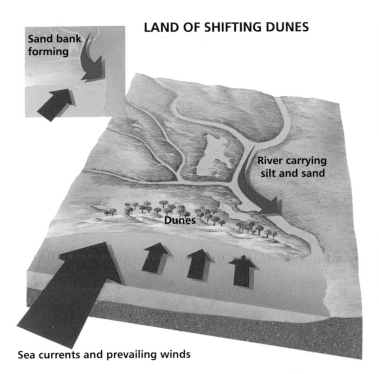

Sand bank forming

River carrying silt and sand

Dunes

Sea currents and prevailing winds

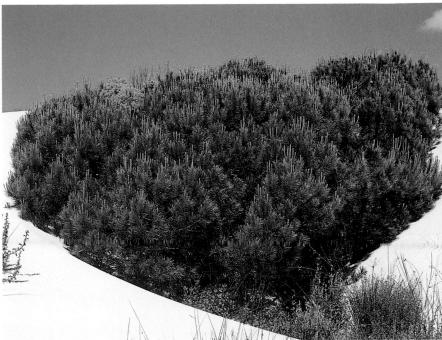

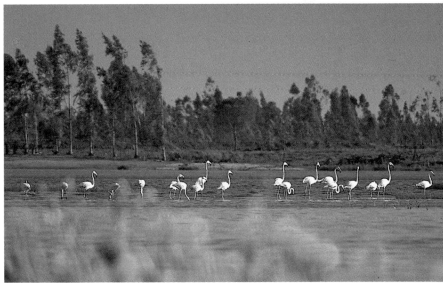

Coto Doñana is an ancient delta, enclosed by deposits of silt and sand. Over centuries the river has washed down huge quantities of soil which clogged all but the main channel and built up a barrier across the delta mouth. Sea currents and prevailing winds have created a beach along the barrier and piled the sand into dunes.

As the shifting dunes move steadily inland, they surround and bury stone pines growing in their path (above right).

Brackish lagoons and mud flats are ideal homes for noisy colonies of flamingos (right).

than 25 pairs of these stealthy hunters roam the park scrubland, preying on rabbits, water birds and deer calves. Wild cats, polecats, otters, foxes and Egyptian mongooses are other mammalian predators in Doñana.

Up until the early 1960s, Coto Doñana was entirely without access roads. The huge wild area, containing heaths and woodlands flanking flood land or muddy marshes according to the season, was unappealing to impatient developers and much too expensive to turn into agricultural land. In 1969 the region became a national park so that this unique environment and its inhabitants would be protected.

Although rich in wildlife and natural terrains, Doñana is a wilderness under a number of serious threats. Wetlands are notoriously susceptible to disruption, having a complex and delicate balance of seasonal water supply, plants and animals. Water flowing southward into the park from the agricultural developments to the north is vulnerable both to diversion and to pollution. In 1986, some 30,000 birds died in the park as a result of an inflow of agricultural pesticides.

Other threats come from the growing pressures of tourism around the park. The dunes at the nearby resort of Matalascanas have been destroyed by people walking on them, and straying wildlife, including rare lynxes, faces a greater risk of being run over by increased local traffic. Summer tourism is also a drain on water resources, just at the time of year when drought is most likely. Doñana is a superb reserve of international importance, but it is also a good example of the warning that erecting a fence around a site is no guarantee of its security and survival.

THE EMPTY QUARTER

"Lying at the heart of southern Arabia is the greatest continuous sand desert in the world"

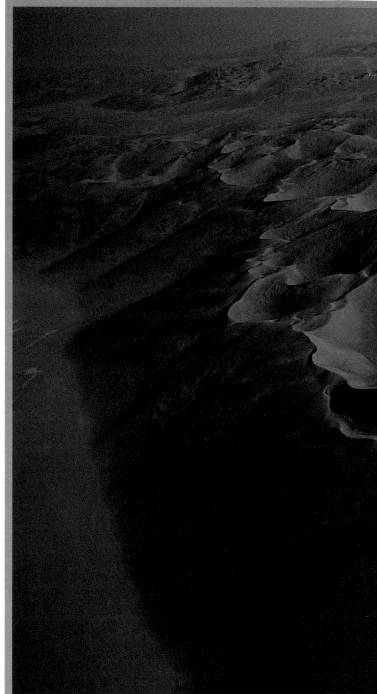

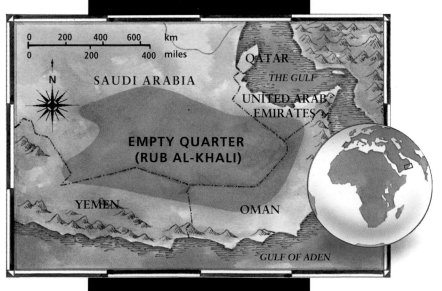

The name could hardly be more expressive. Rub al-Khali, the "Empty Quarter" of Arabia, is the very essence of wilderness. In a part of the world that cradled early civilizations, where the paths of adventurers, traders and wandering peoples have crossed for thousands of years, this region has remained forbidding and

The vast sand sea of the Empty Quarter is so difficult for human travelers to penetrate that, even into this century, much of it remains unexplored.

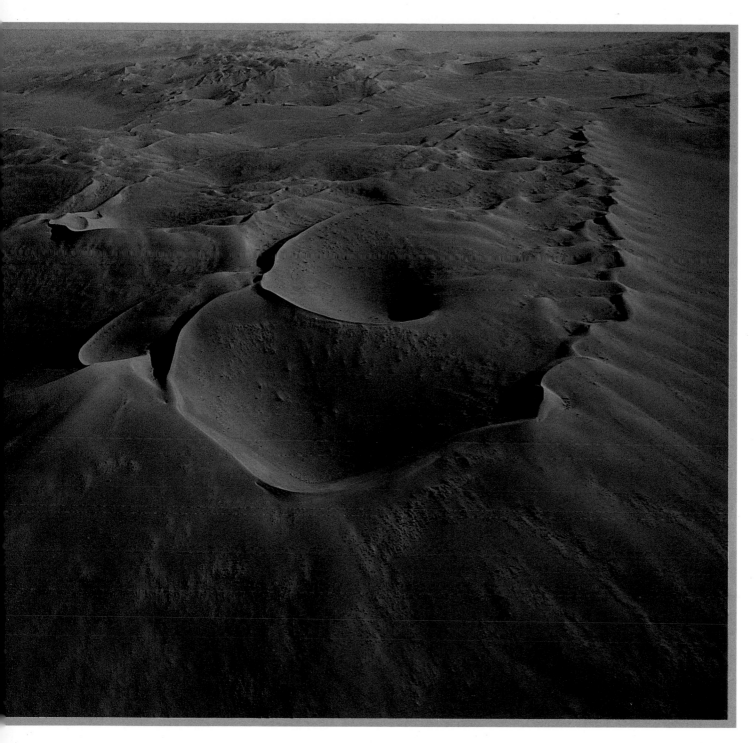

unknown, an empty desert of towering sands and blistering heat. Only scattered Bedouin tribes dared to penetrate this land, but even they could not linger there during the intolerably hot months of summer.

Lying at the heart of southern Arabia, the Rub al-Khali is the greatest continuous sand desert in the world. Up to 300 miles (500 km) wide, it stretches for some 700 miles (1,100 km) across Saudi Arabia east into Oman. Everywhere it is dry, empty and devoid of soil. Across most of the desert, the sands are sculpted into giant, ancient dunes. Between these permanent features, smaller, more mobile dunes may appear, along with the occasional small salt flat nestling in a depression in which, every few years, a puddle of rainfall briefly collects. The area, however, has not always been so arid. Large salt flats near the margins of the Rub al-Khali show where lakes once existed, and probing farther back in geological time, it is clear that conditions here have varied greatly.

Pure sand deserts such as the Rub al-Khali are not as common as is often thought. For so much sand to accumulate in one place there must have been a copious source. The bulk of the sand in the Empty Quarter probably came from volcanic highlands to the west and south. Over the millennia, as the elements gradually weathered away the exposed crystalline rock, fragments were washed downstream onto the lowlands. Winds gathered up the smaller particles and swept them farther into the interior.

Another major source in the past would have been large patches of seabed left high and dry by fluctuations in the level of the ocean to the south and east. Winds driving over the exposed sands would have transported more grains to the accumulations inland.

Those winds blowing in the same prevailing pattern for thousands of

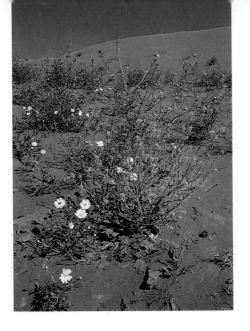

Occasional bouts of heavy rain can bring the desert into bloom. Plants spring to life (above) and, by tapping underground moisture, may stay green for months.

As desert sands absorb the intense midday heat, the surface of the dunes becomes scalding. Desert creatures must save their activity for the cooler hours.

years shaped the sands into the massive dunes that persist today. The formations are most regular in the west, where powerful winds have created a corrugated landscape of parallel ridges and troughs. Toward the center of the Rub al-Khali the pattern becomes less well defined, with more dune ridges running crosswise, while in parts of the east, complicated wind regimes have erected and sculpted huge dunes up to 1,000 feet (330 m) high.

Winds in the Rub al-Khali arm the air with abrasive sand. Daytime temperatures soar above 122°F (50°C) in summer, and no rain may fall on a patch of sand for years. Conversely, warmth escapes into the cloudless sky so fast that, after dark, a winter's night may chill below freezing.

But even this land, empty of resident humans, is far from lifeless.

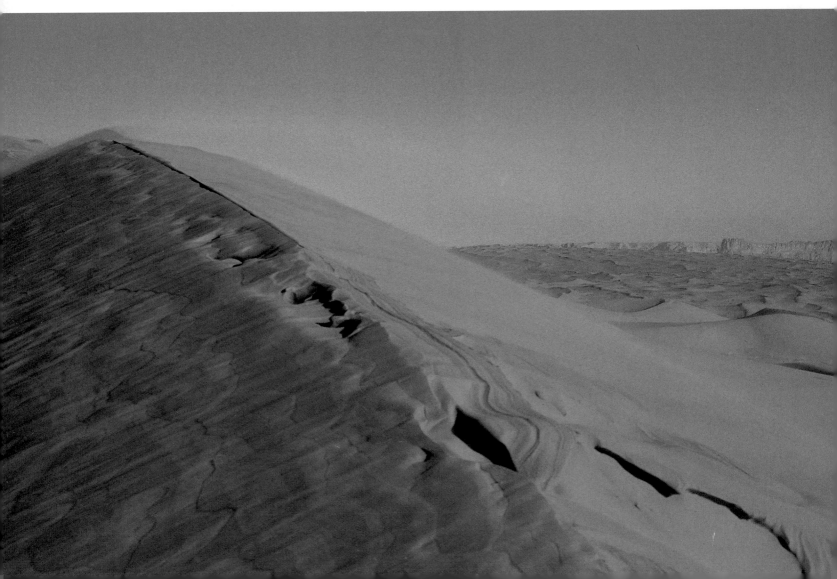

Plants appear here and there, not just as solitary clumps, but thick enough in places to create patches of greenery. At the foot of a dune, there may be small shrubs, saltbushes, tussocks of sedge and short-lived herbs. And, where there are plants, a few animals, such as beetles, butterflies, spiders, scorpions, lizards, larks, gerbils and hares, manage to survive. Still rarer are bustards, sand cats, foxes and gazelles.

One of the principal problems of survival in the desert for any organism is the permanent shortage of water. The ways in which plants and animals cope with drought reveal the sheer adaptability of desert life. Plants have two main strategies. Some are many times more extensive underground than above. They have deep probing roots to tap droplets of moisture hidden deep in the sand, but tiny leaves and stems to minimize water loss through evaporation.

Other plants lie dormant during the long droughts, either as seeds in the sand or as seemingly lifeless, shriveled stems. When a good, steady bout of rain falls, they quickly germinate or burst into greenery, their wide-spreading shallow roots making full use of the moisture before it evaporates. Within a few weeks,

they will have flowered and seeded anew. Shallow-rooted plants also benefit from morning dew.

Some desert insects live in much the same way, lying hidden in the sand in a watertight dormant phase, until stimulated into emergence by heavy rain and fresh plant growth. Larger animals keep active all year and have a remarkable ability to survive without drinking. Herbivores such as rhim gazelle gain enough moisture by eating leaves and roots and by gleaning dew from plants.

Carnivores get most of their water from the body fluids of prey – hoopoe larks, for example, from beetles, sand cats from gerbils and lizards.

Such creatures can get by with so little partly because they are able to conserve moisture. Desert-adapted mammals, for instance, tend to perspire less, urinate less and lose less water vapor when they exhale. For animals and plants simply to survive in the desolate world of the Empty Quarter demands much of nature's evolutionary ingenuity.

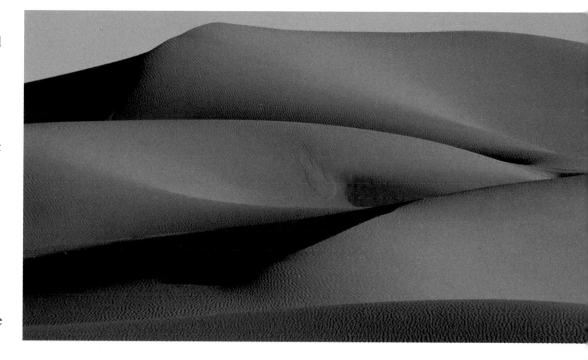

PARALLEL DUNES

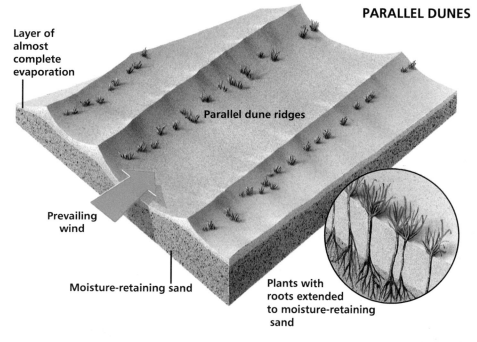

Layer of almost complete evaporation

Parallel dune ridges

Prevailing wind

Moisture-retaining sand

Plants with roots extended to moisture-retaining sand

Occasional rainfall percolates beyond the reach of evaporation, creating a layer of slightly moister sand. At the bases of parallel dunes, where this layer is closer to the surface, hardy plants with deep roots can tap just enough water to survive.

The big dunes of *the Rub al-Khali are permanent desert landmarks (above). Though winds constantly pattern their surfaces and skim grains across their crests, the underlying shape and position of these dunes changes little over the years.*

THE BEDOUIN OF RUB AL-KHALI

If any people can be said to make the Rub al-Khali their home, it is the Bedouin. These hardy nomadic people, for whom the Arabian interior has been a heartland for some 4,000 years, remain the only humans with sufficient knowledge of the dunes and of the perils of the desert to guide travelers in the Empty Quarter.

Bedouin tribes have long lived around the fringes of the zone. They venture into its heart in winter – when temperatures are more bearable – to lead their herds to the patches of scant but fresh pasture, which spring up after the occasional rains. Though the number of Bedouin who lead nomadic lives has been dwindling for decades, a few families, with little but their tents, cooking utensils and livestock, still do so in the Empty Quarter. Clothing consists of long robes and large headcloths to protect them from excessive exposure to the strong sunshine.

The Bedouin move according to the needs of their animals for pasture and for sources of water. In turn, the herds – principally camels, but also sheep and goats – provide them with nourishment in the form of milk products such as curds, buttermilk and cheese, and with meat.

Nomadism in such an open environment requires a flexible form of shelter, and the Bedouin have the perfect solution in their long, low tents of woven camel or goat hair. Easily rolled up for transportation by camel, the tent is secured with ropes over a series of upright poles. The sides can be lifted up by day to improve ventilation or lowered for privacy, warmth at night, or for protection against sandstorms. The design of the tent also reflects the hospitality customary in Bedouin culture. It has an open area to one side for socializing, receiving guests and holding tribal meetings.

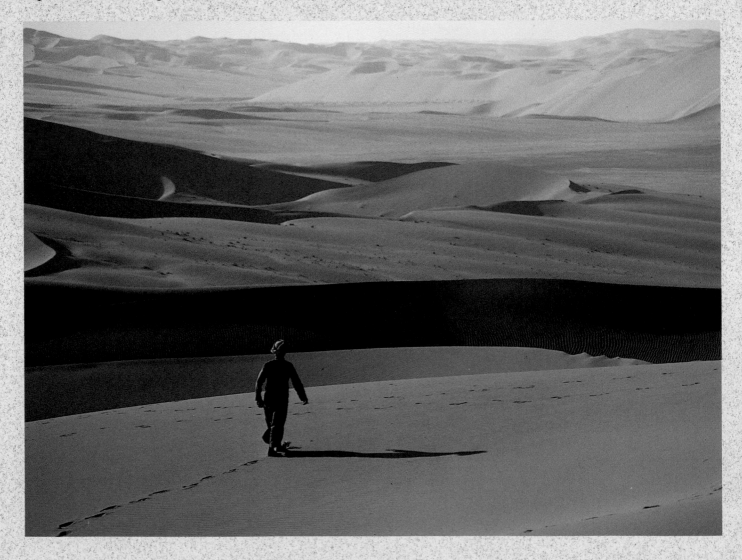

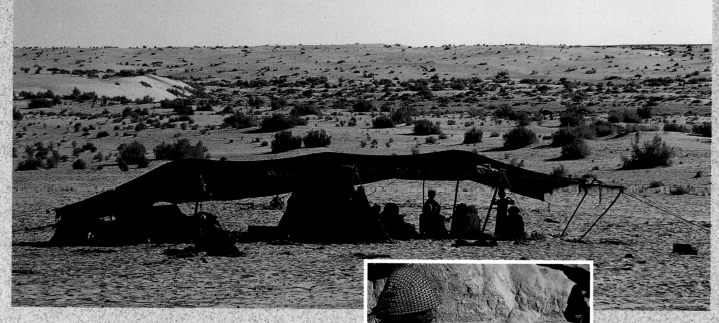

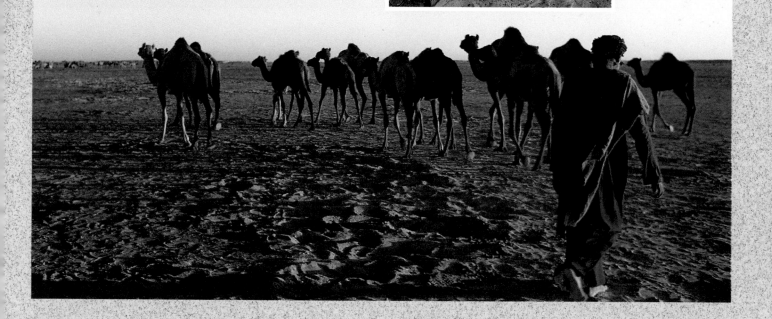

Bedouin men may set out on foot across the sands in the morning to tend their camels, not returning to the shade of their camp until evening (left).

Portable, shady and flexible in construction, the typical Bedouin tent (above) is perfectly suited to a nomadic lifestyle as well as to the harsh environment.

Containers and cooking utensils are among the few material possessions of those Bedouin who still lead traditional nomadic lives (right).

Camels have long been the mainstay of Bedouin tribes, a reliance reflected in the care with which the men tend their herds (below).

THE GOBI DESERT

"One of the world's largest arid zones, the Gobi suffers blistering heat in summer, yet bitter cold in winter"

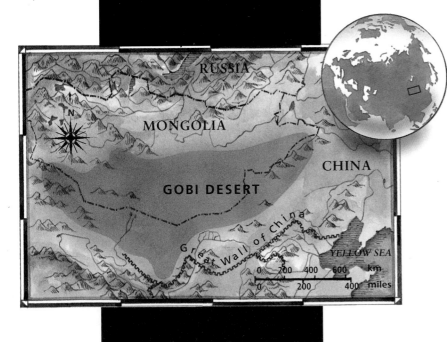

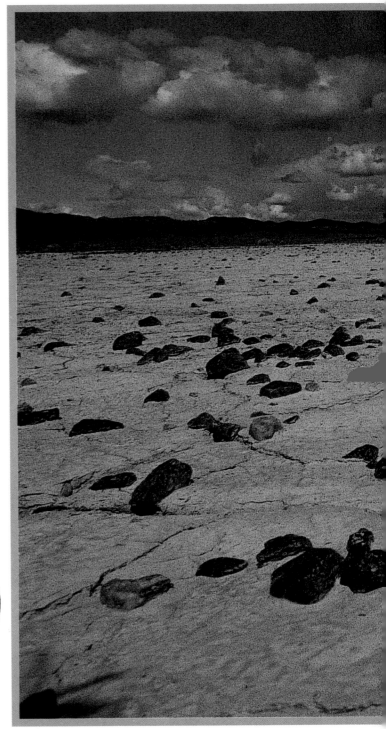

Enormous empty tracts of barren rocks, stone-littered ground and shifting sands, alternating with rolling hills and salt-encrusted depressions, characterize the lonely wilderness of the Gobi Desert. The harsh grandeur of this vast inland region, divided between Mongolia and northern

Set in the heart of the Asian continent, the bleak Gobi Desert comprises a wilderness of sand, gravel and pebble-strewn plains.

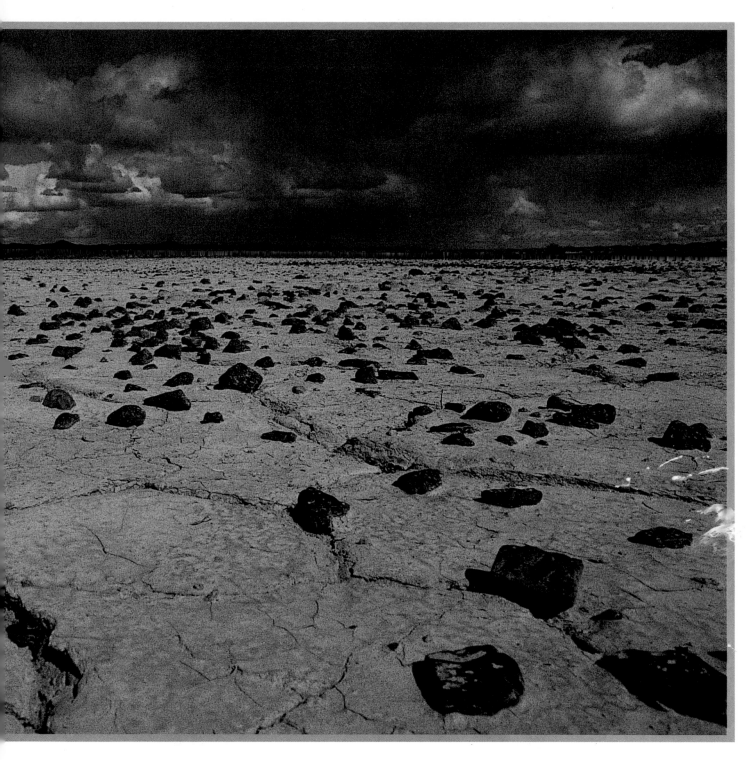

China, is accentuated not just by the aridity of its climate but also by seasonal extremes of temperature that bring blistering heat in summer, yet bitter cold in winter.

Long regarded as a forbidding natural barrier between the Russian steppes and the Chinese heartland, the Gobi Desert is one of the world's largest arid zones. From the east, where it blends in to dry grasslands, to the west, where it connects with other Asian deserts, the Gobi stretches at least 1,000 miles (1,600 km).

With an altitude varying between 2,300 and 5,000 feet (700 and 1,500 m), the Gobi forms a vast upland basin, with no river connection to the outside world. Streams flow into the Gobi from a series of high, fringing mountain ranges, but none flows out. All either dry up in the desert heat, drain into hollows filled by salty lakes or marshes, or disappear underground through coarse sand and gravel.

Subterranean water, beyond the reach of evaporation, is widespread in the Gobi. The ground surface, by contrast, is almost completely dry with little if any soil. In places, the surface is one of smooth, polished rock. Elsewhere, winds have stripped the sand away, but left behind larger stones so that the ground is dotted with pebbles.

Across large areas of the Gobi, in both rocky and sandy landscapes, plant life has scant hold. Usually it is restricted to a few grasses and herbs and stunted drought-resistant shrubs like saxaul and wormwood. Salt-tolerant plants can form more dense cover around the depressions where rainwater collects, and tamarisks may appear wherever their deep roots can tap subterranean water. Around some of the few permanent waters in the desert, oases of poplars and Siberian elms grow.

But the overwhelming impression proffered by the Gobi landscape is one of barren hills and dry plains. Few parts of the desert receive more than 8 inches (200 mm) of rain a year, and that comes in isolated showers. The dryness is mainly a result of the huge distance that prevailing winds from the west and north have to travel overland before they reach the Gobi. After crossing western Eurasia, they have hardly any moisture left to release.

With cloudless skies presenting little barrier to the sun's rays, summer daytime temperatures soar in the Gobi. At midday it can reach 113°F (45°C) in the shade, and rocks on the ground surface may be scalding to touch. The intense heat makes the desert an unwelcoming place and yet, like all deserts, the Gobi is not as empty of life as it may at first seem. Seed-hoarding rodents – mainly gerbils and jerboas – occur wherever there is some vegetation. Jerboas hide underground in their burrows during the heat of the day, waiting to emerge in the cool of night. Geckos – small, nocturnal lizards – employ the same strategy, though they venture out to hunt insects such as beetles.

Winter brings strikingly different conditions. Because of its high

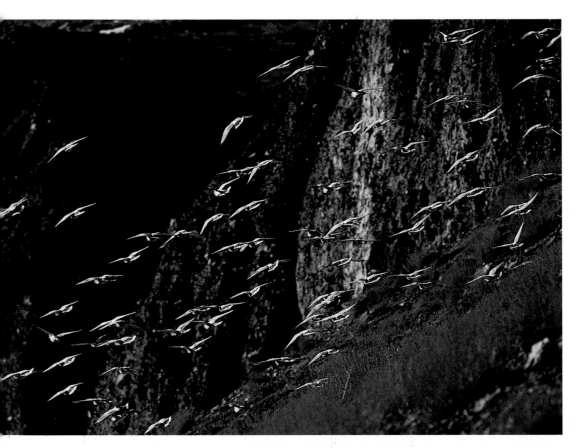

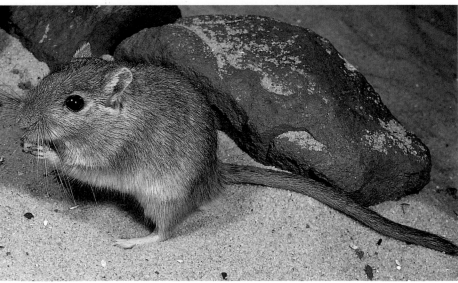

Slopes on the mountain fringes of the Gobi, where rainfall is slightly higher, can support marginally more plants and wildlife than the desert itself. Here a large flock of blue hill pigeons, at home in rugged terrain, takes flight across a steep valley.

The Mongolian gerbil is one of the most abundant animals in the Gobi Desert (left). It forages for seeds, roots and green plant matter.

The Gobi is one of the world's cold deserts. Winter snows can linger in sheltered spots until spring.

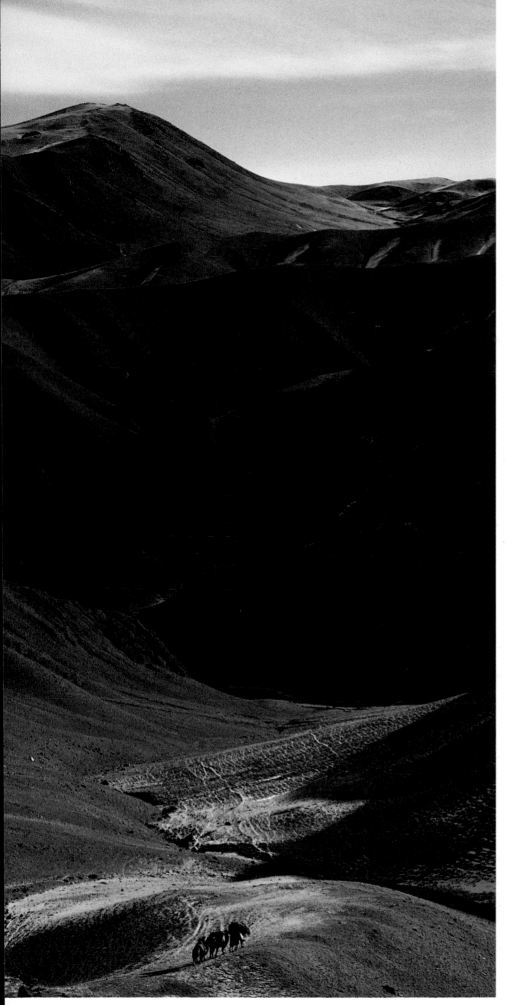

latitude, the Gobi is extremely cold in winter. Strong, chilly winds from the north sweep across the desert, bringing temperatures down at times to -40°F (-40°C). They also whip up violent sandstorms and showers of snow. For months the temperature remains below 32°F (0°C).

Many of the larger mammals that eke a living from the desert have to

> *"Chilly winds whip up violent sandstorms and sometimes bring showers of snow"*

rely on special insulation provided by body fat and thick hair if they are to survive the cold. Pallas's cat has not only long fur, but also a short nose and short legs to minimize the surface area exposed to the elements. The Bactrian camel – the two-humped central Asian species which survives in the wild only in the Gobi Desert – grows an especially long, shaggy coat ready for each winter. Such an adaptation is essential, since an animal of the size of the camel has no hope of finding shelter in the open desert environment.

Several desert birds, including Pallas's sandgrouse, desert wheatears and short-toed larks, opt for migration to avoid the worst weather. Many of them head to arid parts of southern Asia or even north Africa, places where the climatic variations are not quite as extreme as in the extraordinary hot, cold and ever-dry world of the Gobi Desert.

LAKE BAIKAL

"To refer to Baikal as a lake at all is to insult what is patently a great and powerful inland sea"

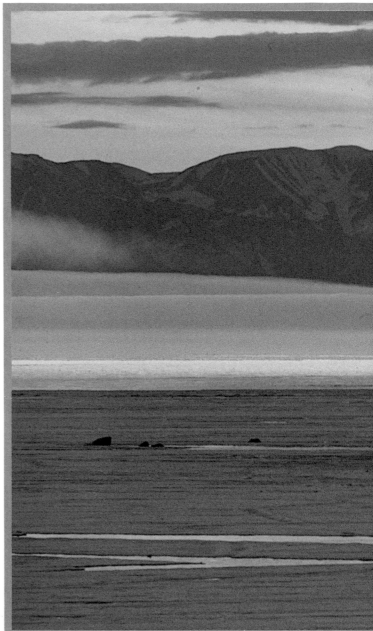

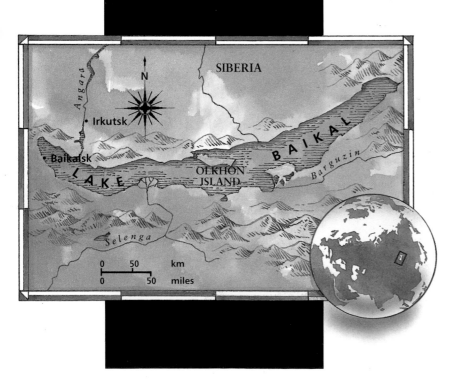

One of Russia's supreme natural treasures, Lake Baikal is set in the vast, sparsely peopled heart of Asia, near the edge of the Mongolian steppe. Stunning mountain backdrops viewed through crystal clear air create a canvas on which the waters paint their changing scenes, from stormy gray, through tranquil blue to the silvery-white glint of winter ice.

Baikal is a lake quite unlike any other: bigger, deeper and older. It fills an enormous trench in the Earth's

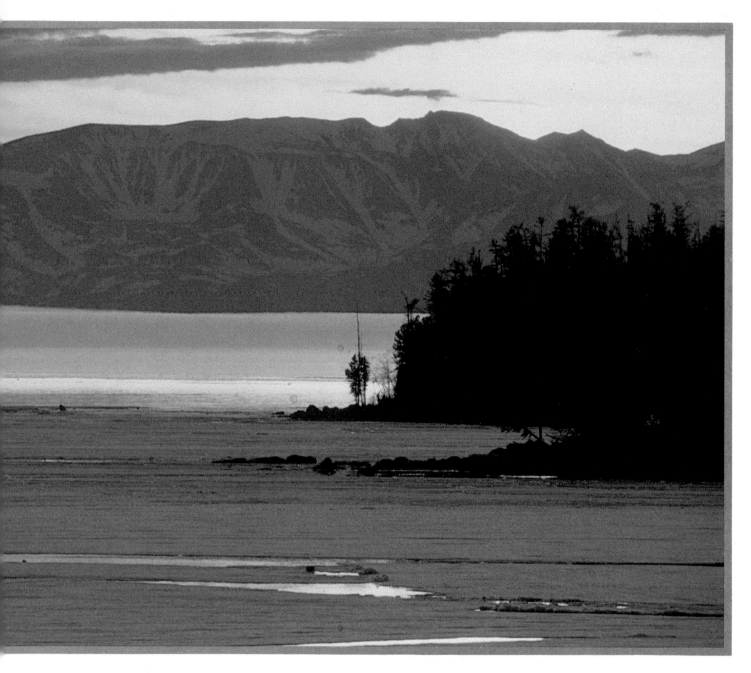

surface, and its deepest portion yet fathomed lies 5,370 feet (1,637 m) beneath the surface. Such depth, given its 395-mile (635-km) length and average width of around 30 miles (50 km), means that it holds more water than any other lake in the world – more than the five Great Lakes combined.

The lake has also been in existence for an extraordinary stretch of time. Estimates suggest that it is 25 million years old – few other lakes on Earth can be dated back more than 20,000 years. During those millions of years, flora and fauna isolated in the lake have had time to evolve myriad new forms unknown elsewhere. Baikal has about 2,500 recorded species of animals and plants, an incomparable 1,500 of which are unique to the lake.

Baikal remains cloaked in mystery and there is still much to learn of its natural history. What is known in no way diminishes the sense of wonder with which it has always been regarded. To the Buryat people who have long lived around Baikal, and

A watery wilderness, Siberia's Lake Baikal is the deepest of all lakes and holds one-fifth of all the world's fresh water. The rugged terrain encircling this great inland sea ranges from windswept mountain peaks to vast swaths of dense coniferous forest.

A RIFT IN THE EARTH'S CRUST

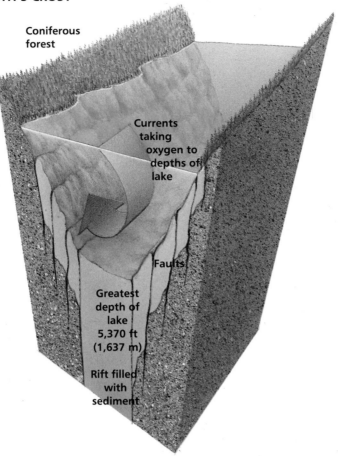

*Lake Baikal lies in
a vast rift valley,
created when
two faults in
the Earth's crust
moved apart. The
rift itself is more
than 5½ miles
(9 km) deep,
much of it filled
with sediment.
Life can live at
greater depths
here than in
other lakes. This
is because the
lake's water
is constantly
circulating,
carrying oxygen
to all parts of it.*

Coniferous forest

Currents taking oxygen to depths of lake

Faults

Greatest depth of lake 5,370 ft (1,637 m)

Rift filled with sediment

On the densely forested eastern
*shores of Baikal, a nature reserve has
been established to protect such rare
Siberian creatures as the sable, a silky-
furred relative of the weasel.*

to generations of Russian settlers in villages and towns along its wild shores, the lake is considered sacred. Indeed, to refer to Baikal as a lake at all is to insult what is patently a great and powerful inland sea.

Baikal's origins lie in the intense geological forces that stress and dislocate sections of the Earth's continental crust, fracturing fault lines and thrusting up mountain blocks. The lake occupies a deep rift valley, a huge chasm of sunken land flanked by rising blocks. To the east and to the north, the wall is especially high, forming snowbound mountain ranges rising 6,500 feet (2,000 m) and more above the lakeside.

Even the water that fills the Baikal chasm is special. More than 300 rivers drain into the lake, bringing with them heavy loads of sediment, along with all sorts of organic detritus and microorganisms. Yet the water that

drains from the lake's only outlet, the Angara River, is almost as clear as distilled water. Water lingers in the deep trough for so long – it has been suggested that incoming water may circulate through the lake for 400 years before it finally flushes out through the Angara – that the finest of sediments settle out, and lake creatures have plenty of opportunity to filter out edible particles and microbes. The lake water is so pure that local people even use it to fill their car batteries.

Winter is hard in Siberia, with temperatures dropping far below zero. Average winter temperatures around Baikal drop to -4°F (-20°C), and the surface of the lake freezes over for months on end. (A short depth below the surface, the water remains constantly cold, but fluid whatever the season.) As soon as the Siberian summer finally completes the thaw, fishing and cargo boats take

readily to the water. But all boat crews remain wary. Fierce winds howling down river valleys can churn up the water within minutes, the strongest creating treacherous waves. In summer dense banks of fog often develop over the water, obscuring all.

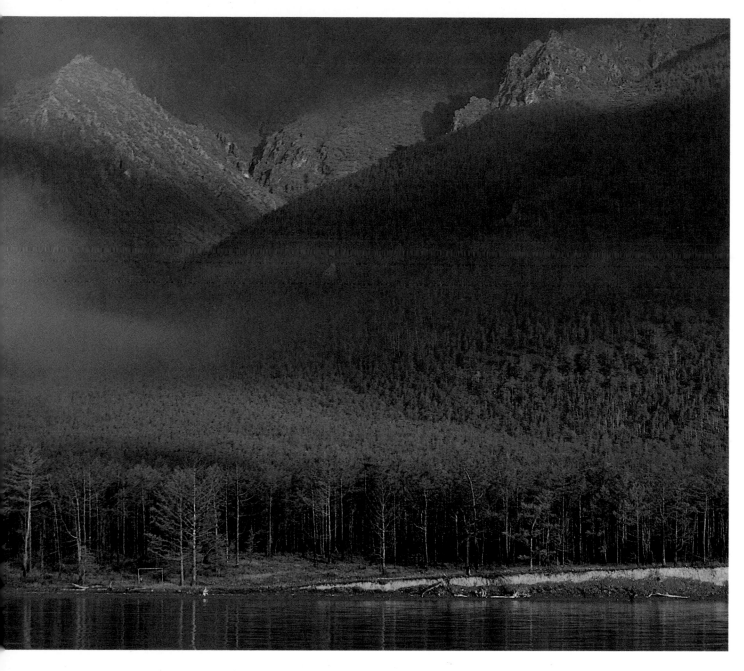

Strong winds and the sinking of chilled surface water each winter may help to explain the extraordinary degree of water circulation within Baikal. Currents take fresh oxygen to the very depths of the lake, sustaining life at all levels. In Africa's tropical Lake Tanganyika, the second-deepest lake in the world, limited circulation makes the lake virtually lifeless below 650 feet (200 m).

Far below the surface of Baikal, by contrast, organisms can survive, as long as they are adapted to the blackness and intense water pressure. More than 50 species of fish live in Lake Baikal, including the curious golomyanka, with its almost transparent body; the sturgeon; the salmon-like omul – an important food fish for the region – and no fewer than 22 species of bullheads.

Shrimp and huge columnar sponges abound in the lake. Both help keep the lake water clean by feeding on organic debris, but the creatures most responsible for Baikal's purity are the legions of tiny epischuras which filter out bacteria and algae. These minute crustaceans crowd in the water at densities of as much as 400,000 per sq. foot (3 million/m²).

Baikal has yet another zoological surprise in store. It is the home of the Baikal seal, the world's only freshwater seal species. Around 70,000 of these mammals live in the lake, feeding on fish and regularly hauling themselves out to rest on tranquil shores and islands. Quite how seals came to reside so far inland is uncertain, but it has been suggested that their ancestors may have migrated from the Arctic up one of the great Siberian rivers during one of the ice ages.

The Baikal seal may be the only mammal living in the lake, but many others dwell in the wild, forested slopes that ring its shores. These forests, dominated around Baikal by larch, birch and pine, are part of the taiga – the vast belt of coniferous forest that stretches across Siberia. This is the realm of sables, brown bears, lynx and elks, of grouse and owls, of crowlike nutcrackers and the black woodpeckers.

To protect such creatures, several reserves and two national parks have been designated on Baikal's shores. The need to protect the lake's natural riches has become ever more pressing as increasing numbers of people have

> *"Fierce winds can churn up the water within minutes, creating towering treacherous waves"*

settled in the region and industrial development has expanded in a way at odds with Baikal's fragile purity. By the 1950s and 1960s, pressure from fishing led to a collapse in the stocks of omul. Logging on the forested slopes increased siltation, and the practice of floating rafts of logs has resulted in many sinking, clogging rivers and bays.

Worse still, effluent from factories and urban waste, some of it carried to the lake from upstream, has brought

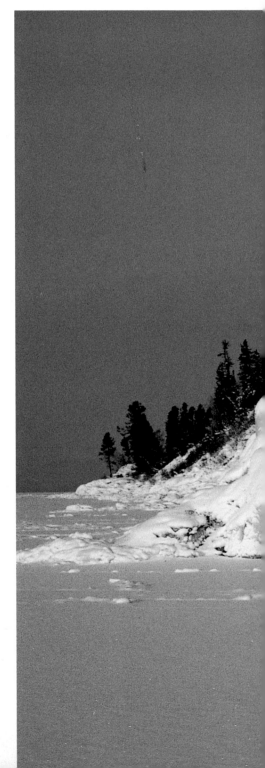

A FOREST OF SPONGES

Baikal water is the purest in the world, and the swaying forest of bright green, freshwater sponges which live on the lake bed at a depth of more than 650 feet (200 m) helps guarantee this purity. As they feed, these sedentary creatures filter tiny organisms such as bacteria and algae from the water, thus preventing it from becoming laden with clogging green slime.

Legions of freshwater shrimp living on the sponges also eat such debris and even clean the filtering pores of the sponges, so increasing their efficiency.

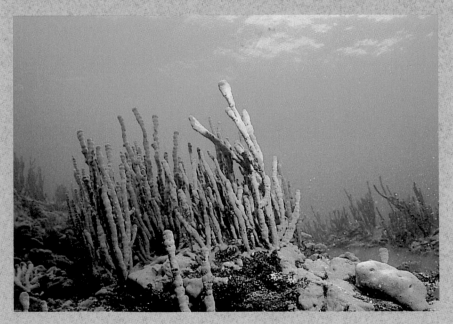

toxic pollution, killing some sections of the lake bed and hampering the recovery of fish stocks. Many polluting sources are to blame, but most notorious is the Baikalsk cellulose plant, which has discharged thousands upon thousands of tons of effluent into the air and water.

Years of protest against the plant and of concern for Baikal's ecosystem in general have at least mitigated some of the damage. Effluents are now treated more thoroughly at Baikalsk than when the plant first opened, and fishing and logging are more closely regulated than before. But most Baikal people feel that much more change is needed.

A lake ecosystem founded on the purity of water that lingers in the basin for hundreds of years simply has no room for industries that pollute or despoil. As local people campaign for their environment, scientists continue to probe for better knowledge of this remarkable watery wilderness. Lake Baikal is still a magnificent jewel of nature, but it is one whose luster could so easily fade.

In winter, when temperatures plummet, Baikal freezes over. But Baikal water is so pure that, although the ice can be more than 3 feet (1 m) thick, it is almost as clear as glass.

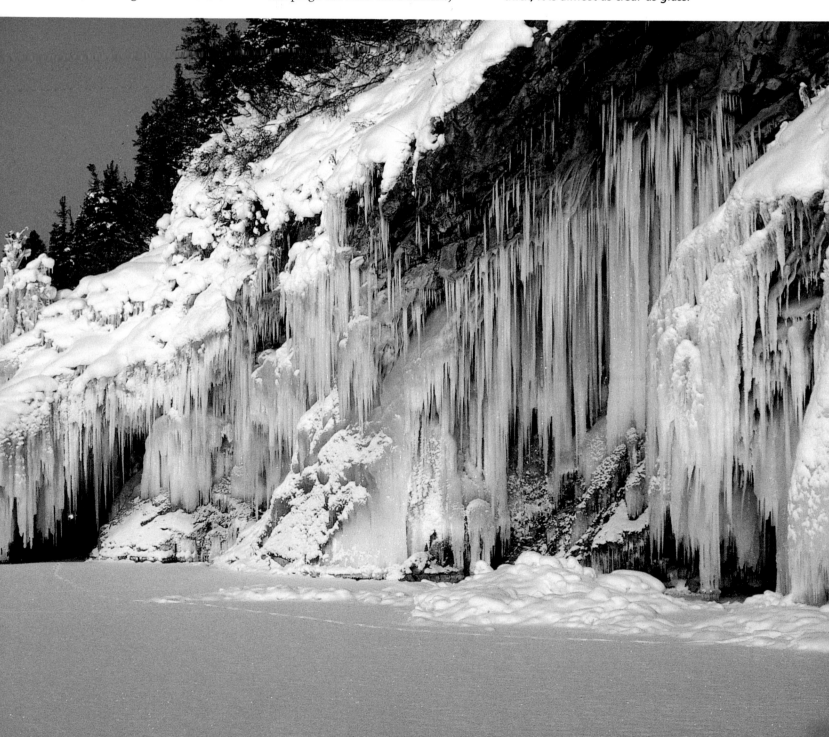

THE FISHERMAN
OF BAIKAL

For the people of Baikal, the lake is more than a vast expanse of water. It is a friend, a provider, even a symbol of spirituality. People's lives are linked to the lake, and they depend on its bounty.

Fish are a vital food source in this harsh Siberian environment, and fishing is a traditional way of life. There are more than 50 sorts of fish in Baikal, but perch, grayling and the salmonlike omul are the bulk of the catch. The omul lives only in Baikal and is a great local delicacy, at its best roasted over an open fire on the lake shores.

But Baikal is volatile and can suddenly change from friend to foe when the mighty storms strike. Winds, such as the *sarma*, can whip up in an instant, lashing the lake's calm waters into a violent frenzy and making the fishermen fear for their lives.

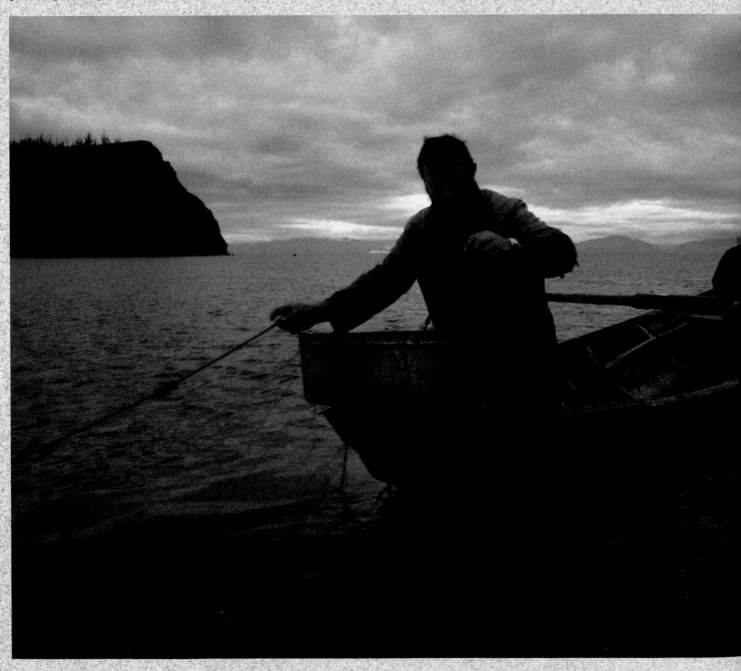

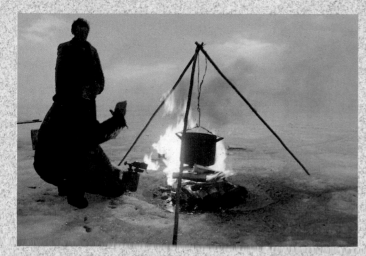

Fishing continues even when Lake Baikal is frozen over in the depths of winter. Fishermen go out onto the ice and cast their nets through holes broken in the surface. Here, some of the day's catch is being cooked over a fire lit on the frozen shores.

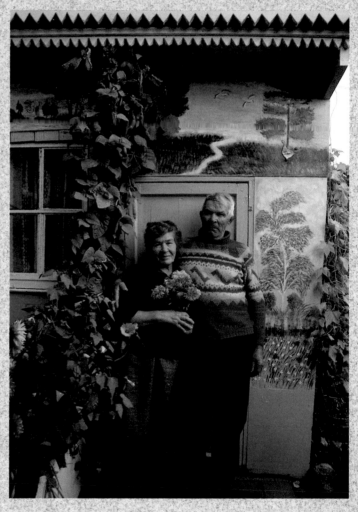

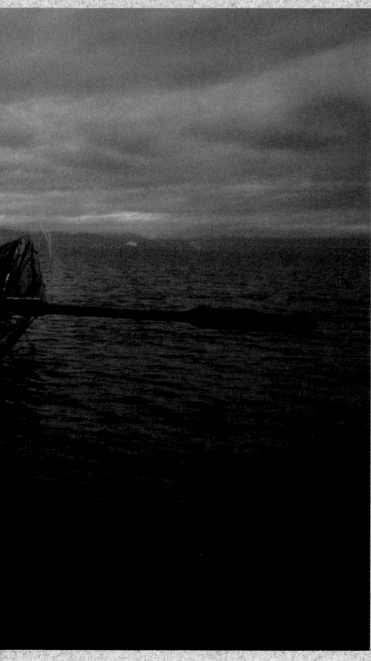

Baikal's deep waters are bitingly cold, and even at the height of summer there are no easy pickings (left). Much of the summer catch is preserved by smoking or salting and is then stored for use in the winter months, when food can be extremely hard to come by.

After a life spent fishing in Baikal's pure waters, this retired fisherman (above) tends his cottage on the shores of the lake that he loves . Over his door is a painting of this "Pearl of Siberia," as the locals call the lake – a constant reminder of its beauty and power.

THE
PAMIRS

"Lines of towering peaks soar above deep ravines carved by torrential rivers"

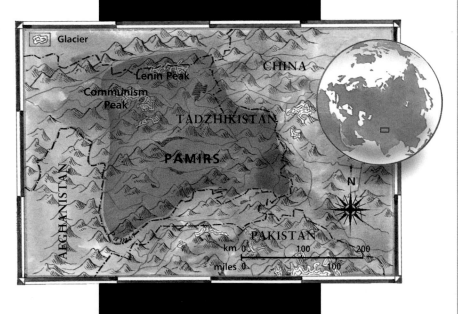

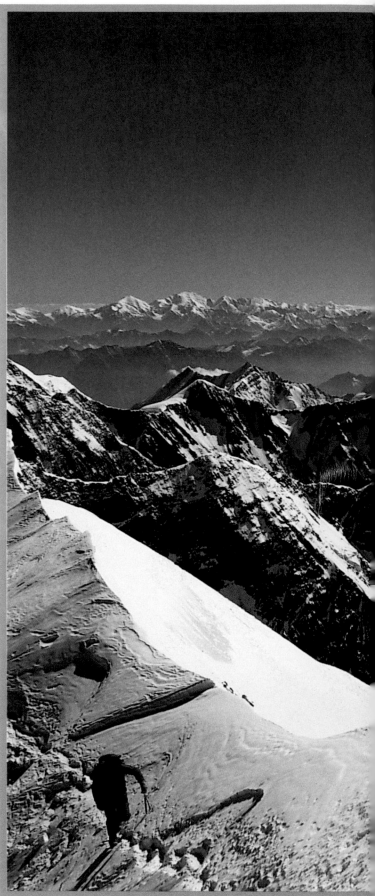

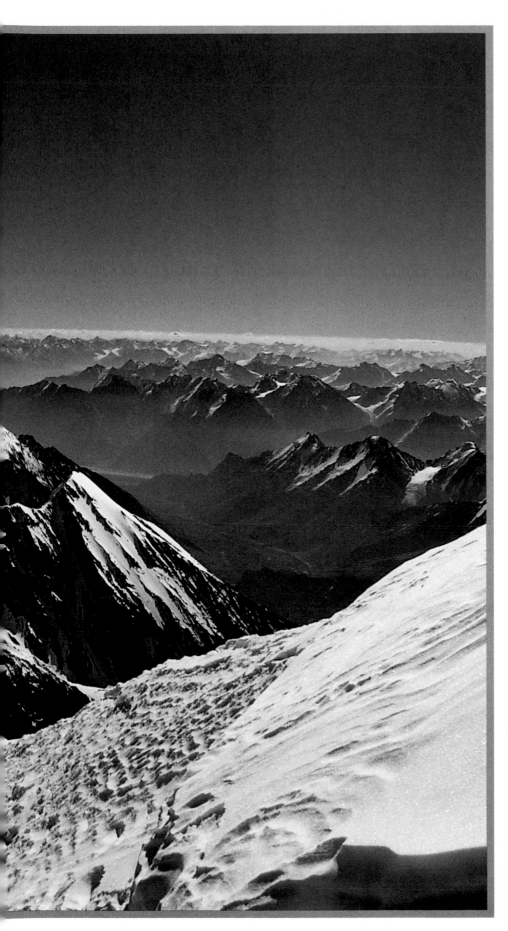

Startling scenic contrasts characterize the mountains of the Pamirs, at the heart of central Asia. In this remote landscape, the scenes juxtaposed by nature are often unexpected. A towering, jagged crest may rise from gentle slopes that lead into a broad, shallow lake; the icy glint of a gray-white glacier may reach out across a sandy brown plain devoid of moisture.

The Pamirs form a great uplifted rectangle of highland at least 155 miles (250 km) across, occupying the eastern half of the Republic of Tadzhikistan. Apart from a series of long, narrow valleys in the west, almost all the land within the Pamirs is more than 10,000 feet (3,000 m) above sea level.

A complex of spectacular ridges – some running west to east, others north to south – raise their peaks much higher still. The tallest, Communism Peak, stands at a mighty 24,590 feet (7,495 m). Like many of the mountain chains, it is mantled with permanent ice descending into valleys as glacier tongues. One of them, the immense Fedchenko glacier, stretches for 48 miles (77 km).

The Pamirs, impressive enough in themselves, stand at the meeting point of several great central Asian ranges: the Himalayas, the Karakorams, the Kunlun, the Tien Shan, the Gissaro-Alai and the Hindu Kush. Where the chains meet, so do their fauna and flora, mixing to give the Pamirs a cross section of life from different quarters. Nevertheless, the wild community is sparse. Cold, dry and stony, the Pamirs present a testing

From the towering summit of Communism Peak, the view stretches across countless crests and ridges in the western Pamirs. Thick yearly deposits of snow on these lofty mountains help to nourish permanent ice caps and as many as 3,000 glaciers.

habitat in which only the most hardy plants and animals can survive.

The tremendous height of the present-day Pamirs is testament to the power of geological movements that have warped and dislocated the entire central Asian mountain system into being. On the evidence of frequent earthquakes in the Pamir region, the mountain-building pressures may still be at work. But the process of uplift is not the only one in action. Erosion, which always works at a faster rate in mountain areas, acts in opposition, constantly wearing down the peaks. Rainfall and frost weather the uplifted rocks; running water and glacier ice, armed with rock fragments, scour slopes and gouge out valleys.

Erosion, on the whole, appears to have been most intense in the western Pamirs. This, along with climatic variations, has given the western and eastern sections of the range strikingly different characters, with a marked contrast in terrain. In the west the valleys tumbling down into the lowlands of Tadzhikistan tend to be

deep and narrow, the high ridges more dramatic in classic Himalayan style. In the east, by unexpected contrast, the relief is one of a high, rolling enclosed plateau, with broad valleys and gentler summits. The east is both drier and colder.

Along the steep, straight valleys of the west, the Pamirs are arguably at their most spectacular. Deep ravines carved by torrential rivers line the valleys that may be 6,500 feet (2,000 m)

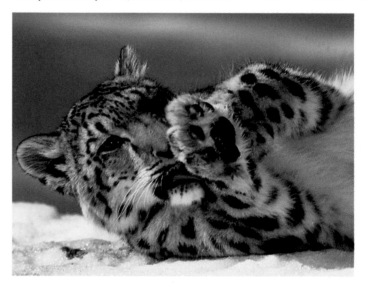

deep. Above them soar lines of towering peaks. While thickets of shrubs cluster in the relative shelter of the valley bottom, the neighboring mountain heights are capped with ice and snow. Bare cliffs and scree predominate on the steep valley slopes, and in some places loose rock deposits dumped by ancient glaciers carpet the valley floors. Heavy falls of rain and snow are deposited on the western mountains, especially during

Thickly furred against the cold, the snow leopard lives among remote crags and ravines, where it hunts mountain goats.

The long-tailed marmot lives beneath the soil in complex burrows and only emerges to feed.

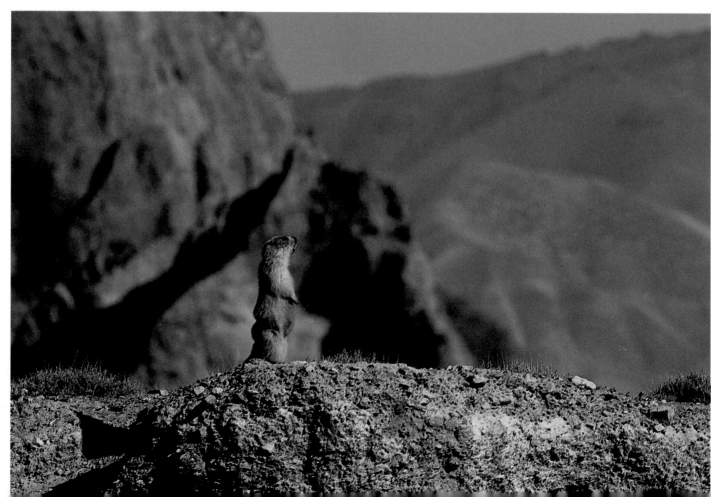

March and April, nourishing the icefields and rivers.

Some hardy animals make their homes on the rugged western slopes. Himalayan snowcocks forage for plant food on the edges of snowfields, making their nests among gray rocks and boulders against which they are well camouflaged. Siberian mountain goats are widespread and may forage at heights of 16,500 feet (5,000 m). Though sure-footed on even the steepest rocky slopes, they cannot always escape from rare and equally agile snow leopards, the elusive big cats of the central Asian mountains. The valleys of the western Pamirs are also home to brown bears, beech martens and mountain weasels.

Life is more difficult still in the eastern Pamirs. Though the terrain is gentler, with broad rounded surfaces and snowbound peaks rarely rising more than 5,000 feet (1,500 m) above the surroundings, the plateau is consistently high, bitterly cold and extremely dry. Average midwinter temperatures are as low as 0°F (–18°C) and yearly precipitation can be below 2½ inches (60 mm), giving the plateau the climate of a cold desert. Much of the ground is bare or lightly spotted with wormwood, cushion plants and steppe grass.

Animals are accordingly few, but admirable in their resistance to hardship. Among the species of mammals that do brave the eastern Pamirs are the argali, magnificent wild sheep that find forage even in winter in the broad valleys, and two well-furred rodents, the long-tailed marmot and the long-eared pika. Several of the birds that live here are those adapted to survive in similar harsh conditions farther to the east, among them Tibetan snowcocks and Tibetan sandgrouse.

Several high lakes enhance the unconventional grandeur of the eastern Pamirs and enliven its wildlife community. The largest of these,

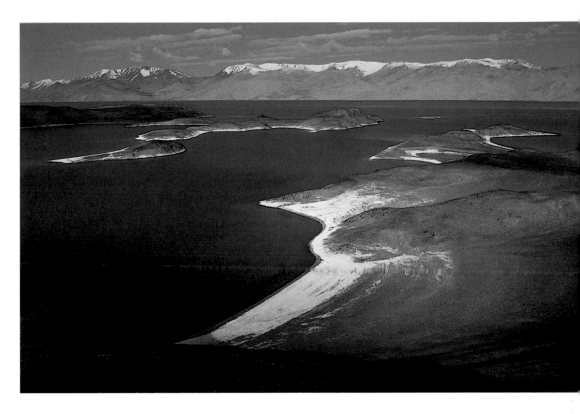

Karakul in the northeast, is about 13,000 feet (4,000 m) above sea level. Though it freezes over in winter, this salt lake supports enough aquatic life in summer to attract nesting terns, gulls and waterfowl in search of food. Bar-headed geese make their nests on islets in the lake. They share their remote havens with colonies of brown-headed gulls, migrants from the coasts and lowlands of India, for which Karakul is the most westerly

Lake Karakul occupies a giant depression high in the eastern Pamirs. The glint of white on its margins shows that it is a salt lake.

breeding site. Strange it may be, but in a land of such contrasts as the eastern Pamirs, it seems fitting that a seagull should choose to breed far inland among some of the highest mountains in the world.

GLACIAL PEAKS AND TROUGHS

Glaciation has left its mark in the dramatic landscapes of the western Pamirs. Erosion by ice has eaten into the mountaintops, creating sharp-ridged, pointed peaks. Massive glaciers have gouged long trough-shaped valleys.

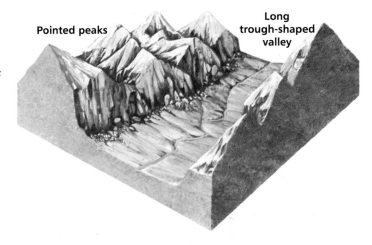

Pointed peaks

Long trough-shaped valley

ROYAL CHITWAN NATIONAL PARK

"Lush greenery, picturesque rivers and lakes, and the distant panorama of the Himalayan peaks"

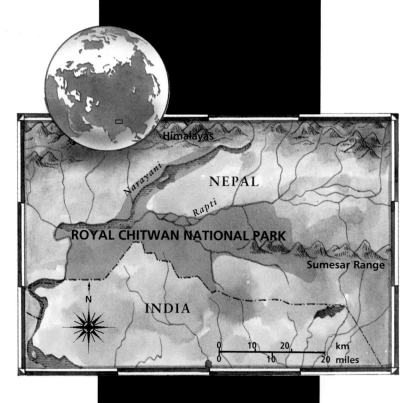

Himalayas

Narayani

NEPAL

Rapti

ROYAL CHITWAN NATIONAL PARK

Sumesar Range

INDIA

N

| 0 | 10 | 20 | km |
| 0 | 10 | | 20 miles |

Hot, humid and with an abundance of wildlife, Royal Chitwan National Park was once a hunting playground of nobility and royalty. Today, it is one of Asia's richest preserves and a vital refuge for

The mighty snow-capped Himalayas look down on the wet lowland wilderness of the Chitwan Park.

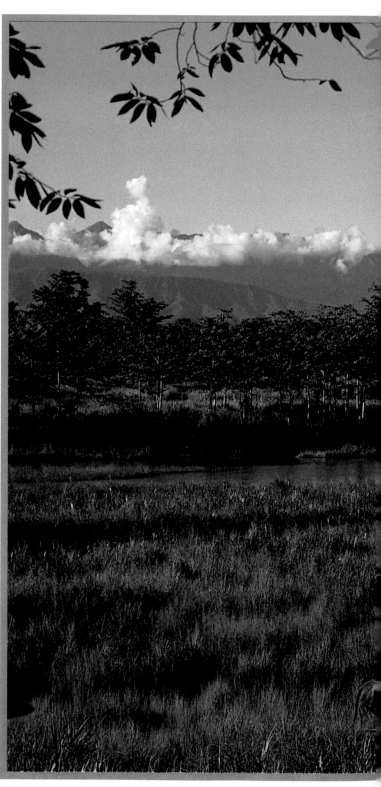

rhinoceroses, tigers and other critically endangered animals.

Chitwan is the best-preserved part of a belt of jungle and swamp that used to run the entire length of southern Nepal. Lying at the base of the great Himalayan chain, beyond its impressive foothills – the Mahabharats – these lowlands soak up both cascading surface water and seepage below ground from the rains that sweep the mountains. Water abounds, forming permanent rivers and marshes and inundating seasonal flood plains during the torrential monsoon peak. The air is stiflingly hot in the summer months, often reaching 100°F (38°C).

The park occupies a central section of this narrow belt. The broad, island-studded Narayani River

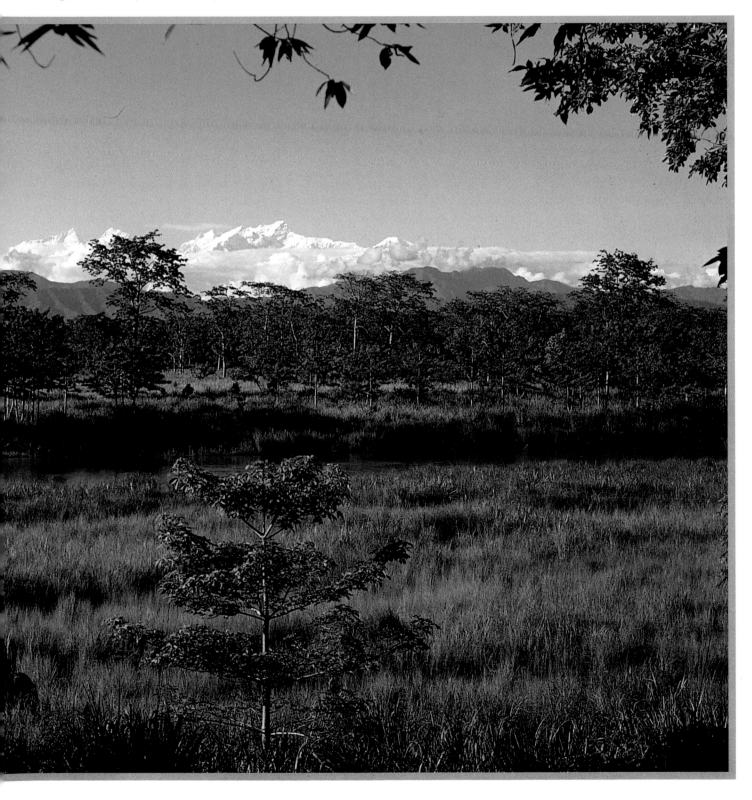

and its winding tributary, the Rapti, form its northern boundary, while the Indian border and another tributary, the Reu River, define the southern frontier. The broad flood plains that surround the rivers lie at about 500 feet (150 m) above sea level. They still have their natural landscapes – swaying rushes and tall grasses on the damp, level ground and strips of forest lining the banks of watercourses. Across the interior of the park rise the Siwalik Hills, a low range in places reaching 2,500 feet (750 m) in altitude.

With its lush greenery, picturesque rivers and lakes and the distant panorama of the Himalayan peaks, Royal Chitwan National Park has a beautiful, tranquil setting. Each of its varied landscapes has a special character of its own, and between them they provide habitats for a delightful diversity of animal life, including about 400 species of birds and at least 70 of butterflies.

The forested hills, deep and inaccessible in the heart of the park, are a rare preserve of seasonal

"Flood plain grasslands are one of the last strongholds of the Indian rhinoceros – a single-horned giant"

tropical forest. This type of forest faces marked climatic changes through the year. Copiously watered during the monsoon, the trees then endure several months of dry season.

The forest habitat that develops differs from tropical rainforest in key respects. Many of the trees, for example, shed leaves during the drought, leaving their crowns bare, and at ground level the forest tends to have

a dry, grassy undergrowth. The interior forests of Chitwan are dominated by sal – magnificent, straight-trunked hardwood trees up to 100 feet (30 m) tall – although chir pine becomes common on the hilltops. The dense habitat the trees create provides sustenance and shelter for rare forest animals, among them sloth bears – curious, long-snouted bears which feed on ants and termites – and herds of gaur – heavily built wild cattle.

Many of the creatures that dwell in the extensive sal forests also occur in the riverside belts of forest on the flood plain. Here a mixture of acacia, shisham, kapok and other tall trees is characteristic. The towering kapok produces a marvelous display of fragrant red flowers in the spring.

Like the interior forests, these belts harbor numerous birds, the more conspicuous among them being Indian peafowls, hornbills, cuckoos and woodpeckers. Two kinds of monkeys, the rhesus macaque and the common langur, are numerous, as are wild boar and axis deer.

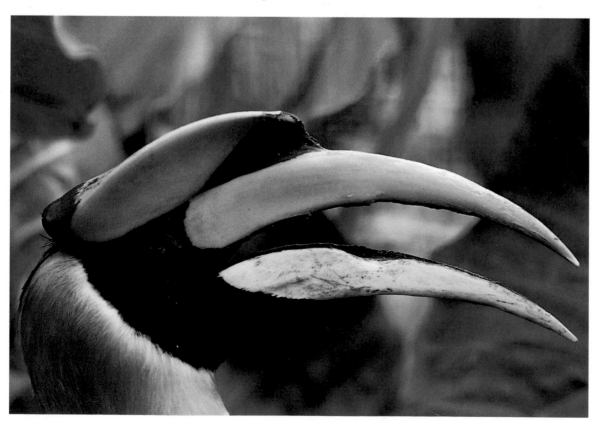

Big, boldly decorated and noisy, the great Indian hornbill hops from branch to branch, plucking fruit.

Rhinoceroses, their horns removed to deter poachers, wallow in the heat of the day to keep cool. In Chitwan they have benefited from the protection of guards and from the conservation of their favored marsh and grassland habitat.

Both boars and deer regularly move out of the riverine forest onto the grasslands. The flat savannas still provide excellent cover, however, because they are dominated by tall, dense grasses. Where elephant grasses predominate, the vegetation may be 20 feet (6 m) high, big enough to conceal not just the stately sambar deer but also the Indian rhinoceros, the second largest of the world's rhinoceros species. Chitwan's flood plain grasslands are among the last strongholds of this single-horned giant. About 350 rhinos, one-quarter of the total remaining population in the wild, live in Chitwan.

All grazing animals other than rhinos have to be wary of attack from tigers. There may be 100 Bengal tigers in the park, most concentrated on the flood plains, where they roam through forest, grassland and marsh in search of game. The marshy beds of rushes and sedge that fringe the rivers, pools and oxbow lakes are also home to semi-aquatic predators such as the marsh crocodile and the Indian python.

For sheer numbers, birds are the most spectacular denizens of the marshes and lakes. Ducks, ibises, egrets, bitterns, herons, storks, hawks and kingfishers search the waters for their various foods such as plant matter, invertebrates, frogs and fish. Adjutant storks and black-necked storks are the largest species, ospreys and fishing eagles the most dramatic as they swoop to the surface to snatch fish in their talons.

Some of the birds present in the park during the winter are migrants, retreating from harsh conditions on their breeding ranges farther north in Asia. The striking Brahminy duck is one of the most abundant, appearing in large numbers on the pools and open rivers.

The big rivers are also home to two rarer but more spectacular creatures. The gharial is a peculiar crocodile, up to 23 feet (7 m) long but with narrow, elongated jaws. The almost dainty snout is excellent for catching fish – minimizing water resistance when the reptile makes its sideways swipe – but is not powerful enough to cope with bigger prey. The Ganges dolphin, one of the few freshwater dolphins in existence, also has a long, toothy snout for grasping fish. It haunts the deeper stretches of water, principally in the Narayani River, and is occasionally spotted as it breaks the water surface. Like so many other rare creatures, dolphins and gharials find precious refuge in this untamed fragment of wild Asia.

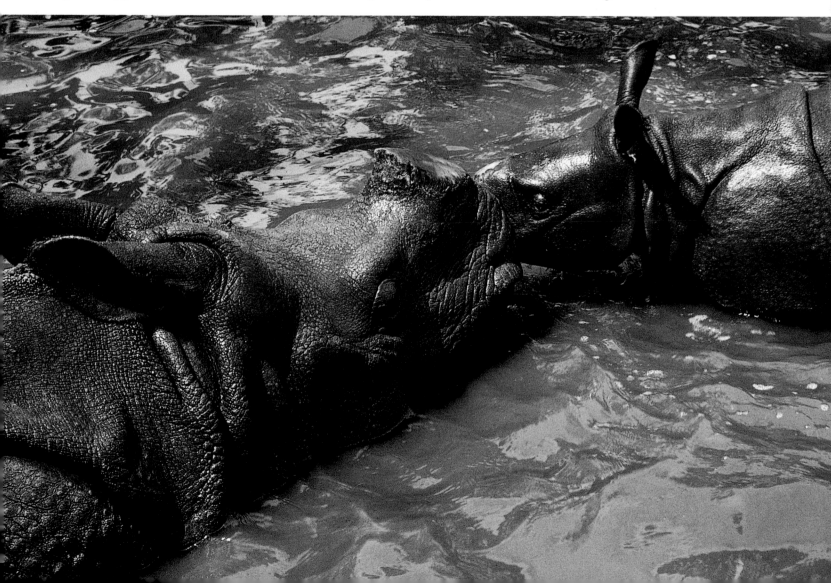

THE
SUNDARBANS

"Here, where land and sea merge, is a place so wild that tigers still rule its forbidding interior"

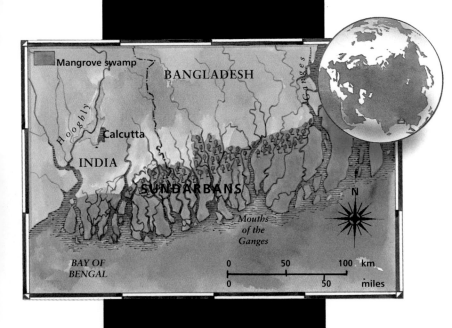

Mangrove swamp
BANGLADESH
Ganges
Hooghly
Calcutta
Ganges
INDIA
SUNDARBANS
N
Mouths of the Ganges
BAY OF BENGAL
0   50   100   km
0   50   miles

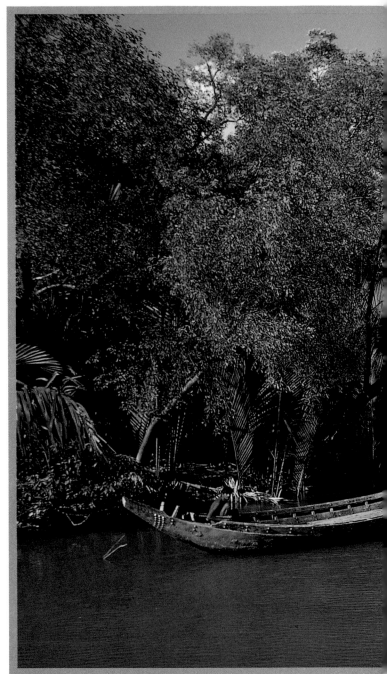

The dense, impenetrable jungle that lines the northern Bay of Bengal is no ordinary forest. At times, beneath the thick foliage there appears a tangle of starkly exposed roots in an ooze of soft mud, divided into islands by shallow, brackish creeks. At other times, the roots, mud and creeks are hidden beneath submerging sea water, leaving only trunks and leaves seemingly sprouting

Built of deposits of silt, clay and sand and shaped by the action of both rivers and tides, the low-lying landscape of the Sundarbans blurs the distinction between land and sea.

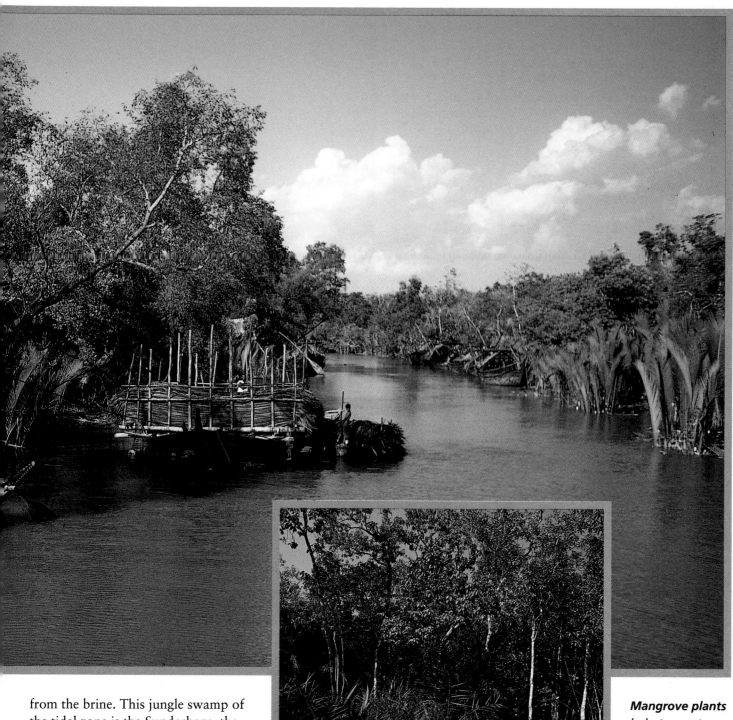

from the brine. This jungle swamp of the tidal zone is the Sundarbans, the biggest mangrove forest in the world. Here, where land and sea merge, is a place so wild that tigers still rule its forbidding interior.

The Sundarbans owes its existence to the great rivers – the Ganges and the Brahmaputra – which, along with other mingling waterways, have built up an enormous delta across southern Bangladesh and adjacent India.

Mangrove plants help to create new land by trapping sediments among their exposed roots. The more silt that accumulates, the higher a patch of swamp becomes.

Copious sediments from the Himalayas have been deposited as the rivers slowed on their approach to the sea and divided into a maze of channels. The seaward margin of the delta forms a tidal plain, a network of channels, mud flats and islands low enough to be inundated by the bay waters when the tide is high. This twice-daily incursion of salt water defines the character of the Sundarbans and sets it apart from the rest of the delta.

The greater adjutant stork, which stands up to 5 feet (1.5 m) tall, is a scavenger. Animal carcasses make up much of its food, but it also preys on small creatures such as frogs and fish.

> "The bulk of the mangrove roots spread beneath the mud, but from them hundreds of rigid projections poke up above the ooze like miniature snorkels"

Stretching for 185 miles (300 km) between the estuaries of the Hooghly River in the west and the Meghna in the east, and reaching at least 18 miles (30 km) inland, the Sundarbans is not just the most extensive but also one of the most varied mangrove belts in the world. Though the drainage pattern of the delta was laid down by river flow, tidal water has taken over to different degrees, creating marked variations in salinity.

In temperate regions of the world, large tidal plains naturally turn into salt marsh. But in the warmth and strong sunshine of the tropics, the habitat that develops is much more lush. Instead of low-growing salt-tolerant plants, a mixture of evergreen shrubs and trees develop, known generally as mangroves. All are specially adapted to cope with the testing conditions of the tidal swamp – repeated immersion in salty water and a soil that is extremely low in oxygen. Special glands on the

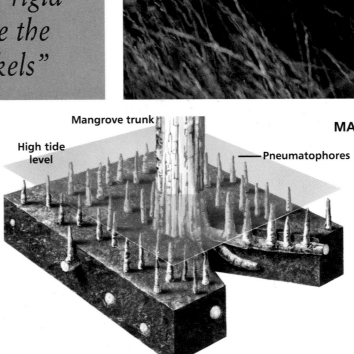

Mangrove trunk

High tide level

Pneumatophores

MANGROVE PLANTS

At low tide, root projections, or pneumatophores, from the sundari mangrove tree are left poking out of the mud. They absorb air through their pores, and oxygen passes down to the roots beneath.

thick, waxy leaves secrete excess salt from the plants, and tiny openings in the bark of the exposed roots absorb oxygen from the air during low tide.

The roots of mangroves are their most extraordinary features. Some of the species in the Sundarbans have peculiar stilt roots that sprout from the trunk and curve down to the surrounding mud, encrusted with oysters and barnacles. In others,

including the widespread sundari that gives the swampland its name, the bulk of the roots spread beneath the mud, but from them hundreds of rigid projections poke up above the ooze like miniature snorkels.

Mangroves are great builders of land. Their roots trap sediments, and as the silt accumulates, the ground beneath the mangroves rises, lessening the degree of tidal immersion.

Throughout the Sundarbans there are patches of soil too high now to be flooded by the normal tide, especially inland where the swamp merges into monsoon forest.

Since different mangrove species have varying tolerances, both of levels of salinity and of flooding, the vegetation of the Sundarbans is far from uniform. Sundari, for example, is the most widespread of some 20 mangrove trees in the region. Since it prefers lower salinity, the plant grows tallest – up to 100 feet (30 m) – along the river estuaries in the east. Salty zones to the west tend to have shrubby mangroves, dominated often by the stilt-rooted goran. Low, deeply flooded areas are usually reserved for slender keora mangroves, while hantal palms may appear in dense groves on high, drier ground.

The mangrove world of the Sundarbans sustains and protects a teeming community of wildlife. At low tide, crabs are the most conspicuous creatures. Fiddler crabs sidle tentatively over the mud, picking at debris and darting back to their holes if danger threatens. Each male fiddler is encumbered with an oversized claw that it snaps loudly on occasion for self-advertisement. Mudskippers are equally curious denizens of the swamps. These small fish can breathe out of water and move over the mud using their front fins as limbs.

When the tide rises, the creeks overflow across the mud and roots. An array of creatures, tolerant of the brackish water, advance into the tangle to take their turn feeding on the rich organic matter of the swamp. Among them are shrimp, lobsters, fishes and river terrapins. Because of the abundance of both food and shelter, mangrove swamps also act as nurseries for a host of marine animals. Planktonic larvae fill the water, and of the 120 species of fish common in the Sundarbans, many

stay here only as juveniles. When full grown, they move out to open sea.

Though protected among the impeding roots and shallows from big predatory sea fish, mangrove fish still risk attack from above. Herons, egrets, kingfishers and fish eagles all hunt in the mangroves. When the mud is exposed, other kinds of birds, such as storks, ibises, sandpipers and stilts, move in to probe for the many

Monitors are large lizards, up to 6½ feet (2 m) long (below). They are good climbers and swimmers and hunt both in the trees and in water for small prey animals and birds' eggs.

The estuarine crocodile often basks on muddy banks, but is also perfectly at home in salt water (bottom). This fearsome giant often lurks with just its eyes and nostrils above the surface.

invertebrates hiding beneath. Flying insects fill the air above, including hordes of mosquitoes and biting flies. The insects provide some of the food for perching birds that forage and nest in the mangrove branches, among them shrikes, mynas and babblers. The trees are also shelter for the Sundarbans' monkeys – rhesus macaques. Some ground animals inhabit the drier parts of the forest but penetrate into the swamp at low tide. They include rodents up to the size of porcupines, groups of wild boar and axis deer.

Many of the ground predators also hunt for prey in the water. Among them are monitor lizards, pythons and fishing cats. The biggest predators of the swamps are those most feared but also most valued by poachers – the mighty estuarine crocodile and the Bengal tiger. For both, the tangled forests and muddy waters of the Sundarbans are a vital refuge.

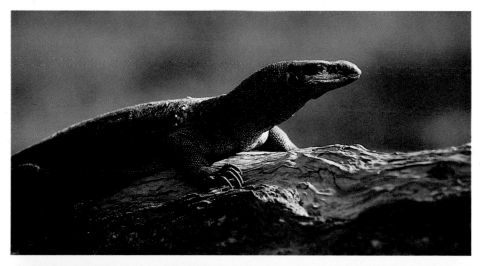

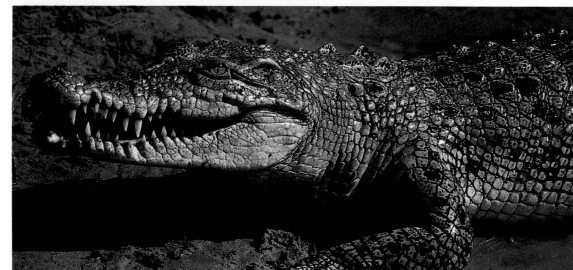

FOOD GATHERERS IN THE SUNDARBANS

There are no permanent villages in the tangled swamps of the Sundarbans, but many thousands of people in India and Bangladesh rely on the region for their living. Harvesters travel into the swamps by boat and move around on foot at low tide as they collect honey and bees' wax and gather grass for matting, reeds for fencing and palm leaves for roofing material. Fishermen make camps in the area and work the waters for weeks on end.

But this wild place, with its healthy population of Bengal tigers, is a dangerous place to be. For years, the annual death toll from tigers has averaged an astonishing 50 to 60. In the past tigers were hunted ruthlessly, partly in response to man-eating.

Today the preferred approach is to reduce the dangers rather than the tiger population. Since the 1980s, some effective deterrents have been tried.

Human dummies have been placed in the forest and wired up to give the tigers a non-lethal shock. People working in the swamps have also been encouraged to wear face masks on the back of the head – tigers prefer to attack from behind unseen, and the masks seem to deter them. In 1987, when 2,500 people tried these masks, nobody wearing one was attacked.

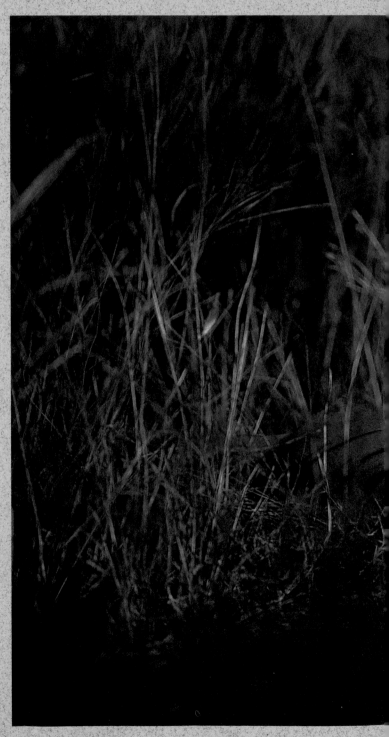

Tiger numbers have been increasing in the Sundarbans in recent decades as a result of strict conservation, and there are now about 500 in total. This represents the largest surviving population in the world. Finding ways to protect people from attack by the animals without turning back the gains of conservation is crucial.

As they go about their work otherwise unprotected, honey-gatherers in the Sundarbans put their faith in a couple of simple ruses designed to ward off tiger attacks. Holding a stick over one shoulder appears to confuse stalking tigers as does wearing a face mask on the back of the head.

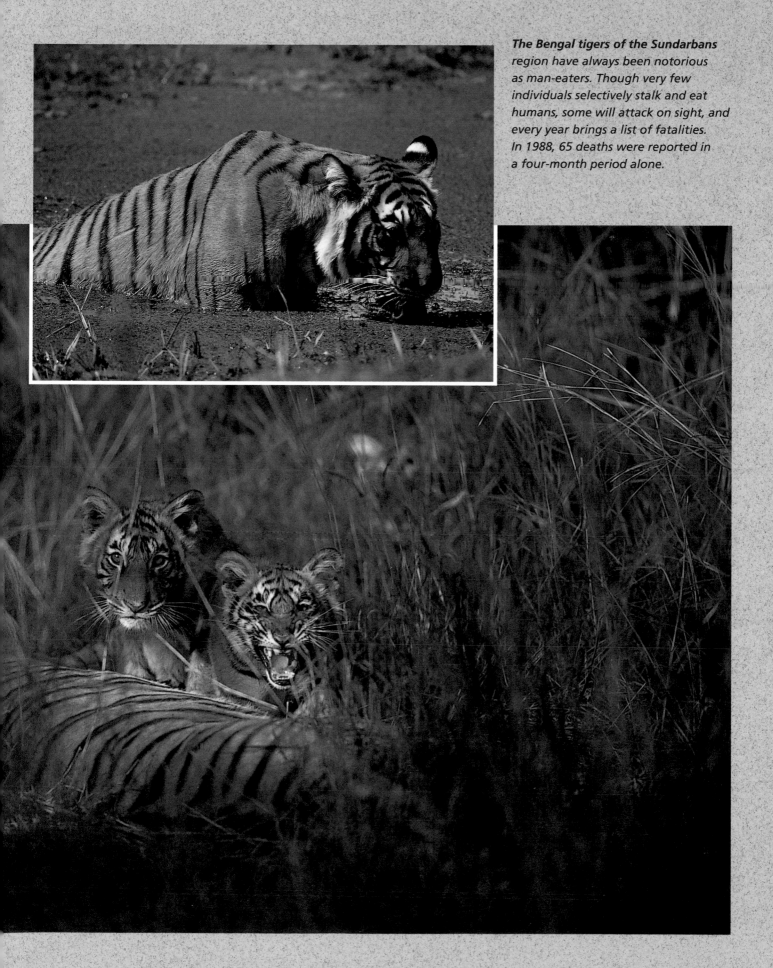

The Bengal tigers of the Sundarbans region have always been notorious as man-eaters. Though very few individuals selectively stalk and eat humans, some will attack on sight, and every year brings a list of fatalities. In 1988, 65 deaths were reported in a four-month period alone.

HIGHLANDS OF IRIAN JAYA

"A land of endless forest, green-clad hills and dramatic mountains, their summits gleaming with snow and ice"

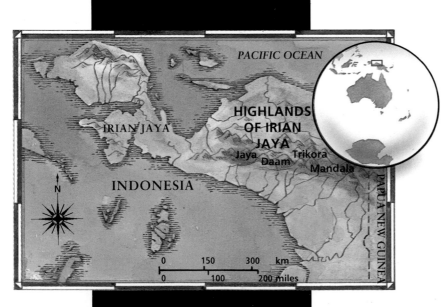

Some of the wildest, least explored territory in all the tropics is contained in Irian Jaya, the western half of the great island of New Guinea. So impenetrable is its rugged, forested interior that, until the advent of air travel, tribes lived there without any contact at all with the outside world. Today, this easternmost province of Indonesia is still a land of endless forest, swamp and green-clad hills, with a chain of dramatic mountain ranges running east-west across its center. The highest peaks reach so far skyward that their summits gleam white with ice and snow.

The steep slopes of the highlands belong to a landscape that is young in geological terms. Indeed, the whole island of New Guinea is a relative newcomer on the world stage. Tectonic collision between two continental plates has literally pushed the island up out of the sea over the last few million years, buckling its central portion into a belt of mountains 100 miles (160 km) wide.

The deformed layers of rock that form most of the highlands today originated as sediments and limestone deposits from the ancient seabed. But these are interspersed with intrusions of volcanic rock, showing that the tensions in the Earth's crust also caused volcanic activity on the surface. There are no active volcanoes now in the mountains – although they do exist on islands close to New Guinea – but the upheavals that pushed the highlands up in the past are almost certainly still at work.

Rugged bare rocks, thin vegetation and glacier-hewn valleys in the central highlands of Irian Jaya contrast greatly with the familiar image of New Guinea as a lush, forest-filled island. The tallest of these mountains soar higher than Mont Blanc and are topped with permanent ice caps.

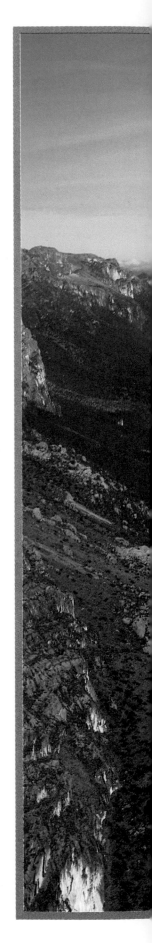

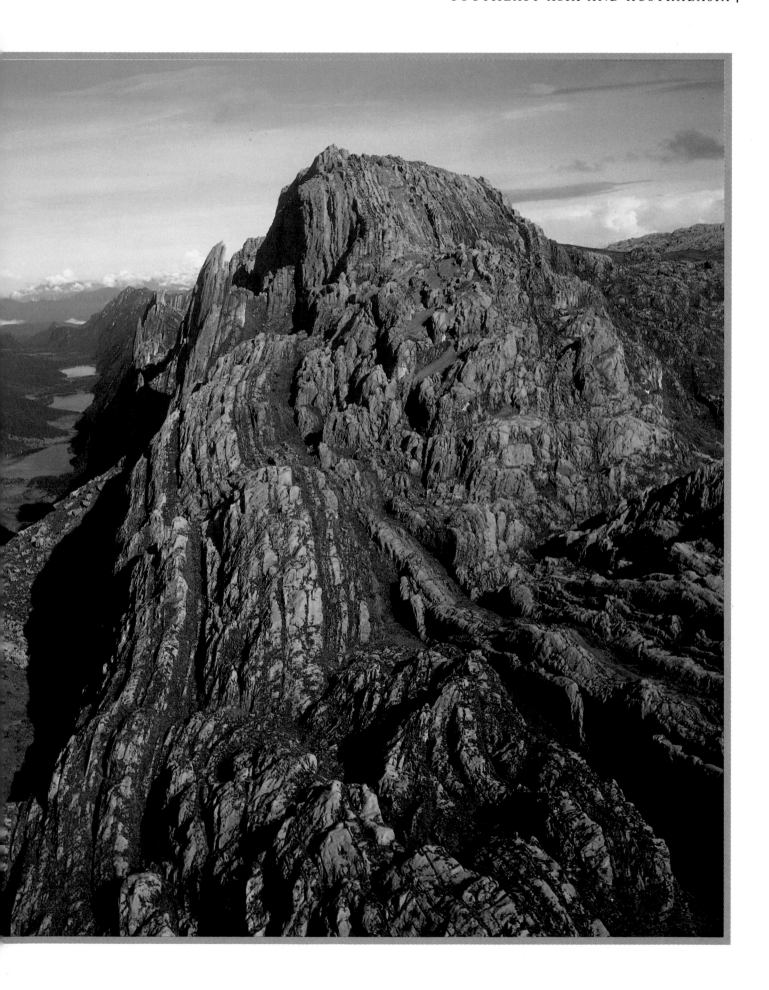

The whole region is frequently rocked by earthquakes.

The foothills, inner valleys and peaks of the Irian Jaya highlands experience widely differing climatic conditions. The contrasts are most sharply defined along the southern rim, where the land rises abruptly from lowland plain to the highest of the peaks. These include Jaya at an altitude of 16,500 feet (5,030 m), Daam at 16,140 feet (4,920 m), Mandala at 15,620 feet (4,760 m) and Trikora at 15,580 feet (4,750 m). From the hot, forest-blanketed lowlands, where temperatures average 80°F (27°C), conditions gradually cool with rising altitude at a rate of about 11°F (6°C) per 3,300 feet (1,000 m). Hence night freezing is common on the high ground, and snow regularly falls in the mountaintops.

The summits of Jaya, Daam and Mandala are all high enough to maintain small but permanent ice caps. These rank as some of the most dramatic of Irian Jaya's natural surprises, since the nearest icefields are in New Zealand and the

"One of the few places in the world where new species of mammals are still being found"

Himalayas, more than 3,000 miles (5,000 km) away. Immediately below these ice caps and across the lesser summits, the landscape becomes one of bare rock and windswept tundra; below that, open, alpine-type meadows stretch across unexpectedly flat mountain plateaus. During the ice ages, most of these landscapes were glaciated – a past evident from the presence of lake-filled depressions, deposits of rock fragments known

as moraines, and other glacial landforms. The retreat of the ice may still be occurring, according to comparison with records from the last century. In fact, ice did not completely disappear from Mount Trikora until the 1940s.

The vegetation of the alpine zone varies considerably with the lay of the land. Tussock grasses and small herbs predominate in many places, with bogs developing on the flatter stretches. In more sheltered sites, and increasingly as altitude drops, there appear luxuriant tree ferns and shrubs, including a rich variety of rhododendrons. Rats, bandicoots and the curious long-nosed echidnas are among the few types of mammals that forage over these high, open habitats. Though the bird life is similarly sparse, several species have their sole home in these remote heights, among them snow mountain quails and orange-cheeked honeyeaters.

Below about 12,300 feet (3,750 m), the meadows and shrubland start to blend into forest on the steep mountain flank. At first, the forest is thin and composed of stunted, elfin trees, many of them conifers and myrtles. Gradually, with descending height, more favorable conditions cause the forest to become denser and richer in tree species. Still, however, there are many gaps in the canopy, often caused by minor landslides on the steep slopes. The spaces are quickly colonized by tangles of bamboo. Throughout this montane forest, humidity is high – often reaching 100 percent in the cool night air. The moist trunks and branches of trees are

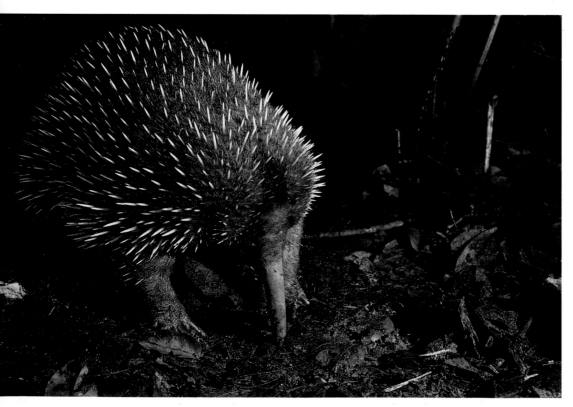

The long-nosed echidna is covered with protective spines similar to those of a porcupine. It searches the forests and mountain grasslands mainly for earthworms, which it hooks onto bristles on the front of its tongue and pulls end-first into its narrow "beak."

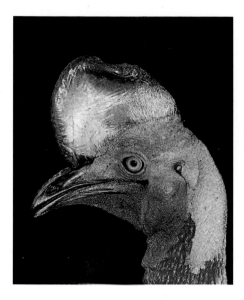

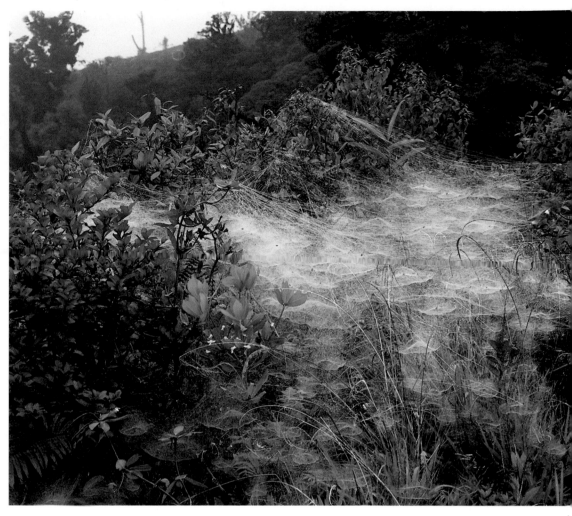

The dwarf cassowary (above) dwells in the mountain forests and feeds mainly on fruit. When threatened or cornered, it is likely to attack, striking out with vicious claws.

A delicate film of spiders' webs stretches between rhododendron bushes below Mount Jaya. The webs are nurseries, giving protection and food to swarms of young spiders.

typically coated with moss, ferns and orchids, and it is common for the forest to be swathed in cloud during the day.

Cloud seldom forms on the warm slopes below 6,600 feet (2,000 m), and it is on these lowest parts of the ranges that the forest starts to resemble lowland tropical rainforest in its structure and diversity. The trees are tall, the canopy closed. "Monkey puzzle" araucarias are among the most distinctive of a wide variety of trees, and there are numerous species of palms and creepers.

From the tree line to the lower slopes, the forests that sweep down the mountainsides burgeon with remarkable creatures. Here giant stick insects and dazzling birdwings – the world's biggest butterflies live. The mountains are the stronghold

of the powerful New Guinea harpy eagle, which often flies below the tree canopy as it hunts for forest prey. Colorful lorikeets and parrots search for fruit in the treetops, their place taken at night by foraging fruit bats.

Much of the animal life of New Guinea has reached the island from nearby Australia rather than from Southeast Asia. Consequently, though the mountain forests have no native deer, monkeys or squirrels, they are home to various marsupial mammals, among them cuscuses, possums, forest wallabies and tree kangaroos. Since many of the tree-dwelling species are nocturnal, they are rarely seen and little is known of their lives.

Given the rugged nature of the terrain and the paucity of scientific investigation in the region, it is perhaps not surprising that these

forests are one of the few places in the world where new species of mammals are still being found. One of the most recent was a variety of tree kangaroo discovered in 1989.

The mountain forests of central Irian Jaya also harbor cassowaries, bowerbirds and birds of paradise, which have their fellow species in northeastern Australia. Birds of paradise, though they are famous for their extraordinary plumage, are much more easily heard than seen as they utter their distinctive calls from high in the canopy. At least 10 species occur at varying heights on the mountain flanks. Halfway up Mount Jaya, a loud crescendo of strange, sputtered noises might sound like radio static, but it is a King of Saxony bird of paradise calling from its perch in this wild, moss-laden forest.

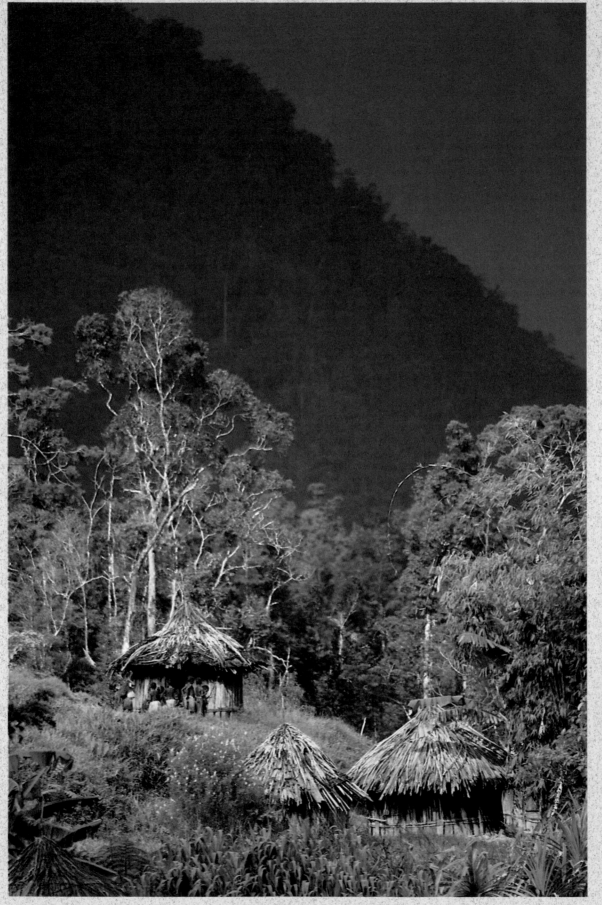

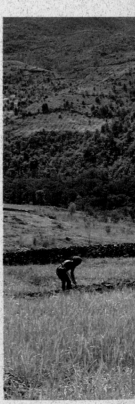

Huts in a Yali *village, set in steep, forested terrain, show the compact, rounded shape and pole-and-thatch construction typical of the homes of highland peoples in Irian Jaya. Roofs hanging low over the walls and false walls behind the door openings help to keep out drafts when the mountain air becomes cool at night.*

PEOPLE OF THE HIGHLAND VALLEYS

Deep in the seemingly formidable mountain barrier that runs the length of central New Guinea lies a series of broad, well-watered, upland valleys. The extent of these valleys was not fully appreciated by the colonial administrations that ruled the island until well into the 20th century, when exploration became more advanced. Neither was the remarkable secret they held. Here, hidden from the outside world, lived hundreds of previously unknown tribes. Some were hunters and gatherers, many cleared small plots in the forest, grew crops for a few years and then left the plots to regenerate. But some – among them the Yali and the Dani people of Irian Jaya – had turned great sections of the valleys into cultivated landscapes, with neat fields and thatch-roofed villages. Evidence suggests that the well-managed farming systems may have been in existence in the valleys for more than 5,000 years.

Today, with the creation of numerous airstrips, most of the estimated 600,000 indigenous highlanders of Irian Jaya have some kind of contact with the exterior world. In some cases, change has overwhelmed their traditions, but many others still lead lives close to those their ancestors have lived for centuries. The huts in which they dwell, the types of implements they use, the few garments they wear, and their customs and rituals follow tradition. Some tribes actively shun outside contact, and a few still engage now and then in intertribal warfare.

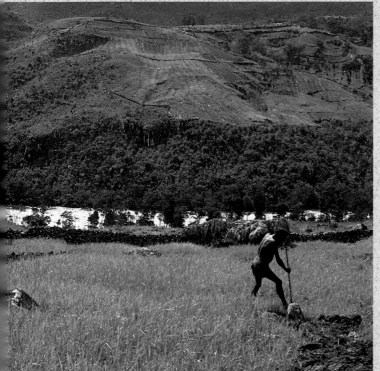

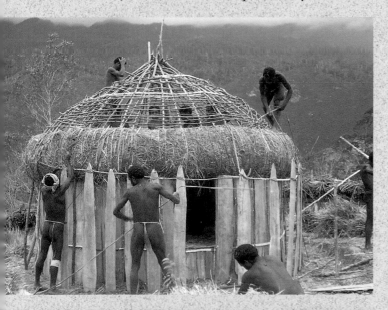

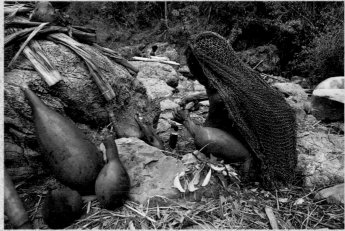

The Dani people have cultivated large stretches of central Irian Jaya for thousands of years (left). Their sophisticated farming system centers on the production of sweet potatoes and on pig-rearing.

Dani men set about building a hut using products of the upland forest – lumber, saplings, vines and palm leaves (above left). The large bolster of grass acts as insulation for a sleeping platform.

Gourds of various shapes are used as storage vessels. The "net-back," a type of headgear extending over the shoulders and back, doubles as a garment and a large bag for carrying crops, piglets and even infants (above).

KRAKATAU

"Scene of the most immense explosions ever recorded on Earth, which changed the face of the entire archipelago"

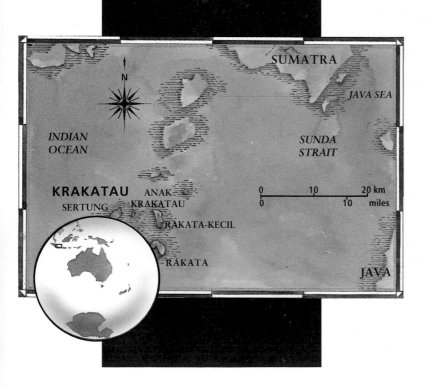

Midway across the Sunda Strait between Java and Sumatra lies an archipelago of four uninhabited islands. Set in a blue tropical sea, the outer three islands display the lush green hue of dense forest. Two are low in profile; the third rises to a sharp crest more than

Where Krakatau tore itself apart more than a century ago, a new volcanic island, Anak Krakatau has already risen from under the sea.

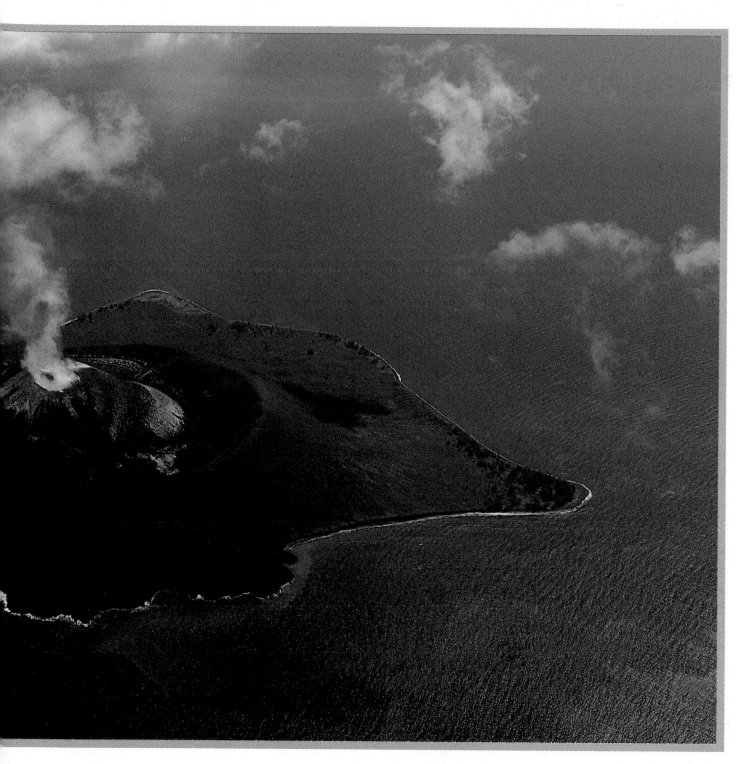

2,625 feet (800 m) high, its inner side forming a dramatically curving cliff. Facing the cliff is the fourth and smallest island – rugged and dark, with a conical mound rising near its center. A thin stream of smoke often trails from its summit.

Though the smoke barely impinges on the serenity of the islands, it is a hint that tranquillity does not always reign there. For these wild remote lands are the volcanic remnants of Krakatau, scene in 1883 of the most immense explosions ever recorded on Earth. The explosions were the climax of a cataclysmic eruption, one so violent that it changed the face of the entire archipelago.

Krakatau's turbulent history is one of repeated rebirth. In prehistoric times, there appears to have been a single giant volcanic cone on the site of Krakatau, built up out of the sea mainly from lava flows pouring from a subterranean reservoir of molten rock, or magma. Most of the top of the cone was destroyed in a huge

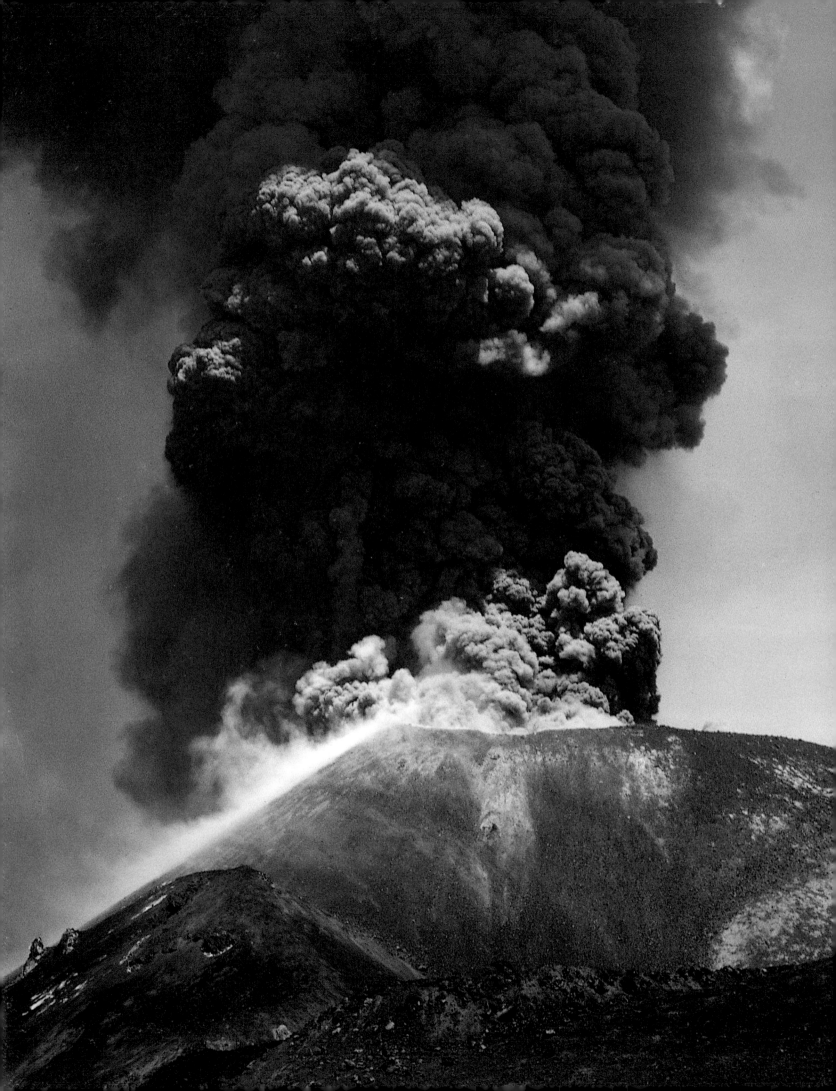

eruption – probably one referred to in a Javanese legend from the year A.D. 416 – leaving a great bowl-shaped crater, or caldera. Only parts of the caldera rim still projected above the sea, forming low islands.

Over the ensuing centuries, magma from the same underground chamber found its way up through one of these islands and developed a new volcanic cone, Rakata. Later, two more cones, known as Danan and Perbuatan, grew from the center of the caldera and merged with Rakata to form one island. Some 4½ miles (7 km) in length, with a distinctive profile, this was the main Krakatau island.

By the 1880s Rakata had ceased activity, and Danan and Perbuatan were mostly quiet. Much of the main island was under thick forest, as were its two low-lying neighbors from the original caldera rim, now known as Sertung and Rakata-kecil.

But in 1883, after several years of frequent earthquakes in the region, Krakatau came vigorously back to life. From late May to August of that year, cycles of eruptions from Krakatau sent enormous ash-laden clouds up to 7 miles (11 km) into the air. First Perbuatan, then vents on Danan, started to emit steam and ash with explosive force. On August 26 the activity came to a head. Increasingly loud explosions from the volcano could eventually be heard all over Java. Thick black ash clouds

doubled in height, and platforms of pumice from the volcano's solid outpourings floated across the strait.

On the morning of the 27th, the eruption reached its climax, with four exceedingly powerful explosions. The third, at 10.20 a.m., was so titanic that it dwarfed even these others. Its force has been estimated as 2,000 times that produced by the bomb

> "During the climax of the eruption two-thirds of the main island disappeared"

THE COLLAPSE OF KRAKATAU
When Krakatau erupted in 1883, Danan and Perbuatan may have caved in first. Rakata's northern slopes were then left without proper support, and this huge section of the cone sheared off and slumped en masse into the sea. In 1927 a new cone, Anak Krakatau, began to rise from the seabed.

dropped on Hiroshima in 1945. The sound could be heard more than 3,000 miles (4,800 km) away, and pressure waves from the blast were detected all over the world. Great boulders were hurled across the Sunda Strait. The ash cloud from the climax towered 50 miles (80 km) high and, as it spread, plunged the whole area into two days of darkness.

But the most devastating effect of the Krakatau eruption was a series of tsunamis, or tidal waves, which swept out across both shores of the strait and into the Java Sea, destroying entire villages and towns. At least 36,000 people lost their lives.

The biggest of the tsunamis overwhelmed the shores of Sumatra and Java shortly after noon on the 27th. It took another day for the eruption of Krakatau finally to run out of steam and, eventually, as the murk and floating pumice cleared, people were able to approach the volcano by boat and see what had happened. What they saw before them was astonishing.

The precise chronology of events is unclear, but during the climax of the eruption, two-thirds of the main island disappeared. Some of it was blown outward, along with huge amounts of pumice and ash from the underlying magma chamber, but most appears to have collapsed below the waves. So much magma had been ejected from beneath that the island had caved in,

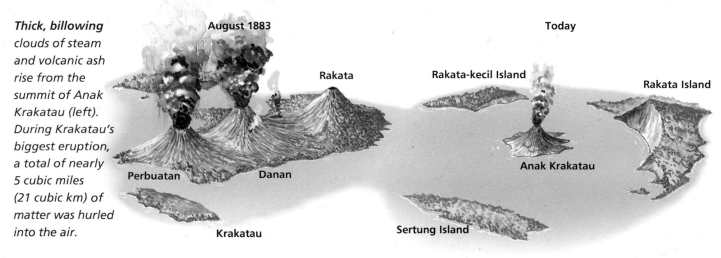

Thick, billowing clouds of steam and volcanic ash rise from the summit of Anak Krakatau (left). During Krakatau's biggest eruption, a total of nearly 5 cubic miles (21 cubic km) of matter was hurled into the air.

August 1883

Rakata

Perbuatan   Danan

Krakatau

Today

Rakata-kecil Island

Rakata Island

Anak Krakatau

Sertung Island

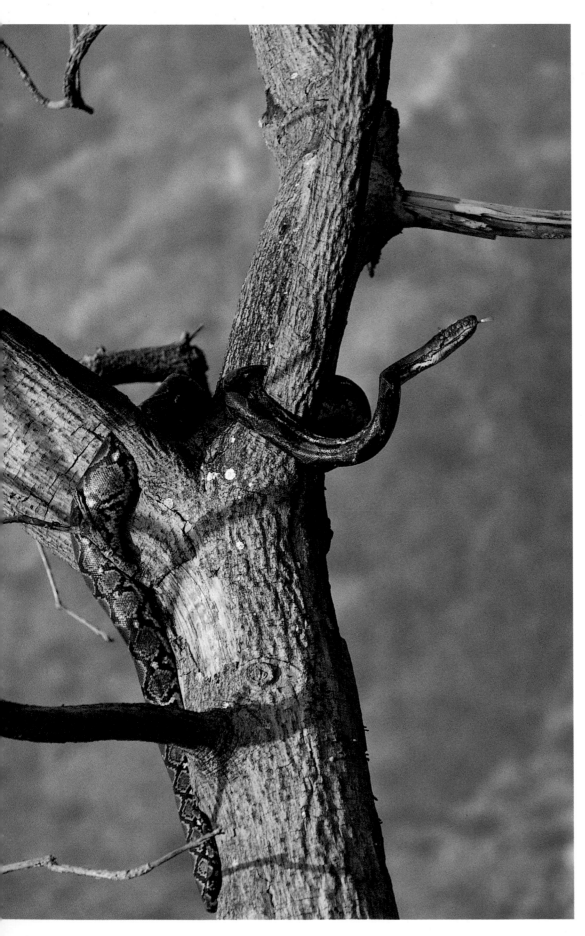

creating a new caldera within the old one, with its floor 1,000 feet (300 m) under the sea.

The collapse of the main island was the most dramatic – but not the only – reshaping of the Krakatau archipelago in 1883. Months of heavy ash falls had smothered Sertung, Rakata-kecil and the remaining southern face of Rakata, accumulating like sandbanks around their old shores, and enlarging Sertung in particular. Meanwhile, Krakatau was preparing for its next rebirth.

In 1927 new volcanic stirrings were detected from the caldera floor. Within a few years, a cinder cone had broken the surface of the sea, and it has continued smoldering, erupting ash and growing ever since. This is the small island in the center of the Krakatau archipelago today. Young, yet already topping 625 feet (190 m) above sea level, it is known as Anak Krakatau, or Child of Krakatau.

The island is for the most part barren. The frequent minor eruptions and the bare surfaces of cinder and ash are hardly welcoming to plants and animals. Yet even there, some plants are managing to grow. A few migratory birds stop to rest on the island, and seabirds feed around its shoreline. If the volcanic activity were to cease, it is certain that more variety of life would become established there. Rakata, Sertung and Rakata-kecil are proof of that.

All plant and animal life on the three outer islands was snuffed out and buried in 1883. Sterile ash covered all. Yet within a few years life, with its remarkable powers of recolonization, was returning to

Land-based animals such as this *reticulated python have managed to recolonize the Krakatau archipelago since the great eruption. Their ancestors may have been swept ashore on rafts of floating debris.*

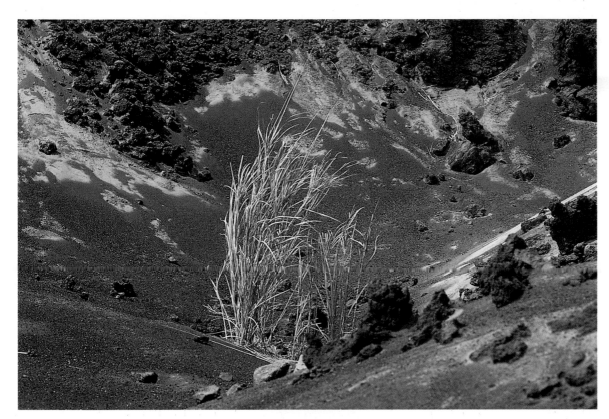

On the harsh, seemingly sterile surface of Anak Krakatau, a few hardy plants have taken root. Grasses, ferns and casuarina bushes all grow on the lower slopes.

The summit of Anak Krakatau is an unstable pile of cinder. Year after year, lava, rock and ash are pushed out of the vent of the volcano during eruptions, raising its cone ever higher.

reclaim them. Hardy pioneering plants like grasses and casuarina appeared first. Many of these prepared the ground – changing its structure and building up soil as they grew and died – and the plants that followed could grow more easily.

The first trees began to spring up, providing more chances for insects, birds, bats and other creatures to find a suitable habitat. By the time Anak Krakatau was emerging, more than 270 species of plants had returned to the outer islands. At least 27 resident landbirds could be seen on Rakata, among them flycatchers, kingfishers and pigeons.

With the rich rainforests of Sumatra and Java only about 25 miles (40 km) away, it was inevitable that certain forms of life would soon reach the islands. Many plant seeds were carried there in the stomachs of birds. Others floated across the sea or drifted in the wind. Butterflies and other flying insects may have made landfall after being swept out to sea on strong winds. Some rodents and

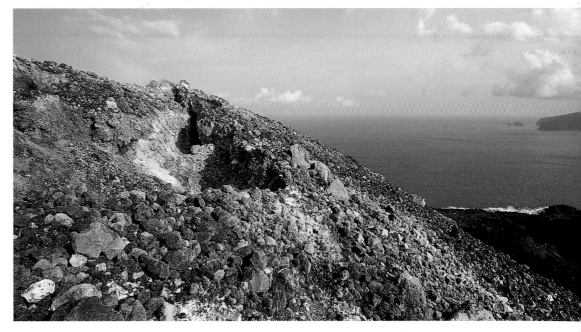

reptiles appear to have floated across by accident on logs and rafts of floating vegetation. Today, the islands have a fairly rich fauna, including pythons, geckos, monitor lizards, rats and fruit bats. In both form and composition, the vegetation in which they now live closely resembles that of a typical rainforest.

But the evidence of the islands' violent past is never far away. Here and there, where the superficial soil layer has been disrupted, it is easy to see the powdery ash left by Krakatau's last explosion. Ultimately, life's hold on these wilderness islands might once again be extinguished. Perhaps Anak Krakatau will see to that.

THE KIMBERLEY PLATEAU

"Soft sandstone hills have been turned into natural sculptures"

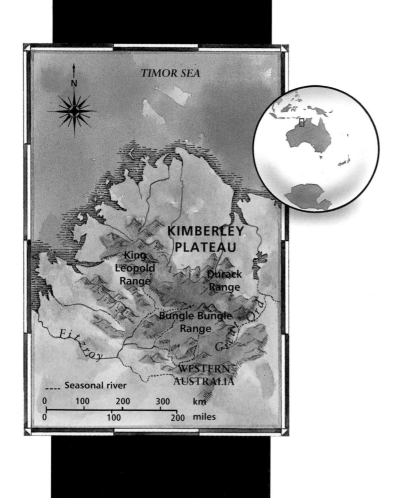

Summer comes suddenly to the Kimberley Plateau, in the far northwest of Australia. By mid-November, the land seems to have contracted after the long months of "the Dry." Red rock shimmers in temperatures which since July have increased to as much as 120°F (49°C), and billabongs – the

Tiger-striped with silica and lichen, the eroded domes of the Bungle Bungle Range glow magically as the sun rises over Kimberley.

pools of water left in empty river beds – provide a last sanctuary for freshwater crocodiles and sawfish. Boab trees living off the moisture in their swollen trunks have shed their leaves in the heat.

Offshore, tropical storms gather force, heralded by banks of bruised clouds and hot winds. They sweep inland over the fragmented shore and mangrove swamps, over stretches of mallee scrub and grassland, and up onto the plateau, where the first of the summer deluges begin.

Paradoxically, although the Kimberley Plateau consists of a whorl of arid mountain ranges flanked to the south and east by the Great Sandy and Gibson deserts, it accounts for more than three-quarters of the water runoff in Western Australia. The summer rains – which average 12 inches (30 cm) a month – pour off the impervious crust of the rock and rush through deep fissures formed by millions of years of rainfall. The engorged Mitchell River, which has

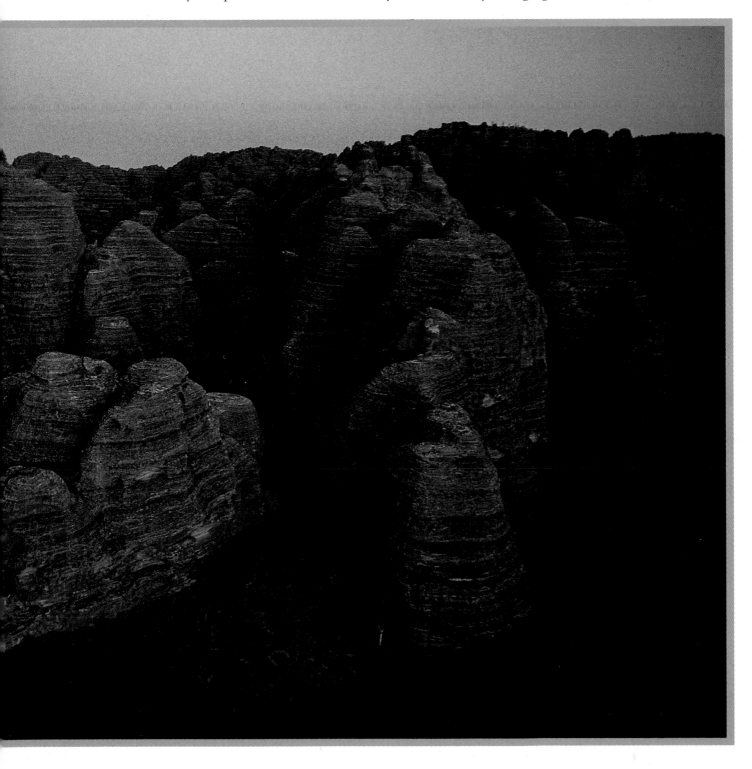

been known to widen from 330 feet (100 m) to 7 miles (11 km) after a few days of rain, rises by as much as 56 feet (17 m). Saltwater crocodiles and stingrays can be found right up to the base of the plateau cliffs, more than 60 miles (100 km) inland.

The Aboriginal name for the Kimberley is "Wandjina," after its creators the Water Spirits, and water is almost wholly responsible for its extraordinary physical geography. The mountains sit on what is known as the Ancient Plateau of Australia, a stable bed of rock which existed long before life on Earth. Some 350 million years, ago these ranges were part of an oceanic bank of limestone and coral far bigger than the Great Barrier Reef. As the sea receded and tectonic forces pushed the mountains upward to heights of more than 3,300 feet (1,000 m), the rain began to do its work, rounding off peaks and scoring the rock with numerous crevices and riverbeds.

Until the Gibb River road was built in 1986 to transport beef from isolated cattle stations, the northern part of the Kimberley Plateau was

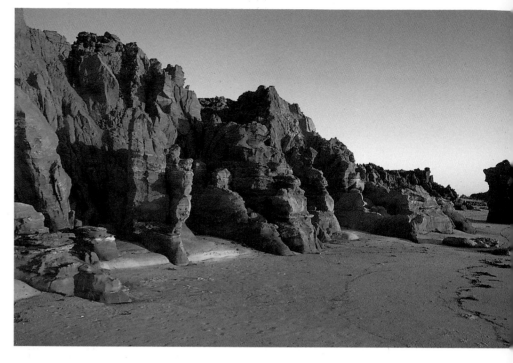

completely inaccessible. Even now the dirt road peters out into nothingness around Mount Elizabeth, and few venture into the interior when faced with the prospect of searing heat and floods. Travelers stick to boat journeys up the coast, to what is known as gorge territory and to natural phenomena such as the

Bungle Bungle sandstone formations.

Some animals, meanwhile, have adapted adroitly to the violent extremes. The wallaroo, a type of kangaroo, reduces water loss by having concentrated urine and no sweat glands. It can survive for two weeks without drinking, keeping cool by licking its forearms and panting.

It is easy to think of the Kimberley as a compact, isolated piece of territory; easy to forget that its 30,000 inhabitants are scattered across an area the size of the Netherlands. The variety of scenery is astounding. The deep red gorges of Windjana and Geikie, studded with gray-green eucalyptus shrubs, and the 2,500-foot (750-m) subterranean cavern at Tunnel Creek – where the Rainbow Serpent is believed by Aborigines to have entered the Earth after the Creation – slice channels through the fossilized limestone of the ancient coral reefs.

To the west, on the low savannas, the only relief from the flatness comes from ungainly boab trees – relatives of the African baobab – thought to have floated over from Madagascar in seed form 75 million years ago.

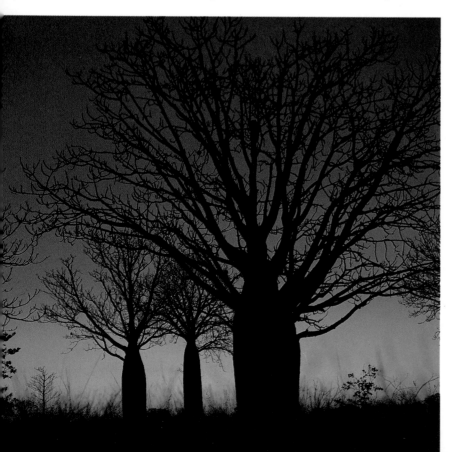

Swollen trunks of boab trees dot the dry savanna near the coast. With their own supply of water in the trunk, the trees can outlive the worst of the summer heat and winter drought, sometimes splitting open in the process.

Tropical storms and powerful ocean tides have fragmented the red coastal rock of the Kimberley Plateau and fashioned it into exotic shapes (left).

Eerily translucent, a ghost bat hangs from the roof of a cave (right). One of the most predatory of all bats, it feeds on birds, lizards and even other bats. It attacks by landing on its victim, wrapping it in its strong wings and delivering a single killing bite to the back of the prey's neck. The ghost bat's sharp teeth have earned its other common name of false vampire bat.

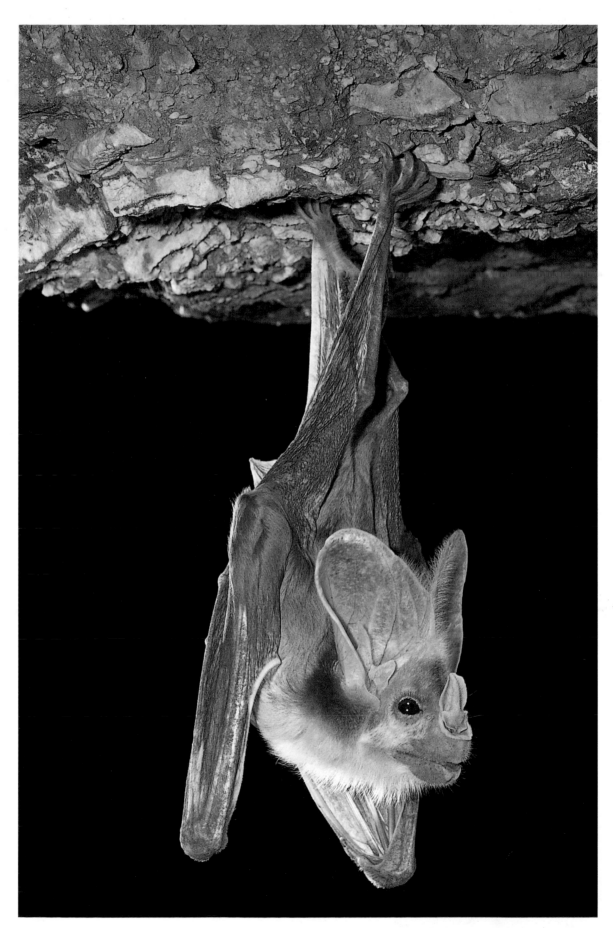

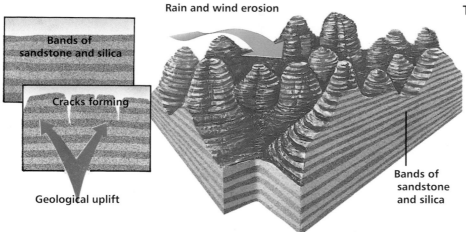

Bands of sandstone and silica

Cracks forming

Geological uplift

Rain and wind erosion

Bands of sandstone and silica

THE BUNGLE BUNGLE MOUNTAINS

Massive forces lifted layers of silica and sandstone on the Kimberley Plateau some one and a half billion years ago, leaving cracks and fissures in the vulnerable rock. Millions of years of wind and water erosion, chiefly from the flash-flooding caused by seasonal downpours, exposed these weaknesses and created the domes and ridges that make up the Bungle Bungle Range.

Miniature ranges of narrow termite mounds are built along strict axes to escape the worst of the sun. But even here water has taken a hand. Whiskey, Nugget, Blackfellow and Bottle Tree creeks, each a tiny thread on the map, are just some of the thousands of watercourses that vein the land, giving rise to small stands of eucalyptus and vine thickets wherever the water supply is permanent. These oases harbor exotic creatures like red-collared lorikeets, death adders and the purple-crowned fairy wren, one of Australia's rarest birds.

Finally, beyond the transitional coastal zone where mangroves survive in brackish, salty conditions – excreting salt from their leaves and supporting a wealth of anerobic life beneath their roots – there are the wide mud flats and racing tides of the Indian Ocean and the Timor Sea. This is a treacherous coast – where water brings life inland, it brings death by the sea. Tides rising by as much as 36 feet (11 m) cover the mud flats faster than a person can walk, sweeping rays and ocean fish into the creeks where "salties" (voracious saltwater crocodiles) wait patiently. Boats caught unawares by whirlpools, vicious ocean currents or cyclones hurtling in toward land, have little hope of survival.

For this reason, the Kimberley coast is rarely seen by humans, except in photographs or the occasional film.

It is spectacularly beautiful. About a quarter of a million wading birds stalk the mud flats, leaving every year on a 1,250-mile (2,000-km) odyssey to Siberia for the breeding season. Mudskipper fish hop rides on fiddler crabs, and red mullet explode out of the water to escape from predators.

Southeast of the main plateau, outside the protective curve of the King Leopold and Durack mountain ranges and below the newly irrigated valleys of the Great Ord River, lies the most dramatic work of the Water

"Modern life has barely grazed the edges of the Kimberley Plateau"

Spirits – the Bungle Bungle Range. Wind and water have turned the soft sandstone hills into monumental natural sculptures, made more dramatic by the stripes of black lichen and orange silica inherent in the rock. On the cliff sides, and hidden in overhangs, are paintings done over thousands of years by Aborigines; tributes to the animals they hunted and the spirits who created them.

No one is allowed to climb the formations; one breach in the thin, hard skin of horizontal quartzite rock on the surface would expose the interior to erosion, and the Bungle Bungles would gradually disappear from the face of the Earth.

Modern life has barely grazed the edges of the Kimberley. There is a brief landscape of rolling pastureland dotted with sheep stations to the south of the Mitchell River, before the desert begins. In the east, millions of acres of grazing have been flooded in the Ord River Irrigation Scheme, which has succeeded in providing a consistent supply of water for agriculture. Aborigines continue to spear and net fish from their remote settlements on the coast. But the heart of the northwest, the plateau and its environs, is still empty; a haunting wilderness visited by the summer rains, baked by the sun and peopled with hardy animals and plants. Kimberley is still Wandjina: the land of the wind and the water.

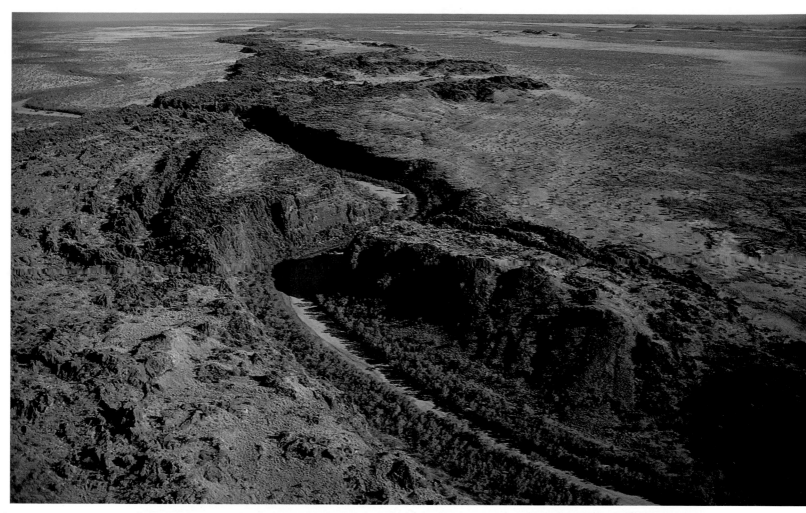

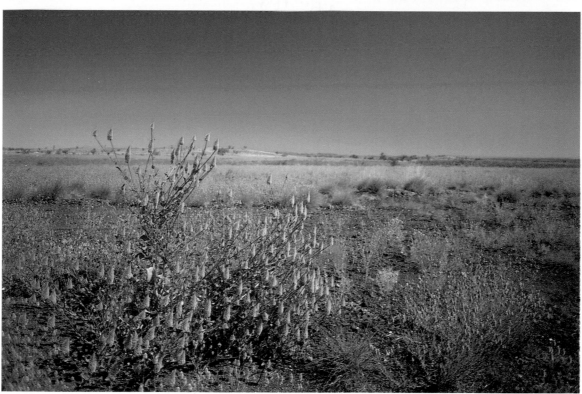

The Windjana Gorge (above) was once part of a limestone and coral bank on the ocean floor.

In the rainy season, the dry plateau springs to life. Seeds sprout and for a time the flat dusty plain fills with the purple and green haze of flowering mulla mulla plants (right).

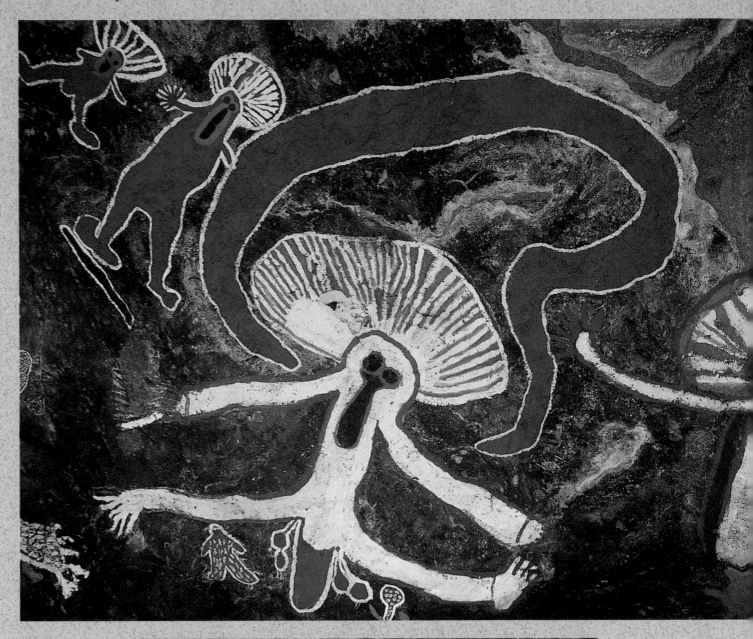

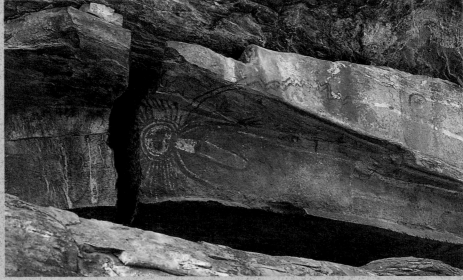

Brilliantly colored in ocher and gypsum, Wandjina figures cavort across a wall in the Dog Cave area of the Kimberley's Napier Range (above). Associated beings in the picture include a python, which represents the Rainbow Serpent.

Ancient paintings of the Wandjina – ancestral beings from sky and sea who formed the landscape and control fertility as well as the elements – still play a significant part in the ceremonial life of Kimberley Aborigines today (left).

ABORIGINAL ART
IN THE KIMBERLEY

The colorful, sedimentary rock walls of the central and northern Kimberley hold the secrets of the ceremonial life and rituals of the Wororra and Ngarinyin Aboriginal peoples. In tunnels, caves and overhangs, paintings in ocher and gypsum – some of them several yards long – have survived changes in climate and in sea levels for as long as 3,000 years.

There are two types of rock paintings in the Kimberley – the older, monochromatic figures known as "Bradshaw figures," after the European who first saw them, and the more famous "Wandjina figures," with stark white bodies, blank eyes and haloes of lines radiating from their heads.

The Wandjina came from the sky and sea, bringing rain and therefore fertility. They were often mouthless, and the lines around their heads may well signify lightning. They are frequently depicted with animal forms and powerful spirits such as the Rainbow Serpent or the Lightning Brothers. Repainted and overpainted by generations of artists, the Wandjina images are still relevant to Aboriginal culture today.

All Aboriginal rock paintings, however remote from modern settlements, are enmeshed in a system of tribal ownership. Repainting – which keeps their influence strong – may not be done by the owners, only by artist kin as dictated by tribal law.

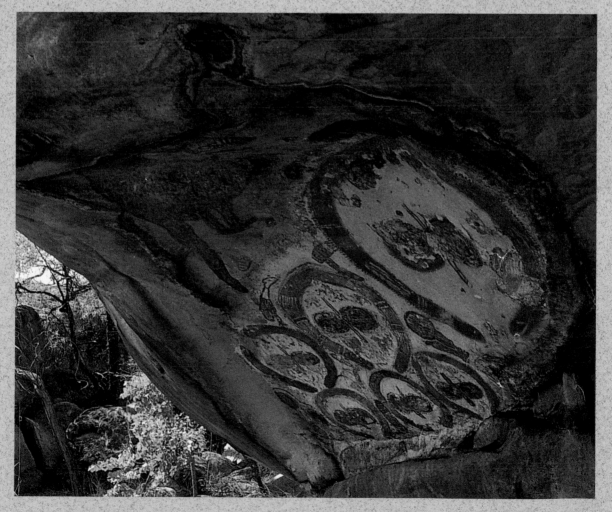

Wandjina figures, such as these on a rocky overhang (right), retain their magic for centuries. They can be repainted to renew their spiritual strength or painted over with new designs, but only by specific artist relatives of their original owners.

CAPE YORK PENINSULA

"One of the most demanding and varied terrains on Earth"

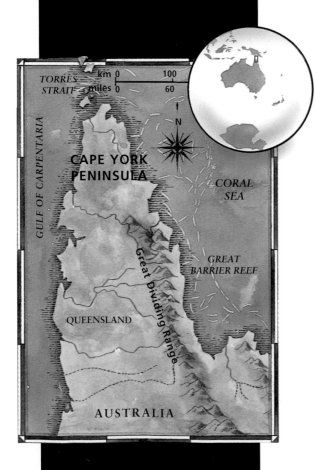

There is only one road to the northeastern peninsula the Australians call simply "The Tip." For six months of the year it is impassable: dry water courses fill with raging currents, rivers appear as if from nowhere and the dirt "washboard" track (so called because of its punishing, runneled surface) turns to mud under the

A strip of sand in a remote bay divides the forests of the Cape York Peninsula from the brilliant waters of the Coral Sea.

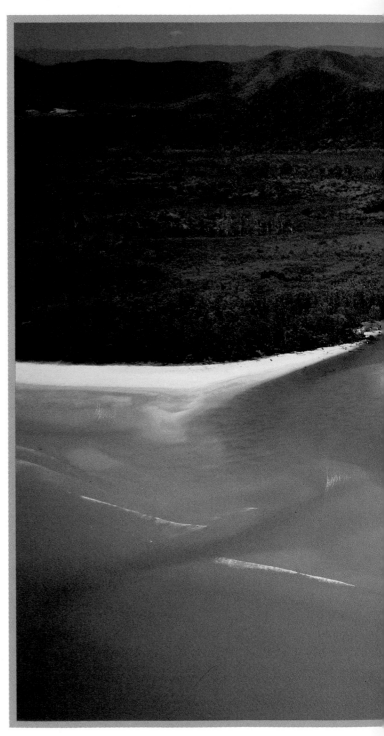

onslaught of tropical storms. Even during the drier months of June to September, it can take days to reach the isolated settlement of Bamaga, at Australia's northernmost point in the state of Queensland.

The Cape York Peninsula, with its 80,000 sq. miles (207,000 km²) of wilderness and its tiny population, occupies a special place in the urban Australian consciousness as the last frontier. The pockets of relict rainforest on the east coast are the sole remaining fragments of Australia as it once was – a land covered by millions of acres of dense forest supporting outsize, primitive plants and animals such as kangaroos. But anthropologically speaking, Cape York should be considered the first frontier, the point at which, around 40,000 years ago, the ancestors of today's Aborigines first crossed from Southeast Asia to populate a new and empty continent.

Today, few people head north over the Mitchell River to explore this remotest area of Queensland. Divided from Asia by the narrow waters of the Torres Strait and split along its length

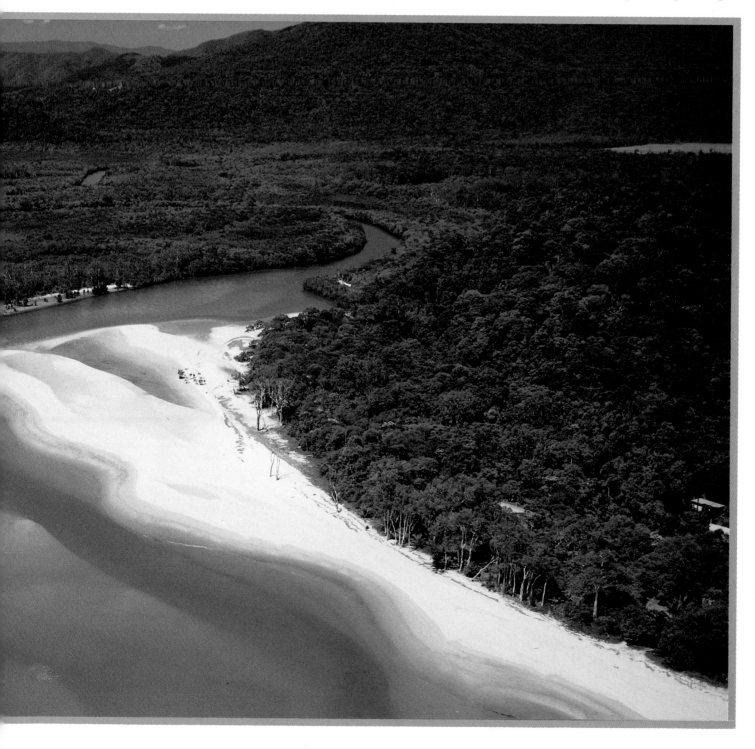

by the fading spine of the Great Dividing Range, the peninsula is markedly different on either side of the mountains. To the west, the wide, tussocky savanna – grazing territory for the hardy cattle known as "scrubmasters" and home to creatures such as native bush cats and agile wallabies – ends in tangled mangrove swamps, desolate beaches and the shallow Gulf of Carpentaria.

By contrast, the narrow strip of land between the eastern foothills of the Great Dividing Range and the Coral Sea on the eastern coast of the peninsula is humid and heavy with vegetation, much of it a continuation of the great Indo-Malaysian rainforest. Giant buttressed trees – their central roots so shallow that the buttresses are vital to counter the weight of the canopy – are hung with lianas, orchids and clinging aroids (members of the lily family).

Every year between November and May, tropical fronts sweep across the peninsula en route to Asia, drenching the eastern forest, replenishing the southern wetlands, and bringing flash-floods to the western savanna. In January, temperatures can climb as high as 95°F (35°C).

The natural life of Cape York, as elsewhere in Australia, is partly the result of the continent's history. Australia was once part of the huge southern landmass known as Gondwana. When, about 160 million years ago, this supercontinent began to split into the separate landmasses of the southern hemisphere, the scattered descendants of Gondwanan species began to evolve in different ways. Among the fauna and flora which developed on the "Australian Ark" – finally isolated millions of years later – were flightless birds, marsupial mammals, the egg-laying mammals known as monotremes, and sclerophylls. These are trees that have developed thick, moisture-retaining cuticles on their narrow leaves. Best known of these is the eucalyptus, a common tree in the rainforests of the Cape York Peninsula.

One resident of the forest, the 6-foot (1.8-m) tall cassowary, a shy, flightless bird, is related to the African ostrich and the South American rhea – both fast-running, flightless birds. The group probably originated in Gondwana before it split up and only later evolved into separate species.

Others, such as birds of paradise, with their spectacular plumage, or the nocturnal sugar glider, a flying possum which skims from tree to tree by means of a parachute-like membrane between its fore and hind limbs, are Southeast Asian in origin. Native Queenslanders include Lumholtz's tree kangaroos – timorous

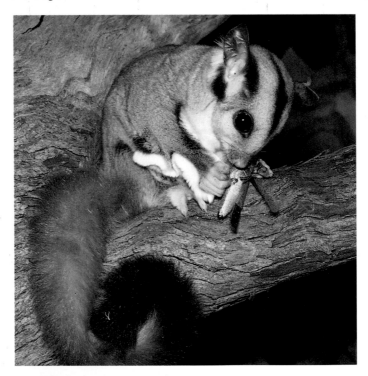

A sugar glider busies itself with its prey high in the forest canopy (left). This little creature can swoop from tree to tree, gliding on the extended membrane of skin between its legs.

Poised for flight, a giant tree frog clings to a vine, using suction pads on its fingers and toes (right).

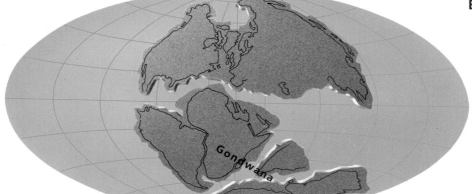

BREAK-UP OF A SUPERCONTINENT
The supercontinent of Gondwana began to fragment some 160 million years ago. As the continental masses slowly drifted apart, each still bore its original flora and fauna. Once parted, these developed into separate species. Marsupials, however, evolved after Africa and India had separated from the others but before the break-up was complete, so they are found only in South America and Australia and as fossils in Antarctica.

*"Pockets of relict rainforest
are the sole remaining fragments of
Australia as it once was"*

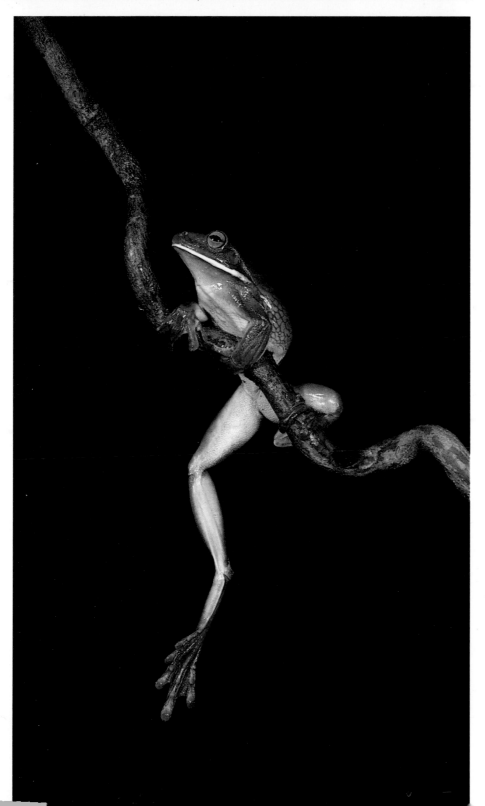

creatures that can drop 45 feet (14 m) from a tree perch down to the ground to escape from danger – and bearded forest dragons – a rare type of lizard.

The peninsula has never welcomed intruders. Its coast is sparsely punctuated with the ruins of gold and pearling towns – eerie testaments to human greed which are gradually being reclaimed by nature. The Aboriginal population has survived, exchanging its semi-nomadic family units for the settlements encouraged by federal government. Even so, the 2,500 Aborigines on the peninsula – including the Torres Strait Islanders – lead an isolated existence; most reserves and communities are far out of reach of the casual visitor.

In the sandstone escarpment at Split Rock, near the town of Laura, Aboriginal history is recorded in the natural "museum" known as the Quinkan Galleries. Dozens of rock art chambers, some 13,000 years old, lie open to the sky, the majority of them off-limits to outsiders. Dugongs, or sea cows – once a valuable source of food – swim across the walls with giant turtles and crocodiles, while scenes of hunting and gathering depict species and ways of life that came and went as sea levels changed.

Cape York's natural wealth has always been the biggest threat to its survival. The iron-rich laterite soil of the west already supplies the world with bauxite, and the ancient but comparatively unfolded peninsular rock contains colossal riches in the form of metals and minerals. The precious area of rainforest on the peninsula has shrunk by three-quarters since European contact. What remains is now under government protection.

But the very remoteness of this wild area may be its salvation. Cape York Peninsula looks likely to remain one of the most demanding and varied terrains on Earth – the first, and last, frontier of Australia.

SOUTH WEST NATIONAL PARK

"Low valleys are blanketed with the world's last great temperate rainforest"

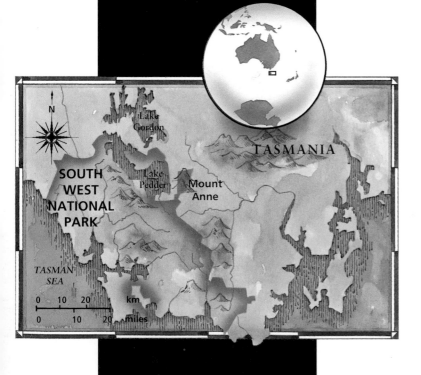

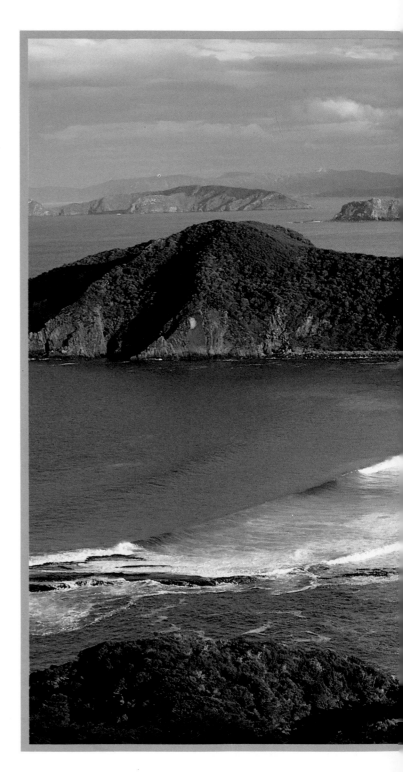

Every few years, in the cool, remote forests of southwest Tasmania, there is a reported sighting of the Tasmanian tiger. It usually comes from a hiker on one of the long, strenuous trails in the 1,740-sq. mile (4,500-km²) wilderness known as the South West National Park, who believes he has glimpsed

Waves roll onto a lonely beach in Tasmania's South West National Park. Violent storms soak the land with 30 inches (750 mm) of rain a year.

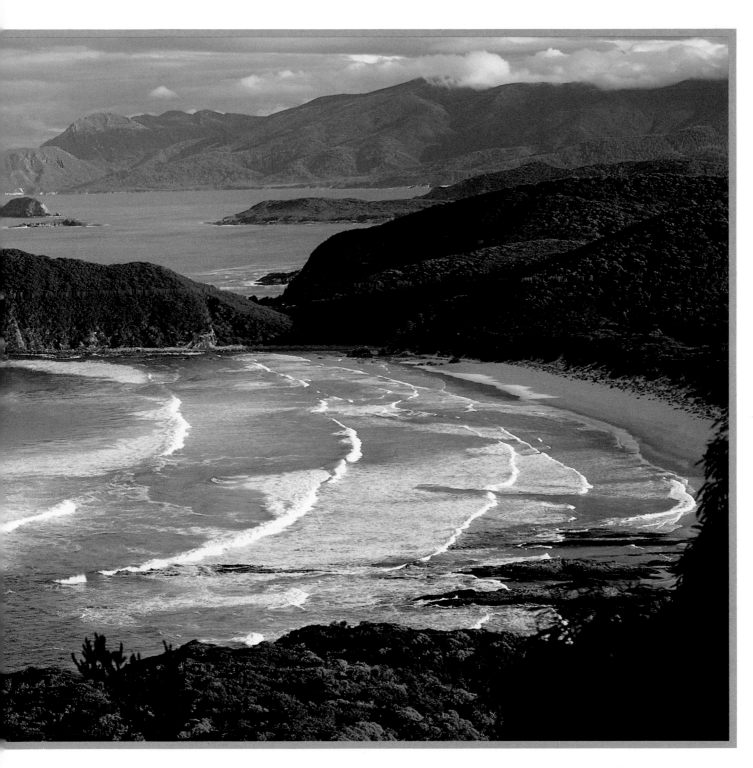

the sloping rump and barred markings of one of the rarest animals on Earth.

If the tiger – in fact, a striped marsupial wolf long thought to be extinct – has survived anywhere, it would be here, among the mountains, rivers and watery sedgelands of Tasmania's loneliest region. The low valleys are blanketed with the world's last great temperate rainforest. Here, stands of gargantuan King Billy and huon pine tower over leatherwood, sassafras and blackwood trees, and clumps of ferns and velvet mosses cluster beneath them.

Temperate rainforest, unlike its tropical relative, is an airy place. Instead of the dozens of tree species with their oversized leaves and flowers and coiled lianas, one species of tree tends to dominate – in this case, the Arctic or tanglefoot beech. This is the only deciduous tree in the forest, which, according to tradition, waits for Anzac Day on April 25 before consuming the landscape in a blaze of autumn colors.

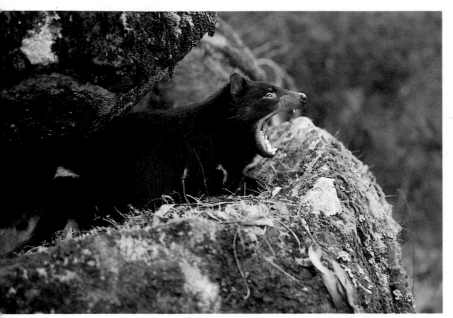

The Tasmanian devil was hunted to extinction on the Australian mainland by dingoes. This stocky marsupial is a scavenger rather than a predator. It has a big head and powerful jaws which can crunch through the bones of carcasses.

"A vicious type of scrub known as "horizontal" has tangled stems that grow vertically for a few yards, then shoot out sideways"

It may appear a gentle wilderness, but southwestern Tasmania is far from defenseless. Large areas have been saved from human intrusion by a vicious type of scrub known as "horizontal" – tangled stems that grow vertically for a few yards and then shoot out sideways, forming a dense tracery of branches which looks solid enough to walk on. Anyone foolish enough to try falls through into the undergrowth – often injuring themselves in the process.

These pockets of unknown territory, together with the more accessible parts of the forest, harbor two-thirds of the many mammal species unique to Tasmania, most of the 14 endemic birds, and several other animals and plants on the verge of extinction.

The island of Tasmania is large – 26,380 sq. miles (68,330 km²) – and shaped like an arrowhead, pointing straight down toward the South Pole from its position 100 miles (160 km) off the southeastern tip of Australia. The island was separated from the mainland 13,000 years ago, during the great melt from the last ice age, and the formation of the Bass Strait marooned dozens of species there to evolve in total isolation.

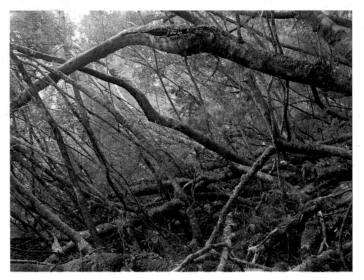

A stand of Tasmania's infamous "horizontal" plant blocks out the light and creates a false floor of branches to trap the unwary. The plant is almost impossible to cut through, even with an axe.

Today Tasmania shares little more than a continental shelf with its estranged parent. Unlike the dry, flat mainland, it is green and mountainous with a consistently wet climate. It lies directly in the path of the Roaring Forties, which bring rain and gales all year round, and during the hot summer it suffers torrential tropical storms from the northwest.

Perhaps because of its remoteness and atypical climate, Tasmanian wildlife tends toward the bizarre. The Tasmanian devil, a nocturnal forest-dweller with black and white markings and sharp claws, produces a blood-curdling scream when cornered. There is a "living fossil" – a species of freshwater shrimp unchanged for 200 million years – still surviving in the frigid alpine tarns, and the improbable red velvet glowworm, which shoots a gluelike substance at its prey from protrusions on each side of its head.

The trees, though slightly less exotic than the animals, are equally impressive. Some of the huon pines – endemic to Tasmania – date from as early as 1,000 years before Christ and are only eclipsed in stature by the soaring trunks of moss-covered King Billies and the pale, lofty swamp gums. The latter, with a height of up

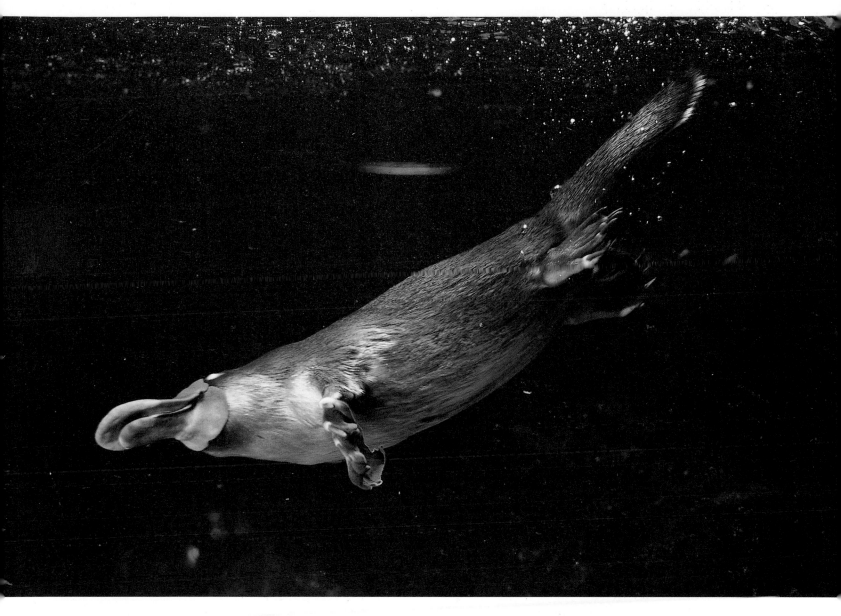

to 312 feet (95 m), is the world's tallest flowering plant.

Complex relationships have developed between fauna and flora. The Tasmanian honeyeater is a bird that feeds off the nectar of eucalyptus blossoms unique to the island. In doing so, the bird picks up pollen on its feathers, cross-fertilizing the trees and ensuring its supply of food for the future. Elusive orange-bellied parrots, of which there are now only about 200, congregate around a single type of tree called *Melaleuca*.

Though protected by law, the Tasmanian wilderness is desperately fragile. Even on designated trails through the open country, with its buttongrass swamps and delicate plants, the most careful walker can spread diseases such as root rot fungus, which attacks plants in moorland and dry eucalyptus forests. The alpine meadows contain more than 300 species of lichens, mosses and ferns which are easily destroyed, and a passionate campaign is under way to restore Lake Pedder, the deepest lake in all Australia, to its natural condition. The lake was flooded for hydroelectricity in 1972, destroying most of its rare fish.

But for the moment it seems that Tasmania's South West National

A duck-billed platypus dives in a freshwater stream, using its sensitive bill to help it find food such as shrimp. Seemingly defenseless, the platypus has a poison spur on each hind foot.

Park, with its eccentric animals, magnificent broadleaf forests and cold seas stocked with bluefin tuna and billfish, remains a safe haven for some of the stranger species on this earth. And perhaps in the deep recesses of the forest, protected by demanding terrain and fierce ramparts of "horizontal," the Tasmanian tiger still hunts its prey in peace.

POOR KNIGHTS ISLANDS

"Winds and strong seas have battered the islands' sides into jagged cliffs which rise straight out of the Pacific Ocean"

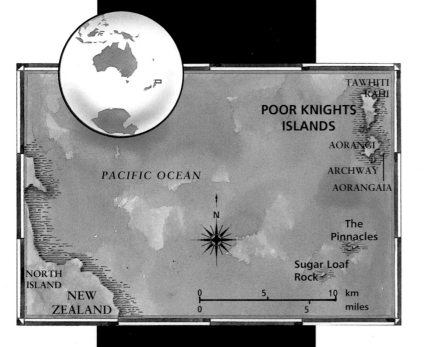

POOR KNIGHTS ISLANDS

TAWHITI RAHI

AORANGI

ARCHWAY

AORANGAIA

The Pinnacles

Sugar Loaf Rock

PACIFIC OCEAN

N

NORTH ISLAND

NEW ZEALAND

0   5   10   km
0   5   miles

Few humans have set foot on Poor Knights Islands in the last century. Most of those who have are scientists camping out for a few days and nights on the small, craggy outcrops perched at the edge of New Zealand's continental shelf, staying only to

Sun streaming through underwater cave entrances at Aorangi Island illuminates a school of pink maomao fish.

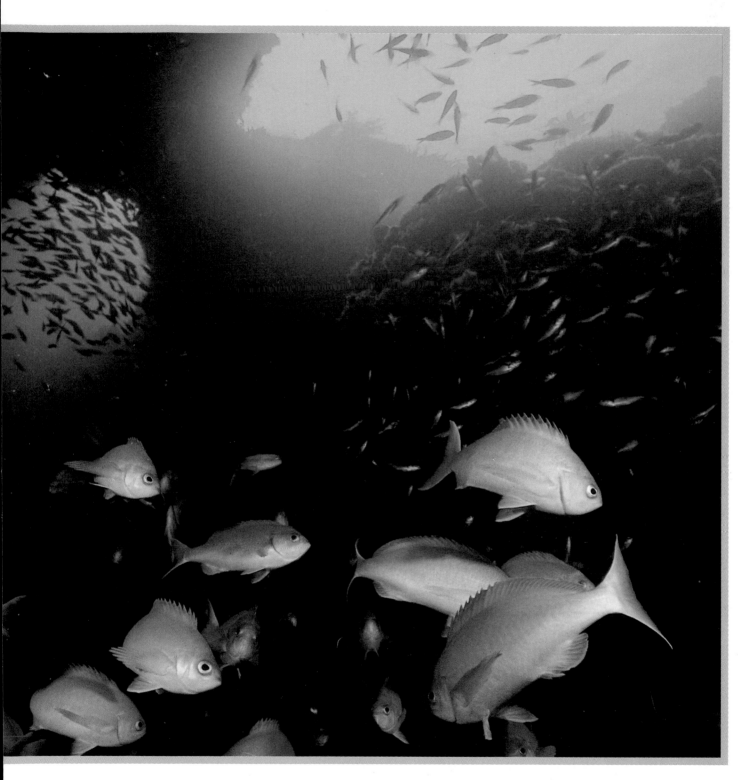

observe the wildlife and the striking rock formations.

A combination of circumstances has made the Poor Knights a natural sanctuary for rare seabirds, insects and a number of reptiles. The islands usually appear on maps as two dots lying about 12 miles (20 km) east of the narrow spit of North Island known as Northland. In fact, there are four islands – Tawhiti Rahi and Aorangi (the two largest), Aorangaia and Archway – and some scattered rock stacks and pinnacles.

Their appearance is forbidding. Northeast winds and strong seas have battered their sides into jagged cliffs, which rise straight out of the Pacific Ocean to a height of 660 feet (200 m). The thin soil of the central plateaus, honeycombed with bird burrows, is surrounded by sparse bands of coastal forest. The climate is unexpectedly mild and subtropical. The islands are

ANCIENT REPTILES

The two largest Poor Knights Islands are famous for their populations of tuataras. These large primitive reptiles look like lizards, but are in fact the only surviving members of an ancient group known as beak-headed reptiles. Destroyed on the mainland by introduced predators such as cats and rats, tuataras thrive in the safety of the islands, feeding on insects such as wetas and beetles.

Tuataras are long-lived. They do not reach sexual maturity until they are about 20 and may live to be 100.

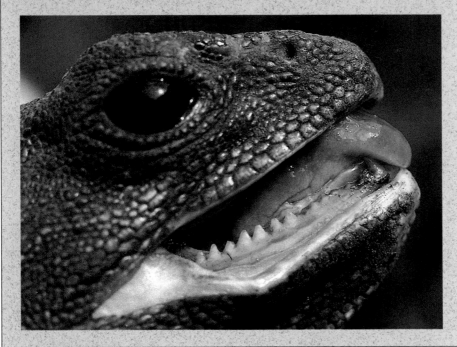

greatly sheltered by the bulk of Northland, and they lie in the path of a warm equatorial current which flows down from northern Queensland and around New Zealand's North Cape. It arrives at the Poor Knights Islands as the East Auckland Current, raising the water temperature by a few degrees and allowing a small pocket of exotic marine life to thrive in otherwise temperate waters.

Perhaps most important, islands such as Poor Knights are the only part of New Zealand that is rat-free. Their inhabitants are safe from the havoc wrought by these killers in the rest of the country. Despite the arrival of Captain Cook's ships, bringing pigs to trade with Maori villagers, no

"Lava tunnels and deep arches shelter rare black coral, and dazzling schools of fish are legendary among divers"

introduced predators reached the islands. The Maoris themselves, who hunted seabirds and their eggs for food, were massacred in a tribal raid from the mainland in 1830, leaving behind only the remains of stone walls and agricultural terracing that now provide homes for birds.

In spite of their small size, the Poor Knights Islands harbor several endemic species. Buller's shearwaters are large seabirds which breed in their thousands on Tawhiti Rahi, where the earth is soft and treacherous with their burrows. When the breeding season is over, the birds migrate as far as Alaska and Chile. They are an aggressive species, and other birds – like the rare Pycroft's petrel and the gray-faced petrel – have been forced to breed away from them in the relative security of Aorangi Island.

Bellbirds, too, breed on Aorangi where they eat the fruit of the hangehange trees, which grow perched on cliffs around the islands. They also eat insects from the tree canopy and nectar from the flowering xeronema lily, another local species.

Giant tree wetas and cave wetas – cricketlike insects which can cover 7 feet (2 m) at a bound – compete for living space in the sparse forests with a poisonous 24-inch (60-cm) long centipede. None of these could have survived if rats and other predators had reached the islands. New Zealand's largest gecko also lives on Poor Knights. A colorful 12-inch (30-cm) long lizard, Duvaucel's gecko, hides under stones or logs during the day and comes out at night to search for berries, nectar and insects to eat.

Tradition has it that when Captain Cook saw the islands in 1760, he christened them Poor Knights because they reminded him of a popular English dish of the time with that name – savory dumplings dipped in egg. But the Poor Knights started life more than nine million years ago as a huge and active volcano; today's tiny islands were once buried under 1,650 feet (500 m) of volcanic debris spewed down the western slopes of the crater. Gradually the cone wore down to mere remnants of rock, smoothed and shaped by the sea into their present form. The sweeping away of softer rock, leaving behind a skeleton of harder stone, created outlandish arches, caves and tunnels. Many are now far below the water level, providing a wide range of habitats and idyllic breeding grounds for marine life.

Where the cliffs emerge vertically from the ocean, they also plummet as much as 400 feet (125 m) to the floor of the continental shelf. Just beyond the shelf, the ocean plunges to far greater depths, producing strong swells and occasionally extremely dangerous currents.

Poor Knights Islands became a marine reserve in 1981. Landing on the islands themselves is now completely forbidden – the delicate balance of the ecology can all too easily be disturbed. Visitors are, however, allowed to explore the waters of the reserve. The "air-bubble caves" (submerged caverns with the roof higher at the back than the front, trapping a pocket of air), lava tunnels as much as 1,300 feet (400 m) long and deep arches are legendary among divers. They shelter clusters of rare black coral and dazzling schools of fish, such as maomao, boarfish and parrot fish. Great trails of red kelp – usually a feature of temperate, rather than subtropical, seas – grow to a size of 200 feet (60 m).

The warm equatorial current brings with it quantities of plankton – food for fish and seabirds alike. Mighty kingfish, weighing up to 80 pounds (36 kg), make their leisurely way through the rocks, caves teem with schools of blue and pink maomao fish and 40-foot (12-m) whale sharks swim ponderously above their shadows. Purple shore crabs, with powerful legs

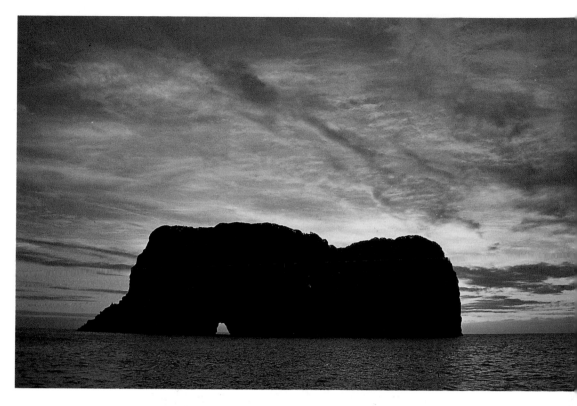

and pincers, scale the rugged cliffs to forage for food among the trees.

Above ground, the only evidence of human occupation is the old 19th-century lighthouse on the north of Tawhiti Rahi and the remains of a Maori population of three or four hundred people. The Poor Knights Islands are left alone, cliff-bound and free of predators, to remain as they have always been, a tiny sliver of New Zealand's past.

Dawn comes to Aorangaia, one of the smaller Poor Knights Islands. Once buried under volcanic material, the remaining rock has been smoothed and weathered by the sea over time.

A mosaic moray eel and a spiny sea urchin strike a threatening note among the fairytale world of cup corals, seaweeds and colorful sponges on the ocean floor (below).

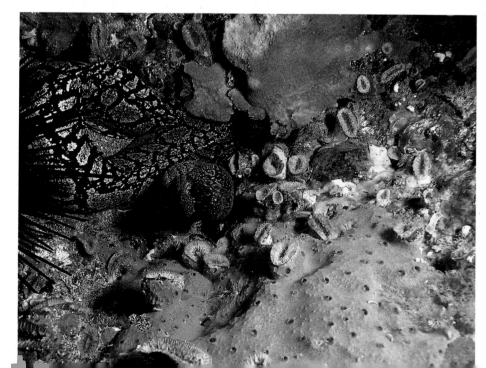

FIORDLAND

"Wild terrain with endless bush, few trails and rich animal life"

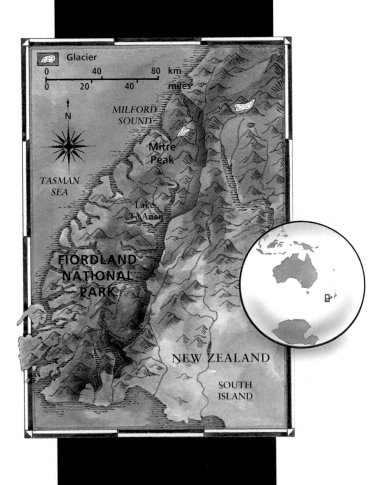

At the southwestern tip of New Zealand, the mighty alps and wild coast of South Island come to a dramatic end. Granite mountains plunge thousands of feet into the cold blue of the Tasman Sea, their slopes so precipitous that they are empty of vegetation. Fur seals raise their heads in sight of the shore, crested penguins dive for fish, and the probing fingers of the Marlborough Sound slide between sheer cliffs, penetrating deep into the haunting coastal region known as Fiordland.

In an already isolated country – New Zealand is about 1,000 miles (1,600 km) from its nearest neighbor – Fiordland is more remote still. Bounded on the north by a jumble of mountain ranges such as the Darrens, the Humboldts, the Stuarts and the Murchisons – their Maori names long since eclipsed by those of explorers and early Scottish settlers – it is wild terrain with endless bush, few trails and a rich variety of animal life. Due south of the Tasman Sea that borders Fiordland's coast, the Southern Ocean stretches away to the Antarctic ice cap.

Fiordland, which covers roughly 3 million acres (1.2 million hectares), was designated as a national park in 1952. The bulk of this beautiful area, named for its resemblance to the fiord coasts of Norway, is a battleground between land and water. After the last ice age, deep troughs gouged in the ancient, metamorphosed gneiss rock by glacial ice were flooded with sea water as the ice retreated. At the same

__Mitre Peak, Fiordland's most famous__ mountain, towers 5,550 feet (1,692 m) above its reflection in the peaceful waters of Milford Sound. The Sounds – inlets carved into the rock by glaciers and flooded by the sea – combine with abundant rainfall to make this one of the wettest places on Earth.

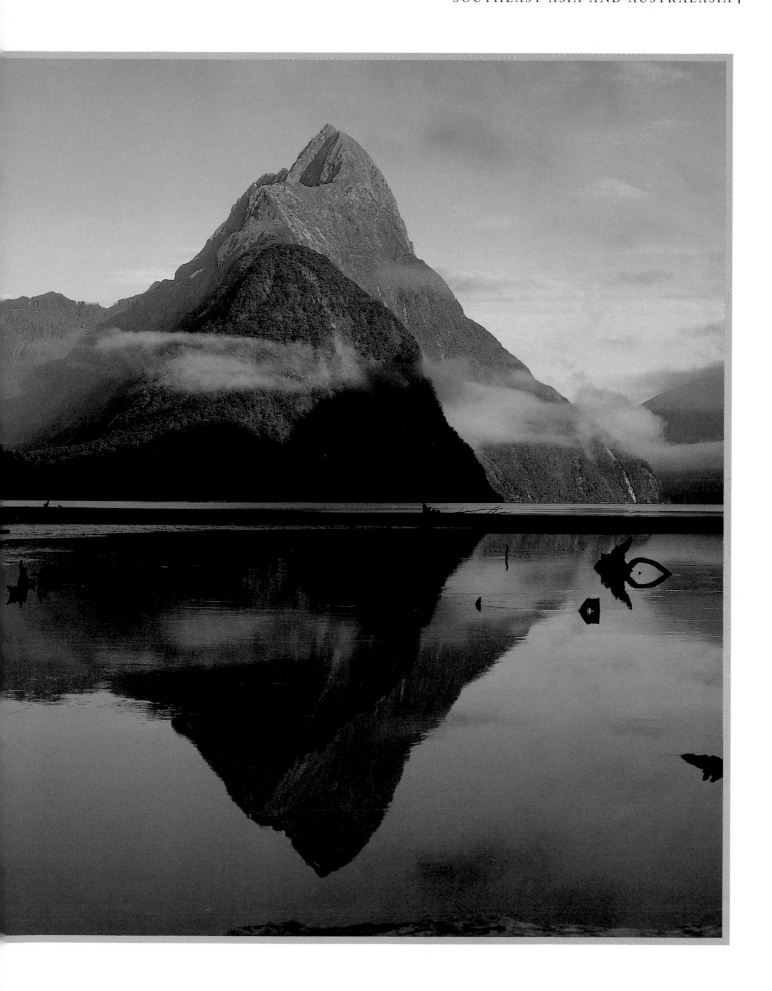

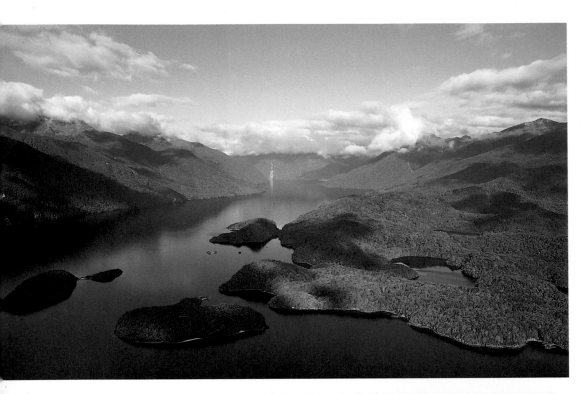

At the heart of Fiordland, Lake Te Anau – once home to a mythical lost tribe of the Maoris – lies like a sheet of glass between the hills (above).

On a rare mist-free day, the icy waters of Sutherland Falls in Fiordland twist nearly 1,800 feet (550 m) down to the valley (right). These dramatic falls are the highest in New Zealand and among the highest in the world.

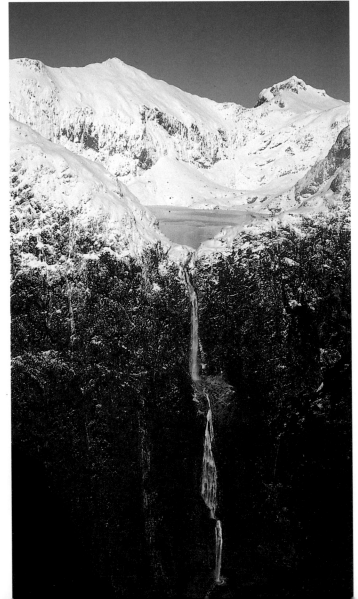

time, meltwaters poured eastward off the mountains and formed a chain of freshwater lakes dammed by glacial debris. These are now a natural barrier between the wild country and the rich pastures of the southern sheep farms. Surrounded and fragmented by water, the nation's biggest protected area seems to be slowly withdrawing from the solid fist of the mainland.

Even without its lakes and encroaching sea, Fiordland could claim to be one of the wettest places on the planet. Prevailing southwest winds dump 236 inches (6,000 mm) of rain on the mountainsides every year. Rain keeps the lowland temperate rainforest in a permanent state of humidity, replenishing lakes and feeding the hundreds of waterfalls that plummet from the cliffs.

New Zealand's isolation has had a profound effect on its flora and fauna. When it parted from other southern landmasses more than 70 million years ago, it took with it a number of flowering plants, but no animals. Living creatures have had to float, fly or swim to reach the islands, and the only endemic land mammals are two species of bats.

A richly forested land, with an equable climate and no serious land predators, New Zealand became a haven for birds. Many large, flightless species evolved – food was plentiful, and there were no enemies from which to escape. One of the largest was the now extinct moa which stood more than 12 feet (3.5 m) high. Today kiwis – New Zealand's national symbol – still forage for food in the Fiordland rainforest, using the nostrils at the tip of their long, curved bills to locate larvae and grubs. Diminutive, flightless birds with vestigial wings and a loose plumage of narrow feathers that resembles coarse hair, kiwis have survived in healthy numbers.

But for many birds, the arrival of human beings was catastrophic. First

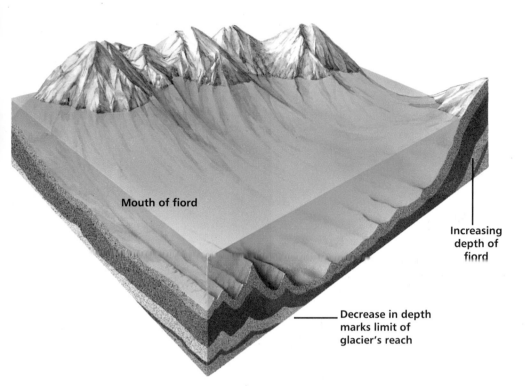

Mouth of fiord

Increasing depth of fiord

Decrease in depth marks limit of glacier's reach

THE NEW ZEALAND FIORDS

When the ice floes finally retreated from the southern tip of New Zealand some 10,000 years ago, they left behind a series of narrow, deep inlets that were eventually flooded by the rising sea. These inlets, or fiords, are typified by a steep-sided, deep channel where the ice scoured its way through the rock. As the fiord approaches the sea, its depth steadily increases. This is because the glacier that created the fiord grew in size as it was fed by side glaciers from tributaries. At the mouth of the fiord, there is a sudden rise in the sea floor, marking the limit of the glacier's reach.

> ## "Towering kauri pines, with their tremendous buttressed trunks and festoons of perching lilies, are hard to tell apart"

came the Maoris, a thousand years ago, who trapped and speared moas, mutton birds and anything else they could catch for food. In 1770 Captain Cook sailed down the coast in the *Endeavour*, and in his wake came sealing and whaling ships with the most dangerous passengers of all – rats, dogs and pigs, which colonized the islands and found the clumsy native birds easy prey.

A century later, settlers hunted creatures they believed to be sheep-killers, including keas – olive green parrots with brilliant vermilion flashes beneath their wings. Keas can still be seen among the snow grass and mountain lilies of the high slopes. They are the only parrots in the world to live above the snowline and are almost certainly carrion-eaters. The birds that managed to survive the onslaught of the early European settlers retreated deep into the forest, along with the Maoris.

Today, no one hiking through the Fiordland bush will meet Maoris – the last sighting of the "lost tribe" of Ngati-Mamoe was in 1870 – or a predator larger than a feral pig.

Certainly no one will die of thirst. The real danger is disorientation: once deep in the temperate rainforest, it is impossible to pinpoint any landmarks and easy to become hopelessly lost among the giant ferns and trees. Towering kauri pines, with their tremendous buttressed trunks and festoons of perching lilies, are hard to tell apart. Farther up in the subalpine forest of arctic beech and conifers, constant heavy rain and mist make the forest floor treacherous. Even the scrubland is thick with sword leaves, spear grass and the poisonous tutu plant.

As a result, large tracts of Fiordland are unexplored. In 1948, a naturalist named Dr. Geoffrey Orbell

was walking in the dense bush around the Murchison Mountains when he saw what he thought was a takahe – a flightless rail with a blue breast, green back and wings, and a large red beak, widely believed to be extinct. He had stumbled across a whole colony, which now numbers more than 300. The site was christened Takahe Valley and is one of the four areas in Fiordland National Park that may not be entered without a permit.

Another flightless rail found in Fiordland is the weka. These voracious birds hunt small creatures as well as feeding on grass and fruit and will even attack other ground-dwelling birds and steal their eggs. Wekas are still relatively common.

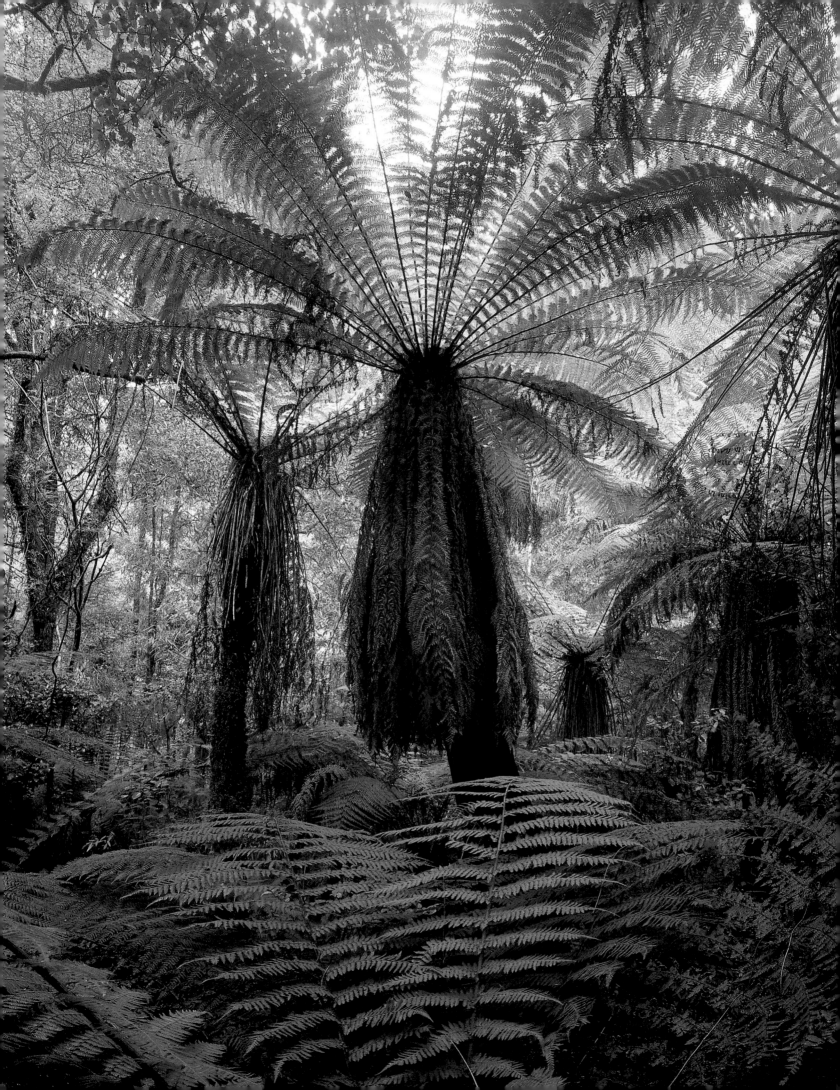

Much rarer are kakapos, the world's largest parrots, found only around the beech forests of the Cleddau Watershed on Milford Sound and on offshore islands. They are agile birds which, although almost flightless, hop and glide along established tracks to feed on grass, ferns and berries. Active at night, kakapos have sensitive bristles around the beak which help them find their way in the dark. Other birds on the danger list are laughing owls, of which there have been no confirmed sightings for 25 years, and kokakos, or wattle birds, which glide from tree to tree and produce a distinctive, sonorous call.

Fiordland's freshwater lakes contain some of the purest water in the world and some of the most awesome sights. On the western shore of Lake Te Anau, a labyrinthine cave system, well known to the Maoris, was discovered at around the time that Orbell found Takahe Valley. Deep inside is a cavern whose walls and roof are covered in glowworms –

"One of the wettest places on the planet where prevailing southwest winds dump a colossal amount of rain every year"

thousands of pinpricks of light scattered through the darkness.

Perhaps the most spectacular scenery in Fiordland is in Milford Sound, which winds inland for 10 miles (16 km), flanked on each side by the world's highest sea cliffs. At times the inlet is so narrow that it seems more like a rock tunnel than a fiord.

Conditions in the fiord are unusual. As the enormous volume of rain that falls yearly on the land filters down through the forests into the fiord, it passes through so much decaying vegetation that it turns the color of tea. When it arrives at the fiord, it does not mix with the salt water, being less dense, but forms a layer 10–13 feet (3–4 m) deep on the surface. The darker color of this top layer of water restricts the penetration of sunlight, and creatures that normally live in deeper water may be found in the first 130 feet (40 m) or so. Such species include sea pens, sea squirts and a huge colony of black coral.

On a calm, sunny day at the head of the sound, the bare walls of Mitre Peak and the spray of Bowen Falls swoop down to meet their mirror images in the still water. This is as far as visiting boats come. They take their photographs and head back to the sea, hoping for a glimpse of a dusky dolphin or even a sperm whale, and leave behind New Zealand's greatest untouched wilderness.

Giant tree ferns, known to the Maoris as mamaku, grow up to 50 feet (15 m) tall in the cool humid forests of Fiordland (left).

One of six species of parrots in New Zealand, the kea (below) uses its long upper bill to tear into carrion, fruit and insects.

The takahe (right) feeds on grass seeds and shoots. The birds are strictly protected, but are still seriously endangered.

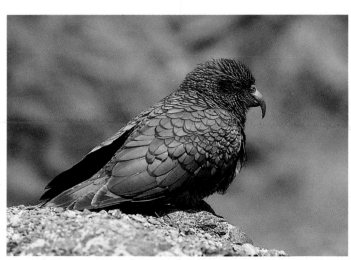

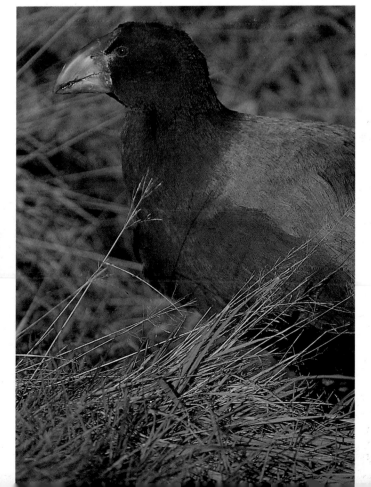

GAZETTEER

Besides the wild places described in depth in this book, there are a number of other sites which can lay claim to wilderness status. A selection of such areas is included in the Gazetteer. Although most of these wildernesses are officially protected as national parks and reserves, many are still under threat. All are priceless. Their loss would be an inestimable tragedy.

POLAR REGIONS

1 Brookes Range ALASKA

Stretching in an unbroken barrier across the top of Alaska, well inside the Arctic Circle, the peaks and ridges of the Brooks Range reach from the Chukchi Sea to the Canadian border and beyond. The mountains represent the northernmost limit of Alaska's trees. There are thickets of willow, spruce and alder in the south-facing valleys, but the north-facing slopes are bare. A profusion of streams and rivers rush down from the mountains toward the sea, crossing a coastal plain patterned with frost polygons and meltwater ponds. The Beaufort Sea once covered this plain, and fossilized coral heads can still be found in the riverbeds.

The Arctic National Wildlife Refuge, which includes the Brooks Range and the coastal plain, covers almost 30,000 sq. miles (78,000 km²). Over 12,400 sq. miles (32,000 km²) of this has been designated a wilderness. Wildlife in the park includes black bears, polar bears and grizzlies, as well as caribou, musk oxen, wolves and porcupines.

2 Northern Yukon National Park CANADA

This 3,860 sq. mile (10,000 km²) park, stretching eastward from the Alaskan border, was established as part-settlement of a land claim with the Inuvialuit people of the region, who have an exclusive right to hunt game within its borders and are involved in the park's planning and management. Bounded on the north by the Beaufort Sea, the park contains coastal, mountain, tundra and taiga zones.

The 150,000-strong caribou herd that lives in the park spends the winter in the southern taiga foraging for food among the trees, sheltered from the worst of the gales and blizzards. They move northward as the weather improves in summer, grazing on the tundra as the frosts melt, and eventually crossing the mountains to calving grounds in the foothills and plains of the coast.

3 Baffin Island CANADA

Some 1,000 miles (1,600 km) long and 500 miles (800 km) wide, Baffin Island faces Greenland across 300 miles (500 km) of Baffin Bay and lies raggedly across the entrance to Hudson Bay. This huge and mountainous island is at the high eastern end of the Canadian Shield, and where it drops abruptly to the sea, it forms the deep fiords on the island's eastern coast which frustrated early attempts to find the North-West Passage. The mountains of eastern Baffin reach altitudes of 7,900 feet (2,400 m) and more.

On the Cumberland Peninsula of the east coast, Auyuittuq National Park is a 8,100 sq. mile (21,000 km²) protected Arctic wilderness of mountain peaks and valleys, glaciers, fiords and rocky shores. Baffin Island is ice-locked for much of the year, but has a rich and varied marine fauna, including ringed, bearded and harp seals. An extensive migratory bird sanctuary on the Great Plain of the Koukdjuak in the west hosts the world's largest goose colony.

4 Greenland

The world's largest island, Greenland is covered with a massive ice cap over 80 percent of its area. With a relatively tiny human population, Greenland is essentially one vast wilderness, and one-third of the island, including all the northeastern coastlands, has been designated a national park.

Most of Greenland's sparse wildlife, like its human inhabitants, stays close to the coastal strips, where there is at least a chance of seeing a little greenery, in the form of mosses, lichens and grasses, in the summer. There are herds of musk oxen and reindeer in the national park area, as well as wandering polar bears, with lemmings and Arctic foxes at the other end of the scale. The fiords and islands of the northeastern coast are home to Greenland seals, common seals and walruses. On the tundra of the Jameson Land peninsula on the east coast, many birds, including long-tailed skua, red-throated divers and whimbrels, breed along the rivers and in the salt marshes. Large numbers of barnacle and pink-footed geese also come here to molt.

5 Svalbard Islands NORWAY

Situated near the 80th parallel, 580 miles (930 km) north of Tromsø, the Svalbard archipelago is high in the Arctic. These nine main islands belong to Norway. While commercial mining exists in part of the group, 45 percent of the total land area is protected by a series of nature reserves and bird sanctuaries.

The name Svalbard means "cold coast," and well over half of the area of these mountainous islands is covered with glaciers and snowfields. However, a warm current of the North Atlantic Drift keeps open a channel through the ice to the western coasts for most of the year. Edgeøya, third largest of the islands, is a reserve favored by denning polar bears. The islands are also a major breeding area for seabirds such as guillemots, fulmars and kittiwakes.

6 South Georgia SOUTHERN OCEAN

The climatic influence of the southern ice cap extends relatively far, compared to that of its northern equivalent, and although the island of South Georgia lies on the 54th parallel, it has permanent snow and ice covering well over half of its area. It is very mountainous, with 13 peaks over 6,600 feet (2,000 m). Snow falls for over 180 days of the year. Gale-force winds are the norm, and in winter the fiords are filled with broken sea ice.

Despite these rigors, South Georgia is something of an oasis in the Southern Ocean, with slopes of green mosses, lichens and tussock grass close to the sea. The island is an important breeding ground for a large number of Antarctic creatures, including huge colonies of Antarctic fur seals and elephant seals. Many species of birds come to South Georgia to find ice-free nesting sites, including macaroni penguins and several types of albatross.

7 Bird Island SOUTHERN OCEAN

Captain Cook named Bird Island when he discovered it in 1775, close to the western end of South Georgia.

NORTH POLE

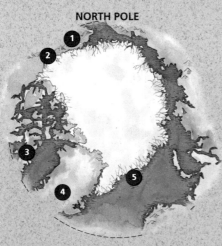

SOUTH POLE

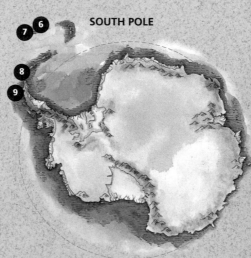

Now, as then, the island's 370 acres (150 ha) can be almost entirely covered, shore to shore, with nesting birds of several species. A small British Antarctic Survey base houses eight or nine scientists, six of whom leave for the winter.

The albatrosses that come to Bird Island, ungainly on land, need grassy or mossy nesting grounds close to steep cliffs, where they can launch themselves easily into the air. The hordes of macaroni penguins prefer to lay their eggs on steep, bare rocky slopes. One particular rock face on Bird Island hosts 80,000 pairs. The only access from the sea is via a narrow channel, full of surging water and haunted by fur seals in search of a penguin meal. The island's petrels live in colonies of burrows. Non-burrowing giant petrels are the island's main scavengers, feeding on the carcasses of penguins that have fallen victim to seals, but also killing smaller birds and chicks.

8 South Shetland Islands SOUTHERN OCEAN

The Antarctic maritime islands of South Shetland are surrounded by pack ice in the winter. This chain of 11 main and many smaller islands is 336 miles (540 km) long. Most are volcanic in origin, and Deception Island, with its classic horseshoe caldera shape, is active, with hot springs and fumaroles. Tourists bathe in the steaming waters, but the bay has been known literally to boil, and major eruptions have occurred this century. King George Island and Livingstone are the largest in the group and house a number of stations manned by nations claiming Antarctic interests.

Close to the Antarctic Peninsula, the South Shetlands have extensive ice fields and glaciers, but also contain some large ice-free areas. Spectacular lichens flourish throughout the group, with some sea cliffs covered with a bright orange mantle. Large colonies of chinstrap, Adélie and gentoo penguins breed here, as do Weddell and elephant seals.

9 Brabant Island ANTARCTICA

Wild and inhospitable Brabant Island, situated close to the Antarctic Peninsula, has ice-covered mountain ranges rising to 8,200 feet (2,500 m) and just a few snow-free areas at midsummer. The island was not explored until the 1980s and was hardly visited before that. Many of the island's rocks show clear volcanic origins, with soaring 660-foot (200-m) cliffs of basaltic columns in places, patchworked with yellow and rust lichens. Elsewhere, in windswept and wet areas, bushy lime-green lichens color the rocks.

The only seals visiting the island in any numbers are Antarctic fur seals. Up to 1,000, mainly bachelor males, are there between January and March. Small numbers of Weddell, crab-eater and leopard seals also appear from time to time. The most common birds are chinstrap penguins, Antarctic fulmars, Cape pigeons, snow petrels, Wilson's storm petrels, blue-eyed shags, kelp gulls and Antarctic terns.

NORTH AND CENTRAL AMERICA

10 Round Island ALASKA, USA

A small extinct volcano of rocky basalt thrust out of the waters of the Bering Sea, Round Island lies 20 miles (32 km) west of Alaska's Nushagak Peninsula. There are no trees on Round Island, but despite its bleak situation, it is green with grass in the summer months and brilliant with flowers such as poppies, wild geraniums and forget-me-nots.

Round Island hosts some species of mice, and also red foxes which prey on them, but by far the most impressive inhabitants are the walruses, which

cram the beaches between June and October. The 10,000 and more walruses spending the summer months on Round Island are all males, a vast bachelor herd that spends the time sunbathing and occasionally swimming off in small groups for a few days to feast on clams and crabs.

11 South Moresby National Park CANADA

Canada's Queen Charlotte Islands are the peaks of an underwater mountain range running parallel to the mainland coast of British Columbia. This archipelago of two large and 150 small islands, warmed by Pacific Ocean currents, receives massive annual rainfalls, and mists often cloak the evergreen rainforests that cover its mountain slopes. The South Moresby National Park, covering 570 sq. miles (1,470 km²) of the second largest island, was founded in 1987 after a long campaign conducted by the native Haida people against commercial logging.

In the dark forests of the park, there are trees possibly 1,000 years old. Some Sitka spruces tower up to 165 feet (50 m) in height, flourishing in the deep, black soil and humid conditions. Other forest giants include western red cedars, western hemlocks and Douglas firs. Wildlife species are often distinct island variants of mainland creatures, including the blue grouse, the northern saw-whet owl and, particularly, large black bears.

12 L'Eau Claire Wilderness CANADA

On the eastern shores of Hudson Bay in northern Quebec, L'Eau Claire Wilderness is a remote and inaccessible swath of rivers, lakes, channels, rapids and streams separating Lac à L'Eau Claire in the east from Richmond Gulf and Hudson Bay in the west. It

is a transition region between the boreal forests of the south and the tundra of the northern Canadian Shield. The region has remained undeveloped due to its harsh winter climate and waterlogged terrain, but is hunted and fished by members of the Cree nation.

The wetlands are breeding grounds for mosquitoes, black flies and horseflies which descend in thick droves on any living creature. The depredations of the blood-sucking insects are capable of killing off old and weak caribou from the herds that migrate across the region. The waters and shores of l'Eau Claire are a paradise for many species of waterbirds, including divers, and favorite fishing and hunting grounds for ospreys and golden eagles.

13 Isle Royale National Park, Lake Superior USA

The largest island in Lake Superior, Isle Royale is 15 miles (24 km) from the Canadian shore, but is technically a part of Michigan, which is 50 miles (80 km) distant. It contains a unique ecological balance between moose and timber wolves, both of which immigrated from Canada, the moose having swum across around 1900, and the wolves having crossed the ice in the big freeze of 1949.

Isle Royale, 45 miles (72 km) long and between 2½ and 5 miles (4 and 8 km) wide, contains 27 lakes and provides a swampy lowland terrain where the moose can feed on water plants in the summer in an environment difficult for the wolves to penetrate. Making do with beavers and the odd moose calf in summer, the wolves' turn comes in winter, when the marshes and lakes freeze over. The two populations thus keep in balance, with about 1,000 moose and some 50 wolves, in three or four packs.

NORTH AND CENTRAL AMERICA

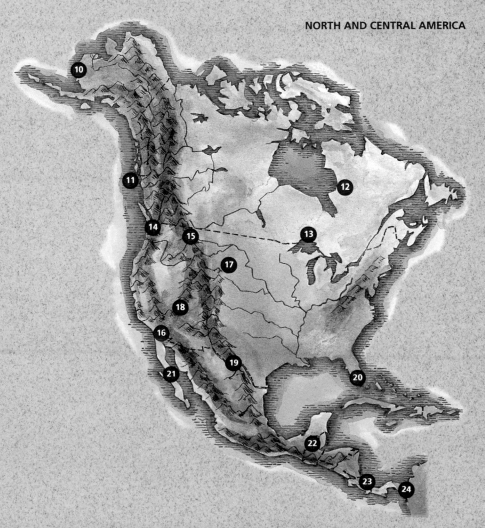

14 Olympic National Park
WASHINGTON, USA

This national park consists of a narrow coastal strip and a large central expanse of the Olympic peninsula, which occupies the most northwesterly point of the contiguous United States. The temperate rainforests of the park suck up the enormous annual rain and snow precipitations falling to the west of the Olympic Mountains. The forests are towering cathedrals of timber, ferns, and trailing festoons and carpets of moss and lichen. Some of the Douglas firs in the lowland forest attain heights of 250 feet (76 m) and more. Occasionally, brilliant flowers relieve the gloom of the forest floor.

Established in 1938 as a refuge for the Roosevelt elk, the park is a remnant of the rainforests that once cloaked almost the entire Pacific coast. In addition to Douglas firs, there are giant Sitka spruces and western hemlocks. A number of icy rivers rush down to the park's coastal strip from the mountains, some carrying spawning salmon in season.

15 The Great Burn IDAHO/MONTANA, USA

Straddling the Idaho-Montana border between the Clearwater and Lolo National Forests, the Great Burn wilderness is a mountainous forest region uniquely and indelibly marked by a great fire that occurred almost a century ago. In August 1910, a drought year in the Idaho and Montana Rockies, gale-force winds fanned a number of small fires and created an inferno which incinerated over 4,600 sq. miles (12,000 km²) of trees. Further fires in succeeding years destroyed seedling growth and prevented regeneration, creating instead large, permanent meadows where once there had been trees.

Now the area known as the Great Burn, covering about 390 sq. miles (1,000 km²), is a diverse mix of mountains, meadows and forested valleys, inhabited by elk, moose, deer and black bears, all of which thrive on the grasses and shrubs which grew up in the new meadows.

16 Yosemite National Park CALIFORNIA, USA

The stunning scenery of the Yosemite National Park in California's Sierra Nevada is in danger of attracting too many visitors, and numbers are being strictly controlled in order to preserve this vast natural wilderness of mountain cliffs, gigantic waterfalls, lakes and forests. Unknown to non-Native Americans until 1833, Yosemite became a state park in 1864 and a national park in 1890.

The park's dramatic rock walls, domes, peaks and spires owe their existence to a combination of movements in the Earth's crust and glacial action. A popular attraction is Yosemite Falls, consisting of an Upper Falls, the world's longest unbroken waterfall at 1,427 feet (435 m), and the Lower Falls beneath, continuing the drop for a further 330 feet (100 m). Yosemite's wildlife includes pumas, black bears, coyotes, mule deer and gray foxes. Pikas and yellow-bellied marmots, both rodents, live among the rocks. Most famous of Yosemite's trees are the majestic redwoods and giant sequoias, which can attain heights of 330 feet (100 m).

17 Badlands SOUTH DAKOTA, USA

The arid and eroded peaks, ridges and gullies of South Dakota's Badlands form a multicolored science fiction landscape that seems hostile and lifeless at first sight, but which is home to a wide variety of creatures and plants. Originating in layers of marine sediment, waterborne mud and volcanic ash, the Badlands today are the result of millions of years of erosion by rain and wind, a process which continues to shape the strange, sculpted terrain.

In and around the most arid gullies and ridges of the Badlands, the most efficient survivors are snakes, bats and rodents. Where the soil is more stable, plants such as prairie golden pea and buffalo grass help to bind it. Agriculture was banned in 1978; since then, prairie grasses have become more established, attracting numbers of the almost extinct pronghorn antelope, America's fastest mammal.

18 Grand Canyon ARIZONA, USA

Possibly the most famous of all American natural landmarks, the Grand Canyon repeatedly reduces new generations of visitors to awed silence. Created over two million years by the abrasive force of the Colorado River working against a giant upheaval in the Earth's crust, the Grand Canyon is today 276 miles (444 km) long. At its most extreme it is 1 mile (1.6 km) deep and 18 miles (29 km) wide. From Lake Powell at its eastern end to Lake Mead in the west, the canyon covers 2,000 sq. miles (5,200 km²).

Despite vast numbers of visitors who descend the steep trails and even raft down the Colorado's rapids, the Grand Canyon remains a true wilderness. The scale and beauty of its cliffs, ravines and empty spaces dwarf all human intrusion. The canyon's great depth creates a wide range of climatic zones, reflected in wildlife populations – from scorpions and lizards on the canyon floor, to gray foxes, herons and deer in fertile side canyons, and the unique Kaibab squirrel in the woods of the North Rim.

19 Big Bend National Park TEXAS, USA

One of the country's least visited national parks, Big Bend occupies over 1,250 sq. miles (3,240 km²) of wild country, embraced within a great curve of the Rio Grande which forms the border between Mexico and the United States. Terrains within the park's confines vary from mountain range and upland desert to lowlands and river environments.

The river banks are particularly rich in wild creatures, with mountain lions, rare Mexican wolves, bobcats, coyotes, collared peccaries and mule deer all coming down to drink. In the Chihuahuan Desert sector of the park live creatures adapted to arid conditions, such as scorpions, lizards, kangaroo rats and black-tailed jackrabbits. The Chisos Mountains soar in the southwest of Big Bend, with several peaks over 7,220 feet (2,200 m) inhabited by high altitude creatures such as Sierra del Carmen whitetail deer and kit foxes.

20 Everglades FLORIDA, USA

The subtropical wilderness of the Florida Everglades covers 33,000 km² (12,750 sq. miles) of the Florida peninsula and contains a mixture of habitats that includes pine forests, mangroves, marshy grasslands and shallow, slow-flowing rivers. The Everglades National Park covers 2,020 sq. miles (5,232 km²) of the tip of the Everglades. This strange, flat area slopes gently south and an 50-mile (80-km) wide river, 6 inches (15 cm) deep flows slowly toward Florida Bay in the rainy season, through expanses of saw grass.

Although threatened by developers and by the water demands of agriculture and the cities, the Everglades is still a refuge for several endangered species such as the Florida panther, the manatee and the loggerhead and green turtles. In the dry season, the alligators of the Everglades dig holes and dredge the clogged channels with their claws and snouts.

21 Baja California MEXICO

The great desert peninsula of Baja California runs parallel to the Mexican northwestern coast for some 800 miles (1,300 km), ranging in width from 30 miles (50 km) to 145 miles (230 km) and forming the western coast of the Gulf of California. The waters on each side of the peninsula are rich in fish and marine life, but the Baja itself is primarily arid, with a wildlife specially adapted to dry, desert conditions. The barren and waterless nature of the Baja has preserved it to a considerable extent from human settlement and exploitation.

Mammals on the Baja include the kangaroo rat, which does not need to drink water, as well as the jackrabbit, the wild burro and several bat species, including the fish-snatching bulldog bat. Mountain ranges run the length of the peninsula, and in the northernmost hills are pumas and wildcats. The birds of the Baja are concentrated around the coast, though the carrion-seeking buzzard thrives in the dry interior, as do several species of rattlesnakes and scorpions.

22 Lacandon Wilderness CHIAPAS, MEXICO

The Lacandon Forest is one of the last great stretches of primeval jungle in Mexico, bounded in the northeast by the Usumacinta River, which forms a border barrier between Mexico and Guatemala. Covering an area of some 2,200 sq. miles (5,700 km²), the forest contains several lakes and a number of tributaries of the Lacuntun River, which eventually joins the Usumacinta to form the forest's southeastern boundary. Dugouts are the only feasible form of transportation within the forest, despite the crocodiles which can reach 25 feet (7 m) in length.

The Lacandon is a true rainforest. The tall trees are draped with orchids and bromeliads, and in the canopy above are noisy macaws and howler monkeys as well as toucans. At a lower level are shrubs and immature trees, and the forest floor itself is moist with rotting leaves and wood.

23 Amistead Biosphere Reserve COSTA RICA

Costa Rica has a particularly diverse flora and fauna which includes elements from both American continents. The country's Amistead Biosphere Reserve in the foothills and uplands of the Cordillera de Talamanca is in fact an assemblage of reserves and protectorates with a total area of 2,257 sq. miles (5,845 km²). The terrain includes glacial lakes, lowland tropical rainforest, subalpine paramo forest, oak stands, high altitude bogs and cloud forest.

The 215 mammal species within the reserve's varied habitats include tapirs, squirrel monkeys, jaguarundi, ocelots and jaguars. Endangered birds under protection include quetzals, orange-breasted falcons and harpy eagles.

24 Kuna Yala Reserve PANAMA

In direct contrast to most threatened indigenous peoples, the 30,000 Kuna Indians of Panama own the land on which they live and grow food. The reserve includes the 350 forested coral islands on which they live, and the narrow coastal plain where they use traditional agricultural methods, as well as hunting and gathering within the forested zone. The Kuna established their reserve in 1938, deliberately distancing themselves from the mainstream of Panamanian society.

In the 1970s, the Kuna were threatened by a new road used by slash-and-burn peasant farmers operating close to the reserve's boundaries. With the aid and advice of concerned organizations, they established the Kuna Wildlands Project, containing four categories of protected territory: a major area restricted to scientific research and controlled tourism; a Kuna agricultural reserve; a Kuna cultural region including the islands and coastal plots; and a restoration strip just outside the reserve, which acts as a buffer zone. The success of this project has encouraged other indigenous groups to follow suit.

SOUTH AMERICA

25 Ciénaga Grande de Santa Marta
COLOMBIA

This mixture of wetland habitats on Colombia's Caribbean coast is situated at the mouth of the Rio Magdalena. Salt lagoons and mangrove swamps line the shore, and further inland is a complex of freshwater lakes, swamp forests and marshes, which can be completely inundated by the Magdalena when the river is in flood. The coastal region itself has a very low rainfall, and the floods are the result of snow melting in the mountains of the Sierra Nevada de Santa Marta.

This 195 sq. miles (500 km²) of wetlands and coastal lagoons is an important feeding, resting and breeding site for migrating waterfowl and resident species. These birds, the shellfish and crustaceans harvested by both birds and humans, and the mangroves lining the lagoons depend on delicate balances between fresh and salt water. Upstream irrigation canals have led to a reduced flow of fresh water from the Rio Magdalena, causing excess salinity in the lagoons and damage to the mangroves. Further damage to the whole ecology of the area will occur unless the freshwater flow is restored.

26 The Llanos VENEZUELA

The Venezuelan Llanos, part of the flood plain of the Orinico and Apure rivers, are lush grassy wetlands for half of the year and a dusty plain for the other half. Extending for 38,600 sq. miles (100,000 km²) in Venezuela, and considerably farther in adjoining Colombia, the Llanos are smoky with frequent forest fires in the dry season, when the wildlife takes refuge in the valley bottoms and along the river banks. Winter rains create a huge marshy territory of rivers and streams, lakes and swamps.

The spectacled caiman, reduced in numbers by poachers, is now making a comeback in the Llanos. The waters are also perilous with red piranhas, electric eels and stingrays. The grasses and scattered palms of the flood plain and the trees of the riverine woodlands provide cover for many creatures, from capybara, white-tailed deer and jaguars, to tree frogs and iguanas. Internationally important as a wading-bird refuge, the wetlands host large breeding colonies of many species of heron, stork and ibis.

27 Maraca BRAZIL

A huge riverine island, Maraca lies some 75 miles (120 km) northwest of Boa Vista, in the northern state of Roraima. Covering an area of about 170 sq. miles (440 km²), Maraca is uninhabited rainforest terrain, with patches of open savanna, seasonally flooded wetlands, creeks and low hills.

Maraca teems with life and represents the forests of the Amazon basin in microcosm, secluded and unspoilt. There are 450 species of birds and almost 50 species of bats. This is no tourist spot. Large and aggressive packs of peccaries patrol the forest, and the nests of hornets and killer bees hang from branches. Jacaré alligators lie submerged in the ponds, and the encircling rivers are home to piranhas, as well as stingrays. Rattlesnakes, boa constrictors and deadly fer-de-lance snakes are common. Mammal life includes jaguars, three-toed sloths, several monkey species, great anteaters, agouti, tree porcupines, tapirs and deer. A Royal Geographical Society project in Maraca has discovered hundreds of species new to science.

28 Chiribiquete National Park COLOMBIA

The park is an outstanding example of sustainable indigenous agriculture at work. Situated on the western edge of the tropical rainforest, against the foothills of the Andes, Chiribiquete covers 3,860 sq. miles (10,000 km²) and is part of the transfer of some traditional forest lands back to Indian ownership. The Colombian government has made the transfer in recognition of the fact that the Indians' agricultural methods are environmentally sound and efficient.

The Indians exist in fairly small family groups, hunting and fishing, and foraging through a wide area for wild produce. In addition, they clear forest gardens, away from the rivers, in which they plant crops including mangoes, papayas, yuccas and peppers. Like most artificially cultivated rainforest soils, these gardens begin to lose their fertility after a couple of years. The Indians then abandon the old gardens and move on to new ones. Over a period of a number of years, the forest gradually recolonizes the area in the same way that it does when a fallen tree creates a clearing.

29 Galápagos Islands PACIFIC OCEAN

The islands, islets, rocks and reefs of the Galápagos archipelago, some 500 miles (800 km) west of the Ecuadorian coast, were made famous by Charles Darwin's visit and subsequent writings. The larger islands, including Isabela with over half of the group's land area, have arid coastal lowlands, dry from low precipitation and dark with volcanic soil. Born of volcanic action only a few million years ago, the islands still have several active peaks. Vegetation ranges from cactuses on the coast to a zone of evergreen forest between 660 feet (200 m) and 1,650 feet (500 m), with ferns and sedges above that.

The Galápagos' flora and fauna must have been conveyed by wind and sea currents, travelling as seeds and eggs on natural vegetation rafts or on the feet and feathers of seabirds. The unique fauna includes giant tortoises, the planet's only marine iguanas, Galápagos fur seals and sea lions, two bat species, many seabirds and many landbirds, including the 13 finch species showing distinct local adaptations, which influenced Darwin's thinking on evolution.

30 Pacaya Samiria National Reserve PERU

The mighty Amazon rises in the Peruvian Andes, and the Pacaya Samiria National Reserve is situated on the Amazon's head-waters, on and around the rivers Pacaya and Samiria and 5,330 sq. miles (13,800 km²) of mixed waterways, oxbow lakes, lagoons, islands and forest. Initially established as a river reserve to protect the paiche, or giant catfish, endangered by overfishing, the enlarged territory is now a refuge for all species of fauna and flora, with a management plan to allow limited and sustainable harvesting by locals for their own needs.

Apart from the huge paiche, stingrays, piranhas and many other fish species, the waters of the reserve contain Amazonian dolphins and caymans. A great variety of creatures inhabits the forests lining the rivers, including wooly and squirrel monkeys, deer, peccaries and two large rodents, the capybara and the paca, both of which are among the sustainable game populations subject to limited hunting.

31 Tambopata-Candamo Reserve PERU

The Peruvian government established this 5,800-sq. mile (15,000-km²) region as an "extractive reserve" for forest products such as rubber and brazil nuts, which can be harvested without harming the ecology of the area and help pay for its management. The reserve stretches from the High Andes down into low jungle, and encompasses the entire watershed of the Tambopata River. Organized ecotourism also contributes to Tambopata's self-sufficiency.

Humans have to share brazil nuts in the reserve with macaws, which have evolved enormously strong beaks to open them. The agouti, a large rodent, also eats the nuts and helps the spread of the plant by burying clusters of uneaten nuts.

32 Lake Titicaca PERU

Legendary birthplace of the Inca nation, at 3,800 m (12,500 feet) high in the Peruvian Andes and almost 3,200 sq. miles (8,300 km²) in area, Lake Titicaca is the world's highest navigable lake. It is fed by snow melt from the surrounding peaks, and the depth varies by 3 feet (1 m) between the wet and dry seasons. Titicaca has only one outlet, the Desaguadero River,

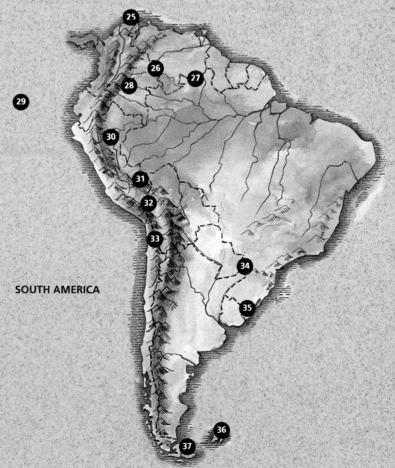

SOUTH AMERICA

which takes about 10 percent of all water leaving the lake. The rest disappears as a result of evaporation, aided by high altitude, strong sunshine and the constant winds of the Altiplano.

In the shallows of the lake grow large areas of the long totora reeds used by the local Indians to build their boats and floating houses. Such a huge area of water, with extensive shallows, is an important winter stopover for migrating North American shorebirds, as well as a permanent home to high Andes waterbird species. Perhaps the most unusual lake dwellers are the frogs, which live on the lake bottom, can breathe through their skin and seldom surface.

33 Atacama-Sechura Desert CHILE

The 1,865-mile (3,000-km) ribbon of the Atacama-Sechura Desert forms a narrow coastal strip overlooked by the massive heights of the Andes. It is one of the most desolate and arid places on Earth, with some regions having a barely measurable 1 mm of precipitation a year. Yet, despite this lack of rain, caused by the rain shadow cast by the Andes, relative humidity can be high, with long periods of fog and cloud. The bleakness is emphasized by the cold, as onshore winds blow in over the icy Humboldt (Peru) Current.

The Humboldt penguins that swim in the cold current are one of the very few forms of life visible in this grim landscape, nesting incongruously under cactus plants at the ocean's edge. In the most arid section of the Atacama, the temperature can drop at sunset from 104°F (40°C) to 32°F (0°C) in an hour. There are a few small rodents and lizards, and the foxes and birds of prey that hunt them, but the overriding character of the Atacama is barrenness, in stark contrast to the rich wildlife on the other side of the mountains.

34 Iguaçu Falls BRAZIL

The great cascade of the Iguaçu Falls pours over the fractured rim of Brazil's Parana Plateau through a sieve of islands covered in vegetation, creating a rank of almost 275 separate falls. The rim over which the wide river plunges is 2½ miles (4 km) in length, and the gorge funneling the waters downstream lies 269 feet (82 m) below the rim. The whole lush region around the falls has long been protected parkland, established by the governments of Argentina and Brazil on their respective sides of the border.

The Iguaçu is South America's third largest river, yet on average it dries up completely every 40 years or so, silencing the cascades for up to a month. Most of the time, the falls thunder over their cliffs of volcanic basalt, in full spate carrying seven times as much water as Niagara and filling the air with a constant mist, encouraging the growth of ferns, mosses and unusual aquatic herbs, which use suckers to cling to the wet rocks.

35 Bañados del Este BRAZIL/URUGUAY

A broad barrier of dunes separates the wetlands of the Brazil-Uruguay coastal border from the Atlantic Ocean, protecting the large, brackish Laguna Merim and its associated freshwater marshes, peat swamps and flood lands. Great flocks of migrating birds breed in these shallow waters, including those coming from farther south during the southern winter and from North America during the southern summer. The entire complex of bodies of water, seasonally flooded grassland and palm savanna covers an area of 4,600 sq. miles (12,000 km²).

Local communities used to harvest coypu in the Bañados for their fur, but the main threat to the area today comes from agriculture and pressure to increase the number of drained areas. Wetlands on both sides of the border have been designated reserves, and numerous coypu still live in the marshes, as well as capybaras.

36 Falkland Islands SOUTH ATLANTIC

Lying 280 miles (450 km) off the Argentine coast, the Falkland Islands are low and windswept, subject to raw westerly gales that keep the vegetation down to shrubs and tussock grass. There are two main islands and numerous offshore islands, and the coasts are rocky and deeply indented with bays and inlets, with cliffs in some places. Some 53 of the offshore islets have been designated reserves.

Due to the lack of trees, the vast numbers of seabirds that come to the Falklands to breed have to nest on or close to the ground. They include shearwaters, black-browed albatrosses and four species of penguins. The bays and inlets of the islands attract populations of southern sea lions, elephant seals and fur seals, all of which were severely depleted in the 19th century, but have now recovered substantially. The most unusual mammal is the sea otter, small numbers of which live among the thick kelp beds around offshore islands.

37 Tierra del Fuego CHILE

The archipelago of Tierra del Fuego is a harsh wilderness of mountainous islands and ragged channels, sculpted by retreating ice and still being eroded by howling westerly gales. Annual rainfall on its western edge is 16 feet (5 m). A graveyard for ships in the days of sail, these inhospitable rocky shores are sometimes fringed with beech forests, although most growth is found on the eastern sides of the islands, out of the icy winds that gust into squalls of 115 mph (100 knots).

The fauna of the region is concentrated in the waters, where the teeming krill supports packed food chains of fish, seabirds, southern sea lions, dolphins and whales. The shoreline rocks are festooned with giant kelp, and the abundant shellfish were once the staple diet of the Yahgan Indians who lived here until the arrival of Europeans caused them all to die through measles. In the eastern tundra-covered plains of the main island of Tierra del Fuego, ducks and geese breed. On the east coast are tidal mud flats used as temporary habitats by birds such as Hudsonian godwits and white-rumped sandpipers which have migrated from Arctic breeding grounds.

AFRICA

38 Banc d'Arguin National Park
MAURITANIA

The Banc d'Arguin is a huge Atlantic coast intertidal wetland system of mud flats, creeks and eelgrass beds. The 3,860-sq. mile (10,000-km²) national park includes the Baie d'Arguin, and the region is a frontier zone between systems, where the Sahara Desert meets the Atlantic Ocean, and the cold Canaries Current from the north meets the much warmer Guinean Current from the south.

The local Imraguen tribespeople fish for migrating mullet in the shallow waters by beating the water with long poles to attract dolphins, which come and drive the fish into the fishermen's nets. The Banc d'Arguin's rich diversity of fauna includes several million migrating shorebirds, including dunlin and bar-tailed godwits, as well as breeding colonies of spoonbills, greater flamingos and great white pelicans. The largest population in the world of the endangered Mediterranean monk seal lives in the park's waters, and marine turtles lay their eggs on the beaches under the protection of camel-mounted wardens.

39 Air and Ténéré National Nature Reserve
NIGER

Covering over 29,730 sq. miles (77,000 km²), or 6 percent of Niger's total area, the Air and Ténéré National Nature Reserve is a hot and arid wilderness of desert and mountain that is a last refuge for many of the creatures of the Sahara and the Sahel that have virtually disappeared elsewhere. It is one of Africa's largest conservation areas, with a small human population, mainly Tuareg nomadic pastoralists.

In the desert portion of the reserve, there are furnacelike areas of shifting dunes where no plants grow, and other areas with a sprinkling of hardy acacia trees. In the Air Mountains, humid mists condense in the cold nights into groundwater, which lies in shallow pools and encourages the growth of palms, as well as Mediterranean-type trees such as wild olives. With its combination of desert and mountain terrains, the reserve contains significant populations of creatures such as ostriches, oryxes, Barbary sheep, gazelles and cheetahs, as well as the endangered Saharan antelope, the addax.

40 Bijagos Archipelago GUINEA BISSAU

The 88 islands and islets of the Bijagos Archipelago cover an area of 3,860 sq. miles (10,000 km²) in an ancient river delta. A tangled web of creeks fringed with mangroves drains the wide mud flats at low tide. Great volumes of fresh water drain down to the sea in the rainy season, and tropical forest comes down to the beach on some islands, interspersed with the palm groves from which the indigenous Bijagos people extract oil and palm wine.

The shallows and mangroves are rich with shellfish, harvested by human islanders, migratory shorebirds, and the otters that swim and fish in and around the creeks. Hippopotamuses in Bijagos have adapted to a beach and saltwater existence, and the tidal creek waters provide a refuge for a large manatee population. Other creatures benefiting from this extensive maze of islands and tidal waterways are four species of marine turtles, two species of crocodiles and two species of dolphins, including the rare Guinean dolphin.

41 Gashaka Gumpti Reserve NIGERIA

Situated close to Nigeria's border with Cameroon, the Gashaka Gumpti Reserve lies in a remote region that combines a rich mixture of uplands, lush rainforest and savanna grasslands. Established in a cooperative effort between central and local government and nearby villages, the management of the reserve maintains a successful balance between wildlife protection and local human demands.

The huge diversity of wildlife in the reserve includes anubis baboons, Ethiopian colobus monkeys and at least six other primates, with the possibility of mountain gorillas in mountain areas so remote they have never been explored. There are leopards and rare golden cats in the rainforest, and plains species include wildebeest, hartebeest, antelopes and gazelles. This abundance of prey animals encourages the leopards that enjoy the reserve's protection.

42 Sudd Swamp and Flood Plain SUDAN

Occupying up to 12,400 sq. miles (32,000 km²) of the basin of the Upper Nile in central Sudan, the Sudd is a humid, rain-drenched wetland where large floating mats of papyrus move slowly on the shallow currents, blocking river channels and spreading the great river's headwaters over a wide area. Once a year, at flood time, the Sudd doubles in area, forcing animals and people to move temporarily to higher ground or into surrounding regions.

Here are some of the biggest gatherings of large mammals left in Africa, in the form of the periodic mass migrations of tiang and white-eared kob antelopes. Here too is the Nile lechwe, an antelope specifically adapted to wetland existence, with elongated hooves that enable it to move through the swamp without sinking. Hippos, crocodiles, giraffes and elephants are all found in the Sudd, which is also Africa's richest wetland bird territory. Threatened by proposed agricultural expansion, the Sudd is of vital importance to the entire Nile ecosystem, as well as being a major wildlife sanctuary.

43 Abijatta-Shalla Lakes National Park
ETHIOPIA

East Africa's major portion of the Great Rift Valley, running from the Red Sea in the north to Lake Manyara, Tanzania, in the south, threads a necklace of lakes, and Ethiopia's Lakes Shalla and Abijatta are among those not too tainted with sodium carbonate to support a varied wildlife.

Separated by a 8,860-foot (2,700-m) mountain ridge, the lakes are very dissimilar in character. Shalla has a depth of 855 feet (260 m), contains the most important island nesting colonies of great white pelicans in the world, but is too deep and steep sided to provide spawning grounds for fish. As a result, the adult pelicans soar up on thermal currents to cross the mountain ridge and go fishing in the shallow waters of Lake Abijatta, returning 24 hours later on the following morning's thermals to feed their young. Hosts of birds, including herons, ibises, kingfishers, cormorants and darters as well as the commuting pelicans, frequent Abijatta's favorite fishing grounds to feast on tilapia and other fish.

44 Ruwenzori Mountains ZAIRE/UGANDA
The upper slopes of the Ruwenzori Mountains are mysterious with mists, festoons of lichen and

gigantic flowering plants. In the zone between approximately 10,830 and 13,125 feet (3,300 and 4,000 m), there are few animals, but plants known as small species in temperate climates exist in gigantic forms specially adapted to survive the extremes of climate. Lobelia and groundsel reach heights of up to 20 feet (6 m), and heathers can grow to tree-size of 40 feet (12 m) and more, stimulated by constant moisture, lack of tree competition, mineral-rich soil, and plenty of ultraviolet radiation.

Between 4,920 and 7,875 feet (1,500 and 2,400 m), the grass-covered foothills of the range change to a canopied rainforest of cedar, camphor and podocarp. Above that is a dense belt of mountain bamboo, superseded at 10,000 feet (3,000 m) by subalpine moorland. Giant flowering plants inhabit the next zone, and above that are the permanent snowfields and glaciers found only here and on neighboring Mounts Kilimanjaro and Kenya.

45 Ngorongoro Crater TANZANIA
Some 2.5 million years ago, a volcano collapsed into a drained subterranean magma chamber forming a caldera, which today is known as the Ngorongoro Crater. The floor of the crater measures 100 sq. miles (260 km²) in area, and is surrounded by a rim some 2,000 feet (610 m) high, making Ngorongoro into a vast natural amphitheater with a floor of savanna grassland. A shallow soda lake lies at the crater's lowest point, where teeming flamingo flocks of both lesser and greater species sift for food.

The animals of Ngorongoro are not prisoners of the crater, and some do leave by old trails over the rim. However, there is little incentive to emigrate, since food is usually plentiful and there is a constant water supply. Elephants and hippos frequent the river fed swamp in the north of the crater, joined in the dry season by gazelles, zebras and wildebeest. Buffaloes, warthogs and ostriches live in the crater, and taking advantage of the plentiful supply of prey animals is a variety of predators, including lions, cheetahs, hyenas, jackals and foxes.

46 Mount Kilimanjaro
TANZANIA

Africa's tallest mountain has a permanent cap of snow and ice despite its proximity to the equator. It has three peaks, and the tallest, Kibo, at 19,341 feet (5,895 m), has a neat circular crater 1½ miles (2.5 km) across. All three peaks are dormant volcanoes, and Kibo may last have erupted within the last few hundred years.

The base of the great mountain is huge, 50 miles (80 km) by 25 miles (40 km), and between 6,235 and 9,845 feet (1,900 and 3,000 m) it is encircled with a zone of thick montane forest. Into this forest of liana-festooned cedars and buttress-rooted podocarp trees come

elephants and Cape buffaloes, bushbuck and duiker, but they are relatively few and far between, and keep quiet and out of sight. Above the forest zone are moorlands of heather, tussock grass and giant groundsel and lobelia. The rocky slopes and valleys above the moors are rough with porous lava. Leopards roam these bleak upper levels, as well as eland, and the strange little rock hyrax, cousin to the elephant, shrieks piercingly in the still air.

47 Etosha National Park NAMIBIA
For most of the year the 2,320 sq. miles (6,000 km²) of the Etosha Pan in the Etosha National Park is dry, and the sun glares off the surface crust of salt. Flamingos and pelicans gather on the highly saline shallows that follow sporadic rain, but beneath the Pan lies a large enough natural reservoir to feed the surrounding pools and springs that deliver water year round.

From all over the greater park area beyond the Pan, the animals home in on the waterholes in the dry season. Magnetized by the scent of water, the herds gather: zebra, giraffe, kudu, gemsbok, wildebeest, hartebeest and elephant. Every so often, summer rains are torrential. Dormant seeds germinate, and the brilliant green of grass and other plant growth covers the clay. The herbivore herds trek off toward the rain and new shoots. Lion families are forced to live on lesser game and birds until the herds return in the winter. Constantly poised in a delicate and perilous balance between survival and death, Etosha remains one of Africa's most magical refuge wildernesses.

48 Madagascar INDIAN OCEAN
Lying 500 miles (800 km) from the coast of southeastern Africa, Madagascar is the fourth largest island in the world, 976 miles (1,570 km) long by 354 miles (569 km) across at the widest point. Hilly woods in the west of the island lead to a central plateau, beyond which, to the east, is a tropical rainforest that catches the rains blowing in from the ocean to the east. In the south there is an arid desert region.

Madagascar is a rare repository of strange and unique creatures, which have developed there in isolation since the island split away from the African mainland 100 million years ago. All the planet's lemurs and half its chameleon species live on the island. Other unique Madagascan creatures include almost 150 species of frogs and 30 species of the unusual, hedgehog-like tenrec family. Many of the island's birds originate from the African mainland, but there are over 40 unique birds, such as the cuckoo roller and the chameleon-eating Madagascan serpent eagle. The island is particularly rich in plants, with an estimated 9,000 species.

49 Kalahari Desert BOTSWANA
With five months of wet summer from October to March, the Kalahari Desert actually receives a much higher average rainfall than a true desert. More rain falls in the north than the south, reflected in vegetation growth: woodland in the north, with ebony, sycamore and baobab; scrubby grassland in the south, with occasional clumps of palms. The rainfall of this semidesert means a wide range of wildlife lives throughout the 100,400-sq. mile (260,000-km²) plateau of the Botswana Kalahari.

The rains form temporary streams and water pans in the depressions between sandy ridges. Because of flooding in the Okavango Delta in the north, many animals migrate south into the temporarily wet desert regions, including springbok, elephants, zebras, wildebeest and buffaloes.

AFRICA

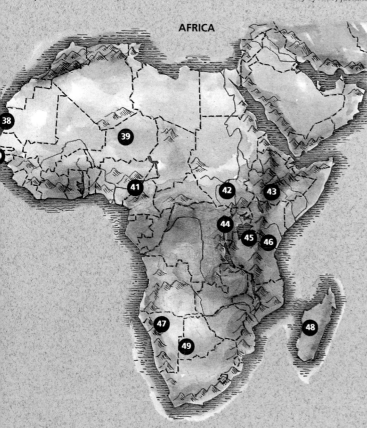

EUROPE

50 Hornstrandir Landscape Reserve
ICELAND

Wild even for Iceland, Hornstrandir is a deeply weathered headland of cliffs and rocky peninsulas in the country's far northwest. Since it is close to the Arctic Circle, the reserve suffers ferocious winters, with heavy, long-lasting snow and winter drift-ice. Summer rains and fogs can also turn into snow storms, and visitors have to approach the 225-sq. mile (580-km²) region either by sea, or on foot over pathless terrain. Hornstrandir is truly one of Europe's most rugged wildernesses, yet it repays the persistent visitor with magnificent scenery and fascinating wildlife.

Ancient lava sheets cover the remains of even more ancient forests, but today Hornstrandir is brilliant with wildflowers in spring and summer, at the same time that the cliffs and ravines of the reserve are acting as nurseries to teeming masses of seabirds. Fulmars, kittiwakes, guillemots, puffins, razorbills and gulls cram every spare inch of space on the ledges, while white-tailed sea eagles and gyrfalcons patrol the bird-cliffs in search of prey.

51 Linnansaari FINLAND

A third of Finland consists of lakes and wetlands, and the small national park of Linnansaari occupies just 3 sq. miles (8 km²) of water and small islands in the large Lake Saimaa, in the country's southeastern lake district. There are many islets in the park, some just rocks, but most thickly wooded with conifers such as spruce and pine as well as deciduous trees like lime, birch and alder. Despite its diminutive size, Linnansaari is a collection of self-contained worlds, with deep inlets and wooded glens, and a lush ground cover of shrubs such as bearberry, bilberry and cowberry.

The lake waters attract goosander, mallards, gulls and black-throated divers, and ospreys breed within the park. The largest island is only 2½ miles (4 km) long. Elk are the largest of the forest fauna, but the most celebrated local mammal is a rare subspecies of Saimaa seal, which may originally have reached the lake from the sea before it was land-locked during the last ice age. It is now one of the world's very few freshwater seals.

52 Hardangervidda NORWAY

Norway's Hardangervidda National Park, in the south of the country, is a harsh, mountainous plateau where few trees grow. The park covers 3,860 sq. miles (10,000 km²) of rocky peaks and icy valleys between 3,935 and 5,575 feet (1,200 and 1,700 m) in altitude, where snow and ice linger on the uplands and on the multitude of lakes for much of the year. The largest herd of wild reindeer in Europe, some 1,400 strong, subsists within the Hardangervidda borders on a diet of mosses, lichens and the dwarf plants of the windy uplands. The region has two climates: a coastal climate in the west where it comes close to the coastal fiords, and a colder inland climate farther east. The region is rich in arctic and subarctic plants, and supports a bird population typifying both arctic and temperate zones, with dotterel and great snipe as well as plovers, wagtails and warblers.

53 Bayerische Wald National Park
GERMANY/CZECHOSLOVAKIA

At over 50 sq. miles (130 km²), with 98 percent tree cover, this is central Europe's largest forest region, a mountainous treescape, rich in plant species, with an abundance of streams, marshes and boggy valleys. A well-organized logging center in the last century, the Bayerische Wald is now a forest in the process of returning to the wild. Streams are re-establishing their ancient courses after having been redirected to act as lumber channels. The drainage ditches dug to facilitate access are now choked with organic debris and vanishing as the forest reclaims its natural form.

Along the Czech border, the park is corrugated with mountain ridges. Spruce is the most common tree at the higher forested levels, merging into mixed colonies of fir, ash, maple, elm, alder, willow and bird cherry farther down. A profusion of woodland and marsh flowers and mosses grows beneath the tree cover and in the meadow clearings and marshes. The rich birdlife includes honey buzzards, pygmy owls and four species of woodpeckers.

54 Höhe Tauern AUSTRIA

The Grossglockner, the loftiest peak in the Austrian Alps at 12,457 feet (3,797 m), dominates the center of Höhe Tauern, Austria's major protected region. Lying in an alpine region of granite, gneiss and schist, Höhe Tauern contains a number of peaks over 10,000 feet (3,000 m). The park has a wealth of breathtaking views and features, from rocky summits streaked with snowfields to thundering waterfalls hundreds of yards high. The Krimml Falls, in the northwest of the park, descend 1,300 feet (400 m) in three great cascades.

With an area of 965 sq. miles (2,500 km²), Höhe Tauern is larger than all the other Austrian reserves put together. There are extensive alpine woodlands along the lower valleys, but the most spectacular wild inhabitants are the great soaring birds of prey which can fully exploit the peaks, cliffs and ravines of the mountain ridges. Golden eagles, griffon vultures and even the rare lammergeier are all visitors to the park.

55 Swiss National Park SWITZERLAND

Situated in the far eastern mountains of the Engadine, adjoining the Italian border, the Swiss National Park was established in 1914 and has a reputation as the best-managed conservation area in Europe. Most of the park lies above 6,500 feet (2,000 m), and it has three major zonal terrains. Evergreen forests, reaching up to a tree line of some 7,550 feet (2,300 m), give way to high alpine meadows, covered in flowers in early summer. Above the meadows are the screes and limestone outcrops of the high peaks and ridges.

The larger carnivores, such as bears, wolves and lynxes, became extinct by the early years of the 20th century, as they did throughout most of the Alps. Ibex and red deer also disappeared, but have returned. Marmots and chamois are common.

56 Saja National Reserve SPAIN

Close to Spain's northern Atlantic coast, in Santander province, the Saja Reserve is named after the Saja River, which is one of several watercourses cutting northward across it to drain eventually into the Atlantic. The reserve also contains the source of the great Ebro River, which runs southeast to enter the Mediterranean. The limestone ridges of the Cordillera Cantabrica in the reserve were once flat plains, but are now tilted on edge. Beech trees have a natural affinity with limestone, and the forests covering most of the reserve are mainly of beech and oak. Some of the trees reach an enormous size, with beeches up to 100 feet (30 m) in height.

Although there are a number of villages within the reserve, the terrains of hill forest, wooded river valley and marshy wetland harbor an exciting range of wildlife, including species that have become extinct elsewhere. Brown bears and wolves survive here, as do populations of boar, wildcat, chamois and roe deer.

57 Pyrenees National Park FRANCE

Stretching along the border with Spain, France's Pyrenees National Park is part of a rugged natural barrier between the two countries. Rocky peaks and grassy uplands predominate, but the park's features also include lakes, waterfalls, glacial basins and thickly forested slopes and valleys. The tree line here is the highest in Europe, with individual trees surviving at altitudes up to 8,530 feet (2,600 m). Mountain pines at high altitude often shelter a dense shrub layer of flowering alpenrose, a species of wild rhododendron. Beechwoods line many of the valleys. In the south and east of the park are the large glacial amphitheaters of the Cirque de Gavarnie and the Cirque de Troumouse. Cirques are ice-worn basins, and the Pyrenean cirques feature cliffs, waterfalls, lakes and flower-filled grass floors. The park is particularly rich in mammal wildlife, with boars, genets, chamois and, rarest of all, brown bears.

58 Ordesa National Park SPAIN

Adjoining a particularly remote sector of the French border which it shares with France's Pyrenees National Park, Spain's Ordesa National Park occupies one of the country's least-known regions. The steep-sided and forested Ordesa Valley formed most of the park's territory from 1918 until 1978, when three further valleys were added, bringing the total area up to 61 sq. miles (157 km²). The highest point in the park is Monte Perdido, at 11,007 feet (3,355 m). The valleys of Ordesa form some of Spain's most isolated environments. Spectacular limestone rock faces and cliffs tower above the forests, and there are many ravines and waterfalls, as well as glaciers and high mountain meadows.

The forests are mainly of Scots pine, mountain pine, beech and silver fir, and their wild inhabitants include otters, wild boars, polecats, Pyrenean ibex and wildcats. The strange, molelike Pyrenean desman hunts in the streams, living in burrows in the banks.

59 Lake Mikri Prespa GREECE

High in the remote mountain borderlands that divide the territories of Greece, Albania and the former Yugoslavia, the shallow waters of Lake Mikri Prespa host one of Europe's most important waterbird populations. The lake is surrounded by extensive reed swamps and marshy lagoons, all forming part of the national park set up by the Greek government in 1971. Mikri Prespa and the adjoining Lake Megali Prespa lie in a bowl-like depression, with a backdrop of gray Albanian mountain peaks. Every spring, torrents of fresh ice-melt recharge the lake waters and flood the surrounding water meadows.

Large colonies of waterbirds breed in the marshes, among them Dalmatian pelicans and white pelicans, both species very rare in Europe. Other waterbirds breeding around the lake include egrets, cormorants, herons, spoonbills, ibises and bitterns. Among the mammals surviving in this inaccessible region are brown bears, wolves, jackals and otters.

60 The Vikos Gorge GREECE

The great chasm of the Vikos Gorge, with its exhilarating views, limestone cliffs and precipitous side canyons, is less well-known than Crete's Samaria Gorge, but is equally impressive, and considerably more difficult to explore. Situated in the mountain territory close to the Albanian border, the gorge contains the source and the upper course of the Voidhomatis River. The icy spring water of

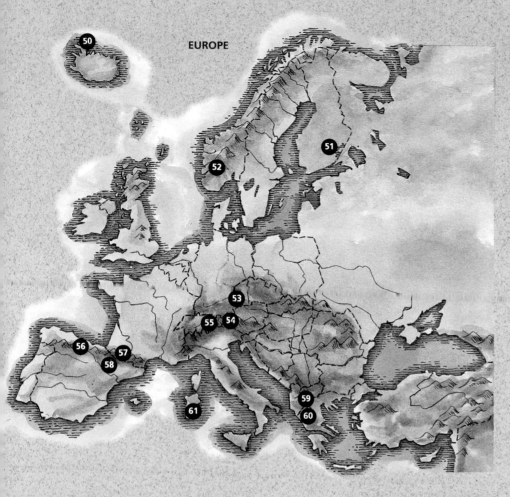

EUROPE

the source bubbles out from the base of astonishing cliffs, soaring upward well over 4,900 feet (1,500 m). The total length of the gorge is a little more than 8 miles (13 km).

Dense coppices of maple, beech and chestnut flank the trail in some upper stretches of the gorge, and where it is joined by the Megas Lakkos Gorge, the Klima spring creates a damp and shadowed environment of ferns, moss and slippery boulders. The region around the gorge still harbors bears, wolves and the European jackal, while golden eagles, Bonelli's eagles, griffon vultures and peregrine falcons haunt the tall cliffs.

61 Gennargentu SARDINIA, ITALY

Sardinia lies 110 miles (180 km) west of the Italian mainland. Much of the island still consists of wild and difficult country, and the Gennargentu National Park, on the eastern coast, occupies some 390 sq. miles (1,000 km²) of Sardinia's wildest terrain. The Gennargentu massif, with several peaks more than 4,900 feet (1,500 m) high, forms the heart of the park, with forest-covered ridges and valleys, and, in the east, dramatic ravines and gorges descending to the Gulf of Orosei.

Large tracts of the Gennargentu territory is made up of maquis, the typical scrubland of the Mediterranean coastlands, consisting of tough shrubs like the strawberry tree and the tree heath, often several yards in height, which are resistant to drought and have replaced the pine and holm-oak forests cleared centuries ago. Maquis is an ideal environment for a variety of creatures, including lizards, snakes, spiders, scorpions and praying mantises. Gennargentu's most celebrated wildlife is its protected mouflon population, which lives within a special reserve in the park.

ASIA

62 Kamchatka EASTERN SIBERIA

Hanging southward for 750 miles (1,200 km) from the eastern end of Siberia, the Kamchatka Peninsula reaches out into the Sea of Okhotsk toward the islands of Japan. Sparsely inhabited, and gloomy with sea fogs much of the time, Kamchatka seems to live in perpetual winter, enlivened by 33 active volcanoes along its length, which add their steam to the low cloud cover. Three of these volcanoes are more than 13,000 feet (4,000 m) high, and one, Klyuchevskaya Sopka, has erupted more than 70 times since 1697, most recently in 1990. Kamchatka contains 400 glaciers and a number of hot springs and geysers.

Vegetation along the rivers flourishes in warm, mineral-rich soil. Each year, salmon migrate up to breeding grounds in the Kamchatka rivers, preyed on by harbor seals along the coast, then by humans. The huge brown bears of the peninsula devour dead and dying fish, exhausted by their migration journey, in preference to catching them, scavenging alongside northern ravens, slaty-backed gulls and the magnificent Steller's sea eagle.

63 Ussuriland SOUTHEASTERN SIBERIA

Plant and animal species of the north meet those from Southeast Asia in Ussuriland, one of Siberia's most diverse wildlife areas. The Sikhote-Alin mountain range, home to the Siberian tiger, runs from north to south for 620 miles (1,000 km) parallel to the coast, with the meadows and wetlands of the Khanka lowland to the southwest.

The northern birch, spruce and pine woods of Ussuriland sustain large populations of birds such as woodpeckers and nutcrackers. Lynxes and wolverines hunt through the trees, which are also the

territory of boars, brown bears and several deer species. At the nature reserve of Kedrovaya Pad, close to the Korean and Chinese borders, the southern character predominates. The forest is brightened and perfumed by flowering shrubs and summer flowers, while large and gorgeous butterflies such as the Maack's swallowtail fly between the trees. Kedrovaya Pad is also a refuge for a few pairs of the extremely rare Amur leopard.

64 Shiretoko National Park JAPAN

Situated on a peninsula at the northeastern end of Hokkaido, Japan's remote, northernmost island, Shiretoko is the country's wildest park. For more than six months of the year, Hokkaido is covered in snow, and winters can be so cold that the inshore waters fill with ice floes, and the rivers and waterfalls that plunge over the peninsula's cliffs freeze solid. During the bitter winter, many seabirds move inland, and at sea the Steller's sea lions move south if inshore ice makes fishing too difficult.

The Shiretoko Peninsula has a spine of volcanic peaks, one of which is still active. Below the volcanic ridge, thick forests encircle the Shiretoko Five Lakes, which are situated in the underlying lava bed. These forests are home to brown bears, foxes and deer. Forestry Bureau plans to log the reserve threatened the habitats of the rare Blakiston's fish owl, a totemic creature to the indigenous Ainu people. Public outcry from all over the country has led to an indefinite postponement of the plan.

65 Astrakhan Reserve VOLGA DELTA, CASPIAN SEA

Lenin created this, the former Soviet Union's first reserve, in 1918, to preserve the Volga Delta from overfishing and bird poachers. Situated at the northern end of the Caspian Sea, the delta is a wildlife oasis set in an enormous area of relatively dry plains and grasslands. Over 250 species of birds use the reserve, many of them fish-eaters. Among the 60 or so mammal species is the Caspian seal.

The channels and streams of the delta are lined with willows, tamarisks and reed beds. The enormous variety of birds feed on the abundant insect, amphibian and fish life. Herons spear frogs, terns trawl the air for insects, and cormorants dive for fish. In the shallows, wild boars dig in the mud with their snouts for roots and snails. There are 100,000 great cormorants in the Astrakhan Reserve, in colonies of 1,000 and more pairs. They build nests of sticks more than 3 feet (1 m) across and fly great distances to catch fish for their young.

66 Tien Shan CHINA/KYRGYZSTAN/KAZAKHSTAN

In Chinese, Tien Shan means "Celestial Mountains," and these border mountains between China and the independent republics of the former Soviet Union have a number of summits over 16,400 feet (5,000 m). The upper reaches of the Tien Shan are covered in perpetual snow and ice, with many glaciers. The foothill plains can be baking hot, but the temperature of the air drops 4°F (2°C) for every 1,000 feet (305 m) of altitude, and the lower slopes are forested with spruce and junipers. Above 9,300 feet (2,800 m) the cold is too severe for forest growth, and juniper scrub eventually gives way to alpine meadow and scree.

Lammergeiers, Himalayan griffons and Eurasian black vultures all ride the air currents of the high ridges in search of carrion. Spring on the southern slopes brings a thaw and the emergence of brilliant bulb flowers, including juno irises and many species of wild tulip, followed by lilies, delphiniums and aconites. Mammal life includes Marco Polo sheep,

Siberian ibex and wild boars, which are found as high as 10,000 feet (3,000 m). Hibernating marmots emerge in the spring, as do brown bears, many of which have very pale fur and white claws.

67 Repetek Biosphere National Reserve
TURKMENISTAN
The Repetek Reserve lies toward the arid edge of the Karakum desert region in southeastern Turkmenistan. The whole area is a stifling, wind-scoured wasteland of sands, dunes and dry clay. At first sight, the land seems lifeless, but on closer inspection it turns out to harbor a thriving variety of desert-adapted flora and fauna. The reserve, covering about 135 sq. miles (350 km²), is a microcosm of the Karakum.

Among the shifting barchan dunes are groups of black saxaul, a deep-rooted and leafless desert tree which grows in groves, usually in low ravines. Camel-thorn, anchored with 100-foot (30-m) tap roots, studs the ridges, and gopherlike susliks inhabit complex colonies in the slopes, preyed on by foxes, jackals and sand cats. Best adapted to the hot sand are the spiders, scorpions, insects and reptiles, including tortoises, monitor lizards, toad-head lizards, and a number of species of snakes – some, like the blunt-nosed and saw-scaled vipers, very poisonous.

68 Dachigam National Park INDIA
Beginning at Marsan Lake, the Daghwan River flows through the Dachigam National Park toward Srinagar, collecting tributaries as it goes. The whole park, tucked up tight against India's northern border, is a catchment area for Srinagar's drinking-water supply. Dachigam is only 54 sq. miles (140 km²) in area, but it manages to incorporate most of the habitats of the fertile and mountainous Himalayan approaches within its borders, from riverine forests to bare rock and alpine scrub.

In the winter, the snow lies thick, and many high-altitude birds move down to where food is available. Endangered hangul deer, for which the park is the world's major refuge, move to the shelter of the lower valleys. In spring, the Himalayan black bears come out of hibernation, and the short summer sees the alpine meadows ablaze with alpine flowers.

69 Arjin Shan Reserve, CHINA
In addition to being one of the world's largest nature reserves, at 17,375 sq. miles (45,000 km²), Arjin Shan is also one of the last of the real wildernesses – remote, uninhabited and virtually inaccessible. The reserve consists of an enormous relatively flat plain, containing large freshwater and saline lakes, and encircled by a towering ring of snow-covered peaks. The lowest part of the reserve is at 10,170 feet (3,100 m), and its highest point is the peak of Wu-lu-k'o-mu-shih at 25,338 feet (7,723 m).

Arjin Shan is one of the last places left in Asia where large herds of hoofed mammals can travel unimpeded across the great areas necessary for them to find sufficient grazing. Herds of Tibetan antelope and wild ass move across the plain, congregating on the shores of the lakes when there is enough grass to crop. In the mountains are the herds of hardy high altitude feeders, like wild yak and Tibetan gazelle. Higher up still, among the rocks of the high meadows, forage ibex and blue sheep. Naturally, predators are also part of the system, and the reserve has wolves, lynxes and snow leopards.

70 Wolong Nature Reserve, SOUTHERN CHINA
The Wolong Nature Reserve is warm and wet, with misty mountains, ravinelike river valleys, and several forest zones climbing the slopes. Evergreen forests

form the lowest zone, with a band of broadleaved trees above them, merging into a final swathe of conifers up to the tree line. The highest peaks are well over 19,700 feet (6,000 m), so there are considerable uplands of bare, rocky terrain. The torrential downpours of the summer monsoons turn earth to mud and loosen rocks already destabilized by frost and the region's frequent earthquakes. The resultant mud and rock avalanches leave livid scars in the mountain forests, which are soon recolonized by bamboo and shrubs.

Wolong's most famous denizen is the giant panda, and the reserve hosts China's largest population of this endangered species, with up to 70 individuals. The reserve also contains other rarities, such as the tree-climbing red panda, the clouded leopard and the golden monkey. Brilliant plumage is common among the reserve's birds, such as Temminck's tragopan and the Chinese monal.

71 Asir National Park SAUDI ARABIA
Saudi Arabia's southwestern Asir province flanks the Red Sea. Here, the Asir mountain range plunges to the ribbon of coastal plain known as the Tihamah. The 10,000-foot (3,000-m) scarp stands in the path of the northwest monsoons, and each year enough rain falls to convert the dry beds of the region's rivers into roaring torrents for a while. The Asir National Park contains mountains, juniper woodlands, humid scrub plains and bakingly hot beaches.

A land bridge once existed between Africa and Saudi Arabia, and many of the species in the park have African origins, including baboons, jackals, hyraxes and jerboas. Among the birds are African bearded vultures, Nile Valley sunbirds, gray hornbills and Bataleur eagles. The park is an important refuge in Saudi Arabia, where the popularity of hunting has pushed some species, such as the Arabian bustard, almost to extinction. The park is also on a major migratory route between Europe and eastern Africa used by over 200 species, including swallows, warblers and birds of prey.

72 Thar Desert NORTHWEST INDIA/PAKISTAN
Covering 270,270 sq. miles (700,000 km²) in the states of Rajasthan and Gujarat, the Thar Desert straddles the long northwestern border with Pakistan. The variety of desert habitats is large, with static and mobile dunes, rocky pavements and outcrops, and salt flats. The desert is not plantless, and there are large areas of seewan grass, as well as both wiry and succulent shrubs, and sparse trees.

Many of the desert creatures have extraordinary abilities to conserve water. The wild asses can hold reserves of water in their bodies for when it is needed and can survive extreme dehydration. The chinkara gazelle can go entirely without water, producing metabolic water from its food. The desert is not an attractive habitat for most humans, so the wildlife of the Thar is still diverse, with large numbers of birds and insects as well as mammals such as foxes and jackals. The Indian wolf has suffered at the hands of shepherds, having turned to sheep as prey when antelope numbers fell due to overhunting by humans.

73 Sagarmatha National Park NEPAL
Famous as the Everest park, Sagarmatha contains a stupendous collection of peaks, with seven summits over 23,000 feet (7,000 m), including the 29,078-foot (8,863-m) Everest. This is the park at the top of the world. It is situated in northeastern Nepal, and its northern boundary coincides with the Tibetan border. The Dudh Kosi River, and its tributaries, which eventually join up with the Ganges system,

draws its headwaters from the park's four main glaciers via deeply carved valleys.

With its lower boundary at 9,334 feet (2,845 m), Sagarmatha contains relatively few mammals. Those that do inhabit the park include Himalayan musk deer, Asiatic black bears, snow leopards and red pandas, as well as wooly hares, Tibetan water shrews and short-tailed moles. An important high altitude breeding ground for birds, Sagarmatha contains 36 species which breed in the park, such as blood pheasants, Tibetan snowcocks and Himalayan monals. To offset the effects of tourism, special no-go areas are being established where all human activity is forbidden.

74 Kaziranga National Park ASSAM, NORTHEASTERN INDIA
Kaziranga lies on the banks of the Brahmaputra River, and once a year, as the monsoons swell the waters to a raging flood, wildlife and people have to escape to high ground. The retreating river leaves extensive shallow swamps behind it, and these characterize the park, together with flat plains of elephant grass, and patches of evergreen forest. Kaziranga has been a reserve since 1926, when it was established to protect its rhinos from extinction.

The forest patches and tall elephant grass provide ideal stalking country for the good-sized tiger population in Kaziranga. Prey animals are plentiful, but tourist visitors wisely travel by elephant to view the wildlife rather than run the risk of encountering tigers. In addition to the tame riding elephants, the park contains large herds of migrating wild elephants. Other common inhabitants include buffaloes, swamp deer, gaurs, leopard cats and otters. The park is also rich in birds of prey, with several species of fishing eagles commonly seen.

75 Xishuangbanna Nature Reserve
SOUTHEASTERN CHINA
The 770 sq. miles (2,000 km²) of the Xishuangbanna Nature Reserve in Yunnan province lie within a tropical rainforest and house an exceptional variety of plants, some 50 percent of which are on China's protected list. The forest of the reserve is dense and luxuriant, with lianas, parasitic plants and other creepers trailing from the high canopy. Some trees, like the lofty fig, a type of banyan, also have aerial roots which grow down from the branches.

The reserve is not all solid forest, and rivers create open corridors. There are also outcrops of limestone, with unusual narrow pinnacles, and caves. Yet the vigor of the rainforest never ceases in the search for more space, and trees grow even on the exposed rocks, clinging to fissures and hanging onto boulders with nets of encircling roots. Asian elephants, gaurs and Hoolock gibbons all live within the reserve, and many species of animals and birds may have originally evolved in the region.

76 Khao Yai National Park THAILAND
One of the Asian mainland's last unexploited tropical forests, the 837 sq. mile (2,168 km²) Khao Yai National Park, once a refuge for bandits, remains one of the few reserves where the visitor can see tigers, leopard cats, Malaysian sun bears and gibbons in the wild, using trails that were made by wild elephants rather than park rangers. The terrain is mountainous, and in fact Khao Yai is part of the Phanom Dongrek range, with three peaks over 4,000 feet (1,200 m) in the park, and an upland rainfall that averages 120 inches (3,000 mm). Despite the torrential rains of July to October, there is a dry season that begins in November, during which all but the very largest water courses dry out completely.

The varied forest gleams with flowers, as well as such birds as scarlet minivets, green magpies, blue-winged leaf-birds and vernal hanging parrots. Hornbills and mynas feed on the fruit of strangling fig trees, which are also a vital food source for many other forest creatures, including gibbons, macaques, palm civets and certain bats.

77 Wilpattu National Park SRI LANKA

Largest of Sri Lanka's reserves, Wilpattu covers 508 sq. miles (1,316 km²) in the northwest of the island and is bounded by the sea on its western side. All across the park are the shallow basinlike pans known as *villus*, built many centuries ago by local princes as a form of irrigation, for Sri Lanka has no natural lakes, and the water table is deep beneath the surface. The *villus* have become the focus for wildlife within the park. Habitats vary, with sand dunes, dry thornbush terrain and deep forested regions.

Wilpattu is famous for its leopards and also has a bear population. Bears can sometimes be seen devouring ants from the park's many anthills, especially after rain. No elephants are resident within park boundaries, but migrating herds of 30 or more pass through, avoiding human contact as much as possible, and hiding out in the forest during the day. In this dry terrain, the *villus* are an irresistible magnet to wildlife such as barking deer and mouse deer, which in turn attract leopards.

SOUTHEAST ASIA/AUSTRALASIA

78 Iglit Baco National Park PHILIPPINES

Population density and the lumber industry have destroyed much of the Philippines' wild forest land, but difficulty of terrain and a flood-ridden rainy season for half of the year have helped the Iglit Baco National Park in the center of the island of Mindoro to avoid the worst depredations. Several tribal communities live within the park, hunting and practicing shifting rice cultivation. The western region of the park is mainly grassland, while in the eastern portion, evergreen forest and dry-season deciduous trees and shrubs predominate.

The mountainous center of the park, dominated by the 8,163-foot (2,488-m) Mount Baco, contains extensive grasslands riven by steep canyons and ravines. The endemic tamarau, a miniature water buffalo-like herbivore only 3 feet (1 m) high, lives in the mountain grasslands as well as in swampy lowland areas. Other mammals include prickly porcupines, wild pigs, deer and monkeys. Endemic Philippine birds, such as the tarictic hornbill and the yellow-breasted fruit dove, share the park with parrots, doves, swifts and kingfishers.

79 Kinabalu National Park EAST MALAYSIA

The multiple granite peaks of Mount Kinabalu tower above the Kinabalu National Park in the Malaysian state of Sabah in northern Borneo, a few degrees north of the equator. Visitors to this luxuriously forested park, intent on climbing Borneo's highest mountain, pass through several distinct zones of forest growth on the ascent.

First, there is a lowland region of lumber trees, where the rare rafflesia, the world's largest flower, is sometimes found. Above 4,000 feet (1,200 m) is a zone of mixed montane forest, rich in oaks and conifers. Brilliant rhododendrons, and some of Kinabalu's thousand species of orchids grow here, alongside carnivorous pitcher plants. Tree ferns and climbing bamboos flourish in the mossy environment of the next zone of cloud forest, up to 10,830 feet (3,300 m), after which comes the open summit

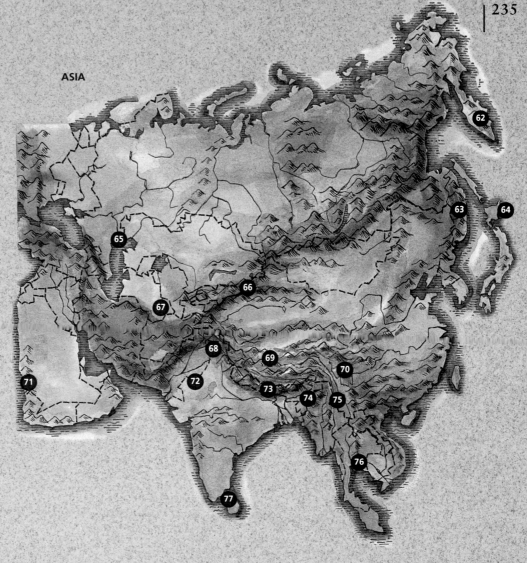

region of granite slabs up to 13,455 feet (4,100 m). With a reputation as one of the best managed parks in the region, Kinabalu has over 300 bird species and 100 mammal species as well as its unique flora.

80 Mulu National Park SARAWAK, EAST MALAYSIA

Mulu is an extraordinary forest environment which can be entered only by means of long boat voyages up a series of rivers. The park has mountains, caves, alluvial forests, surreal landscapes of sandstone pinnacles, and a stupendous annual rainfall of between 25 and 200 inches (600 and 5,000 mm). But, there is a grave threat hanging over Mulu – that of the logging companies. They have already stripped out the lumber along the river banks. Penan tribespeople who live in the park barricaded logging roads and created international publicity in an attempt to halt wholesale logging in the late 1980s, but the loggers have strong political support, and the logging continues.

In the meantime, Mulu is still a wildlife enthusiast's dream, with almost every bird known to exist in Borneo, as well as several primates, such as macaques, leaf monkeys and Bornean gibbons. There is also a huge bat population centered on a number of caverns, and other mammals include sun bears, slow loris, western tarsiers and yellow-throated martens.

81 Mount Leuser National Park SUMATRA, INDONESIA

This great national park, covering 3,860 sq. miles (10,000 km²) of Indonesia's westernmost island, of international importance as a major refuge of the

endangered Sumatran two-horned rhinoceros, and for its vital rehabilitation centers for orphaned orangutans. It has a long history of protection. The range of habitats includes coastal forest on Sumatra's west coast, mountain highlands which include the 11,093-foot (3,381-m) Mount Leuser, and extensive riverine terrains on both banks of the great River Alas which bisects the park.

The richness of Leuser's fauna is hard to exaggerate. In addition to the rare rhino, the forests conceal tigers, clouded leopards and barking deer, as well as primates including Thomas's leafmonkeys, long-tailed macaques, orangutans and siamang gibbons. The rare Sumatra elephant prefers the river valleys, where there are salt licks, and the valleys are also home to otters, hog badgers and leopard cats. In all, there are 176 mammal species, some 320 bird species, 194 reptile species and 52 amphibian species.

82 Komodo National Park LESSER SUNDAS, INDONESIA

The climate of the Lesser Sundas is relatively arid, with sparse tree cover on the uplands. The islands of the group lie in Australia's rain shadow and receive rain only between November and March. Komodo National Park consists of three islands, Komodo, Rinca and Padar, and is the home of the planet's heaviest lizard, the Komodo dragon.

Virtually unknown outside its home islands until the early 20th century, the Komodo dragon is a giant monitor lizard which can reach 10 feet (3 m) in length and weigh 330 pounds (150 kg). It preys on a variety of creatures, including deer, feral water buffaloes, pigs and horses, all of which thrive in the park's savanna woodland and open grassland. The park lies in an overlap area between Asia and Australia, with species typical of both continents, notably among the bird population. Australian species such as sulfur-crested cockatoos and friar birds share terrain with Asian jungle fowls and monarch flycatchers.

83 Central and Southern Highlands PAPUA NEW GUINEA

Despite the encroachment of mining and logging, Papua New Guinea still retains most of its rugged wild landscape, especially in the mountains. Below 10,000 feet (3,000 m) are mid-montane forests, with animals and plants that have adapted to survive only here and can live neither higher up nor lower down. In the misty, overcast environment live several of the bird-of-paradise species in which the island is so rich. The plant life includes great beech trees closely related to beeches in New Zealand and South America, survivors from the break-up of ancient Gondwana. Brilliant color among the trees comes from mosses, fungi and many of New Guinea's 2,500 species of orchids.

Above 10,000 feet (3,000 m), the upper montane begins, with thick banks of wet moss everywhere. Bowerbird species build their bowers up here, decorated with shells and feathers, and canopies of orchid stems. Above the moss forest is a zone of subalpine grassland and stunted woodland, where wild dogs and spotted marsh harriers hunt small rodents and mountain wallabies graze.

84 Kakadu National Park AUSTRALIA

Aboriginal peoples have inhabited Arnhem Land in Australia's Northern Territory for over 30,000 years, and Aboriginal organizations own half of the area of the Kakadu National Park on the Arnhem coast, taking part in management decisions for Australia's largest and most diverse preserve. The park incorporates freshwater marshes, tidal estuaries, salt flats and mangrove swamps on offshore islands.

Kakadu teems with birdlife, dominated in peak periods by 8-foot (2.5-m) magpie geese. Other wetland inhabitants include huge saltwater crocodiles. In the dry season, saltwater tides penetrate the flood plain of the rivers that cross and define the park, carrying saltwater fish, including sharks, up to 20 miles (30 km) inland. Freshwater crocodiles and long-necked turtles inhabit creeks and ponds.

85 Great Barrier Reef AUSTRALIA

The largest system of coral reefs in the world, the Great Barrier Reef stretches for more than 1,250 miles (2,000 km) down the Queensland coast, a vast complex of 2,900 separate reefs and over 500 islands and islets. Growing threats from tourism, the oil industry and agricultural effluvia led in 1975 to the creation of the Great Barrier Reef Marine National Park, covering 98.5 percent of the reef's area.

The reef is a huge and complex ecosystem, containing 400 species of corals, which have suffered serious inroads from population explosions of the crown-of-thorns starfish in recent years. Seagrass beds shelter large populations of dugong, which, along with all sea turtles, are fully protected within the park. Over 240 species of birds nest on the coral cays, including terns, white-bellied sea eagles, reef herons and ospreys. At least 1,500 species of fish and 4,000 species of mollusks help make the reef one of the world's most important marine biospheres.

86 The Olgas CENTRAL AUSTRALIA

Formed from a conglomerate of granite, gneiss and volcanic rocks, and resisting the erosion that over millions of years pared back the plain around them, the Olgas are a group of some 30 massive rocky domes covering an area of 13½ sq. miles (35 km²), several of which are over 1,650 feet (500 m) in height. In the steep clefts and chasms dividing the red domes are shaded rock pools, oases of life festooned with vines and sheltering lizards, snakes, birds and small mammals. Gum trees grow in the creek beds in some of the ravines, alongside mosses, ferns, yellow-flowered cassia and acacia bushes.

The sheer, curving sides of the individual domes are bare, though some are crowned with spinifex. The Olgas, like nearby Uluru (Ayer's Rock), are a sacred site of the Aborigines, who believe a sacred serpent sleeps in a cavern inside Mount Olga, the largest of the domes. The serpent's breath is the wind that sometimes howls through the gorges.

87 The Simpson Desert CENTRAL AUSTRALIA

The great red dunes of the Simpson Desert run in parallel lines, some as much as 75 miles (120 km) long. More than 1,000 of these dune ridges range across the desert, up to 130 feet (40 m) high, and with corridors 330 feet to ½ mile (100 m to 1 km) wide between them. Covering over 56,000 sq. miles (145,000 km²), it is one of the driest regions of Australia.

With savage daytime temperatures and little shade, the Simpson hosts specially adapted populations which leave their tracks in the sand overnight. The sand goanna preys on small marsupial mammals, insects, scorpions, birds and other reptiles. The most common vegetation is spinifex, growing in sparse and spiny clumps. After the rare rain showers, desert flowers bloom profusely, then die quickly, leaving their seeds lying dormant until the next rain. Some birds, like the black-faced wood swallow, begin their breeding cycles the moment it rains.

88 Lake Eyre CENTRAL AUSTRALIA

South of the Simpson Desert, Lake Eyre is situated on top of the planet's largest artesian system, the Lake Eyre Basin, draining an area of 425,000 sq. miles (1.1 million km²). Four major rivers drain into the lake, yet it is arid and apparently waterless most of the time, forming a huge salt flat of about 2,320 sq. miles (6,000 km²), most of which lies 50 feet (15 m) below sea level. Creatures living in this glaring blast furnace have extraordinary survival techniques.

The eggs of the brine shrimp can remain for years in suspended animation until rain starts their brief life cycle. The lizards known as Lake Eyre dragons hibernate in burrows in the salt crust and use their eyelids as sun visors. A few times a century, an errant tropical cyclone dumps quantities of water into the lake's huge drainage basin, flooding vast areas of salt flat. In 1974, the lake experienced its biggest floods in perhaps 500 years, covering an area of 350 sq. miles (900 km²) to a depth of 13–16 feet (4–5m). During the rare floods, many birds, including cockatoos, ducks, waders and pelicans, gravitate to the lake from all over the continent.

89 The Snares Islands NEW ZEALAND

Some 125 miles (200 km) southwest of New Zealand's South Island lie the Snares, a group of small islands. The two largest in the group are North East Island, of 692 acres (280 ha), and Broughton Island, of 119 acres (48 ha). Protected by wild and rocky coasts and formidable seas, the Snares are an important bird sanctuary. A forest of *Olearia*, or giant tree daisy, and tussock meadows cover much of the main islands, which have floors of black peat riddled with the burrows of some six million sooty shearwaters.

The islands have three unique species of landbird: the Snares black tit, the Snares fernbird and the Snares snipe. Other landbirds include silver-eyes, redpolls, blackbirds, thrushes and gray warblers. The seabirds dominate the islands' fauna, with a large population of 80,000 Snares crested penguins. New Zealand fur seals live on the main islands and the islets of the Western Chain. A small bachelor herd of Hooker's sea lions visits annually, as do a few elephant seals. The Snares have never suffered the introduction of species associated with humans, such as rats and cats, and have thus avoided the destruction of native species that such introductions have brought to many islands.

SOUTHEAST ASIA AND AUSTRALASIA

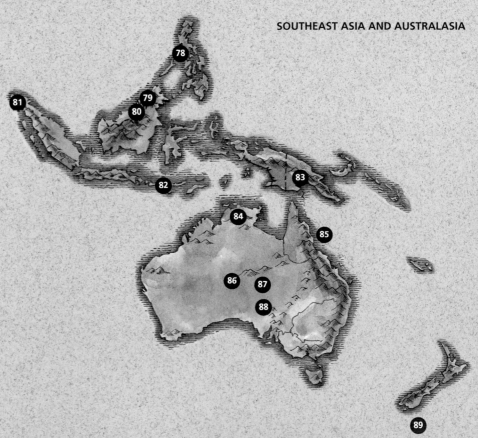

Photographic credits

l = left, *r* = right, *t* = top,
c = center, *b* = bottom

1 Eric Lawrie/Royal Geographical Society; 2/3 Thomas Kitchin/Tom Stack & Associates; 4 Paul McCormick/The Image Bank; 5 Anthony Bannister/NHPA; 6 Peter Davey/Bruce Coleman; 6/7 Hans Christian Heap/Planet Earth Pictures; 7 Ben Osborne/Oxford Scientific Films; 10/12 Nikita Ovsyanikov/Planet Earth Pictures; 13t Daniel Cox/Oxford Scientific Films; 13b Francisco Erize/Bruce Coleman; 14/15 Bryan & Cherry Alexander; 16 Jim Brandenburg/ Zefa Picture Library; 17 Jim Brandenburg/Planet Earth Pictures; 18/19 Jim Brandenburg/Zefa Picture Library; 19t Jim Brandenburg/NHPA; 19b Jim Brandenburg/Zefa Picture Library; 20/21 Jill Ranford/Ffotograff; 22 Martin W. Grosnick/Ardea; 23 Richard & Julia Kemp/Survival Anglia; 24/25 D. Parer & E. Parer-Cook/Ardea; 26/27 Ben Osborne/ Oxford Scientific Films; 28/29 Colin Monteath/Mountain Camera; 30/31 J.E. Pasquier/ Rapho; 32 Paul McCormick/The Image Bank; 33t John Shaw/Tom Stack & Associates; 33b John Eastcott/Planet Earth Pictures; 34 Steve Kaufman/Peter Arnold; 34/35 Douglas T. Cheeseman Jr./Peter Arnold; 36/37 Stephen Krasemann/NHPA; 38/39 Julian Pottage/Robert Harding Picture Library; 41t Patti Murray/Oxford Scientific Films; 41b Survival Anglia; 42l Erwin & Peggy Bauer/ Bruce Coleman; 42/43 Daniel J. Cox/Oxford Scientific Films; 44/45 Tom Mangelsen; 46 Tom Ulrich/ Oxford Scientific Films; 47t Tom Mangelsen; 47b Frank Schneidermeyer/Oxford Scientific Films; 48/49 David Muench; 50 Jen & Des Bartlett/Bruce Coleman; 51t M.P. Kahl/Bruce Coleman; 51b Charlie Ott/Bruce Coleman; 52/53 David Muench; 54/55 David Muench; 55/56 John Shaw/NHPA; 57 David A. Ponton/Planet Earth Pictures; 58/59 Dieter & Mary Plage/Bruce Coleman; 60t Kevin Schafer/NHPA; 60b/61 Michael Fogden/Oxford Scientific Films; 62/63 Ivor Edmonds/Planet Earth Pictures; 64 Chris Prior/Planet Earth Pictures; 65 James H. Carmichael/The Image Bank; 66/67 Tony Morrison/South American Pictures; 69 Kimball Morrison/South American Pictures; 71 Adrian Warren/Ardea; 72/73 André Bärtschi/Planet Earth Pictures; 74 Stephen Dalton/NHPA; 75t K.W. Fink/Ardea; 75b André Bärtschi/Planet Earth Pictures; 76 Partridge Productions/Oxford

Scientific Films; 77 Kevin Schafer/ Tom Stack & Associates; 78 Robin Hanbury-Tenison/Robert Harding Picture Library; 78/79 Thomas Kelly/Impact; 79 Victor Englebert/ Select Photo Agency; 80/81 Carlos G.E. Velha/The Image Bank; 82t Luiz Claudio Marigo/Bruce Coleman; 82b George Gainsburgh/ NHPA; 83 Richard Matthews/ Planet Earth Pictures; 84/85 Eric Lawrie/Royal Geographical Society; 86t Gunter Ziesler/Bruce Coleman; 86b François Gohier/ Ardea; 87 Roger Few; 88/89 Tony Morrison/South American Pictures; 89t Tony Morrison/South American Pictures; 89b John Bulmer/Comstock; 90/92 Richard Matthews/Planet Earth Pictures; 93t Richard Coomber/Planet Earth Pictures; 93b Richard Matthews/ Planet Earth Pictures; 94/95 Bernadette Waters/Planet Earth Pictures; 96 Julie Bergada/Aspect Picture Library; 97 Konrad Wothe/Oxford Scientific Films; 98/99 Boireau/Rapho; 100 Mike Brown/Oxford Scientific Films; 101l Boireau/Rapho; 101r G.K. Brown/Ardea; 102/104l Keith Scholey/Planet Earth Pictures; 104/105 Owen Newman/Oxford Scientific Films; 106/107 Jonathan Scott/Planet Earth Pictures; 108 Stephen Krasemann/Peter Arnold; 108/109 Rafi Ben-Shahar/Oxford Scientific Films; 110/111 Peter Davey/Bruce Coleman; 112 Mirella Ricciardi/Colorific!; 112/113t Brian Boyd/Colorific!; 112/113b Jonathan Scott/Planet Earth Pictures; 114/115 John Newby/WWF International; 115 Anthony Bannister/Oxford Scientific Films; 116 Nick Gordon/ Ardea; 117 Jacques Jangoux; 118/119 Anthony Bannister/ NHPA; 120 Carol Farneti/Planet Earth Pictures; 121 Mike Rosenberg/Oxford Scientific Films; 122 Richard Packwood/Oxford Scientific Films; 122/123 E.A. Janes/NHPA; 123 Carol Farneti/ Planet Earth Pictures; 124 Anthony Bannister/NHPA; 124/125 Tom Nebbia/Aspect Picture Library; 125 Nigel Dennis/ NHPA; 126/127 Peter Johnson/ NHPA; 128 Anthony Bannister/ Oxford Scientific Films; 129 Antoinette Jaunet/Aspect Picture Library; 130 Anthony Bannister/NHPA; 131t David Hughes/Bruce Coleman; 131b Michael Fogden/Oxford Scientific Films; 132/133 Bengt Olof Olsson/ Bildhuset; 134 Ferrero/Labat/ Ardea; 135t Johnny Johnson/Bruce Coleman; 135b John Noble/ Wilderness Photographic Library; 136 Pelle Stackman/Tiofoto AB; 137 Robert Harding Picture Library; 138/141 David Paterson; 142/143 L. Campbell/Scotland in

Focus; 143t Alan & Sandy Carey/ Oxford Scientific Films; 143b Gordon Langsbury/Bruce Coleman; 144/145 Bomford & Borkowski/Survival Anglia; 146/147l David Woodfall/NHPA; 147r Hans Reinhard/Zefa Picture Library; 148/149 Ivor Edmonds/ Planet Earth Pictures; 150 David Hughes/Robert Harding Picture Library; 151t Nigel Dennis/NHPA; 151b Hervé Berthoule/Explorer; 152/153 Francisco J. Erize/Bruce Coleman; 154 Jose Luis Gonzalez Grande/Bruce Coleman; 155t Ian Beames/Ardea; 155b Robert Frerck/Robert Harding Picture Library; 156/157 Comstock; 158/159 Hans Christian Heap/ Planet Earth Pictures; 160/161t Comstock; 161c Robin Constable/ Hutchison Library; 161b Alan Keohane/Impact; 162/164t Joel Bennett/Survival Anglia; 164b Michael Leach/NHPA; 165 Joel Bennett/Survival Anglia; 166/167 Tony Allen/Oxford Scientific Films; 168/169 Richard Kirby; 170 Doug Allan/Oxford Scientific Films; 170/171 John Hartley/ NHPA; 172/173 Sarah Leen/ Matrix/Colorific!; 174/175 Colin Monteath/Mountain Camera; 176t Tim Davis/Oxford Scientific Films; 176b/177 Martyn Colbeck/Oxford Scientific Films; 178/179 Mike Price/Bruce Coleman; 180 Paolo Koch/Okapia; 181 Rod Williams/ Bruce Coleman; 182/183 Ann & Bury Peerless; 183 Duncan Maxwell/Robert Harding Picture Library; 184 Rod Williams/Bruce Coleman; 185t Dieter & Mary Plage/Survival Anglia; 185b/186l Carlo Dani & Ingrid Jeske/Natural Science Photos; 186/187 Anup Shah/Planet Earth Pictures; 187 Gunter Ziesler/Bruce Coleman; 188/189 Gerald Cubitt; 190 D. Parer & E. Parer-Cook/Auscape; 191l Alain Compost/Bruce Coleman; 191r Gerald Cubitt; 192 Bryan & Cherry Alexander; 192/193 Adrian Arbib/Royal Geographical Society; 193l J. Riley/Hedgehog House; 193r Robert Harding Picture Library; 194/195 Comstock; 196/199 Dieter & Mary Plage/Survival Anglia; 200/201 Sam Abell/ National Geographic Society; 202 Robert Harding Picture Library; 202 John Lythgoe/Planet Earth Pictures; 203 Jean-Paul Ferrero/ Auscape; 205t Reg Morrison/ Auscape; 205b Jan Taylor/NHPA; 206 Purdy & Matthews/Planet Earth Pictures; 206/207 D. Parer & E. Parer-Cook/Ardea; 207 Purdy & Matthews/Planet Earth Pictures; 208/209 Natural Images/ NHPA; 210 Belinda Wright/ Oxford Scientific Films; 211 Jean-Paul Ferrero/Auscape; 212/213 Richard Packwood/

Oxford Scientific Films; 214t John Cancalosi/Bruce Coleman; 214b/215 Jean-Paul Ferrero/Ardea; 216/217 Darryl Torckler/ Hedgehog House; 218 G.R. Roberts; 219t Darryl Torckler/ Hedgehog House; 219b Kim Westerskou/Hedgehog House; 220/221 Superstock; 222t Frances Furlong/Survival Anglia; 222b Norman Tomalin/Bruce Coleman; 224 Tom Till/Auscape; 225l Tom Ulrich/Oxford Scientific Films; 225r John Cancalosi/Bruce Coleman

Illustration credits

Maps throughout: **Andrew Farmer**

Diagrams: **Gary Hincks, Janos Marffy, Richard Bonson and Andrew Farmer**

Editorial director **Ruth Binney**
Managing editor **Lindsay McTeague**
Text editor **Isabella Raeburn**
DTP **Pennie Jelliff**
Production **Sarah Hinks**
Kate Waghorn
Coordinator **Tim Probart**

Typeset by **Millions Design**
Origination by **CLG**, Verona, Italy

If the publishers have unwittingly infringed copyright in any illustration reproduced, they would pay an appropriate fee on being satisfied to the owner's title.